MW01265479

OTHER TITLES OF INTEREST

CODING AND REIMBURSEMENT

CPT Coders Choice®, Thumb Indexed
CPT & HCPCS Coding Made Easy!
HCPCS Coders Choice®
Health Insurance Carrier Directory
ICD-9-CM, Coders Choice®, Thumb Indexed
ICD-9-CM Coding Made Easy!
Medicare Compliance Manual
Medical Fees in the United States
Medicare Rules & Regulations
Reimbursement Manual for the Medical Office
The Coder's Handbook

PRACTICE MANAGEMENT

Computerizing Your Medical Office
Effective Laboratory Supervision
Encyclopedia of Practice and Financial Management
Managing Medical Office Personnel
Marketing Healthcare
Marketing Strategies for Physicians
Medical Practice Handbook
Medical Staff Privileges
On-Line Systems: How to Access and Use Databases
Patient Satisfaction
Performance Standards for the Laboratory
Physician's Office Laboratory
Professional and Practice Development
Promoting Your Medical Practice
Remodeling Your Professional Office
Starting in Medical Practice

AVAILABLE FROM YOUR LOCAL MEDICAL BOOKSTORE OR BY CALLING 1-800-MED-SHOP

CPT·PLUS!

MILLENNIUM EDITION

A Comprehensive Guide
To Current Procedural
Terminology

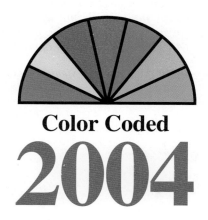

Color Coded
2004

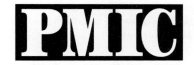

ISBN 1-57066-288-6

Practice Management Information Corporation
4727 Wilshire Boulevard
Los Angeles, California 90010
1-800-MED-SHOP
http://pmiconline.com/

Printed in China

INTRODUCTION

CPT® PLUS! 2004 is an enhanced CPT® coding resource which includes all official CPT 2004 codes and complete descriptions plus comprehensive CPT coding instructions, full-color anatomical illustrations, a unique color-coding system to help identify CPT codes subject to special coding rules, and a new and improved alphabetic index.

The CPT coding system includes over 7,900 codes and descriptions for reporting medical services, procedures, supplies and materials. Accurate CPT coding provides an efficient method of communicating medical services and procedures among health care providers, health care facilities, and third party payers and enhances the health care provider's control of the reimbursement process.

The CPT coding system is revised annually by the American Medical Association (AMA). Each year hundreds of additions, changes and deletions are made the CPT coding system. These changes become effective on January 1st. CPT is required by federal law for all health insurance claim forms filed with Medicare, Medicaid, CHAMPUS and Federal Employee Health Plans and is accepted or required by all other third party payers.

CPT® PLUS! 2004 provides valuable instructions, coding tips, and other information to help providers maximize reimbursement while minimizing audit liability. Our objective is to make CPT coding faster, easier and more accurate for medical office, healthcare facility and third party payer coding and billing staff, while setting a new standard for CPT coding references.

James B. Davis, Publisher

DISCLAIMER

This publication is designed to offer basic information regarding coding and reporting of medical services, supplies and procedures using the CPT coding system. The information presented is based on a thorough analysis of the CPT coding system and the experience and interpretations of the editors. Though all of the information has been carefully researched and checked for accuracy and completeness, neither the editors nor the publisher accept any responsibility or liability with regard to errors, omissions, misuse or misinterpretation.

CONTENTS

CPT CODING FUNDAMENTALS

CPT® is an acronym for Current Procedural Terminology. Physicians' Current Procedural Terminology, Fourth Edition, known as CPT-4 or more commonly CPT, is a systematic listing of codes and descriptions which classify medical services and procedures. CPT codes are used by physicians, hospitals, and other health care professionals, to report specific medical, surgical and diagnostic services and procedures for statistical and third party payment purposes.

The CPT coding system is maintained by the American Medical Association (AMA) and a revised edition of the CPT book is published each fall. The new CPT codes become effective on January 1st of the following year. The revisions in each new edition are prepared by the CPT Editorial Panel with the assistance of physicians representing all specialties of medicine.

A thorough understanding of the CPT coding system is essential in order to provide accurate reporting of medical services and procedures, maximize payments from third parties, minimize denials, rejections and reductions from third parties, and to protect the medical practice from audit liability.

KEY POINTS REGARDING THE CPT CODING SYSTEM

- *CPT codes describe medical procedures, services and supplies.*

- *All CPT codes are five digit codes.*

- *CPT codes are mandated by federal law for Medicare, Medicaid, CHAMPUS and Federal Employee Health Plan (FEHP) reporting and are accepted or required by all other third party payers.*

- *CPT codes are self-definitive, eg. with the exception of CPT codes for unlisted procedures and/or the few CPT codes which include the term specify in the description, each CPT code number represents the universal definition of the service or procedure.*

- *CPT codes are revised and updated annually by the AMA and the revisions become effective each January 1st. Hundreds of CPT codes are added, changed or deleted each year. All health care professionals, third party payers, and health care facilities must maintain copies of the current code books.*

- *Accurate CPT coding provides an efficient method of communicating medical, surgical and diagnostic services and procedures among health care professionals, health care facilities, and third party payers.*

- *Accurate CPT coding enhances the health care provider's control of the reimbursement process.*

1

STRUCTURE OF THE CPT CODING SYSTEM

The CPT coding system includes over 7,900 codes and definitions for medical services, procedures and diagnostic tests. Each procedure or service is identified by a five digit code, followed by the definition.

The CPT coding system is divided into eight **SECTIONS**. The seven sections of are:

Evaluation and Management	99201-99499
Anesthesiology	00100-01999, 99100-99140
Surgery	10021-69990
Radiology	70010-79999
Pathology and Laboratory	80048-89356
Medicine	90000-99199, 99500-99602
Category II Performance Measurement	0001F-0011F
Category III Emerging Technology	0001T-0061T

Each section of the CPT book includes subsections with anatomic, procedural, condition, or descriptor subheadings. The Evaluation and Management (E/M) section is presented first because 1) these codes are used by virtually all health care providers and 2) are the most frequently used CPT codes.

HOW TO USE THE CPT CODING SYSTEM

A provider or coder using the CPT coding system first chooses the name and associated code of the procedure or service which most accurately identifies and describes the service(s) performed. The provider or coder then chooses names and codes for additional services or procedures. If necessary, modifiers are chosen and added to the selected service and procedure codes. All services or procedures coded must also be documented in the patient's medical record.

According to CPT, "The listing of a service or procedure and its code number in a specific section of the CPT book does not restrict its use to a specific specialty group. Any procedure or service in any section of the CPT coding system may be used to designate the services rendered by any qualified physician or other qualified health care professional."

The codes and descriptions listed in the CPT coding system are those that are generally consistent with contemporary medical practice and being performed by health care professionals in clinical practice. Inclusion in the CPT coding system does not represent endorsement by the American Medical Association of any particular diagnostic or therapeutic procedure. In addition, inclusion or exclusion of a procedure does not imply any health insurance coverage or reimbursement policy.

CPT FORMAT AND CONVENTIONS

DESCRIPTIONS

The descriptions associated with CPT codes have been developed by the AMA to provide complete descriptions of medical services and procedures.

Many CPT descriptions include the definition of basic procedures followed by supplemental descriptions for variations or modifications of the basic procedure. In the CPT coding book, the basic procedure description ends with a semicolon (;), followed by the additional description.

If a CPT description includes the same basic procedure as the preceding listing, the basic procedure is not listed. Only the supplemental description is listed, preceded by an indentation. For example:

25100   Arthrotomy, wrist joint; with biopsy

25105   with synovectomy

SYMBOLS

● *A filled BLACK CIRCLE preceding a CPT code indicates that the code is new to this revision of the CPT coding system. A symbol key appears on all left-hand pages.*

▲ *A filled BLACK TRIANGLE preceding a CPT code indicates that there is a revision to the description. Wherever possible, the revised text is identified with underlining.*

( ) *CPT codes enclosed within parenthesis have been deleted from the CPT coding system and should no longer be used.*

+ *A bold plus sign preceding a CPT code indicates that the code is an "add-on" code and must be listed in addition to the main CPT code.*

⊘ *This symbol preceding a CPT code indicates that the code is exempt from the use of modifier -51.*

Note that a CPT code may be preceded by the add-on, star symbol or modifier-51 exempt symbol, in addition to new or changed code symbols.

COLOR CODING

Separate procedure. A procedure or service that is normally performed as an integral component of a total service or procedure. CPT codes identified as separate procedure codes should not be coded in addition to the basic procedure code of which it is considered an integral component.

However, if the procedure or service that is usually designated as a separate procedure is performed independently or is considered to be unrelated or distinct from other procedures or services provided at that time, the separate procedure may be coded by itself. The modifier -59 should be added to the separate procedure code to indicate that the procedure is not considered to be a component of another procedure, but is a distinct, independent procedure.

Unlisted code. Descriptions include the term "unlisted." Use only when a CPT code which specifically describes the service or procedure is unavailable. A report is usually required by third party payers.

Nonspecific code. Descriptions include the term "specify" instructing the coder to include additional information such as the quadrant, the nerve, the muscle, the level of spine, the number of joints, the type of study, the method of dosimetry, the hormone, the receptor, the assay method, the type of kit, the material injected, the type of tests, the number of tests, the doses provided.

CCI comprehensive code. Indicates codes identified as comprehensive codes in the Comprehensive Coding Initiative, revised annually. Per CMS rules, all identifiable component procedures are included in the comprehensive code and should not be billed separately to Medicare.

ITALICIZED AND NON-ITALICIZED TEXT

Italicized text is used throughout this publication to distinguish information authored, contributed or otherwise provided by PMIC.

Non-italicized text is used to distinguish information reproduced verbatim from CPT 2004, published by the American Medical Association.

SECTION OVERVIEWS

Specific guidelines are presented at the beginning of each of the six sections of the CPT coding system. The guidelines define items that are necessary to interpret and report the procedures and services contained in that section. CPT guidelines also provide explanations regarding terms that apply only to a particular section.

CODING & BILLING ISSUES

Most billing, coding and reporting issues involving the CPT® coding system apply generally to all medical specialties and professions. However, there are some specialty specific issues defined in each section of the CPT coding system that apply only to the specific medical specialty represented.

SUPPORTING DOCUMENTATION

Documentation in the patient's medical report must clearly support the procedures, services and supplies coded on the health insurance claim form. Most medical chart reviewers take the position that if something is not documented in the medical record, then the service or procedure was not performed and therefore is not subject to reimbursement.

If a medical practice is selected for an audit by Medicare or other third party payer, the accuracy and completeness of the documentation of the medical records, or lack thereof, will have a significant impact on the outcome of the audit. The current emphasis on "fraud" and "abuse" by Medicare, Medicaid and private third party payer necessitates a review of documentation by all health care professionals.

SPECIAL MEDICARE CONSIDERATIONS

To satisfy Medicare requirements, there must be sufficient documentation in the medical record to verify the services coded and the level of care required. Section 1833(e) of Title XVIII, Social Security Act requires "available information that documents a claim." If there is no documentation to justify the services or level of care, the claim cannot be considered for Medicare benefits.

If there is insufficient documentation to support claims that have already been paid by Medicare, the reimbursement will be considered an overpayment and a refund will be requested by Medicare. Medicare has the authority to review any information, including medical records, when such information pertains to a Medicare claim.

UNLISTED PROCEDURES OR SERVICES

There are services or procedures performed by health care professionals that are not found in the CPT coding system. These services or procedures may be either new procedures which have not yet been assigned a CPT code or simply a variation of a procedure which precludes using the existing CPT code. Each

---

5

section of the CPT coding system includes codes for reporting these unlisted procedures.

Unlisted procedure codes should not be coded unless the coder has reviewed the CPT coding system carefully to ensure that a more specific code is not available. If a specific CPT code is not located, check for HCPCS codes that may be reportable.

As a rule, a report needs to be enclosed with the health insurance claim form when reporting unlisted procedure codes. Because unlisted procedure codes are subject to manual medical review, payment is usually slower than for normal processing time.

CPT ADDITIONS, CHANGES, AND DELETIONS

Each year hundreds of codes are added, changed or deleted from the CPT coding system. A summary of these changes is found in Appendix B of the CPT code book which provides a quick reference for coding review. In addition to the appendix, these modifications are identified throughout the CPT code book.

ADDITIONS TO THE CPT CODING SYSTEM

New codes are added to the CPT coding system each year. New CPT codes are identified with a small black circle placed to the left of the code number. Examples of new codes found in CPT 2004 include:

- **01173**   Anesthesia for open repair of fracture disruption of pelvis or column fracture involving acetabulum

- **0060T**   Electrical impedence scan of breast, bilateral (risk assessment device for breast cancer)

CHANGES TO CPT CODE DEFINITIONS

Each year the definitions of many CPT codes are revised. CPT codes with changed definitions are identified with a small black triangle placed to the left of the code number. Examples of CPT codes with changed definitions in CPT 2004 include:

▲ **20240**   Biopsy, bone, open; superficial (eg, ilium, sternum, spinous process, ribs, trochanter of femur)

▲ **37785**   Ligation, division, and/or excision of varicose vein cluster(s), one leg

The only way to determine exactly what part of the definition has been changed is to compare the current changed definition with the definition from the previous edition of the CPT code book.

DELETIONS FROM THE CPT CODING SYSTEM

Each year some CPT codes are deleted. Deleted CPT codes, and references to replacement codes, are enclosed within parenthesis. Examples of CPT codes deleted from CPT 2004 include:

(47134   deleted 2004 edition. To report, use 47140)

(61862   deleted 2004 edition. To report, see 61867-61868)

NEW SECTIONS AND SUB-SECTIONS

New sections and subsections are frequently added to the CPT coding system to reflect changes in technology or medical practice and to provide additional code sequences for special purposes. Examples of new sub-sections added to CPT 2004 include:

Category II Performance Measurement   0001F-0011F

CATEGORY II PERFORMANCE MEASUREMENT CODES

Category II, Performance Measurement CPT codes, are designed to facilitate outcomes research. This new section was introduced in the 2004 CPT updates. Category II codes include the letter "F" as the fifth digit of the five digit CPT code. These codes are optional, and are not a substitute for Category I codes.

CATEGORY III EMERGING TECHNOLOGY CODES

Emerging technology codes are temporary codes for emerging technology, services and procedures. These codes are designed to permit data collection and assessment of new technologies. All Category III codes include the letter "T" as the fifth digit of the five digit CPT code. The inclusion of a specific service or procedure in this section does not imply or endorse clinical efficacy, safety, or applicability to clinical practice.

CPT 2004 ADDITIONS, CHANGES, AND DELETIONS

Following is a summary listing all additions, deletions, and revisions applicable to CPT 2004 codes. The descriptors of the codes listed as "grammatical change" have not been substantially changed, but involve placement of the semicolon, or other punctuation, or a similar minor change.

EVALUATION AND MANAGEMENT

99293 Terminology revised

99294 Terminology revised

99295 Terminology revised

99296 Terminology revised

ANESTHESIA

00528 Terminology revised

00529 Code added

00544 Code deleted

01173 Code added

01958 Code added

SURGERY-INTEGUMENTARY

10040 Starred procedure designation removed

10060 Starred procedure designation removed

10080 Starred procedure designation removed

10120 Starred procedure designation removed

10140 Starred procedure designation removed

10160 Starred procedure designation removed

11000 Starred procedure designation removed

11100 Terminology revised

11200 Starred procedure designation removed

11300 Starred procedure designation removed

11305 Starred procedure designation removed

11310 Starred procedure designation removed

11730 Starred procedure designation removed

11900 Starred procedure designation removed

11901 Starred procedure designation removed

12001 Starred procedure designation removed

12002 Starred procedure designation removed

12004 Starred procedure designation removed

12011 Starred procedure designation removed

12013 Starred procedure designation removed

12031 Starred procedure designation removed

12032 Starred procedure designation removed

12041 Starred procedure designation removed

12051 Starred procedure designation removed

15786 Starred procedure designation removed

16020 Starred procedure designation removed

16025 Starred procedure designation removed

17000 Starred procedure designation removed

17110 Starred procedure designation removed

17250	Starred procedure designation removed		**20600**	Starred procedure designation removed
17260	Starred procedure designation removed		**20605**	Starred procedure designation removed
17270	Starred procedure designation removed		**20610**	Starred procedure designation removed
17280	Starred procedure designation removed		**20650**	Starred procedure designation removed
17340	Starred procedure designation removed		**20665**	Starred procedure designation removed
17360	Starred procedure designation removed		**20670**	Starred procedure designation removed
17380	Starred procedure designation removed		**20982**	Code added
19000	Starred procedure designation removed		**21100**	Starred procedure designation removed
19100	Starred procedure designation removed		**21315**	Starred procedure designation removed
			21355	Starred procedure designation removed

SURGERY-MUSCULOSKELETAL

20000	Starred procedure designation removed		**21685**	Code added
20206	Starred procedure designation removed		**22532**	Code added
			22533	Code added
20240	Terminology revised		**22534**	Code added
20500	Starred procedure designation removed		**23700**	Starred procedure designation removed
20501	Starred procedure designation removed		**24640**	Starred procedure designation removed
20520	Starred procedure designation removed		**26010**	Starred procedure designation removed
20525	Starred procedure designation removed		**26011**	Starred procedure designation removed
20550	Terminology revised		**26356**	Terminology revised
20551	Terminology revised		**26357**	Terminology revised
20552	Terminology revised		**27086**	Starred procedure designation removed

9

27256	Starred procedure designation removed
27257	Starred procedure designation removed
27275	Starred procedure designation removed
27570	Starred procedure designation removed
27605	Starred procedure designation removed
27860	Starred procedure designation removed
28001	Starred procedure designation removed
28002	Starred procedure designation removed
28190	Starred procedure designation removed
28630	Starred procedure designation removed
28635	Starred procedure designation removed
28660	Starred procedure designation removed
28665	Starred procedure designation removed

SURGERY-RESPIRATORY

30000	Starred procedure designation removed
30020	Starred procedure designation removed
30200	Starred procedure designation removed
30210	Starred procedure designation removed
30300	Starred procedure designation removed

30560	Starred procedure designation removed
30801	Starred procedure designation removed
30901	Starred procedure designation removed
30903	Starred procedure designation removed
30905	Starred procedure designation removed
30906	Starred procedure designation removed
31000	Starred procedure designation removed
31002	Starred procedure designation removed
31622	Terminology revised
31625	Terminology revised
31628	Terminology revised
31629	Terminology revised
31632	Code added
31633	Code added
32000	Starred procedure designation removed
32400	Starred procedure designation removed
32420	Starred procedure designation removed
32960	Starred procedure designation removed

SURGERY-CARDIOVASCULAR

33010	Starred procedure designation removed
33011	Starred procedure designation removed

33310	Terminology revised	**36534**	Code deleted
34805	Code added	**36535**	Code deleted
35510	Code added	**36536**	Code deleted
35512	Code added	**36537**	Code deleted
35522	Code added	**36555**	Code added
35525	Code added	**36556**	Code added
35697	Code added	**36557**	Code added
36000	Starred procedure designation removed	**36558**	Code added
		36560	Code added
36400	Terminology revised	**36561**	Code added
36405	Starred procedure designation removed	**36563**	Code added
36410	Terminology revised	**36565**	Code added
36415	Starred procedure designation removed	**36566**	Code added
		36568	Code added
36440	Starred procedure designation removed	**36569**	Code added
		36570	Code added
36470	Starred procedure designation removed	**36571**	Code added
36471	Starred procedure designation removed	**36575**	Code added
		36576	Code added
36488	Code deleted	**36578**	Code added
36489	Code deleted	**36580**	Code added
36490	Code deleted	**36581**	Code added
36491	Code deleted	**36582**	Code added
36493	Code deleted	**36583**	Code added
36510	Starred procedure designation removed	**36584**	Code added
36530	Code deleted	**36585**	Code added
36531	Code deleted	**36589**	Code added
36532	Code deleted	**36590**	Code added
36533	Code deleted	**36595**	Code added

11

36596	Code added
36597	Code added
36600	Starred procedure designation removed
36660	Starred procedure designation removed
36838	Code added
37765	Code added
37766	Code added
37785	Terminology revised
38208	Terminology revised
38209	Terminology revised
38300	Starred procedure designation removed

SURGERY-DIGESTIVE SYSTEM

40800	Starred procedure designation removed
40804	Starred procedure designation removed
41000	Starred procedure designation removed
41005	Starred procedure designation removed
41250	Starred procedure designation removed
41251	Starred procedure designation removed
41252	Starred procedure designation removed
41800	Starred procedure designation removed
42000	Starred procedure designation removed
42300	Starred procedure designation removed

42310	Starred procedure designation removed
42320	Starred procedure designation removed
42400	Starred procedure designation removed
42650	Starred procedure designation removed
42660	Starred procedure designation removed
42700	Starred procedure designation removed
43237	Code added
43238	Code added
43242	Terminology revised
43259	Terminology revised
43450	Starred procedure designation removed
43752	Terminology revised
43760	Starred procedure designation removed
45900	Starred procedure designation removed
45905	Starred procedure designation removed
45915	Starred procedure designation removed
46030	Starred procedure designation removed
46050	Starred procedure designation removed
46080	Starred procedure designation removed
46320	Starred procedure designation removed

12

46500	Starred procedure designation removed
46900	Starred procedure designation removed
46910	Starred procedure designation removed
47000	Starred procedure designation removed
47133	Grammatical revision
47134	Code deleted
47140	Code added
47141	Code added
47142	Code added
48102	Starred procedure designation removed
49080	Starred procedure designation removed
49081	Starred procedure designation removed
49180	Starred procedure designation removed
49400	Starred procedure designation removed
49420	Starred procedure designation removed

SURGERY-URINARY

50200	Starred procedure designation removed
50390	Starred procedure designation removed
50398	Starred procedure designation removed
50688	Starred procedure designation removed
51000	Starred procedure designation removed
51005	Starred procedure designation removed
51600	Starred procedure designation removed
51700	Starred procedure designation removed
51705	Starred procedure designation removed
51710	Starred procedure designation removed
53500	Code added
53600	Starred procedure designation removed
53601	Starred procedure designation removed
53620	Starred procedure designation removed
53621	Starred procedure designation removed
53660	Starred procedure designation removed
53661	Starred procedure designation removed

SURGERY-MALE GENITAL

54050	Starred procedure designation removed
54055	Starred procedure designation removed
54200	Starred procedure designation removed
55000	Starred procedure designation removed
55100	Starred procedure designation removed

SURGERY-FEMALE GENITAL

56405	Starred procedure designation removed
56420	Starred procedure designation removed
56605	Starred procedure designation removed
56606	Starred procedure designation removed
56720	Starred procedure designation removed
57020	Starred procedure designation removed
57100	Starred procedure designation removed
57150	Starred procedure designation removed
57160	Starred procedure designation removed
57400	Starred procedure designation removed
57410	Starred procedure designation removed
57425	Code added
57452	Starred procedure designation removed
57454	Starred procedure designation removed
57500	Starred procedure designation removed
57511	Starred procedure designation removed
57800	Starred procedure designation removed
58100	Starred procedure designation removed

58300	Starred procedure designation removed
58340	Terminology revised
58350	Starred procedure designation removed

SURGERY-MATERNITY CARE AND DELIVERY

59000	Starred procedure designation removed
59020	Starred procedure designation removed
59030	Starred procedure designation removed
59070	Code added
59072	Code added
59074	Code added
59076	Code added
59897	Code added

SURGERY-NERVOUS SYSTEM

60000	Starred procedure designation removed
60100	Starred procedure designation removed
61000	Starred procedure designation removed
61001	Starred procedure designation removed
61020	Starred procedure designation removed
61026	Starred procedure designation removed
61050	Starred procedure designation removed
61055	Starred procedure designation removed

61070	Starred procedure designation removed
61105	Starred procedure designation removed
61107	Starred procedure designation removed
61210	Starred procedure designation removed
61537	Code Added
61538	Terminology revised
61539	Terminology revised
61540	Code added
61543	Terminology revised
61566	Code added
61567	Code added
61862	Code deleted
61863	Code added
61864	Code added
61867	Code added
61868	Code added
62268	Starred procedure designation removed
62269	Starred procedure designation removed
62270	Starred procedure designation removed
62272	Starred procedure designation removed
62280	Starred procedure designation removed
62281	Starred procedure designation removed
62282	Starred procedure designation removed
62284	Starred procedure designation removed
62290	Starred procedure designation removed
62291	Starred procedure designation removed
63101	Code added
63102	Code added
63103	Code added
63173	Terminology revised
64400	Starred procedure designation removed
64402	Starred procedure designation removed
64405	Starred procedure designation removed
64408	Starred procedure designation removed
64410	Starred procedure designation removed
64412	Starred procedure designation removed
64413	Starred procedure designation removed
64415	Starred procedure designation removed
64417	Starred procedure designation removed
64418	Starred procedure designation removed
64420	Starred procedure designation removed
64421	Starred procedure designation removed
64425	Starred procedure designation removed

64430	Starred procedure designation removed	**65430**	Starred procedure designation removed
64435	Starred procedure designation removed	**65435**	Starred procedure designation removed
64445	Starred procedure designation removed	**65780**	Code added
64449	Code added	**65781**	Code added
64450	Starred procedure designation removed	**65782**	Code added
64505	Starred procedure designation removed	**65800**	Starred procedure designation removed
64508	Starred procedure designation removed	**65805**	Starred procedure designation removed
64510	Starred procedure designation removed	**66020**	Starred procedure designation removed
64517	Code added	**66030**	Starred procedure designation removed
64520	Starred procedure designation removed	**67500**	Starred procedure designation removed
64530	Starred procedure designation removed	**67515**	Starred procedure designation removed
64680	Terminology revised	**67700**	Starred procedure designation removed
64681	Code added	**67710**	Starred procedure designation removed

SURGERY-EYE/ADNEXA

65205	Starred procedure designation removed	**67715**	Starred procedure designation removed
65210	Starred procedure designation removed	**67810**	Starred procedure designation removed
65220	Starred procedure designation removed	**67820**	Starred procedure designation removed
65222	Starred procedure designation removed	**67825**	Starred procedure designation removed
65270	Starred procedure designation removed	**67840**	Starred procedure designation removed
65410	Starred procedure designation removed	**67850**	Starred procedure designation removed
		67912	Code added

16

67916	Terminology revised		**70558**	Code added
67917	Terminology revised		**70559**	Code added
67923	Terminology revised		**72270**	Terminology revised
67924	Terminology revised		**75860**	Terminology revised
68135	Starred procedure designation removed		**75998**	Code added
			76082	Code added
68200	Starred procedure designation removed		**76083**	Code added
68371	Code added		**76085**	Code deleted
68440	Starred procedure designation removed		**76362**	Terminology revised
			76375	Terminology revised
68801	Starred procedure designation removed		**76394**	Terminology revised
68810	Starred procedure designation removed		**76490**	Code deleted
			76514	Code added
68840	Starred procedure designation removed		**76831**	Terminology revised
			76872	Terminology revised
68850	Starred procedure designation removed		**76937**	Code added
			76940	Code added

SURGERY-AUDITORY SYSTEM

69000	Starred procedure designation removed		**78800**	Terminology revised
			78802	Terminology revised
69020	Starred procedure designation removed		**78804**	Code added
			79100	Terminology revised
69420	Starred procedure designation removed		**79400**	Terminology revised
69421	Starred procedure designation removed		**79403**	Code added
69433	Starred procedure designation removed			

PATHOLOGY AND LABORATORY

RADIOLOGY

			83716	Terminology revised
70250	Terminology revised		**84155**	Terminology revised
70260	Terminology revised		**84156**	Code added
70557	Code added		**84157**	Code added
			84160	Terminology revised

17

84165	Terminology revised	**89268**	Code added
85055	Code added	**89272**	Code added
85396	Code added	**89280**	Code added
87040	Terminology revised	**89281**	Code added
87045	Terminology revised	**89290**	Code added
87046	Terminology revised	**89291**	Code added
87070	Terminology revised	**89335**	Code added
87075	Terminology revised	**89342**	Code added
87269	Code added	**89343**	Code added
87272	Terminology revised	**89344**	Code added
87328	Terminology revised	**89346**	Code added
87329	Code added	**89350**	Code deleted
87660	Code added	**89352**	Code added
88112	Code added	**89353**	Code added
88312	Terminology revised	**89354**	Code added
88342	Terminology revised	**89355**	Code deleted
88358	Terminology revised	**89356**	Code added
88361	Code added	**89360**	Code deleted
89055	Terminology revised	**89365**	Code deleted
89220	Code added	**89399**	Code deleted
89225	Code added		

MEDICINE

89230	Code added	**90655**	Code added
89235	Code added	**90657**	Terminology revised
89240	Code added	**90658**	Terminology revised
89250	Terminology revised	**90659**	Code deleted
89251	Terminology revised	**90693**	Terminology revised
89252	Code deleted	**90698**	Code added
89256	Code deleted	**90703**	Terminology revised
89258	Terminology revised	**90704**	Terminology revised

18

90705	Terminology revised		**99562**	Code deleted
90706	Terminology revised		**99563**	Code deleted
90707	Terminology revised		**99564**	Code deleted
90708	Terminology revised		**99565**	Code deleted
90715	Code added		**99566**	Code deleted
90718	Terminology revised		**99567**	Code deleted
90727	Terminology revised		**99568**	Code deleted
90733	Terminology revised		**99569**	Code deleted
90734	Code added		**99601**	Code added
91110	Code added		**99602**	Code added
95990	Terminology revised			

CATEGORY II

95991	Code added
97537	Terminology revised
97755	Code added
99024	Terminology revised
99025	Code deleted
99050	Terminology revised
99512	Terminology revised
99551	Code deleted
99552	Code deleted
99553	Code deleted
99554	Code deleted
99555	Code deleted
99556	Code deleted
99557	Code deleted
99558	Code deleted
99559	Code deleted
99560	Code deleted
99561	Code deleted

0001F	Code added
0002F	Code added
0003F	Code added
0004F	Code added
0005F	Code added
0006F	Code added
0007F	Code added
0008F	Code added
0009F	Code added
0010F	Code added
0011F	Code added

CATEGORY III EMERGING TECHNOLOGY CODES

0001T	Terminology revised
0002T	Code deleted
0025T	Code deleted
0044T	Terminology revised
0045T	Code added

19

0046T   Code added

0047T   Code added

0048T   Code added

0049T   Code added

0050T   Code added

0051T   Code added

0052T   Code added

0053T   Code added

0054T   Code added

0055T   Code added

0056T   Code added

0057T   Code added

0058T   Code added

0059T   Code added

0060T   Code added

0061T   Code added

STARRED PROCEDURES

Starred procedure designation was removed from CPT 2004.

INSTRUCTIONAL NOTES

Notes found in the CPT coding system give instructions for using codes. When selecting a code, look for instructions in the section guidelines for any additional information necessary to code accurately. Also, instructional notes take the form of parenthetical statements and paragraphs, which may appear at the beginning of subsections, headings and subheadings, or above and below the code itself.

DEFINITION OF NEW AND ESTABLISHED PATIENT

Solely for the purposes of distinguishing between new and established patients, professional services are those face-to-face services rendered by a physician and coded by a specific cpt code(s). A new patient is one who has not received any professional services from the physician or another physician of the same specialty who belongs to the same group practice, within the past three years.

An established patient is one who has received professional services from the physician or another physician of the same specialty who belongs to the same group practice, within the past three years.

In the instance where a physician is on call for or covering for another physician, the patient's encounter will be classified as it would have been by the physician who is not available.

No distinction is made between new and established patients in the emergency department. Evaluation and Management services in the emergency department category may be coded for any new or established patient who presents for treatment in the emergency department.

PLACE (LOCATION) OF SERVICE

The CPT coding system makes specific distinctions for place (location) of service for CPT codes defined in the evaluation and management section. The place of service may have considerable impact on reimbursement. The following list gives CPT code ranges for some specific places of service:

Office [or Other Outpatient] Services	*99201-99215*
Hospital [Inpatient] Services	*99221-99239*
Emergency Department	*99281-99288*
Nursing Facility Services	*99301-99316*
Domiciliary, Rest Home, or Custodial Care Services	*99321-99333*
Home Services	*99341-99353*

21

HOSPITAL CARE

Hospital services frequently cause reimbursement problems for health care professionals. The three most common coding errors are:

- *More than one physician submits an initial hospital care code for the same patient.*

- *Follow-up hospital visits are coded incorrectly.*

- *Concurrent care visits by multiple specialists are coded improperly.*

If more than one physician is involved in the process of hospitalizing a patient, for example, surgeon and internist, the physicians must decide which is going to actually admit the patient and report the admission services on the health insurance claim form. If both do, the first health insurance claim form to arrive will be processed and paid, and the second will be rejected.

There are valid reasons for visiting a patient more than once daily while hospitalized, however, many physicians and even some insurance billers do not know that subsequent hospital visit codes are for "daily" services. When a physician visits the patient twice in one day, providing a brief level of service each time, the physician or insurance biller may incorrectly report two hospital visit services for the same day, instead of a higher level code incorporating both visits.

Reporting multiple hospital visits provided on the same day separately on the health insurance claim form usually results in either the entire claim being returned for clarification, or the second visit being denied as an apparent duplication. Unfortunately, insurance billers who are unclear on the proper coding of same day hospital visits may simply accept the rejection without question and write-off the unpaid visit as uncollectible.

The CPT coding system clearly defines subsequent hospital care as "per day", meaning daily services. If the physician visits the patient twice in one day, providing the equivalent of "brief" services each time, report the service using the appropriate evaluation and management code that defines the cumulative level of service provided.

HOSPITAL DISCHARGE

The CPT codes for hospital discharge services are evaluation and management code 99238 and 99239, defined as Hospital Discharge Day Management. Hospital discharge services include final examination of the patient, discussion of the hospital stay, instructions for continuing care, and preparation of discharge records. Many health insurance companies do not recognize and/or do not reimburse this CPT code.

Options for the use of these codes include the use of one of the other hospital daily services codes from the evaluation and management series 99231-99233 and perhaps using a code that has a higher value than the routine hospital visit.

REFERRAL

A referral is the transfer of the total care or specific portion of care of a patient from one physician to another. A referral is not a request for consultation. If a patient is referred to the physician for total care or a portion of their care, use evaluation and management visit codes, and other CPT codes if appropriate, to report the services provided. If a patient is sent to the physician for a consultation, use evaluation and management consultation codes to report the services provided.

SEPARATE OR MULTIPLE PROCEDURES

It is appropriate to designate multiple procedures that are rendered on the same date by separate entries. For example: if a proctosigmoidoscopy was performed in addition to a hospital visit, the proctosigmoidoscopy would be considered a SEPARATE procedure and listed in addition to the hospital visit on the health insurance claim form. Another example would be individual medical psychotherapy rendered in addition to a brief subsequent hospital service. In this instance, both services would be coded.

SUPPLIES AND MATERIALS SUPPLIED BY THE PHYSICIAN

The CPT coding system includes specific codes for identifying certain supplies and materials provided by the physician. These supply codes are used to report supplies and materials that are not included in the definition of the basic service.

CPT CODES FOR SUPPLIES AND MATERIALS

92390-92396 Supply of spectacles, contact lenses, low vision aids and ocular prosthesis.

95144-95170 Provision of antigens for allergen immunotherapy.

96545 Provision of chemotherapy agent.

99070 Supplies and materials (except spectacles) provided by the physician.

99071 Educational supplies, such as books, tapes, and pamphlets, provided by the physician for the patient's education at cost to physician.

78990 & 79900 Diagnostic and therapeutic radiopharmaceuticals.

PURCHASED DIAGNOSTIC SERVICES

It is common for physicians to bill patients and health insurance companies for diagnostic services that were procured or ordered on behalf of the patient but not actually provided by the ordering physician. It is also common for the ordering physician to "mark-up" the fee for the purchased service prior to billing. This is referred to as global billing.

Medical equipment companies, particularly those offering electrocardiography, pulmonary diagnostic equipment, and other diagnostic equipment, have used this global billing concept in the past as a method of selling physicians a new "profit center" for their practice. Some even provided technicians, who were not employees of the practice, to perform the diagnostic tests in the physicians office. OBRA 1987 placed severe restrictions on global billing of certain diagnostic tests as of March 1, 1988.

The Medicare regulations apply to diagnostic tests other than clinical laboratory tests including, but not limited to: EKGs, EEGs, cardiac monitoring, X-rays and ultrasound. Global billing is allowed only when the billing physician personally performs or supervises the diagnostic procedure. To qualify under the supervision definition, the person performing the test must be an employee or the physician or group. Ownership interest in an outside supplier does not meet the supervision requirement.

Billing for purchased services under the new requirement is complicated. The provider must provide the supplier's name, address, provider number and net charge on the health insurance claim form. In addition, a HCPCS Level III modifier must be coded to indicate that the service was purchased. Billing for global services usually will also require a HCPCS Level III modifier to indicate that the service was not purchased. This requirement does not apply to the professional component of these services if provided separately.

Providers should discontinue billing for the technical component of diagnostic services that were not provided or supervised by the provider as defined in this regulation for the following reasons:

1. *The provider is no longer making any profit on these procedures;*

2. *Operating costs are higher due to the increased reporting requirements; and*

3. *Risk of audit liability is increased if these services are not coded properly.*

UNBUNDLING

Unbundling is defined as reporting multiple CPT codes when one CPT code is sufficient. For example, it is considered unbundling if incidental surgical procedures are coded separately, or office visits for uncomplicated follow-up care are separately coded. This practice often happens unintentionally. However, most third-party payers currently have software in place to catch unbundling when it occurs. When physicians continually break out or itemize services in this manner, they often find themselves under close scrutiny and even the focus of an audit by the insurance company. It is most important to know the guidelines to prevent unbundling when coding and billing for services and/or procedures.

This page intentionally left blank.

CPT MODIFIERS

The CPT® coding system includes two-digit modifier codes which are used to report that a service or procedure has been "altered or modified by some specific circumstance" without altering or modifying the basic definition or CPT code.

The proper use of CPT modifiers can speed up claim processing and increase reimbursement, while the improper use of CPT modifiers may result in claim delays or claim denials. In addition, using certain CPT modifiers, for example -22, too frequently may trigger a claims audit.

CPT MODIFIERS

-21   Prolonged evaluation and management services

When the face-to-face or floor/unit service(s) provided is prolonged or otherwise greater than that usually required for the highest level of evaluation and management service within a given category, it may be identified by adding modifier '-21' to the evaluation and management code number. A report may also be appropriate.

-22   Unusual procedural services

When the service(s) provided is greater than that usually required for the listed procedure, it may be identified by adding modifier '-22' to the procedure number. A report may also be appropriate.

This modifier is not to be used to report procedure(s) complicated by adhesion formation, scarring, and/or alteration of normal landmarks due to late effects of prior surgery, irradiation, infection, very low weight (ie, neonates and infants less than 10kg) or trauma.

Modifier -22 is frequently abused and misused. Some physicians routinely add modifier -22 to CPT procedure codes with the expectation that higher reimbursement will be forthcoming. Many third party payers routinely ignore an undocumented modifier -22 on health insurance claim forms for the same reason.

In most cases, it is more appropriate to choose a CPT code of a higher value than to use modifier -22. If the provider reports modifier -22, documentation in the form of a cover letter or report must be provided with the health insurance claim form to explain the situation or circumstances that make the procedure(s) unusual.

-23   Unusual anesthesia

Occasionally, a procedure, which usually requires either no anesthesia or local anesthesia, because of unusual circumstances must be done under general anesthesia. This circumstance may be reported by adding the modifier '-23' to the procedure code of the basic service.

-24   Unrelated evaluation and management service by the same physician during a postoperative period

The physician may need to indicate that an evaluation and management service was performed during a postoperative period for a reason(s) unrelated to the original procedure. This circumstance may be reported by adding the modifier '-24' to the appropriate level of E/M service.

-25   Significant, separately identifiable evaluation and management service by the same physician on the same day of a procedure or other service

The physician may need to indicate that on the day a procedure or service identified by a CPT code was performed, the patient's condition required a significant, separately identifiable E/M service above and beyond the other service provided or beyond the usual preoperative and postoperative care associated with the procedure that was performed. The E/M service may be prompted by the symptom or condition for which the procedure and/or service was provided. As such, different diagnoses are not required for reporting of the E/M services on the same date. This circumstance may be reported by adding the modifier '-25' to the appropriate level of E/M service.

Note: This modifier is not used to report an E/M service that resulted in a decision to perform surgery. See modifier '-57.'

-26   Professional component

Certain procedures are a combination of a physician component and a technical component. When the physician component is reported separately, the service may be identified by adding the modifier '-26' to the usual procedure number.

-27   Multiple outpatient hospital evaluation and management encounters on the same date

For hospital outpatient reporting purposes, utilization of hospital resources related to separate and distinct E/M encounters performed in multiple outpatient hospital settings on the same date may be reported by adding the modifier '-27' to each appropriate level outpatient and/or emergency department E/M code(s).

This modifier provides a means of reporting circumstances involving evaluation and management services provided by physician(s) in more than one (multiple) outpatient hospital setting(s) (eg, hospital emergency department, clinic).

Note: This modifier is not to be used for physician reporting of multiple E/M services performed by the same physician on the same date. For physician reporting of all outpatient evaluation and management services provided by the same physician on the same date and performed in multiple outpatient setting(s) (eg, hospital emergency department, clinic), see Evaluation and Management, Emergency Department, or Preventive Medicine Services codes.

-32 Mandated services

Services related to mandated consultation and/or related services (eg, PRO, third party payer, governmental, legislative or regulatory requirement) may be identified by adding the modifier '-32' to the basic procedure.

Occasionally a consultation and/or related service may be mandated by a third party (eg, peer review organization, third party payer, governmental, legislative or regulatory requirement).

HCPCS modifier -SF is reported instead of CPT modifier -32 if the patient is a Medicare patient.

-47 Anesthesia by surgeon

Regional or general anesthesia provided by the surgeon may be reported by adding the modifier '-47' to the basic service. (This does not include local anesthesia.)

Note: Modifier '-47' would not be used as a modifier for the Anesthesia procedures.

-50 Bilateral procedure

Unless otherwise identified in the listings, bilateral procedures that are performed at the same operative session, should be identified by adding the modifier '-50' to the appropriate five digit code.

This modifier is reported when bilateral procedures requiring a separate incision are performed during the SAME operative session. Proper reporting of this modifier on the CMS1500 health insurance claim form requires the CPT procedure code to be listed two times: first with no modifier, and the second time with modifier -50.

This modifier may not be used if the definition of the basic procedure code includes the term "bilateral."

29

-51   Multiple procedures

When multiple procedures, other than E/M services, are performed at the same session by the same provider, the primary procedure or service may be reported as listed. The additional procedure(s) or service(s) may be identified by appending the modifier '-51' to the additional procedure or service code(s).

Note: This modifier should not be appended to designated "add-on" codes.

-52   Reduced services

Under certain circumstances a service or procedure is partially reduced or eliminated at the physician's discretion. Under these circumstances the service provided can be identified by its usual procedure number and the addition of the modifier '-52' signifying that the service is reduced. This provides a means of reporting reduced services without disturbing the identification of the basic service.

Note: For hospital outpatient reporting of a previously scheduled procedure/ service that is partially reduced or canceled as a result of extenuating circumstances or those that threaten the well-being of the patient prior to or after administration of anesthesia, see modifiers '-73' and '-74' (see modifiers approved for ASC hospital outpatient use).

The intended use of this modifier is to report the reduction of a service without affecting provider profiles maintained by health insurance companies.

Modifier -52 is another frequently misused modifier. Some medical practices mistakenly use modifier -52 to mean "reduced fee" and use it as a discounting method. Not only is this incorrect, the provider may seriously damage their provider profile with health insurance companies. The proper use for modifier -52 is to report that a service was not completed, or some part of a multiple-part service was not performed. A fee reduction may be in order as well; however that is not the primary purpose of the modifier.

-53   Discontinued procedure

Under certain circumstances, the physician may elect to terminate a surgical or diagnostic procedure. Due to extenuating circumstances or those that threaten the well being of the patient, it may be necessary to indicate that a surgical or diagnostic procedure was started but discontinued. This circumstance may be reported by adding the modifier '-53' to the code reported by the physician for the discontinued procedure.

Note: This modifier is not used to report the elective cancellation of a procedure prior to the patient's anesthesia induction and/or surgical preparation in the operating suite. For hospital outpatient/ambulatory surgery center (ASC) reporting of a previously scheduled procedure/service that is partially reduced or cancelled as a result of extenuating circumstances or those that threaten the well-being of the patient prior to or after administration of anesthesia, see modifiers '-73' and '-74' (see modifiers approved for ASC hospital outpatient use).

-54 Surgical care only

When one physician performs a surgical procedure and another provides preoperative and/or postoperative management, surgical services may be identified by adding the modifier '-54' to the usual procedure number.

-55 Postoperative management only

When one physician performed the postoperative management and another physician performed the surgical procedure, the postoperative component may be identified by adding the modifier '-55' to the usual procedure number.

-56 Preoperative management only

When one physician performed the preoperative care and evaluation and another physician performed the surgical procedure, the preoperative component may be identified by adding the modifier '-56' to the usual procedure number.

-57 Decision for surgery

An evaluation and management service that resulted in the initial decision to perform the surgery may be identified by adding the modifier '-57' to the appropriate level of E/M service.

-58 Staged or related procedure or service by the same physician during the postoperative period

The physician may need to indicate that the performance of a procedure or service during the postoperative period was: a) planned prospectively at the time of the original procedure (staged); b) more extensive than the original procedure; or c) for therapy following a diagnostic surgical procedure. This circumstance may be reported by adding the modifier '-58' to the staged or related procedure.

Note: This modifier is not used to report the treatment of a problem that requires a return to the operating room.

-59 Distinct Procedural Service

Under certain circumstances the physician may need to indicate that a procedure or service was distinct or independent from other services performed on the same day. Modifier '-59' is used to identify procedures/services that are not normally reported together, but are appropriate under the circumstances. This may represent a different session or patient encounter, different procedure or surgery, different site or organ system, separate incision/excision, separate lesion, or separate injury (or area of injury in extensive injuries) not ordinarily encountered or performed on the same day by the same physician.

However, when another already established modifier is appropriate it should be used rather than modifier '-59.' Only if no more descriptive modifier is available, and the use of modifier '-59' best explains the circumstances, should modifier '-59' be used.

-62 Two surgeons

When two surgeons work together as primary surgeons performing distinct part(s) of a procedure, each surgeon should report his/her distinct operative work by adding the modifier '-62' to the procedure code and any associated add-on code(s) for that procedure as long as both surgeons continue to work together as primary surgeons.

Each surgeon should report the co-surgery once using the same procedure code. If additional procedure(s) (including add-on procedure(s) are performed during the same surgical session, separate code(s) may also be reported with the modifier '-62' added.

Note: If a co-surgeon acts as an assistant in the performance of additional procedure(s) during the same surgical session, those services may be reported using separate procedure code(s) with the modifier '-80' or modifier '-82' added, as appropriate.

-63 Procedure performed on infants less than 4 kg

Procedures performed on neonates and infants up to a present body weight of 4 kg may involve significantly increased complexity and physician work commonly associated with these patients. This circumstance may be reported by adding the modifier '-63' to the procedure number.

Note: Unless otherwise designated, this modifier may only be appended to procedures/services listed in the 20000-69999 code series. Modifier '-63' should not be appended to any CPT codes listed in the Evaluation and Management Services, Anesthesia, Radiology, Pathology/Laboratory, or Medicine sections.

-66 Surgical team

Under some circumstances, highly complex procedures (requiring the concomitant services of several physicians, often of different specialties, plus other highly skilled specialy trained personnel, various types of complex equipment) are carried out under the "surgical team" concept. Such circumstances may be identified by each participating physician with the addition of the modifier '-66' to the basic procedure number used for reporting services.

-73 Discontinued out-patient hospital/ambulatory surgery center (ASC) procedure prior to the administration of anesthesia

Due to extenuating circumstances or those that threaten the well being of the patient, the physician may cancel a surgical or diagnostic procedure subsequent to the patient's surgical preparation (including sedation when provided, and being taken to the room where the procedure is to be performed), but prior to the administration of anesthesia (local, regional block(s) or general). Under these circumstances, the intended service that is prepared for but cancelled can be reported by its usual procedure number and the addition of the modifier '-73.'

Note: The elective cancellation of a service prior to the administration of anesthesia and/or surgical preparation of the patient should not be reported. For physician reporting of a discontinued procedure, see modifier '-53.'

-74 Discontinued out-patient hospital/ambulatory surgery center (ASC) procedure after administration of anesthesia

Due to extenuating circumstances or those that threaten the well being of the patient, the physician may terminate a surgical or diagnostic procedure after the administration of anesthesia (local, regional block(s), general) or after the procedure was started (incision made, intubation started, scope inserted, etc.). Under these circumstances, the procedure started but terminated can be reported by its usual procedure number and the addition of the modifier '-74.'

Note: The elective cancellation of a service prior to the administration of anesthesia and/or surgical preparation of the patient should not be reported. For physician reporting of a discontinued procedure, see modifier '-53.'

-76 Repeat procedure by same physician

The physician may need to indicate that a procedure or service was repeated subsequent to the original procedure or service. This circumstance may be reported by adding the modifier '-76' to the repeated procedure/service.

-77   Repeat procedure by another physician

The physician may need to indicate that a basic procedure or service performed by another physician had to be repeated. This situation may be reported by adding modifier '-77' to the repeated procedure/service.

-78   Return to the operating room for a related procedure during the postoperative period

The physician may need to indicate that another procedure was performed during the postoperative period of the initial procedure. When this subsequent procedure is related to the first, and requires the use of the operating room, it may be reported by adding the modifier '-78' to the related procedure. (For repeat procedures on the same day, see '-76.')

-79   Unrelated procedure or service by the same physician during the postoperative period

The physician may need to indicate that the performance of a procedure or service during the postoperative period was unrelated to the original procedure. This circumstance may be reported by using the modifier '-79.' (For repeat procedures on the same day, see '-76.')

-80   Assistant surgeon

Surgical assistant services may be identified by adding the modifier '-80' to the usual procedure number(s).

-81   Minimum assistant surgeon

Minimum surgical assistant services are identified by adding the modifier '-81' to the usual procedure number.

-82   Assistant surgeon (when qualified resident surgeon not available)

The unavailability of a qualified resident surgeon is a prerequisite for use of modifier '-82' appended to the usual procedure code number(s).

-90   Reference (outside) laboratory

When laboratory procedures are performed by a party other than the treating or reporting physician, the procedure may be identified by adding the modifier '-90' to the usual procedure number.

-91   Repeat clinical diagnostic laboratory test

In the course of treatment of the patient, it may be necessary to repeat the same laboratory test on the same day to obtain subsequent (multiple) test results. Under these circumstances, the laboratory test performed can be identified by its usual procedure number and the addition of modifier '-91.'

Note: This modifier may not be used when tests are rerun to confirm initial results; due to testing problems with specimens or equipment; or for any other reason when a normal, one-time, reportable result is all that is required.

This modifier may not be used when other code(s) describe a series of tests results (eg, glucose tolerance tests, evocative/suppression testing). This modifier may only be used for laboratory test(s) performed more than once on the same day on the same patient.

-99 Multiple modifiers

Under certain circumstances two or more modifiers may be necessary to completely delineate a service. In such situations modifier '-99' should be added to the basic procedure, and other applicable modifiers may be listed as part of the description of the service.

ANESTHESIA PHYSICAL STATUS MODIFIERS

P1 A normal healthy patient

P2 A patient with mild systemic disease

P3 A patient with severe systemic disease

P4 A patient with severe systemic disaease that is a constant threat to life

P5 A moribund patient who is not expected to survive without the operation

P6 A declared brain-dead patient whose organs are being removed for donor purposes

HCPCS MODIFIERS

HCPCS modifiers, defined and managed by The Centers for Medicare and Medicaid Services (CMS), are two digit modifier codes which may be either alpha (all letters) or alphanumeric (letters plus numbers). Some HCPCS modifiers may be used with CPT codes to modify procedures and services on health insurance claim forms filed for Medicare patients. See the most current edition of HCPCS for a complete list.

This page intentionally left blank.

ANATOMICAL ILLUSTRATIONS

A fundamental knowledge and understanding of basic human anatomy and physiology is a prerequisite for accurate CPT© procedure coding. While a comprehensive treatment of anatomy and physiology is beyond the scope of this text, the large scale, full color anatomical illustrations on the following pages are designed to facilitate the procedure coding process for both beginning and experienced coders.

The illustrations provide an anatomical perspective of procedure coding by providing a side-by-side view of the major systems of the human body and a corresponding list of the most common CPT procedural categories used to report medical, surgical and diagnostic services performed on the illustrated system.

The CPT procedural categories listed on the left facing page of each anatomical illustration are code ranges only and should not be used for coding. These categories are provided as "pointers" to the appropriate section of CPT, where the definitive code may be found.

PLATE 1. SKIN AND SUBCUTANEOUS TISSUE - MALE

**SKIN, SUBCUTANEOUS AND
ACCESSORY STRUCTURES**

Incision and Drainage	10040-10180
Excision—Debridement	11000-11044
Paring or Cutting	11055-11057
Biopsy	11100-11101
Removal of Skin Tags	11200-11201
Shaving of Lesions	11300-11313
Excision-Benign Lesions	11400-11471
Excision-Malignant Lesions	11600-11646

Nails	11719-11765

Repair (Closure)

Repair-Simple	12001-12021
Repair-Intermediate	12031-12057
Repair-Complex	13100-13160
Adjacent Tissue Transfer	14000-14350
Free Skin Grafts	15000-15400
Flaps (Skin and/or Deep Tissues)	15570-15999
Burns	16000-16036

Destruction

Destruction, Benign or Premalignant Lesions	17000-17250
Destruction, Malignant Lesions	17260-17286
Mohs' Micrographic Surgery	17304-17310
Other Destruction Procedures	17340-17999

Laboratory Services

Skin Tests, Immunology	86485-86586
Skin Tests, Allergy	95010-95199

Visit and Medicine Services

E/M Services	99201-99499
Special Dermatological Procedures	96900-96999

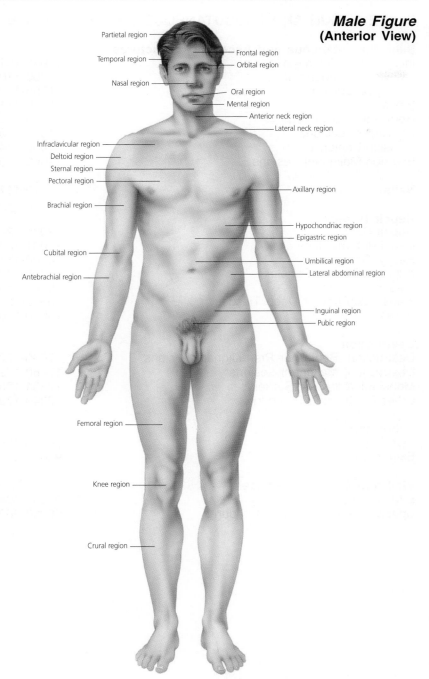

Male Figure
(Anterior View)

Partietal region

Temporal region

Nasal region

Frontal region

Orbital region

Oral region

Mental region

Anterior neck region

Lateral neck region

Infraclavicular region

Deltoid region

Sternal region

Pectoral region

Brachial region

Axillary region

Hypochondriac region

Epigastric region

Cubital region

Antebrachial region

Umbilical region

Lateral abdominal region

Inguinal region

Pubic region

Femoral region

Knee region

Crural region

©Practice Management Information Corp., Los Angeles, CA

39

PLATE 2. SKIN AND SUBCUTANEOUS TISSUE - FEMALE

Skin, Subcutaneous and Accessory Structures

Incision and Drainage	10040-10180
Excision-Debridement	11000-11044
Paring or Cutting	11055-11057
Biopsy	11100-11101
Removal of Skin Tags	11200-11201
Shaving of Lesions	11300-11313
Excision-Benign Lesions	11400-11471
Excision-Malignant Lesions	11600-11646

Nails   11719-11765

Repair (Closure)

Repair-Simple	12001-12021
Repair-Intermediate	12031-12057
Repair-Complex	13100-13160
Adjacent Tissue Transfer	14000-14350
Free Skin Grafts	15000-15400
Flaps (Skin and/or Deep Tissues)	15570-15999
Burns	16000-16036

Destruction

Destruction, Benign or Premalignant Lesions	17000-17250
Destruction, Malignant Lesions	17260-17286
Mohs' Micrographic Surgery	17304-17310
Other Destruction Procedures	17340-17999

Laboratory Services

Skin Tests, Immunology	86485-86586
Skin Tests, Allergy	95010-95199

Visit and Medicine Services

E/M Services	99201-99499
Special Dermatological Procedures	96900-96999

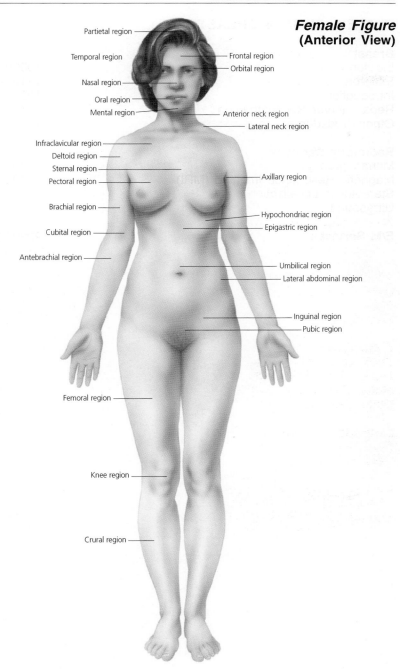

Female Figure
(Anterior View)

Partietal region
Temporal region
Frontal region
Orbital region
Nasal region
Oral region
Mental region
Anterior neck region
Lateral neck region
Infraclavicular region
Deltoid region
Sternal region
Pectoral region
Axillary region
Brachial region
Hypochondriac region
Epigastric region
Cubital region
Antebrachial region
Umbilical region
Lateral abdominal region
Inguinal region
Pubic region
Femoral region
Knee region
Crural region

©Practice Management Information Corp., Los Angeles, CA

41

PLATE 3. FEMALE BREAST

Breast
Incision	19000-19030
Excision	19100-19272
Introduction	19290-19295
Repair and/or Reconstruction	19316-19396
Other Procedures	19499

Radiology Services
Mammography	76082-76092
Magnetic Resonance Imaging (MRI)	76093-76094
Stereotactic Localization	76095
Ultrasound	76645

E/M Services   99201-99499

Female Breast

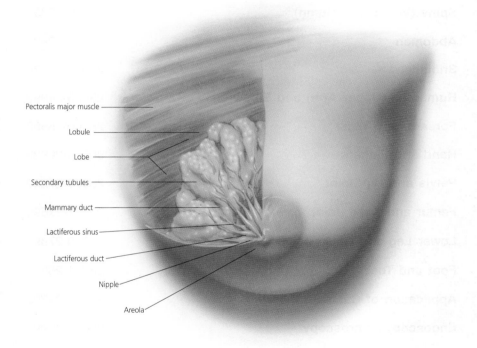

Pectoralis major muscle

Lobule

Lobe

Secondary tubules

Mammary duct

Lactiferous sinus

Lactiferous duct

Nipple

Areola

PLATE 4. MUSCULAR SYSTEM AND CONNECTIVE TISSUE - ANTERIOR VIEW

General	20000-20999
Head	21010-21499
Neck (Soft Tissues) and Thorax	21501-21899
Back and Flank	21920-21935
Spine (Vertebral Column)	22100-22899
Abdomen	22900-22999
Shoulder	23000-23929
Humerous (Upper Arm) and Elbow	23930-24999
Forearm and Wrist	25000-25999
Hand and Fingers	26010-26989
Pelvis and Hip Joint	26990-27299
Femur and Knee Joint	27301-27599
Lower Leg and Ankle Joint	27600-27899
Foot and Toes	28001-28899
Application of Casts/Strapping	29000-29799
Endoscopy/Arthroscopy	29800-29999
E/M Services	99201-99499

Muscular System
(Anterior View)

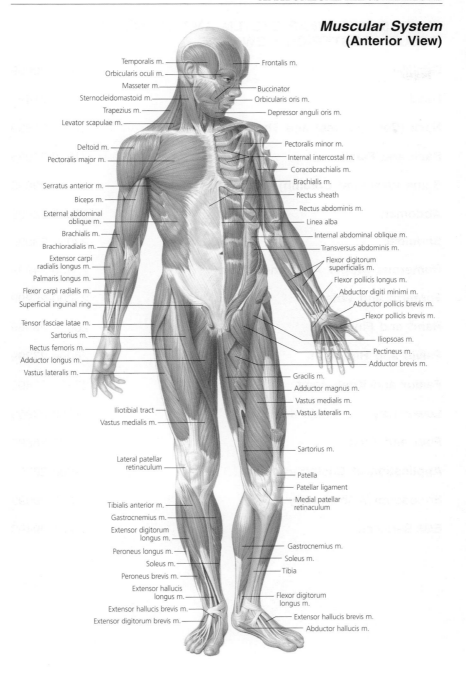

Temporalis m.
Orbicularis oculi m.
Masseter m.
Sternocleidomastoid m.
Trapezius m.
Levator scapulae m.

Frontalis m.
Buccinator
Orbicularis oris m.
Depressor anguli oris m.

Deltoid m.
Pectoralis major m.

Pectoralis minor m.
Internal intercostal m.
Coracobrachialis m.
Brachialis m.
Rectus sheath
Rectus abdominis m.
Linea alba
Internal abdominal oblique m.
Transversus abdominis m.
Flexor digitorum superficialis m.
Flexor pollicis longus m.
Abductor digiti minimi m.
Abductor pollicis brevis m.
Flexor pollicis brevis m.
Iliopsoas m.
Pectineus m.
Adductor brevis m.

Serratus anterior m.
Biceps m.
External abdominal oblique m.
Brachialis m.
Brachioradialis m.
Extensor carpi radialis longus m.
Palmaris longus m.
Flexor carpi radialis m.
Superficial inguinal ring
Tensor fasciae latae m.
Sartorius m.
Rectus femoris m.
Adductor longus m.
Vastus lateralis m.

Gracilis m.
Adductor magnus m.
Vastus medialis m.
Vastus lateralis m.

Iliotibial tract
Vastus medialis m.

Sartorius m.

Lateral patellar retinaculum

Patella
Patellar ligament
Medial patellar retinaculum

Tibialis anterior m.
Gastrocnemius m.
Extensor digitorum longus m.
Peroneus longus m.
Soleus m.
Peroneus brevis m.
Extensor hallucis longus m.
Extensor hallucis brevis m.
Extensor digitorum brevis m.

Gastrocnemius m.
Soleus m.
Tibia

Flexor digitorum longus m.
Extensor hallucis brevis m.
Abductor hallucis m.

PLATE 5. MUSCULAR SYSTEM AND CONNECTIVE TISSUE - POSTERIOR VIEW

General	20000-20999
Head	21010-21499
Neck (Soft Tissues) and Thorax	21501-21899
Back and Flank	21920-21935
Spine (Vertebral Column)	22100-22899
Abdomen	22900-22999
Shoulder	23000-23929
Humerous (Upper Arm) and Elbow	23930-24999
Forearm and Wrist	25000-25999
Hand and Fingers	26010-26989
Pelvis and Hip Joint	26990-27299
Femur and Knee Joint	27301-27599
Lower Leg and Ankle Joint	27600-27899
Foot and Toes	28001-28899
Application of Casts/Strapping	29000-29799
Endoscopy/Arthroscopy	29800-29999
E/M Services	99201-99499

Muscular System
(Posterior View)

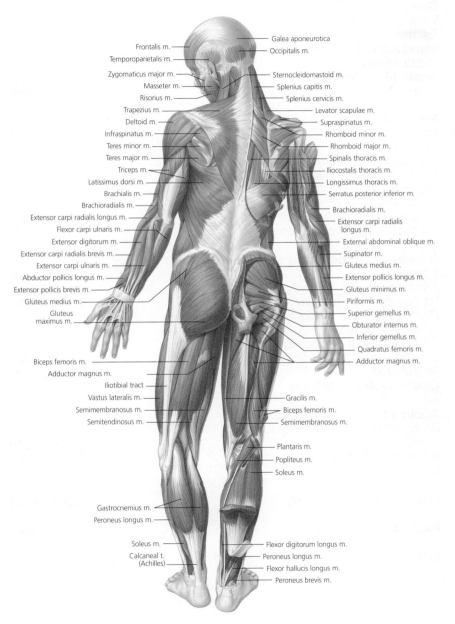

Frontalis m.
Temporoparietalis m.
Zygomaticus major m.
Masseter m.
Risorius m.
Trapezius m.
Deltoid m.
Infraspinatus m.
Teres minor m.
Teres major m.
Triceps m.
Latissimus dorsi m.
Brachialis m.
Brachioradialis m.
Extensor carpi radialis longus m.
Flexor carpi ulnaris m.
Extensor digitorum m.
Extensor carpi radialis brevis m.
Extensor carpi ulnaris m.
Abductor pollicis longus m.
Extensor pollicis brevis m.
Gluteus medius m.
Gluteus maximus m.
Biceps femoris m.
Adductor magnus m.
Iliotibial tract
Vastus lateralis m.
Semimembranosus m.
Semitendinosus m.
Gastrocnemius m.
Peroneus longus m.
Soleus m.
Calcaneal t. (Achilles)

Galea aponeurotica
Occipitalis m.
Sternocleidomastoid m.
Splenius capitis m.
Splenius cervicis m.
Levator scapulae m.
Supraspinatus m.
Rhomboid minor m.
Rhomboid major m.
Spinalis thoracis m.
Iliocostalis thoracis m.
Longissimus thoracis m.
Serratus posterior inferior m.
Brachioradialis m.
Extensor carpi radialis longus m.
External abdominal oblique m.
Supinator m.
Gluteus medius m.
Extensor pollicis longus m.
Gluteus minimus m.
Piriformis m.
Superior gemellus m.
Obturator internus m.
Inferior gemellus m.
Quadratus femoris m.
Adductor magnus m.
Gracilis m.
Biceps femoris m.
Semimembranosus m.
Plantaris m.
Popliteus m.
Soleus m.
Flexor digitorum longus m.
Peroneus longus m.
Flexor hallucis longus m.
Peroneus brevis m.

PLATE 6. MUSCULAR SYSTEM - SHOULDER AND ELBOW

General
Wound exploration - Trauma	20100-20103
Excision	20150-20251
Introduction or Removal	20500-20694
Replantation	20802-20838
Grafts of Implants	20900-20938
Other	20950-20999

Shoulder
Incision	23000-23044
Excision	23065-23222
Introduction or Removal	23330-23350
Fracture and/or Dislocation	23500-23680
Manipulation	23700
Arthrodesis	23800-23802
Amputation	23900-23921
Other/Unlisted Procedures	23929

Humerous (Upper Arm) and Elbow
Incision	23930-24006
Excision	24065-24155
Introduction or Removal	24160-24220
Repair, Revision and/or Reconstruction	24300-24498
Fracture and/or Dislocation	24500-24685
Arthrodesis	24800-24802
Amputation	24900-24940
Other/Unlisted Procedure	24999

Application of Casts/Strapping
Body and Upper Extremity Casts and Strapping	29000-29280
Removal or Repair	29700-29750
Other	29799

Endoscopy/Arthroscopy
29805-29838

Radiology Services
73000-73225

E/M Services
99201-99499

Shoulder and Elbow
(Anterior View)

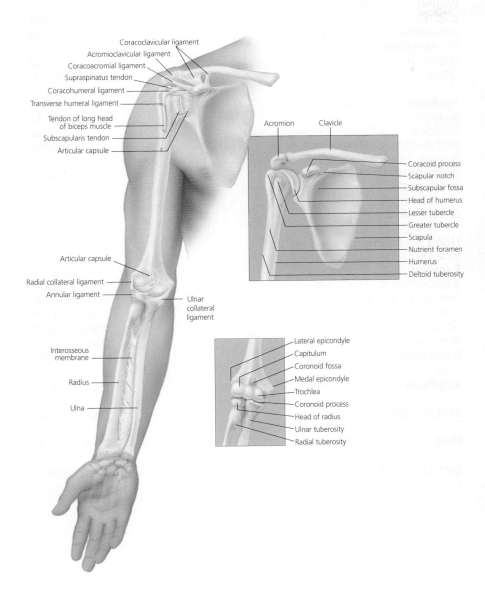

Coracoclavicular ligament
Acromioclavicular ligament
Coracoacromial ligament
Supraspinatus tendon
Coracohumeral ligament
Transverse humeral ligament
Tendon of long head of biceps muscle
Subscapularis tendon
Articular capsule

Acromion
Clavicle

Coracoid process
Scapular notch
Subscapular fossa
Head of humerus
Lesser tubercle
Greater tubercle
Scapula
Nutrient foramen
Humerus
Deltoid tuberosity

Articular capsule
Radial collateral ligament
Annular ligament
Ulnar collateral ligament

Interosseous membrane
Radius
Ulna

Lateral epicondyle
Capitulum
Coronoid fossa
Medal epicondyle
Trochlea
Coronoid process
Head of radius
Ulnar tuberosity
Radial tuberosity

©Scientific Publishing Ltd., Rolling Meadows, IL

49

PLATE 7. MUSCULAR SYSTEM - HAND AND WRIST

General

Wound exploration - Trauma	20100-20103
Excision	20105-20251
Introduction or Removal	20500-20694
Replantation	20802-20838
Grafts of Implants	20900-20938
Other	20950-20999

Forearm and Wrist

Incision	25000-25040
Excision	25065-25240
Introduction or Removal	25246-25259
Repair, Revision and/or Reconstruction	25260-25492
Fracture and/or Dislocation	25500-25695
Arthrodesis	25800-25830
Amputation	25900-25931
Other/Unlisted Procedure	25999

Hand and Fingers

Incision	26010-26080
Excision	26100-26262
Introduction or Removal	26320
Repair, Revision, and/or Reconstruction	26340-26596
Fracture and/or Dislocation	26600-26785
Arthrodesis	26820-26863
Amputation	26910-26952
Other/Unlisted Procedure	26989

Application of Casts/Strapping	29000-29280
Endoscopy/Arthroscopy	29840-29848
Radiology Services	73000-73225
E/M Services	99201-99499

Hand and Wrist

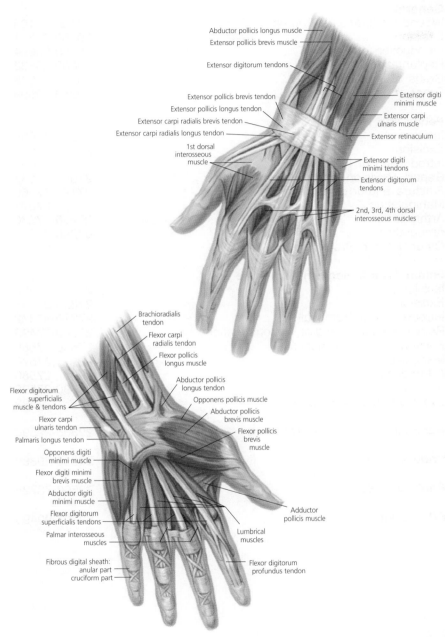

Abductor pollicis longus muscle
Extensor pollicis brevis muscle
Extensor digitorum tendons
Extensor pollicis brevis tendon
Extensor pollicis longus tendon
Extensor carpi radialis brevis tendon
Extensor carpi radialis longus tendon
1st dorsal interosseous muscle
Extensor digiti minimi muscle
Extensor carpi ulnaris muscle
Extensor retinaculum
Extensor digiti minimi tendons
Extensor digitorum tendons
2nd, 3rd, 4th dorsal interosseous muscles

Brachioradialis tendon
Flexor carpi radialis tendon
Flexor pollicis longus muscle
Abductor pollicis longus tendon
Flexor digitorum superficialis muscle & tendons
Opponens pollicis muscle
Abductor pollicis brevis muscle
Flexor carpi ulnaris tendon
Flexor pollicis brevis muscle
Palmaris longus tendon
Opponens digiti minimi muscle
Flexor digiti minimi brevis muscle
Abductor digiti minimi muscle
Flexor digitorum superficialis tendons
Adductor pollicis muscle
Palmar interosseous muscles
Lumbrical muscles
Fibrous digital sheath: anular part cruciform part
Flexor digitorum profundus tendon

PLATE 8. MUSCULOSKELETAL SYSTEM - HIP AND KNEE

General

Wound exploration - Trauma	20100-20103
Excision	20150-20251
Introduction or Removal	20500-20694
Replantation	20802-20838
Grafts of Implants	20900-20938
Other	20950-20999

Pelvis and Hip Joint

Incision	26990-27036
Excision	27040-27080
Introduction or Removal	27086-27096
Repair, Revision, and/or Reconstruction	27097-27187
Fracture and/or dislocation	27193-27266
Manipulation	27275
Arthrodesis	27280-27286
Amputation	27290-27295
Other/Unlisted Procedure	27299

Femur (Thigh Region) and Knee Joint

Incision	27301-27320
Excision	27323-27365
Introduction or Removal	27370-37372
Repair, Revision, and/or Reconstruction	27380-27499
Fracture and/or Dislocation	27500-27566
Manipulation	27570
Arthrodesis	27580
Amputation	27590-27598
Other/Unlisted Procedure	27599

Application of Casts/Strapping   29305-29590

Endoscopy/Arthroscopy   29850-29889

Radiology Services   73500-73725

E/M Services   99201-99499

Hip and Knee
(Anterior View)

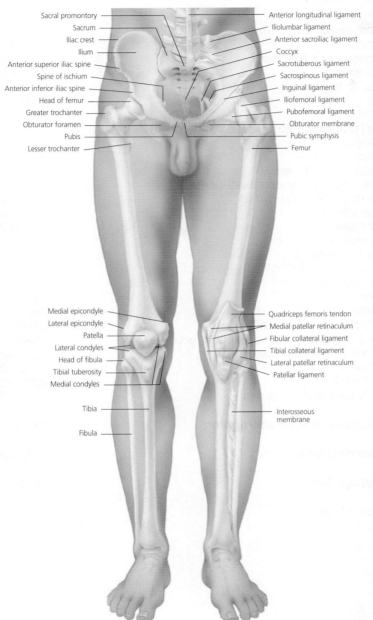

Sacral promontory
Sacrum
Iliac crest
Ilium
Anterior superior iliac spine
Spine of ischium
Anterior inferior iliac spine
Head of femur
Greater trochanter
Obturator foramen
Pubis
Lesser trochanter

Anterior longitudinal ligament
Iliolumbar ligament
Anterior sacroiliac ligament
Coccyx
Sacrotuberous ligament
Sacrospinous ligament
Inguinal ligament
Iliofemoral ligament
Pubofemoral ligament
Obturator membrane
Pubic symphysis
Femur

Medial epicondyle
Lateral epicondyle
Patella
Lateral condyles
Head of fibula
Tibial tuberosity
Medial condyles

Tibia

Fibula

Quadriceps femoris tendon
Medial patellar retinaculum
Fibular collateral ligament
Tibial collateral ligament
Lateral patellar retinaculum
Patellar ligament

Interosseous membrane

©Scientific Publishing Ltd., Rolling Meadows, IL

PLATE 9. MUSCULOSKELETAL SYSTEM - FOOT AND ANKLE

General
Wound exploration - Trauma	20100-20103
Excision	20150-20251
Introduction or Removal	20500-20694
Replantation	20802-20838
Grafts of Implants	20900-20938
Other	20950-20999

Leg (Tibia and Fibula) and Ankle Joint
Incision	27600-27612
Excision	27613-27647
Introduction or Removal	27648
Repair, Revision and/or Reconstruction	27650-27745
Fracture and/or Dislocation	27750-27848
Manipulation	27860
Arthrodesis	27870-27871
Amputation	27880-27889
Other Procedures	27892-27899

Foot and Toes
Incision	28001-28035
Excision	28043-28175
Introduction or Removal	28190-28193
Repair, Revision, and/or Reconstruction	28200-28360
Fracture and/or Dislocation	28400-28675
Arthrodesis	28705-28760
Amputation	28800-28825
Other/Unlisted Procedures	28899

Application of Casts/Strapping	29305-29590
Endoscopy/Arthroscopy	29891-29999
Radiology Services	73500-73725
E/M Services	99201-99499

Foot and Ankle

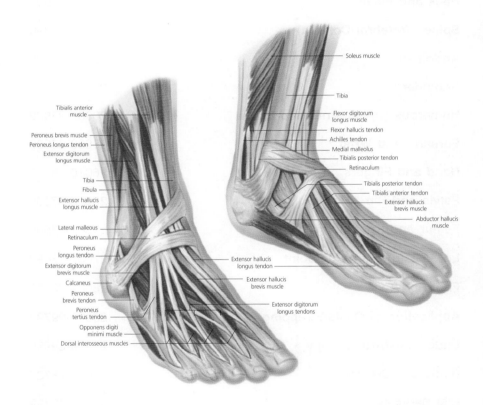

Soleus muscle

Tibia

Flexor digitorum longus muscle

Flexor hallucis tendon

Achilles tendon

Medial malleolus

Tibialis posterior tendon

Retinaculum

Tibialis anterior muscle

Peroneus brevis muscle

Peroneus longus tendon

Extensor digitorum longus muscle

Tibia

Fibula

Extensor hallucis longus muscle

Lateral malleous

Retinaculum

Peroneus longus tendon

Extensor digitorum brevis muscle

Calcaneus

Peroneus brevis tendon

Peroneus tertius tendon

Opponens digiti minimi muscle

Dorsal interosseous muscles

Extensor hallucis longus tendon

Extensor hallucis brevis muscle

Extensor digitorum longus tendons

Tibialis posterior tendon

Tibialis anterior tendon

Extensor hallucis brevis muscle

Abductor hallucis muscle

PLATE 10. SKELETAL SYSTEM - ANTERIOR VIEW

General	20100-20999
Head	21010-21499
Neck (Soft Tissues) and Thorax	21501-21899
Back and Flank	21920-21935
Spine (Vertebral Column)	22100-22899
Abdomen	22900-22999
Shoulder	23000-23929
Humerous (Upper Arm) and Elbow	23930-24999
Forearm and Wrist	25000-25999
Hand and Fingers	26010-26989
Pelvis and Hip Joint	26990-27299
Femur and Knee Joint	27301-27599
Lower Leg and Ankle Joint	27600-27899
Foot and Toes	28001-28899
Application of Casts/Strapping	29000-29799
Endoscopy/Arthroscopy	29800-29999
Radiology Services	70010-73725
E/M Services	99201-99499

Skeletal System
(Anterior View)

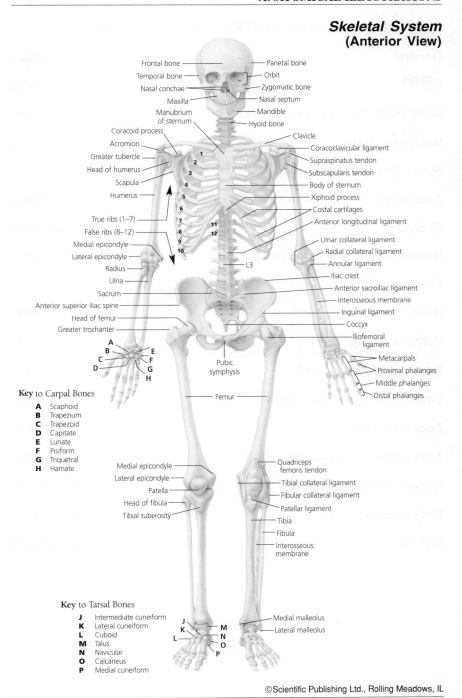

Frontal bone
Temporal bone
Nasal conchae
Maxilla
Manubrium of sternum
Coracoid process
Acromion
Greater tubercle
Head of humerus
Scapula
Humerus
True ribs (1–7)
False ribs (8–12)
Medial epicondyle
Lateral epicondyle
Radius
Ulna
Sacrum
Anterior superior iliac spine
Head of femur
Greater trochanter

Parietal bone
Orbit
Zygomatic bone
Nasal septum
Mandible
Hyoid bone
Clavicle
Coracoclavicular ligament
Supraspinatus tendon
Subscapularis tendon
Body of sternum
Xiphoid process
Costal cartilages
Anterior longitudinal ligament
Ulnar collateral ligament
Radial collateral ligament
Annular ligament
Iliac crest
Anterior sacroiliac ligament
Interosseous membrane
Inguinal ligament
Coccyx
Iliofemoral ligament
Metacarpals
Proximal phalanges
Middle phalanges
Distal phalanges

L3

Pubic symphysis

Femur

Key to Carpal Bones

A	Scaphoid
B	Trapezium
C	Trapezoid
D	Capitate
E	Lunate
F	Pisiform
G	Triquetral
H	Hamate

Medial epicondyle
Lateral epicondyle
Patella
Head of fibula
Tibial tuberosity

Quadriceps femoris tendon
Tibial collateral ligament
Fibular collateral ligament
Patellar ligament
Tibia
Fibula
Interosseous membrane

Key to Tarsal Bones

J	Intermediate cuneiform
K	Lateral cuneiform
L	Cuboid
M	Talus
N	Navicular
O	Calcaneus
P	Medial cuneiform

Medial malleolus
Lateral malleolus

©Scientific Publishing Ltd., Rolling Meadows, IL

PLATE 11. SKELETAL SYSTEM - POSTERIOR VIEW

General	20100-20999
Head	21010-21499
Neck (Soft Tissues) and Thorax	21501-21899
Back and Flank	21920-21935
Spine (Vertebral Column)	22100-22899
Abdomen	22900-22999
Shoulder	23000-23929
Humerous (Upper Arm) and Elbow	23930-24999
Forearm and Wrist	25000-25999
Hand and Fingers	26010-26989
Pelvis and Hip Joint	26990-27299
Femur and Knee Joint	27301-27599
Lower Leg and Ankle Joint	27600-27899
Foot and Toes	28001-28899
Application of Casts/Strapping	29000-29799
Endoscopy/Arthroscopy	29800-29999
Radiology Services	70010-73725
E/M Services	99201-99499

Skeletal System
(Posterior View)

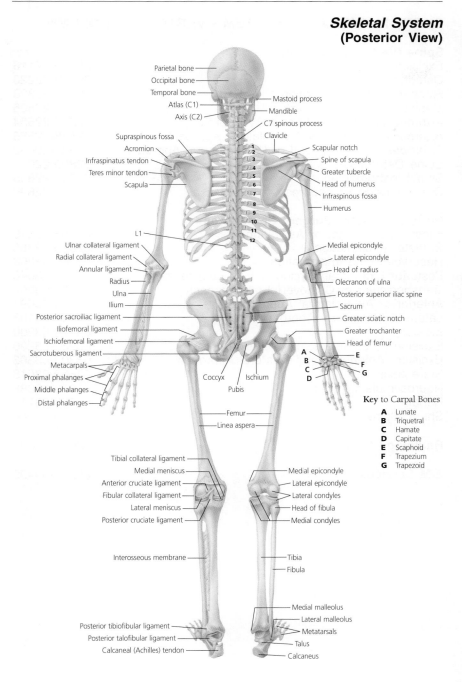

Parietal bone
Occipital bone
Temporal bone
Atlas (C1)
Axis (C2)
Supraspinous fossa
Acromion
Infraspinatus tendon
Teres minor tendon
Scapula
L1
Ulnar collateral ligament
Radial collateral ligament
Annular ligament
Radius
Ulna
Ilium
Posterior sacroiliac ligament
Iliofemoral ligament
Ischiofemoral ligament
Sacrotuberous ligament
Metacarpals
Proximal phalanges
Middle phalanges
Distal phalanges

Mastoid process
Mandible
C7 spinous process
Clavicle
Scapular notch
Spine of scapula
Greater tubercle
Head of humerus
Infraspinous fossa
Humerus
Medial epicondyle
Lateral epicondyle
Head of radius
Olecranon of ulna
Posterior superior iliac spine
Sacrum
Greater sciatic notch
Greater trochanter
Head of femur

A
B
C
D
E
F
G

Coccyx   Ischium
Pubis

Femur
Linea aspera

Tibial collateral ligament
Medial meniscus
Anterior cruciate ligament
Fibular collateral ligament
Lateral meniscus
Posterior cruciate ligament

Medial epicondyle
Lateral epicondyle
Lateral condyles
Head of fibula
Medial condyles

Interosseous membrane

Tibia
Fibula

Medial malleolus
Lateral malleolus
Metatarsals
Talus
Calcaneus

Posterior tibiofibular ligament
Posterior talofibular ligament
Calcaneal (Achilles) tendon

Key to Carpal Bones

A   Lunate
B   Triquetral
C   Hamate
D   Capitate
E   Scaphoid
F   Trapezium
G   Trapezoid

©Scientific Publishing Ltd., Rolling Meadows, IL

59

PLATE 12. SKELETAL SYSTEM - VERTEBRAL COLUMN

Spine (Vertebral Column)
Excision	22100-22116
Osteotomy	22210-22226
Fracture and/or Dislocation	22305-22328
Manipulation	22505
Arthrodesis-Lateral Extracavitary Approach	22532-22534
Arthrodesis-Anterior or Anterolateral Approach	22548-22585
Arthrodesis-Posterolateral or Posterolateral Approach	22590-22632
Spine Deformity	22800-22819
Spinal Instrumentation	22840-22855
Other/Unlisted Procedures	22899

Nervous System Surgery Procedures
Injection, Drainage, or Aspiration	62263-62319
Catheter Implantation	62350-62355
Reservoir/Pump Implantation	62360-62368
Posterior Extradural Laminotomy or Laminectomy	63001-63048
Transpedicular or Costovertebral Approach	63055-63066
Anterior or Anterolateral Approach	63075-63091
Lateral Extracavitary Approach	63101-63103
Incision	63170-63200
Excision by Laminectomy of Lesion	63250-63290
Excision, Anterior or Anterolateral Approach	63300-63308
Stereotaxis	63600-63615
Neurostimulators (Spinal)	63650-63688
Repair	63700-63710
Shunt, Spinal CSF	63740-63746

Radiology Services
72010-72295

E/M Services
99201-99499

Vertebral Column
(Lateral View)

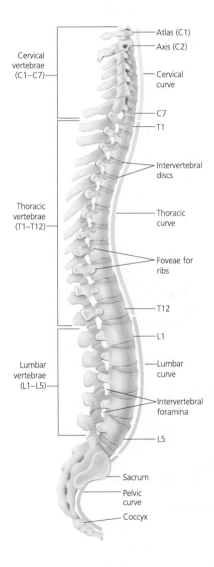

Atlas (C1)

Axis (C2)

Cervical
vertebrae
(C1–C7)

Cervical
curve

C7

T1

Intervertebral
discs

Thoracic
vertebrae
(T1–T12)

Thoracic
curve

Foveae for
ribs

T12

L1

Lumbar
vertebrae
(L1–L5)

Lumbar
curve

Intervertebral
foramina

L5

Sacrum

Pelvic
curve

Coccyx

PLATE 13. RESPIRATORY SYSTEM

Nose

Incision	30000-30020
Excision	30100-30160
Introduction	30200-30220
Removal of Foreign Body	30300-30320
Repair	30400-30630
Destruction	30801-30802
Other	30901-30999

Accessory Sinuses

Incision	31000-31090
Excision	31200-31230
Endoscopy	31231-31294
Other	31299

Larynx

Excision	31300-31420
Introduction	31500-31502
Endoscopy	31505-31579
Repair	31580-31590
Destruction	31595
Other	31599

Trachea and Bronchi

Incision	31600-31614
Endoscopy	31615-31656
Introduction	31700-31730
Repair	31750-31830

Lungs and Pleura

Incision	32000-32225
Excision	32310-32540
Endoscopy	32601-32665
Repair	32800-32820
Lung Transplantation	32850-32854
Surgical Collapse Therapy; Thoracoplasty	32900-32960

Radiology Services/Chest   71010-71555

E/M Services   99201-99499

Respiratory System

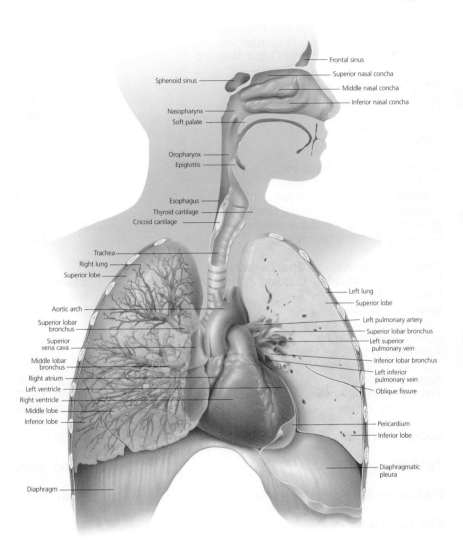

Frontal sinus
Superior nasal concha
Sphenoid sinus
Middle nasal concha
Inferior nasal concha
Nasopharynx
Soft palate
Oropharynx
Epiglottis
Esophagus
Thyroid cartilage
Cricoid cartilage
Trachea
Right lung
Superior lobe
Left lung
Superior lobe
Aortic arch
Left pulmonary artery
Superior lobar bronchus
Superior lobar bronchus
Left superior pulmonary vein
Superior vena cava
Inferior lobar bronchus
Middle lobar bronchus
Right atrium
Left inferior pulmonary vein
Left ventricle
Oblique fissure
Right ventricle
Middle lobe
Inferior lobe
Pericardium
Inferior lobe
Diaphragmatic pleura
Diaphragm

©Scientific Publishing Ltd., Rolling Meadows, IL

PLATE 14. HEART AND PERICARDIUM

General
Pericardium	33010-33050
Cardiac Tumor	33120-33130
Pacemaker or Defibrillator	33200-33249
Electrophysiologic Operative Procedures	33250-33261
Patient Activated Event Recorder	33282-33284
Wounds of the Heart and Great Vessels	33300-33335

Cardiac Valves
Aortic Valve	33400-33417
Mitral Valve	33420-33430
Tricuspid Valve	33460-33468
Pulmonary Valve	33470-33478

Coronary Artery Bypass
Coronary Artery Anomalies	33500-33506
Venous Grafting for Bypass	33510-33516
Combined Arterial-Venous Grafting	33517-33530
Arterial Grafting for Bypass	33533-33545
Coronary Endarterectomy	33572

Repair of Anomalies and Defects
Single Ventricle/Other Cardiac Anomalies	33600-33619
Septal Defect	33641-33697
Sinus of Valsalva	33702-33722
Total Anomalous Pulmonary Venous Drainage	33730-33732
Shunting Procedures	33735-33767
Transposition of the Great Vessels	33770-33781
Truncus Arteriosus	33786-33788
Aortic Anomalies	33800-33853
Thoracic Aortic Aneurysm	33860-33877
Pulmonary Artery	33910-33924

Heart/Lung Transplant
33930-33945

Cardiac Assist
33960-33980

Radiology Services/Heart
75552-75556

E/M Services
99201-99499

Heart
(External View)

Left common carotid artery
Brachiocephalic artery
Left subclavian artery
Aortic arch
Ligamentum arteriosum
Superior vena cava
Left pulmonary artery
Ascending aorta
Pulmonary trunk
Left auricle
Right coronary artery
Circumflex artery
Right atrium
Great cardiac vein
Right ventricle
Anterior descending (interventricular) artery
Anterior cardiac vein
Left ventricle
Right marginal artery
Small cardiac vein
Apex

Heart
(Internal View)

Superior vena cava
Right pulmonary artery branches
Left pulmonary artery
Aorta
Pulmonary trunk
Left pulmonary veins
Right pulmonary veins
Left atrium
Pulmonary semilunar valve
Aortic semilunar valve
Right atrium
Bicuspid (left AV) valve
Tricuspid (right AV) valve
Left ventricle
Papillary muscle
Interventricular septum
Chordae tendineae
Inferior vena cava
Myocardium
Right ventricle
Trabeculae carneae

PLATE 15. CIRCULATORY SYSTEM

Embolectomy/Thrombectomy
Arterial, With or Without Repair
Venous, Direct or w/Catheter

34001-34203
34401-34490

Venous Reconstruction

34501-34530

Repair
Endovascular Repair of Aneurysm
Direct Repair of Aneurysm
Repair Arteriovenous Fistula
Repair Blood Vessel Other Than for Fistula

34800-34900
35001-35162
35180-35190
35201-35286

Thromboendarterectomy

35301-35390

Transluminal Angioplasty

35450-35476

Transluminal Atherectomy

35480-35495

Bypass Graft
Vein
In-situ Vein
Composite Grafts

35500-35572
35582-35587
35681-35683

Transposition and Exploration/Revision
Arterial Transposition
Exploration/Revision

35691-35697
35700-35907

Vascular Injection Procedures
Intravenous
Intra-Arterial/Intra-Aortic
Venous
Arterial
Intraosseous

36000-36015
36100-36299
36400-36597
36600-36660
36680

Cannulization or Shunt and Other Procedures
Intervascular Cannulization or Shunt
Portal Decompression Procedures
Transcatheter Procedures
Intravascular Ultrasound Services
Ligation and Other Procedures

36800-36870
37140-37183
37195-37209
37250-37251
37565-37799

Radiology Services

75600-75996

E/M Services

99201-99499

Vascular System

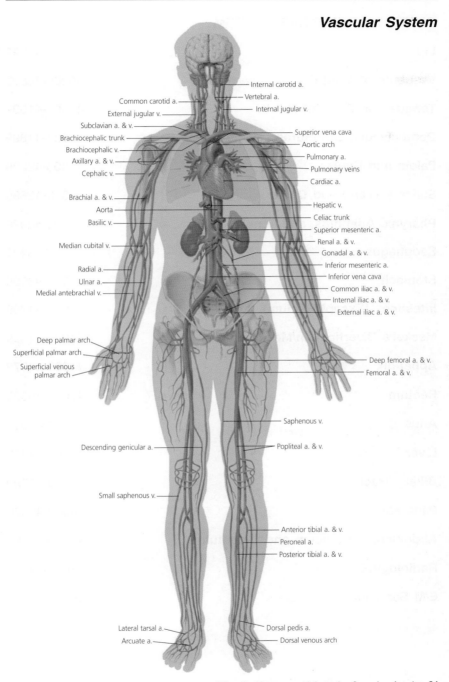

- Internal carotid a.
- Vertebral a.
- Common carotid a.
- Internal jugular v.
- External jugular v.
- Subclavian a. & v.
- Brachiocephalic trunk
- Superior vena cava
- Brachiocephalic v.
- Aortic arch
- Axillary a. & v.
- Pulmonary a.
- Cephalic v.
- Pulmonary veins
- Cardiac a.
- Brachial a. & v.
- Hepatic v.
- Aorta
- Celiac trunk
- Basilic v.
- Superior mesenteric a.
- Median cubital v.
- Renal a. & v.
- Gonadal a. & v.
- Radial a.
- Inferior mesenteric a.
- Ulnar a.
- Inferior vena cava
- Medial antebrachial v.
- Common iliac a. & v.
- Internal iliac a. & v.
- External iliac a. & v.
- Deep palmar arch
- Superficial palmar arch
- Superficial venous palmar arch
- Deep femoral a. & v.
- Femoral a. & v.
- Saphenous v.
- Descending genicular a.
- Popliteal a. & v.
- Small saphenous v.
- Anterior tibial a. & v.
- Peroneal a.
- Posterior tibial a. & v.
- Lateral tarsal a.
- Dorsal pedis a.
- Arcuate a.
- Dorsal venous arch

PLATE 16. DIGESTIVE SYSTEM

Lips	40490-40799
Vestibule of Mouth	40800-40899
Tongue and Floor of Mouth	41000-41599
Dentoalveolar Structures	41800-41899
Palate and Uvula	42000-42299
Salivary Gland and Ducts	42300-42699
Pharynx, Adenoids, and Tonsils	42700-42999
Esophagus	43020-43499
Stomach	43500-43999
Intestines (Except Rectum)	44005-44799
Meckel's Diverticulum/Mesentery	44800-44899
Appendix	44900-44979
Rectum	45000-45999
Anus	46020-46999
Liver	47000-47399
Biliary Tract	47400-47999
Pancreas	48000-48999
Abdomen, Peritoneum and Omentum	49000-49999
Radiology Services	74000-74363
E/M Services	99201-99499

Digestive System

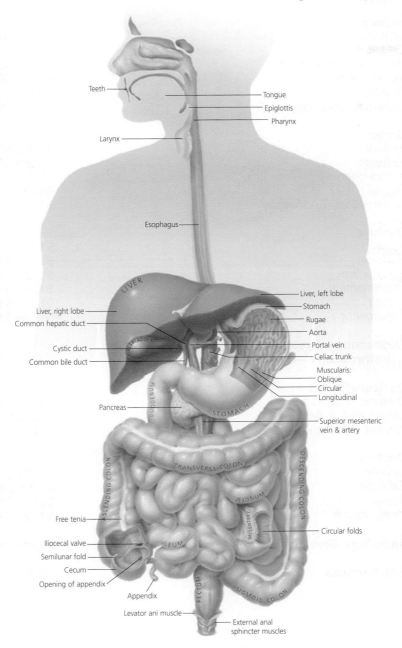

Teeth

Tongue

Epiglottis

Pharynx

Larynx

Esophagus

LIVER

Liver, left lobe

Stomach

Rugae

Liver, right lobe

Common hepatic duct

Aorta

Portal vein

Cystic duct

Celiac trunk

Common bile duct

Muscularis:
Oblique
Circular
Longitudinal

Pancreas

STOMACH

Superior mesenteric
vein & artery

ASCENDING COLON

DESCENDING COLON

TRANSVERSE COLON

JEJUNUM

Free tenia

MESENTERY

Circular folds

Iliocecal valve

ILEUM

Semilunar fold

Cecum

Opening of appendix

RECTUM

Appendix

SIGMOID COLON

Levator ani muscle

External anal
sphincter muscles

PLATE 17. GENITOURINARY SYSTEM

Kidney

Incision	50010-50135
Excision	50200-50290
Renal Transplantation	50300-50380
Introduction	50390-50398
Repair	50400-50540
Laparoscopy/Endoscopy	50541-50580

Ureter

Incision	50600-50630
Excision	50650-50660
Introduction	50684-50690
Repair	50700-50940
Laparoscopy/Endoscopy	50945-50980

Bladder

Incision	51000-51080
Excision	51500-51597
Introduction	51600-51720
Urodynamics	51725-51798
Repair	51800-51980
Laparoscopy	51990-51992

Endoscopy—Cystoscopy— Urethroscopy—Cystourethroscopy   52000-52010

Transurethral Surgery

Urethra and Bladder	52204-52318
Ureter and Pelvis	52320-52355
Vesical Neck and Prostate	52400-52700

Urethra

Incision	53000-53085
Excision	53200-53275
Repair	53400-53520
Manipulation	53600-53665

Radiology Services   74400-74485

E/M Services   99201-99499

Urinary System

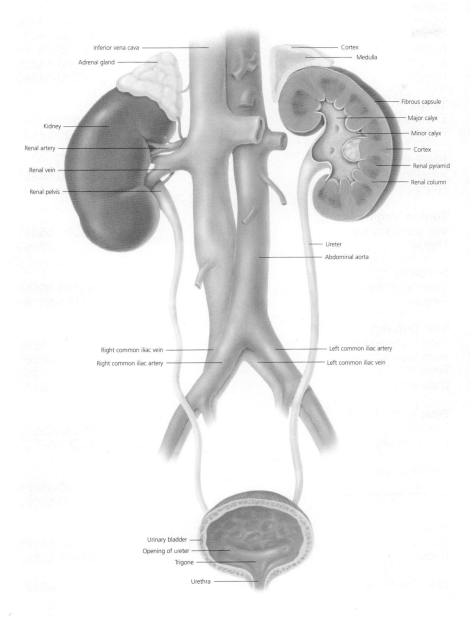

Inferior vena cava
Adrenal gland
Cortex
Medulla
Fibrous capsule
Kidney
Major calyx
Renal artery
Minor calyx
Renal vein
Cortex
Renal pelvis
Renal pyramid
Renal column
Ureter
Abdominal aorta
Right common iliac vein
Left common iliac artery
Right common iliac artery
Left common iliac vein
Urinary bladder
Opening of ureter
Trigone
Urethra

PLATE 18. MALE REPRODUCTIVE SYSTEM

Penis
Incision	54000-54015
Destruction	54050-54065
Excision	54100-54164
Introduction	54200-54250
Repair	54300-54440

Testis
Excision	54500-54560
Repair	54600-54680

Epididymis
Incision/Excision	54700-54861
Repair	54900-54901

Tunica Vaginalis
Incision/Excision	55000-55041
Repair	55060

Scrotum
Incision/Excision	55100-55150
Repair	55175-55180

Vas Deferens
Incision/Excision	55200-55250
Introduction	55300
Repair	55400
Suture	55450

Spermatic Cord
Excision	55500-55540
Laparoscopy	55550-55559

Seminal Vesicles
Incision	55600-55605
Excision	55650-55680

Prostate
Incision	55700-55725
Excision	55801-55865

E/M Services
	99201-99499

Male Reproductive System

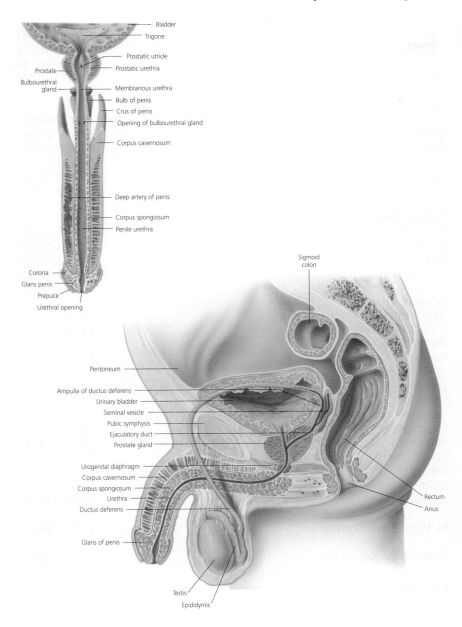

PLATE 19. FEMALE REPRODUCTIVE SYSTEM

Vulva, Perineum and Introitus

Incision	56405-56441
Destruction	56501-56515
Excision	56605-56740
Repair	56800-56810

Vagina

Incision	57000-57023
Destruction	57061-57065
Excision	57100-57135
Introduction	57150-57180
Repair	57200-57335
Manipulation	57400-57415

Cervix Uteri

Endoscopy	57452-57461
Excision	57500-57556
Repair	57700-57720
Manipulation	57800-57820

Corpus Uteri

Excision	58100-58294
Introduction	58300-58353
Repair	58400-58540
Laparoscopy/Hysteroscopy	58545-58579

Oviduct

Incision	58600-58615
Laparoscopy	58660-58679
Excision	58700-58720
Repair	58740-58770

Ovary

Incision	58800-58825
Excision	58900-58960

In Vitro Fertilization   58970-58976

Radiology Services   74710-74775

E/M Services   99201-99499

Female Reproductive System

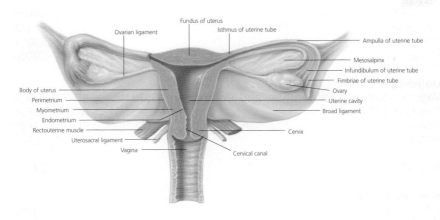

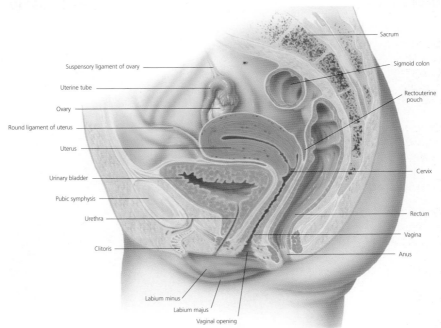

PLATE 20. PREGNANCY, CHILDBIRTH AND THE PUERPERIUM

Antepartum Services

Antepartum Services	59000-59076
Excision	59100-59160
Introduction	59200
Repair	59300-59350

Delivery

Vaginal Delivery, Antepartum and Postpartum Care	59400-59430
Cesarean Delivery	59510-59525
Delivery after Previous Cesarean Delivery	59610-59622
Abortion	59812-59857

Radiology Services
59400-59430

Radiology Services	74710-74775

E/M Services

E/M Services	99201-99499
Newborn Care	99431-99440

Female Reproductive System: Pregnancy
(Lateral View)

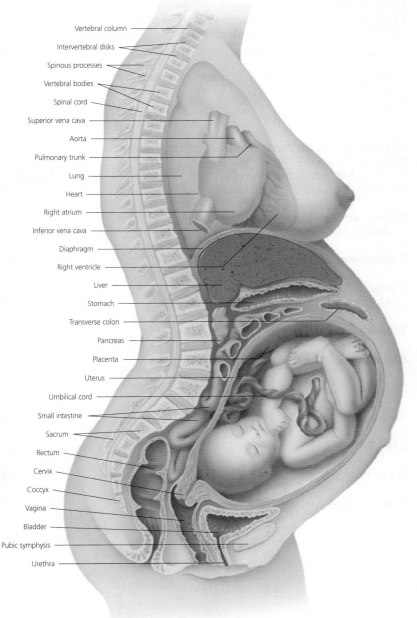

Vertebral column

Intervertebral disks

Spinous processes

Vertebral bodies

Spinal cord

Superior vena cava

Aorta

Pulmonary trunk

Lung

Heart

Right atrium

Inferior vena cava

Diaphragm

Right ventricle

Liver

Stomach

Transverse colon

Pancreas

Placenta

Uterus

Umbilical cord

Small intestine

Sacrum

Rectum

Cervix

Coccyx

Vagina

Bladder

Pubic symphysis

Urethra

PLATE 21. NERVOUS SYSTEM - BRAIN

Skull, Meninges, and Brain
Injection, Drainage, or Aspiration   61000-61070
Twist Drill, Burr Hole(s), or Trephine   61105-61253
Craniectomy or Craniotomy   61304-61576

Surgery of Skull Base Approach Procedures
Anterior Cranial Fossa   61580-61586
Middle Cranial Fossa   61590-61592
Posterior Cranial Fossa   61595-61598

Surgery of Skull Base Definitive Procedures
Base of Anterior Cranial Fossa   61600-61601
Base of Middle Cranial Fossa   61605-61613
Base of Posterior Cranial Fossa   61615-61616

Repair and/or Reconstruction of Surgical Defects of Skull Base
                                                      61618-61619

Endovascular Therapy   61623-61626

Surgery for Aneurysm, Arterio-Venous Malformation or Vascular Disease
                                                      61680-61711

Stereotaxis   61720-61795

Neurostimulators (Intra-Cranial)   61850-61888

Repair   62000-62148

Neuroendoscopy   62160-62165

CSF Shunt   62180-62258

Radiology Services   70010-70559

E/M Services   99201-99499

Brain
(Base View)

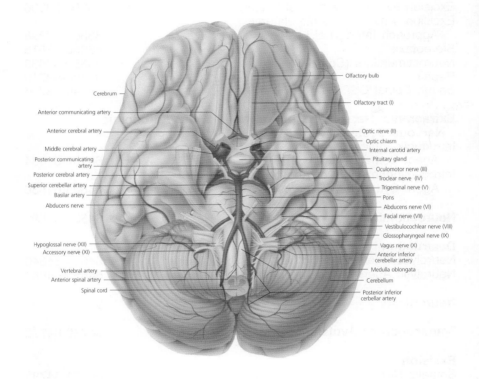

Olfactory bulb
Cerebrum
Olfactory tract (I)
Anterior communicating artery
Anterior cerebral artery
Optic nerve (II)
Optic chiasm
Middle cerebral artery
Internal carotid artery
Posterior communicating artery
Pituitary gland
Posterior cerebral artery
Oculomotor nerve (III)
Superior cerebellar artery
Troclear nerve (IV)
Basilar artery
Trigeminal nerve (V)
Abducens nerve
Pons
Abducens nerve (VI)
Facial nerve (VII)
Vestibulocochlear nerve (VIII)
Glossopharyngeal nerve (IX)
Hypoglossal nerve (XII)
Vagus nerve (X)
Accessory nerve (XI)
Anterior inferior cerebellar artery
Vertebral artery
Medulla oblongata
Anterior spinal artery
Cerebellum
Spinal cord
Posterior inferior cerebellar artery

PLATE 22. NERVOUS SYSTEM

Spine and Spinal Cord

Injection, Drainage or Aspiration	62263-62319
Catheter Implantation	62350-62368
Posterior Extradural Laminotomy or Laminectomy	63001-63048
Transpedicular or Costovertebral Approach	63055-63066
Anterior or Anterolateral Approach	63075-63091
Incision	63170-63200
Excision by Laminectomy of Lesion	63250-63290
Excision, Anterior or Anterolateral Approach Intraspinal Lesion	63300-63308
Stereotaxis	63600-63615
Neurostimulators (Spinal)	63650-63688
Repair	63700-63710
Shunt, Spinal CSF	63740-63746

Extracranial Nerves, Peripheral Nerves and Autonomic Nervous System

Introduction/Injection of Anesthetic Agent Somatic Nerves	64400-64484
Introduction/Injection of Anesthetic Agent Sympathetic Nerves	64505-64530

Neurostimulators
64550-64595

Destruction

Neurolytic Agent Somatic Nerves	64600-64640
Neurolytic Agent Sympathetic Nerves	64680-64681

Neuroplasty
64702-64727

Transection or Avulsion
64732-64772

Excision

Somatic Nerves	64774-64795
Sympathetic Nerves	64802-64823

Neurorrhaphy

Without Nerve Graft	64831-64876
With Nerve Graft	64885-64907

E/M Services
99201-99499

Nervous System

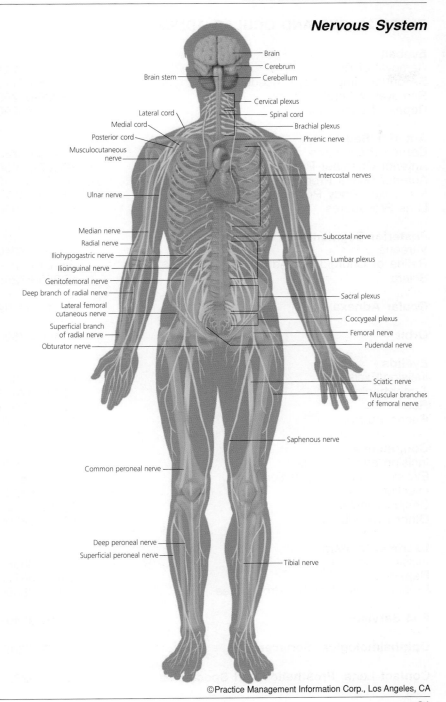

- Brain
- Cerebrum
- Cerebellum
- Brain stem
- Cervical plexus
- Lateral cord
- Spinal cord
- Medial cord
- Brachial plexus
- Posterior cord
- Phrenic nerve
- Musculocutaneous nerve
- Intercostal nerves
- Ulnar nerve
- Median nerve
- Radial nerve
- Subcostal nerve
- Iliohypogastric nerve
- Ilioinguinal nerve
- Lumbar plexus
- Genitofemoral nerve
- Deep branch of radial nerve
- Sacral plexus
- Lateral femoral cutaneous nerve
- Coccygeal plexus
- Superficial branch of radial nerve
- Femoral nerve
- Obturator nerve
- Pudendal nerve
- Sciatic nerve
- Muscular branches of femoral nerve
- Saphenous nerve
- Common peroneal nerve
- Deep peroneal nerve
- Superficial peroneal nerve
- Tibial nerve

PLATE 23. EYE AND OCULAR ADNEXA

Eyeball

Removal of Eye	65091-65114
Secondary Implant(s) Procedures	65125-65175
Removal of Foreign Body	65205-65265
Repair of Laceration	65270-65290

Anterior Segment

Cornea Procedures	65400-65782
Anterior Chamber Procedures	65800-66030
Anterior Sclera Procedures	66130-66250
Iris, Ciliary Body Procedures	66500-66770
Lens Procedures	66820-66990

Posterior Segment

Vitreous	67005-67040
Retina or Choroid Procedures	67101-67228
Sclera	67250-67255

Ocular Adnexa   67311-67399

Orbit   67400-67599

Eyelids

Incision/Excision	67700-67850
Tarsorrhaphy	67875-67882
Repair	67900-67924
Reconstruction	67930-67975

Conjunctiva

Incision and Drainage	68020-68040
Excision and/or Destruction	68100-68135
Injection	68200
Conjunctivoplasty	68320-68340
Other Procedures	68360-68399

Lacrimal System

Incision/Excision	68400-68550
Repair	68700-68770
Probing and/or Related Procedures	68801-68850

E/M Services   99201-99499

Ophthalmological Services   92002-92287

Contact Lens, Prosthetics and Spectacles   92310-92396

Right Eye
(Horizontal Section)

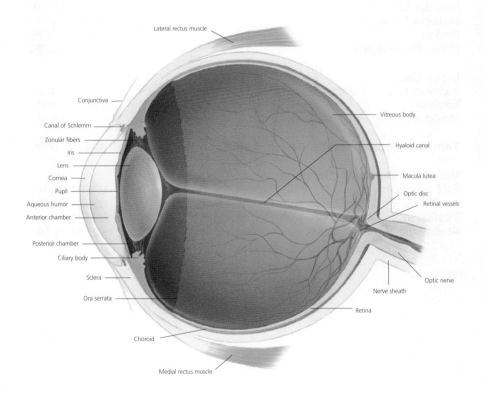

Lateral rectus muscle

Conjunctiva

Canal of Schlemm

Zonular fibers

Iris

Lens

Cornea

Pupil

Aqueous humor

Anterior chamber

Posterior chamber

Ciliary body

Sclera

Ora serrata

Choroid

Medial rectus muscle

Vitreous body

Hyaloid canal

Macula lutea

Optic disc

Retinal vessels

Optic nerve

Nerve sheath

Retina

©Scientific Publishing Ltd., Rolling Meadows, IL

PLATE 24. AUDITORY SYSTEM

External Ear

Incision	69000-69090
Excision	69100-69155
Removal of Foreign Body	69200-69222
Repair	69300-69320

Middle Ear

Introduction	69400-69410
Incision/Excision	69420-69554
Repair	69601-69676
Other Procedures	69700-69799

Inner Ear

Incision and/or Destruction	69801-69840
Excision	69905-69915
Introduction	69930

Temporal Bone, Middle Fossa Approach   69950-69970

Visit and Medicine Services

E/M Services	99201-99499
Vestibular Function Tests with Observation	92531-92534
Vestibular Function Tests with Recording	92541-92548
Audiologic Function Tests	92551-92597

The Ear

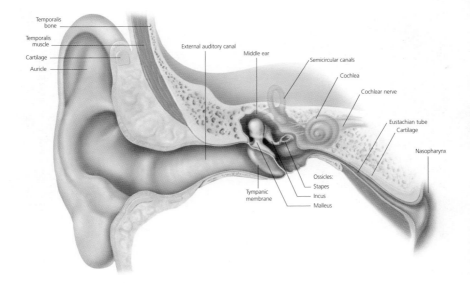

EVALUATION & MANAGEMENT GUIDELINES

EVALUATION AND MANAGEMENT (E/M) SERVICES OVERVIEW

The first section of the CPT coding system is the evaluation and management (E/M) section, which includes procedure codes for visits and special care services. Within each subsection, the CPT codes are arranged first by patient category, then by the level of service.

The evaluation and management section of the CPT coding system includes codes for reporting visits, consultations, prolonged service, case management services, preventive medicine services, newborn care, and special services. The section is divided into categories such as office visits, hospital visits and consultations. Most of the categories are further divided into two or more subcategories.

The subcategories for evaluation and management services are further classified into levels of service that are identified by specific codes. The level of service classification is important because the physician work required to provide the service varies by the type of service, the place of service, and the patient's clinical status.

The basic format of the evaluation and management service codes and definitions is the same for most categories.

- *A unique five-digit CPT code number is listed*

- *The place and/or type of service is specified, for example "office consultation"*

- *The content of the service is defined, eg. "comprehensive history and comprehensive examination"*

- *The nature of the presenting problem(s) usually associated with a given level is described.*

- *The time typically required to provide the service is specified.*

EVALUATION AND MANAGEMENT SERVICES SUBSECTIONS

The Evaluation and Management section of the CPT book is divided into the following subsections:

87

Office or Other Outpatient Services	99201-99215
Hospital Observation Services	99217-99220
Hospital Inpatient Services	99221-99239
Consultations	99241-99275
Emergency Department Services	99281-99288
Pediatric Critical Care Patient Transport	99289-99290
Critical Care Services	99291-99292
Inpatient and Pediatric Critical Care Services	99293-99294
Inpatient Neonatal Critical Care	99295-99296
Intensive (Non-Critical) Low Birth Weight Services	99298-99299
Nursing Facility Services	99301-99316
Domiciliary, Rest Home or Custodial Care Services	99321-99333
Home Services	99341-99350
Prolonged Services	99354-99360
Case Management Services	99361-99373
Care Plan Oversight Services	99374-99380
Preventive Medicine Services	99381-99429
Newborn Care Services	99431-99440
Special Evaluation and Management Services	99450-99456
Other Evaluation and Management Services	99499

All of these subsections have extensive notes that should be reviewed carefully prior to selecting codes for services located within the section.

EVALUATION AND MANAGEMENT SERVICES GUIDELINES

In addition to the information presented in the introduction, several other items unique to the Evaluation and Management codes are defined or identified in the guidelines.

CLASSIFICATION OF EVALUATION AND MANAGEMENT SERVICES

The Evaluation and Management section is divided into broad categories such as office visits, hospital visits, and consultations. Most of the categories are further divided into two or more subcategories (subsections) of evaluation and management services. For example, there are two subcategories of office visits (new patient and established patient) and there are two subcategories of hospital visits (initial and subsequent).

The subcategories of evaluation and management services are further classified into levels of evaluation and management services that are identified by specific codes. This classification is important because the nature of physician work varies by type of service, place of service, and the patient's status.

The basic format of the levels of evaluation and management services is the same for most categories. First, a unique code number is listed. Second, the place and/or type of service is specified, eg, office consultation. Third, the content of the service is defined, eg, comprehensive history and comprehensive examination. Fourth, the nature of the presenting problem(s) usually associated with a given level is described. Fifth, the time typically required to provide the service is specified.

DEFINITIONS OF COMMONLY USED TERMS

Certain key words and phrases are used throughout the Evaluation and Management section. The following definitions are intended to reduce the potential for differing interpretations and to increase the consistency of reporting by physicians in differing specialties.

NEW AND ESTABLISHED PATIENT

Solely for the purposes of distinguishing between new and established patients, professional services are those face-to-face services rendered by a physician and coded by a specific CPT code(s). A new patient is one who has not received any professional services from the physician or another physician of the same specialty who belongs to the same group practice, within the past three years.

An established patient is one who has received professional services from the physician or another physician of the same specialty who belongs to the same group practice, within the past three years.

In the instance where a physician is on call for or covering for another physician, the patient's encounter will be classified as it would have been by the physician who is not available.

No distinction is made between new and established patients in the emergency department. Evaluation and Management services in the emergency department category may be coded for any new or established patient who presents for treatment in the emergency department.

CHIEF COMPLAINT

A concise statement describing the symptom, problem, condition, diagnosis or other factor that is the reason for the encounter, usually stated in the patient's words.

CONCURRENT CARE

Concurrent care is the provision of similar services, eg, hospital visits, to the same patient by more than one physician on the same day. When concurrent care is provided, no special reporting is required. Modifier '-75' has been deleted.

COUNSELING

Counseling is a discussion with a patient and/or family concerning one or more of the following areas:

- diagnostic results, impressions, and/or recommended diagnostic studies;

- prognosis;

- risks and benefits of management (treatment) options;

- instructions for management (treatment) and/or follow-up;

- importance of compliance with chosen management (treatment) options;

- risk factor reduction; and

- patient and family education. (For psychotherapy, see 90804-90857)

FAMILY HISTORY

A review of medical events in the patient's family that includes significant information about:

- the health status or cause of death of parents, siblings, and children;

- specific diseases related to problems identified in the chief complaint or history of the present illness, and/or system review;

- diseases of family members which may be hereditary or place the patient at risk.

HISTORY OF PRESENT ILLNESS

A chronological description of the development of the patient's present illness from the first sign and/or symptom to the present. This includes a description of location, quality, severity, timing, context, modifying factors and associated signs and symptoms significantly related to the presenting problem(s).

LEVELS OF EVALUATION AND MANAGEMENT SERVICES

Within each category or subcategory of evaluation and management service, there are three to five levels of evaluation and management services available for reporting purposes. Levels of evaluation and management services are not interchangeable among the different categories or subcategories of service. For example, the first level of evaluation and management services in the subcategory of office visit, new patient, does not have the same definition as the first level of evaluation and management services in the subcategory of office visit, established patient.

The levels of evaluation and management services include examinations, evaluations, treatments, conferences with or concerning patients, preventive pediatric and adult health supervision, and similar medical services, such as the determination of the need and/or location for appropriate care. Medical screening includes the history, examination, and medical decision making required to determine the need and/or location for appropriate care and treatment of the patient (eg, office and other outpatient setting, emergency department, nursing facility, etc.). The levels of evaluation and management services encompass the wide variations in skill, effort, time, responsibility and medical knowledge required for the prevention or diagnosis and treatment of illness or injury and the promotion of optimal health. Each level of evaluation and management services may be used by all physicians.

The descriptors for the levels of evaluation and management services recognize seven components, six of which are used in defining the levels of evaluation and management services. These components are:

- history;

- examination;

- medical decision making;

- counseling;

- coordination of care;

- nature of presenting problem; and

- time.

The first three of these components (history, examination, and medical decision making) are considered the key components in selecting a level of evaluation and management services. (See "determine the extent of history obtained")

The next three components (counseling, coordination of care, and the nature of the presenting problem) are considered contributory factors in the majority of encounters. Although the first two of these contributory factors are important evaluation and management services, it is not required that these services be provided at every patient encounter.

Coordination of care with other providers or agencies without a patient encounter on that day is coded using the case management codes.

The final component, time, is discussed in detail.

Any specifically identifiable procedure (ie, identified with a specific cpt code) performed on or subsequent to the date of initial or subsequent "Evaluation and management services" should be coded separately. The actual performance and/or interpretation of diagnostic tests/studies ordered during a patient encounter are not included in the levels of evaluation and management services. Physician

91

performance of diagnostic tests/studies for which specific CPT codes are available may be coded separately, in addition to the appropriate evaluation and management code. The physician's interpretation of the results of diagnostic tests/studies (ie, professional component) with preparation of a separate distinctly identifiable signed written report may also be coded separately, using the appropriate CPT code with the modifier '-26' appended.

The physician may need to indicate that on the day a procedure or service identified by a CPT code was performed, the patient's condition required a significant separately identifiable evaluation and management service above and beyond other services provided or beyond the usual preservice and postservice care associated with the procedure that was performed. The evaluation and management service may be caused or prompted by the symptoms or condition for which the procedure and/or service was provided. This circumstance may be coded by adding the modifier '-25' to the appropriate level of evaluation and management service. As such, different diagnoses are not required for reporting of the procedure and the evaluation and management services on the same date.

NATURE OF PRESENTING PROBLEM

A presenting problem is a disease, condition, illness, injury, symptom, sign, finding, complaint, or other reason for encounter, with or without a diagnosis being established at the time of the encounter. The evaluation and management codes recognize five types of presenting problems that are defined as follows:

Minimal: a problem that may not require the presence of the physician, but service is provided under the physician's supervision.

Self-limited or minor: a problem that runs a definite and prescribed course, is transient in nature, and is not likely to permanently alter health status or has a good prognosis with management/compliance.

Low severity: a problem where the risk of morbidity without treatment is low; there is little to no risk of mortality without treatment; full recovery without functional impairment is expected.

Moderate severity: a problem where the risk of morbidity without treatment is moderate; there is moderate risk of mortality without treatment; uncertain prognosis or increased probability of prolonged functional impairment.

High severity: a problem where the risk of morbidity without treatment is high to extreme; there is a moderate to high risk of mortality without treatment or high probability of severe, prolonged functional impairment.

PAST HISTORY

A review of the patient's past experiences with illnesses, injuries, and treatments that includes significant information about:

- prior major illnesses and injuries;

- prior operations;

- prior hospitalizations;

- current medications;

- allergies (eg, drug, food);

- age appropriate immunization status;

- age appropriate feeding/dietary status.

SOCIAL HISTORY

An age appropriate review of past and current activities that includes significant information about:

- marital status and/or living arrangements;

- current employment;

- occupational history;

- use of drugs, alcohol, and tobacco;

- level of education;

- sexual history;

- other relevant social factors

SYSTEM REVIEW (REVIEW OF SYSTEMS)

An inventory of body systems obtained through a series of questions seeking to identify signs and/or symptoms which the patient may be experiencing or has experienced. For the purposes of CPT the following elements of a system review have been identified:

- Constitutional symptoms (fever, weight loss, etc.)

- Eyes

- Ears, nose, mouth, throat

- Cardiovascular

- Respiratory

- Gastrointestinal

- Genitourinary

- Musculoskeletal

- Integumentary (skin and/or breast)

93

- Neurological

- Psychiatric

- Endocrine

- Hematologic/lymphatic

- Allergic/immunologic

The review of systems helps define the problem, clarify the differential diagnosis, identify needed testing, or serves as baseline data on other systems that might be affected by any possible management options.

TIME

The inclusion of time in the definitions of levels of evaluation and management services has been implicit in prior editions of CPT. The inclusion of time as an explicit factor beginning in CPT 1992 is done to assist physicians in selecting the most appropriate level of evaluation and management services. It should be recognized that the specific times expressed in the visit code descriptors are averages, and therefore represent a range of times which may be higher or lower depending on actual clinical circumstances.

Time is not a descriptive component for the emergency department levels of evaluation and management services because emergency department services are typically provided on a variable intensity basis, often involving multiple encounters with several patients over an extended period of time. Therefore, it is often difficult for physicians to provide accurate estimates of the time spent face-to-face with the patient.

Studies to establish levels of evaluation and management services employed surveys of practicing physicians to obtain data on the amount of time and work associated with typical evaluation and management services. Since "work" is not easily quantifiable, the codes must rely on other objective, verifiable measures that correlate with physicians' estimates of their "work". It has been demonstrated that physicians' estimations of intraservice time (as explained on the next page), both within and across specialties, is a variable that is predictive of the "work" of evaluation and management services. This same research has shown there is a strong relationship between intra-service time and total time for evaluation and management services. Intra-service time, rather than total time, was chosen for inclusion with the codes because of its relative ease of measurement and because of its direct correlation with measurements of the total amount of time and work associated with typical evaluation and management services.

Intra-service times are defined as face-to-face time for office and other outpatient visits and as unit/floor time for hospital and other inpatient visits. This distinction is necessary because most of the work of typical office visits takes place during the face-to-face time with the patient, while most of the work of typical hospital visits takes place during the time spent on the patient's floor or unit.

Face-to-face time (office and other outpatient visits and office consultations): for coding purposes, face-to-face time for these services is defined as only that time that the physician spends face-to-face with the patient and/or family. This includes the time in which the physician performs such tasks as obtaining a history, performing an examination, and counseling the patient.

Physicians also spend time doing work before or after the face-to-face time with the patient, performing such tasks as reviewing records and tests, arranging for further services, and communicating further with other professionals and the patient through written reports and telephone contact.

This non-face-to-face time for office services—also called pre- and post-encounter time—is not included in the time component described in the evaluation and management codes. However, the pre- and post-face-to-face work associated with an encounter was included in calculating the total work of typical services in physician surveys.

Thus, the face-to-face time associated with the services described by any evaluation and management code is a valid proxy for the total work done before, during, and after the visit.

Unit/floor time (hospital observation services, inpatient hospital care, initial and follow-up hospital consultations, nursing facility): for reporting purposes, intra-service time for these services is defined as unit/floor time, which includes the time that the physician is present on the patient's hospital unit and at the bedside rendering services for that patient. This includes the time in which the physician establishes and/or reviews the patient's chart, examines the patient, writes notes and communicates with other professionals and the patient's family.

In the hospital, pre- and post-time includes time spent off the patient's floor performing such tasks as reviewing pathology and radiology findings in another part of the hospital.

This pre- and post-visit time is not included in the time component described in these codes. However, the pre- and post-work performed during the time spent off the floor or unit was included in calculating the total work of typical services in physician surveys. Thus, the unit/floor time associated with the services described by any code is a valid proxy for the total work done before, during, and after the visit.

UNLISTED SERVICE

An evaluation and management service may be provided that is not listed in this section of CPT. When reporting such a service, the appropriate "Unlisted" code may be used to indicate the service, identifying it by "Special Report", as discussed in the following paragraph. The "Unlisted Services" and accompanying codes for the evaluation and management section are as follows:

99429   Unlisted preventive medicine service
99499   Unlisted evaluation and management service

SPECIAL REPORT

An unlisted service or one that is unusual, variable, or new may require a special report demonstrating the medical appropriateness of the service. Pertinent information should include an adequate definition or description of the nature, extent, and need for the procedure; and the time, effort, and equipment necessary to provide the service. Additional items which may be included are complexity of symptoms, final diagnosis, pertinent physical findings, diagnostic and therapeutic procedures, concurrent problems, and follow-up care.

CLINICAL EXAMPLES

Clinical examples of the codes for evaluation and management services are included in the CPT code book to assist physicians in understanding the meaning of the descriptors and selecting the correct code. The clinical examples are listed in Appendix C of the CPT code book. Each example was developed by physicians in the specialties shown.

The same problem, when seen by physicians in different specialties, may involve different amounts of work. Therefore, the appropriate level of encounter should be coded using the descriptors rather than the examples.

The examples have been tested for validity and approved by the CPT editorial panel. Physicians were given the examples and asked to assign a code or assess the amount of time and work involved. Only those examples that were rated consistently have been included in Appendix C.

INSTRUCTIONS FOR SELECTING A LEVEL OF EVALUATION AND MANAGEMENT SERVICE

IDENTIFY THE CATEGORY AND SUBCATEGORY OF SERVICE

The categories and subcategories of codes available for reporting evaluation and management services are shown in Table 1 on the following page.

Table 1: Categories and subcategories of service

Category/subcategory	Code Numbers
Office or other outpatient services	
New patient	99201-99205
Established patient	99211-99215
Hospital observation discharge services	99217
Hospital observation services	99218-99220
Hospital observation or inpatient care services	
(including admission and discharge services)	99234-99236
Hospital inpatient services	
Initial hospital care	99221-99223
Subsequent hospital care	99231-99233
Hospital discharge services	99238-99239
Consultations	
Office consultations	99241-99245
Initial inpatient consultations	99251-99255
Follow-up inpatient consultations	99261-99263
Confirmatory consultations	99271-99275
Emergency department services	99281-99288
Pediatric patient transport	99289-99290
Critical care services	
Adult (over 24 months of age)	99291-99292
Pediatric	99293-99294
Neonatal	99295-99296
Intensive Care (Low Birth Weight)	99298-99299
Nursing facility services	
Comprehensive nursing facility assessments	99301-99303
Subsequent nursing facility care	99311-99313
Nursing facility discharge services	99315-99316
Domiciliary, rest home or custodial care services	
New patient	99321-99323
Established patient	99331-99333
Home services	
New patient	99341-99345
Established patient	99347-99350
Prolonged services	
With direct patient contact	99354-99357
Without direct patient contact	99358-99359
Standby services	99360
Case management services	
Team conferences	99361-99362
Telephone calls	99371-99373
Care plan oversight services	99374-99380
Preventive medicine services	
New patient	99381-99387
Established patient	99391-99397
Individual counseling	99401-99404
Group counseling	99411-99412
Other	99420-99429
Newborn care	99431-99440
Special E/M services	99450-99456
Other E/M services	99499

REVIEW THE REPORTING INSTRUCTIONS FOR THE SELECTED CATEGORY OR SUBCATEGORY

Most of the categories and many of the subcategories of service have special guidelines or instructions unique to that category or subcategory. Where these are indicated, eg, "Inpatient Hospital Care," special instructions will be presented preceding the levels of evaluation and management services.

REVIEW THE LEVEL OF EVALUATION AND MANAGEMENT SERVICE DESCRIPTORS AND EXAMPLES IN THE SELECTED CATEGORY OR SUBCATEGORY

The descriptors for the levels of evaluation and management services recognize seven components, six of which are used in defining the levels of evaluation and management services. These components are:

- history;
- examination;
- medical decision making;
- counseling;
- coordination of care;
- nature of presenting problem; and
- time.

The first three of these components (ie, history, examination, and medical decision making) should be considered the key components in selecting the level of evaluation and management services. An exception to this rule is in the case of visits which consist predominantly of counseling or coordination of care.

The nature of the presenting problem and time are provided in some levels to assist the physician in determining the appropriate level of E/M service.

DETERMINE THE EXTENT OF HISTORY OBTAINED

The extent of the history is dependent upon clinical judgment and on the nature of presenting problems(s). The levels of evaluation and management services recognize four types of history that are defined as follows:

Problem focused: chief complaint; brief history of present illness or problem.

Expanded problem focused: chief complaint; brief history of present illness; problem pertinent system review.

Detailed: chief complaint; extended history of present illness; problem pertinent system review extended to include a review of a limited number of additional systems; pertinent past, family, and/or social history directly related to the patient's problems.

98

Comprehensive: chief complaint; extended history of present illness; review of systems which is directly related to the problem(s) identified in the history of the present illness plus a review of all additional body systems; complete past, family, and social history.

The comprehensive history obtained as part of the preventive medicine evaluation and management service is not problem-oriented and does not involve a chief complaint or present illness. It does, however, include a comprehensive system review and comprehensive or interval past, family, and social history as well as a comprehensive assessment/history of pertinent risk factors.

DETERMINE THE EXTENT OF EXAMINATION PERFORMED

The extent of the examination performed is dependent on clinical judgment and on the nature of the presenting problem(s). The levels of evaluation and management services recognize four types of examination that are defined as follows:

Problem focused: a limited examination of the affected body area or organ system.

Expanded problem focused: a limited examination of the affected body area or organ system and other symptomatic or related organ system(s).

Detailed: an extended examination of the affected body area(s) and other symptomatic or related organ system(s).

Comprehensive: a general multi-system examination or a complete examination of a single organ system. Note: the comprehensive examination performed as part of the preventive medicine evaluation and management service is multisystem, but its extent is based on age and risk factors identified.

For the purposes of these CPT definitions, the following body areas are recognized:

- Head, including the face
- Neck
- Chest, including breasts and axilla
- Abdomen
- Genitalia, groin, buttocks
- Back
- Each extremity

For the purposes of these CPT definitions, the following organ systems are recognized:

- Eyes
- Ears, nose, mouth, and throat

- Cardiovascular

- Respiratory

- Gastrointestinal

- Genitourinary

- Musculoskeletal

- Skin

- Neurologic

- Psychiatric

- Hematologic/lymphatic/immunologic

DETERMINE THE COMPLEXITY OF MEDICAL DECISION MAKING

Medical decision making refers to the complexity of establishing a diagnosis and/or selecting a management option as measured by:

- the number of possible diagnoses and/or the number of management options that must be considered;

- the amount and/or complexity of medical records, diagnostic tests, and/or other information that must be obtained, reviewed, and analyzed; and

- the risk of significant complications, morbidity, and/or mortality, as well as comorbidities, associated with the patient's presenting problems(s), the diagnostic procedure(s) and/or the possible management options.

Four types of medical decision making are recognized: straightforward; low complexity; moderate complexity; and high complexity. To qualify for a given type of decision making, two of the three elements in Table 2 below must be met or exceeded.

Table 2: Complexity of Medical Decision Making

Number of diagnoses or management options	Amount and/or complexity of data to be reviewed	Risk of complications and/or morbidity or mortality	Type of decision making
Minimal	Minimal or none	Minimal	**Straightforward**
Limited	Limited	Low	**Low complexity**
Multiple	Moderate	Moderate	**Moderate complexity**
Extensive	Extensive	High	**High complexity**

Comorbidities/underlying diseases, in and of themselves, are not considered in selecting a level of evaluation and management services unless their presence significantly increases the complexity of the medical decision making.

SELECT THE APPROPRIATE LEVEL OF EVALUATION AND MANAGEMENT SERVICES BASED ON THE FOLLOWING

1.   For the following categories/subcategories, all of the key components, (ie, history, examination, and medical decision making), must meet or exceed the stated requirements to qualify for a particular level of evaluation and management service: office, new patient; hospital observation services; initial hospital care; office consultations; initial inpatient consultations; confirmatory consultations; emergency department services; comprehensive nursing facility assessments; domiciliary care, new patient; and home, new patient.

2.   For the following categories/subcategories, two of the three key components (ie, history, examination, and medical decision making) must meet or exceed the stated requirements to qualify for a particular level of evaluation and management services: office, established patient; subsequent hospital care; follow-up inpatient consultations; subsequent nursing facility care; domiciliary care, established patient; and home, established patient.

3.   When counseling and/or coordination of care dominates (more than 50%) the physician/patient and/or family encounter (face-to-face time in the office or other outpatient setting or floor/unit time in the hospital or nursing facility), then time may be considered the key or controlling factor to qualify for a particular level of evaluation and management services. This includes time spent with parties who have assumed responsibility for the care of the patient or decision making whether or not they are family members (eg, foster parents, person acting in locum parentis, legal guardian). The extent of counseling and/or coordination of care must be documented in the medical record.

OTHER DEFINITIONS OF NATURE OF THE PRESENTING PROBLEM

In addition to the above five specific definitions found in the CPT coding system, there are other definitions found in the E.M Service codes used to report Subsequent Hospital Care and Follow-Up Inpatient Consultations. See Table 3 for these additional definitions.

DIAGNOSTIC TESTS OR STUDIES

The performance of diagnostic tests or studies for which specific CPT codes are available is not included in the levels of evaluation and management services. Any diagnostic tests or studies performed by the physician for which specific CPT codes are available should be coded separately, in addition to the appropriate evaluation and management service code.

Table 3: Other Definitions of Nature of Presenting Problems

Evaluation and Management Codes	Nature of Presenting Problem(s) Defined	Equivalent To
99231 or 99261	Stable, recovering or improving	Self-limited or minor
99232 or 99262	Inadequate response or minor complication	Low to moderate severity
99233 or 99263	Significant complication or new problem	Moderate to high severity

EVALUATION AND MANAGEMENT SERVICES MODIFIERS

Evaluation and management services may be modified under certain circumstances. When applicable, the modifying circumstance should be identified by reporting the appropriate modifier code in addition to the basic service. Modifiers which may be used with evaluation and management service codes are:

-21 Prolonged evaluation and management services

-24 Unrelated evaluation and management service by the same physician during a postoperative period

-25 Significant, separately identifiable evaluation and management service by the same physician on the same day of the procedure or other service

-32 Mandated services

-52 Reduced services

-57 Decision for surgery

HOW TO CHOOSE EVALUATION AND MANAGEMENT CODE(S)

Choosing the correct evaluation and management service code to report is a nine step process. The most important steps, in terms of both reimbursement and audit liability, are verifying compliance and documentation.

1.   Identify the Category of Service

Where was the patient seen and what category of services were provided?

☐   *Office or Other Outpatient Services*

- ☐ *Hospital Observation Services*
- ☐ *Hospital Inpatient Services*
- ☐ *Consultations*
- ☐ *Emergency Department Services*
- ☐ *Pediatric Patient Transport*
- ☐ *Critical Care Services*
- ☐ *Neonatal Intensive Care*
- ☐ *Nursing Facility Services*
- ☐ *Domiciliary, Rest Home or Custodial Care Services*
- ☐ *Home Services*
- ☐ *Prolonged Services*
- ☐ *Standby Services*
- ☐ *Case Management Services*
- ☐ *Care Plan Oversight Services*
- ☐ *Preventive Medicine Services*
- ☐ *Special or Other E/M Services*

2. *Identify the Subcategory of Service*

Is the patient a new patient or established patient?
Is the service initial care, subsequent care or follow-up?

- ☐ *New Patient*
- ☐ *Established Patient*
- ☐ *Initial Care*
- ☐ *Subsequent Care*
- ☐ *Follow-up*

3. *Determine the Extent of History Obtained*

What level of history was taken on this patient?

- ☐ *Problem Focused*
- ☐ *Expanded Problem Focused*
- ☐ *Detailed*
- ☐ *Comprehensive*

4. *Determine the Extent of Examination Performed*

What level of physician examination was performed?

- ☐ *Problem Focused*
- ☐ *Expanded Problem Focused*
- ☐ *Detailed*
- ☐ *Comprehensive*

5. *Determine the Complexity of Medical Decision Making*

What level of medical decision making was required?

☐ *Straightforward*
☐ *Low Complexity*
☐ *Moderate Complexity*
☐ *High Complexity*

6.   Record the Approximate Amount of Time

How much time was spent either face-to-face with the patient for office visits and consults, or unit or floor time for hospital care, hospital consults, and nursing facilities?

If counseling and/or coordination of care exceeds 50 percent of the total face-to-face physician/patient encounter, then TIME is considered to be the key or controlling factor which qualifies the choice of a particular level of evaluation and management service. The extent of counseling and/or coordination of care must be documented in the medical record.

7.   Verify Compliance with Reporting Requirements

All Three Key Components Required

To report services for new patients, initial care, office or confirmatory consultations, emergency department services, and comprehensive nursing facility assessments, all three key components must meet or exceed the stated requirements.

☐ *History component met or exceeded*
☐ *Examination component met or exceeded*
☐ *Medical decision making component met or exceeded*

Two of Three Key Components Required

To report services to established patients, subsequent or follow-up care, two of the three key components must meet or exceed the stated requirements.

☐ *History component met or exceeded; and/or*
☐ *Examination component met or exceeded; and/or*
☐ *Medical decision making component met or exceeded*

8.   Verify Documentation

Make sure that the medical record includes proper documentation of the history, examination, medical decision making, the nature of the problem(s), the approximate amount of time, and when appropriate, the extent of counseling and/or coordination of care.

9.   Assign the Code

The following is an example of the code selection process.

EXAMPLE OF THE CODE SELECTION PROCESS

1. Category of Service	*Office*
2. Subcategory	*New patient*
3. History	*Problem focused*
4. Examination	*Problem focused*
5. Medical Decision Making	*Straightforward*
6. Intra-service Time	*10 minutes*
7. Key Components	*Met or exceeded*
8. Documentation	*Met or exceeded*
9. Assign the Code	***99201***

EVALUATION AND MANAGEMENT SERVICES DOCUMENTATION GUIDELINES

Documentation in the medical record of all services provided is critical for reimbursement and audit liability. If the provider reported a service or procedure on the health insurance claim form but did not document it, or document it completely, in the patient's medical records, from the point of view of Medicare or private health insurance company auditors, the service was not performed, can't be reported, and therefore will not be paid for.

Millions of dollars are reclaimed from physicians and other medical professionals annually by Medicare and other third party payers because the medical record documentation does not support the services and procedures reported. Providers can protect their medical practices from audit liability by following the most current documentation guidelines published by CMS.

The following documentation guidelines for evaluation and management services were developed jointly by the American Medical Association (AMA) and CMS. The stated goal of CMS in publishing these guidelines is to provide physicians and health insurance claims reviewers with advice about preparing or reviewing documentation for evaluation and management services.

In developing and testing the validity of these guidelines, special emphasis was placed on assuring that they:

- *are consistent with the clinical descriptors and definitions contained in CPT,*

105

- *would be widely accepted by clinicians and minimize any changes in record-keeping practices; and*

- *would be interpreted and applied uniformly by users across the country.*

WHAT IS DOCUMENTATION AND WHY IS IT IMPORTANT?

Medical record documentation is required to record pertinent facts, findings, and observations about an individual's health history including past and present illnesses, examinations, tests, treatments, and outcomes. The medical record chronologically documents the care of the patient and is an important element contributing to high quality care. The medical record facilitates:

- *the ability of the physician and other medical professionals to evaluate and plan the patient's immediate treatment, and to monitor his/her health care over time;*

- *communication and continuity of care among physicians and other medical professionals involved in the patient's care;*

- *accurate and timely claims review and payment;*

- *appropriate utilization review and quality of care evaluations; and*

- *collection of data that may be useful for research and education.*

An appropriately documented medical record can reduce many of the hassles associated with claims processing and may serve as a legal document to verify the care provided, if necessary.

WHAT DO THIRD PARTY PAYERS WANT AND WHY?

Because payers have a contractual obligation to enrollees, they may require reasonable documentation that services are consistent with the insurance coverage provided. They may request information to validate:

- *the site of service;*

- *the medical necessity and appropriateness of the diagnostic and/or therapeutic services provided; and/or*

- *that services provided have been accurately reported.*

GENERAL PRINCIPLES OF MEDICAL RECORD DOCUMENTATION

The principles of documentation listed below are applicable to all types of medical and surgical services in all settings. For evaluation and management (E/M) services, the nature and amount of physician work and documentation varies by type of service, place of service and the patient's status. The general principles listed below may be modified to account for these variable circumstances in providing evaluation and management services.

1. *The medical record should be complete and legible.*

2. *The documentation of each patient encounter should include:*

   - *the reason for the encounter as well as relevant history, physical examination findings and prior diagnostic test results;*

   - *an assessment, clinical impression or diagnosis;*

   - *a plan for care; and*

   - *the date and legible identity of the observer.*

3. *If not documented, the rationale for ordering diagnostic and other ancillary services should be easily inferred.*

4. *Past and present diagnoses should be accessible to the treating and/or consulting physician.*

5. *Appropriate health risk factors should be identified.*

6. *The patient's progress, response to and changes in treatment, and revision of diagnosis should be documented.*

7. *CPT and ICD-9-CM codes reported on the health insurance claim form or patient billing statement should be supported by the documentation in the medical record.*

DOCUMENTATION OF EVALUATION AND MANAGEMENT SERVICES

This section provides definitions and documentation guidelines for the three key components of evaluation and management services and for visits which consist predominately of counseling or coordination of care. The three key components—history, examination, and medical decision making—appear in the descriptors for office and other outpatient services, hospital observation services, hospital inpatient services, consultations, emergency department services, nursing facility services, domiciliary care services, and home services. Note that Documentation Guidelines are identified by the symbol •DG.

The E/M descriptors recognize seven components which are used in defining the levels of service. These components are:

- *History*

- *Examination*

- *Medical decision making*

- *Counseling*

- *Coordination of care*

- *Nature of presenting problem*

- *Time*

The first three (i.e., history, examination and medical decision making) are the key components in selecting the level of evaluation and management services. However, with visits that consist predominantly of counseling or coordination of care, <u>time</u> is the key or controlling factor to qualify for a particular level of evaluation and management service.

Because the level of evaluation and management service is dependent on two or three key components, performance and documentation of one component (e.g., examination) at the highest level does not necessarily mean that the encounter in its entirety qualifies for the highest level of evaluation and management service.

These documentation guidelines for evaluation and management services reflect the needs of the typical adult population. For certain groups of patients, the recorded information may vary slightly from that described here.

Specifically, the medical records of infants, children, adolescents and pregnant women may have additional or modified information recorded in each history and examination area.

As an example, newborn records may include under history of the present illness, the details of the mother's pregnancy and the infant's status at birth; social history focused on family structure; family history focused on congenital anomalies and hereditary disorders in the family. In addition, the content of a pediatric examination will vary with the age and development of the child. Although not specifically defined in these documentation guidelines, these patient group variations on history and examination are appropriate.

DOCUMENTATION OF HISTORY

The levels of evaluation and management services are based on four types of history (Problem Focused, Expanded Problem Focused, Detailed, and Comprehensive). Each type of history includes some or all of the following elements:

- *Chief complaint*

- *History of present illness*

- *Review of systems*

- *Past, family and/or social history*

The extent of history of present illness, review of systems and past, family and/or social history that is obtained and documented is dependent upon clinical judgement and the nature of the presenting problem(s).

108

Present History	Review of Systems	Past, Family or Social History	Type of History
Brief	N/A	N/A	Problem Focused
Brief	Problem Pertinent	N/A	Expanded Problem Focused
Extended	Extended	Pertinent	Detailed
Extended	Complete	Complete	Comprehensive

The above chart shows the progression of the elements required for each type of history. To qualify for a given type of history all three elements in the table must be met. (A chief complaint is indicated at all levels.)

●*DG:* The chief complaint, review of systems and past, family and/or social history may be listed as separate elements of history, or they may be included in the description of the history of the present illness.

●*DG:* A review of systems and/or a past, family and/or social history obtained during an earlier encounter does not need to be re-recorded if there is evidence that the physician reviewed and updated the previous information. This may occur when a physician updates his or her own record or in an institutional setting or group practice where many physicians use a common record. The review and update may be documented by:

● describing any new review of systems and/or past, family and/or social history information or noting there has been no change in the information; and

● noting the date and location of the earlier review of systems and/or past, family and/or social history.

●*DG:* The review of systems and/or past, family and/or social history may be recorded by ancillary staff or on a form completed by the patient. To document that the physician reviewed the information, there must be a notation supplementing or confirming the information recorded by others.

●*DG:* If the physician is unable to obtain a history from the patient or other source, the record should describe the patient's condition or other circumstance which precludes obtaining a history.

Definitions and specific documentation guidelines for each of the elements of history are listed below.

CHIEF COMPLAINT

The chief complaint is "a concise statement describing the symptom, problem, condition, diagnosis, or other factor that is the reason for the encounter, usually stated in the patient's words."

●*DG:* *The medical record should clearly reflect the chief complaint.*

HISTORY OF PRESENT ILLNESS

The history of present illness is "a chronological description of the development of the patient's present illness from the first sign and/or symptom to the present." *It includes the following elements:*

● *Location*

● *Quality*

● *Severity*

● *Duration*

● *Timing*

● *Context*

● *Modifying factors*

● *Associated signs and symptoms*

Brief *and* **extended** *history of present illnesses are distinguished by the amount of detail needed to accurately characterize the clinical problem(s). A* **brief** *history of present illness consists of one to three elements of the history of present illness.*

●*DG:* *The medical record should describe at least one to three elements of the present illness (history of present illness).*

An **extended** *history of present illness consists of at least four elements of the history of present illness or the status of at least three chronic or inactive conditions.*

●*DG:* *Medical record should describe at least four elements of the present illness (history of present illness), or the status of at least three chronic or inactive conditions.*

REVIEW OF SYSTEMS

A review of systems is "an inventory of body systems obtained through a series of questions seeking to identify signs and/or symptoms which the patient may be experiencing or has experienced." *For purposes of review of systems, the following systems are recognized:*

- *Constitutional symptoms (e.g., fever, weight loss)*
- *Eyes*
- *Ears, Nose, Mouth, Throat*
- *Neck*
- *Cardiovascular*
- *Respiratory*
- *Gastrointestinal*
- *Genitourinary*
- *Musculoskeletal*
- *Integumentary (skin and/or breast)*
- *Neurological*
- *Psychiatric*
- *Endocrine*
- *Hematologic/Lymphatic*
- *Allergic/Immunologic*

A **problem pertinent** review of systems inquires about the system directly related to the problem(s) identified in the history of present illness.

●*DG:* The patient's positive responses and pertinent negatives for the system related to the problem should be documented.

An **extended** review of systems inquires about the system directly related to the problem(s) identified in the history of present illness and a limited number of additional systems.

●*DG:* The patient's positive responses and pertinent negatives for two to nine systems should be documented.

A **complete** review of systems inquires about the system(s) directly related to the problem(s) identified in the history of present illness plus all additional body systems.

●*DG:* At least ten organ systems must be reviewed. Those systems with positive or pertinent negative responses must be individually documented. For the remaining systems, a notation indicating all other systems are negative is permissible. In the absence of such a notation, at least ten systems must be individually documented.

PAST, FAMILY AND/OR SOCIAL HISTORY

The past, family and/or social history consists of a review of the following areas:

- *Past history: the patient's past experiences with illnesses, operations, injuries and treatments.*

- *Family history: a review of medical events in the patient's family, including diseases which may be hereditary or place the patient at risk.*

- *Social history: an age appropriate review of past and current activities.*

For certain categories of evaluation and management services that include only an interval history, it is not necessary to record information about the past, family and/or social history. Those categories are subsequent hospital care, follow-up inpatient consultations and subsequent nursing facility care.

*A **pertinent** past, family and/or social history is a review of the history area(s) directly related to the problem(s) identified in the history of present illness.*

•*DG:* At least one specific item from any of the three history areas must be documented for a pertinent past, family and/or social history

*A **complete** past, family and/or social history is of a review of two or all three of the past, family and/or social history areas, depending on the category of the evaluation and management service. A review of all three history areas is required for services that by their nature include a comprehensive assessment or reassessment of the patient. A review of two of the three history areas is sufficient for other services.*

•*DG:* At least one specific item from two of the three history areas must be documented for a complete past, family and/or social history for the following categories of evaluation and management services: office or other outpatient services, established patient; emergency department; domiciliary care, established patient; and home care, established patient.

•*DG:* At least one specific item from each of the three history areas must be documented for a complete past, family and/or social history for the following categories of evaluation and management services: office or other outpatient services, new patient; hospital observation services; hospital inpatient services, initial care; consultations; comprehensive nursing facility assessments; domiciliary care, new patient; and home care, new patient.

DOCUMENTATION OF EXAMINATION

The levels of E/M services are based on four types of examination:

- *Problem Focused* — "a limited examination of the affected body area or organ system."

- *Expanded Problem Focused* — "a limited examination of the affected body area or organ system and any other symptomatic or related body organ system(s)."

- *Detailed* — "an extended examination of the affected body area(s) and other symptomatic or related organ system(s)."

- *Comprehensive* — "a general multi-system examination, or complete examination of a single organ system."

These types of examinations have been defined for general multi-system and the following single organ systems:

- *Cardiovascular*

- *Ears, Nose, Mouth and Throat*

- *Eyes*

- *Genitourinary (Female)*

- *Genitourinary (Male)*

- *Hematologic/Lymphatic/Immunologic*

- *Musculoskeletal*

- *Neurological*

- *Psychiatric*

- *Respiratory*

- *Skin*

A general multi-system examination or a single organ system examination may be performed by any physician regardless of specialty. The type (general multi-system or single organ system) and content of examination are selected by the examining physician and are based upon clinical judgement, the patient's history, and the nature of the presenting problem(s).

The content and documentation requirements for each type and level of examination are summarized below and described in detail in tables beginning on page 116. In the tables, organ systems and body areas recognized by CPT for purposes of describing examinations are shown in the left column. The content, or individual elements, of the examination pertaining to that body area or organ system are identified by bullets (●) in the right column.

113

Parenthetical examples, (e.g., ...), have been used for clarification and to provide guidance regarding documentation. Documentation for each element must satisfy any numeric requirements (such as "Measurement of any three of the following seven...") included in the description of the element. Elements with multiple components but with no specific numeric requirement (such as "Examination of liver and spleen") require documentation of at least one component. It is possible for a given examination to be expanded beyond what is defined here. When that occurs, findings related to the additional systems and/or areas should be documented.

●*DG:* Specific abnormal and relevant negative findings of the examination of the affected or symptomatic body area(s) or organ system(s) should be documented. A notation of "abnormal" without elaboration is insufficient.

●*DG:* Abnormal or unexpected findings of the examination of any asymptomatic body area(s) or organ system(s) should be described.

●*DG:* A brief statement or notation indicating "negative" or "normal" is sufficient to document normal findings related to unaffected area(s) or asymptomatic organ system(s).

GENERAL MULTI-SYSTEM EXAMINATIONS

To qualify for a given level of multi-system examination, the following content and documentation requirements should be met:

- *Problem Focused Examination — should include performance and documentation of one to five elements identified by a bullet (●) in one or more organ system(s) or body area(s).*

- *Expanded Problem Focused Examination — should include performance and documentation of at least six elements identified by a bullet (●) in one or more organ system(s) or body area(s).*

- *Detailed Examination — should include at least six organ systems or body areas. For each system/area selected, performance and documentation of at least two elements identified by a bullet (●) is expected. Alternatively, a detailed examination may include performance and documentation of at least twelve elements identified by a bullet (●) in two or more organ systems or body areas.*

- *Comprehensive Examination — should include at least nine organ systems or body areas. For each system/area selected, all elements of the examination identified by a bullet (●) should be performed, unless specific directions limit the content of the examination. For each area/system, documentation of at least two elements identified by a bullet is expected.*

SINGLE ORGAN SYSTEM EXAMINATIONS

Variations among single organ system examinations in the organ systems and body areas identified in the left columns and in the elements of the examinations described in the right columns reflect differing emphases among specialties. To qualify for a given level of single organ system examination, the following content and documentation requirements should be met:

- *Problem Focused Examination — should include performance and documentation of one to five elements identified by a bullet (●), whether in a box with a shaded or unshaded border.*

- *Expanded Problem Focused Examination — should include performance and documentation of at least six elements identified by a bullet (●), whether in a box with a shaded or unshaded border.*

- *Detailed Examination — examinations other than the eye and psychiatric examinations should include performance and documentation of at least twelve elements identified by a bullet (●), whether in box with a shaded or unshaded border.*

  Eye and psychiatric examinations should include the performance and documentation of at least nine elements identified by a bullet (●), whether in a box with a shaded or unshaded border.

- *Comprehensive Examination — should include performance of all elements identified by a bullet (●), whether in a shaded or unshaded box. Documentation of every element in each box with a shaded border and at least one element in each box with an unshaded border is expected.*

Documentation of every element in each box with a shaded border and at least one element in each box with an unshaded border is expected.

GENERAL MULTI-SYSTEM EXAMINATION

SYSTEM/BODY AREA	ELEMENTS OF EXAMINATION
Constitutional	• *Measurement of any three of the following seven vital signs: 1) sitting or standing blood pressure, 2) supine blood pressure, 3) pulse rate and regularity, 4) respiration, 5) temperature, 6) height, 7) weight (May be measured and recorded by ancillary staff)* • *General appearance of patient (e.g., development, nutrition, body habitus, deformities, attention to grooming)*
Eyes	• *Inspection of conjunctivae and lids* • *Examination of pupils and irises (e.g., reaction to light and accommodation, size and symmetry)* • *Ophthalmoscopic examination of optic discs (e.g., size, C/D ratio, appearance) and posterior segments (e.g., vessel changes, exudates, hemorrhages)*
Ears, Nose, Mouth, Throat	• *External inspection of ears and nose (e.g., overall and appearance, scars, lesions, masses)* • *Otoscopic examination of external auditory canals and tympanic membranes* • *Assessment of hearing (e.g., whispered voice, finger rub, tuning fork)* • *Inspection of nasal mucosa, septum and turbinates* • *Inspection of lips, teeth and gums* • *Examination of oropharynx: oral mucosa, salivary glands, hard and soft palates, tongue, tonsils and posterior pharynx*
Neck	• *Examination of neck (e.g., masses, overall appearance, symmetry, tracheal position, crepitus)* • *Examination of thyroid (e.g., enlargement, tenderness, mass)*

Respiratory

- *Assessment of respiratory effort (e.g., intercostal retractions, use of accessory muscles, diaphragmatic movement)*
- *Percussion of chest (e.g., dullness, flatness, hyperresonance)*
- *Palpation of chest (e.g., tactile fremitus)*
- *Auscultation of lungs (e.g., breath sounds, adventitious sounds, rubs)*

Cardiovascular

- *Palpation of heart (e.g., location, size, thrills)*
- *Auscultation of heart with notation of abnormal sounds and murmurs*

Examination of:

- *Carotid arteries (e.g., pulse amplitude, bruits)*
- *Abdominal aorta (e.g., size, dbruits)*
- *Femoral arteries (e.g., pulse amplitude, bruits)*
- *Pedal pulses (e.g., pulse amplitude)*
- *Extremities for edema and/or varicosities*

Chest (Breasts)

- *Inspection of breasts (e.g., symmetry, nipple discharge)*
- *Palpation of breasts and axillae (e.g., masses or lumps, tenderness)*

Gastrointestinal (Abdomen)

- *Examination of abdomen with notation of presence of masses or tenderness*
- *Examination of liver and spleen*
- *Examination for presence or absence of hernia*
- *Examination (when indicated) of anus, perineum and rectum, including sphincter tone, presence of hemorrhoids, rectal masses*
- *Obtain stool sample for occult blood test when indicated*

Genitourinary Male

- *Examination of the scrotal contents (e.g., hydrocele, spermatocele, tenderness of cord, testicular mass)* continued

117

- *Examination of the penis*
- *Digital rectal examination of prostate gland (e.g., size, symmetry, nodularity, tenderness)*

Genitourinary Female

- *Pelvic examination (with or without specimen collection for smears and cultures), including:*
- *Examination of external genitalia (e.g., general appearance, hair distribution, lesions) and vagina (e.g., general appearance, estrogen effect, discharge, lesions, pelvic support, cystocele, rectocele)*
- *Examination of urethra (e.g., masses, tenderness, scarring)*
- *Examination of bladder (e.g., fullness, masses, tenderness)*
- *Cervix (e.g., general appearance, lesions, discharge)*
- *Uterus (e.g., size, contour, position, mobility, tenderness, consistency, descent or support)*
- *Adnexa/parametria (e.g., masses, tenderness, organomegaly, nodularity)*

Lymphatic

Palpation of lymph nodes in two or more areas:

- *Neck*
- *Axillae*
- *Groin*
- *Other*

Musculoskeletal

- *Examination of gait and station*
- *Inspection and/or palpation of digits and nails (eg clubbing, cyanosis, inflammatory conditions, petechiae, ischemia, infections, nodes)*
- *Examination of joints, bones and muscles of one or more of the following six areas: 1) head and neck; 2) spine, ribs and pelvis; 3) right upper extremity; 4) left upper extremity; 5) right lower extremity; and 6) left lower*

EVALUATION & MANAGEMENT GUIDELINES

extremity. The examination of a given area includes:

- *Inspection and/or palpation with notation of presence of any misalignment, asymmetry, crepitation, defects, tenderness, masses, effusions*

- *Assessment of range of motion with notation of any pain, crepitation or contracture*

- *Assessment of stability with notation of any dislocation (luxation), subluxation or laxity*

- *Assessment of muscle strength and tone (e.g., flaccid, cog wheel, spastic) with notation of any atrophy or abnormal movements*

Skin

- *Inspection of skin and subcutaneous tissue (e.g., rashes, lesions, ulcers)*

- *Palpation of skin and subcutaneous tissue (e.g., induration, subcutaneous nodules, tightening)*

Neurologic

- *Test cranial nerves with notation of any deficits*

- *Examination of deep tendon reflexes with notation of pathological reflexes (e.g., Babinski)*

- *Examination of sensation (e.g., by touch, pin, vibration, proprioception)*

Psychiatric

- *Description of patient's judgment and insight*

  Brief assessment of mental status including:

- *Orientation to time, place and person*

- *Recent and remote memory*

- *Mood and affect (e.g., depression, anxiety, agitation)*

119

CONTENT AND DOCUMENTATION REQUIREMENTS

Level of Exam	Perform and Document:
Problem Focused	One to five elements identified by a bullet.
Expanded Problem Focused	At least six elements identified by a bullet.
Detailed	At least two elements identified by a bullet from each of six areas/systems OR at least twelve elements identified by a bullet in two or more areas/systems.
Comprehensive	Perform all elements identified by a bullet in at least nine organ systems or body areas and document at least two elements identified by a bullet from each of nine areas/systems.

CARDIOVASCULAR EXAMINATION

SYSTEM/BODY AREA	ELEMENTS OF EXAMINATION
Constitutional	• *Measurement of any three of the following seven vital signs: 1) sitting or standing blood pressure, 2) supine blood pressure, 3) pulse rate and regularity, 4) respiration, 5) temperature, 6) height, 7) weight (May be measured and recorded by ancillary staff)* • *General appearance of patient (e.g., development, nutrition, body habitus, deformities, attention to grooming)*
Head and Face	
Eyes	• *Inspection of conjunctivae and lids (e.g., xanthelasma)*
Ears, Nose, Mouth and Throat	• *Inspection of teeth, gums and palate* • *Inspection of oral mucosa with notation of presence of pallor or cyanosis*
Neck	• *Examination of jugular veins (e.g., distension; a, v or cannon a waves)* • *Examination of thyroid (e.g., enlargement, tenderness, mass)*
Respiratory	• *Assessment of respiratory effort (e.g., intercostal retractions, use of accessory muscles, diaphragmatic movement)* • *Auscultation of lungs (e.g., breath sounds, adventitious sounds, rubs)*
Cardiovascular	• *Palpation of heart (e.g., location, size and forcefulness of the point of maximal impact; thrills; lifts; palpable S3 or S4)* • *Auscultation of heart including sounds, abnormal sounds and murmurs*

continued

	• *Measurement of blood pressure in two or more extremities when indicated (e.g., aortic dissection, coarctation)*
	Examination of:
	• *Carotid arteries (e.g., waveform, pulse amplitude, bruits, apical-carotid delay)*
	• *Abdominal aorta (e.g., size, bruits)*
	• *Femoral arteries (e.g., pulse amplitude, bruits)*
	• *Pedal pulses (e.g., pulse amplitude)*
	• *Extremities for peripheral edema and/or varicosities*

Chest (Breasts)

Gastrointestinal (Abdomen)	• *Examination of abdomen with notation of presence (Abdomen) of masses or tenderness*
	• *Examination of liver and spleen*
	• *Obtain stool sample for occult blood from patients who are being considered for thrombolytic or anticoagulant therapy*

Genitourinary

Lymphatic

Musculoskeletal	• *Examination of the back with notation of kyphosis or scoliosis*
	• *Examination of gait with notation of ability to undergo exercise testing and/or participation in exercise programs*
	• *Assessment of muscle strength and tone (e.g., flaccid, cog wheel, spastic) with notation of any atrophy and abnormal movements*

Extremities	• *Inspection and palpation of digits and nails (e.g., clubbing, cyanosis, inflammation, petechiae, ischemia, infections, Osler's nodes)*
Skin	• *Inspection and/or palpation of skin and subcutaneous tissue (e.g., stasis dermatitis, ulcers, scars, xanthomas)*
Neurological/Psychiatric	*Brief assessment of mental status including:* • *Orientation to time, place and person* • *Mood and affect (e.g., depression, anxiety, agitation)*

CONTENT AND DOCUMENTATION REQUIREMENTS

Level of Exam	*Perform and Document:*
Problem Focused	*One to five elements identified by a bullet.*
Expanded Problem Focused	*At least six elements identified by a bullet.*
Detailed	*At least twelve elements identified by a bullet.*
Comprehensive	*Perform all elements identified by a bullet; document every element in each box with a shaded border and at least one element in each box with an unshaded border.*

EAR, NOSE AND THROAT EXAMINATION

SYSTEM/BODY AREA	ELEMENTS OF EXAMINATION
Constitutional	• *Measurement of any three of the following seven vital signs: 1) sitting or standing blood pressure, 2) supine blood pressure, 3) pulse rate and regularity, 4) respiration, 5) temperature, 6) height, 7) weight (May be measured and recorded by ancillary staff)* • *General appearance of patient (e.g., development, nutrition, body habitus, deformities, attention to grooming)* • *Assessment of ability to communicate (e.g., use of sign language or other communication aids) and quality of voice*
Head and Face	• *Inspection of head and face (e.g., overall appearance, scars, lesions and masses)* • *Palpation and/or percussion of face with notation of presence or absence of sinus tenderness* • *Examination of salivary glands* • *Assessment of facial strength*
Eyes	• *Test ocular motility including primary gaze alignment*
Ears, Nose, Mouth and Throat	• *Otoscopic examination of external auditory canals and tympanic membranes including pneumo-otoscopy with notation of mobility of membranes* • *Assessment of hearing with tuning forks and clinical speech reception thresholds (e.g., whispered voice, finger rub)* • *External inspection of ears and nose (e.g., overall appearance, scars, lesions and masses)* • *Inspection of nasal mucosa, septum and turbinates*

continued

- *Inspection of lips, teeth and gums*
- *Examination of oropharynx: oral mucosa, hard and soft palates, tongue, tonsils and posterior pharynx (e.g., asymmetry, lesions, hydration of mucosal surfaces)*
- *Inspection of pharyngeal walls and pyriform sinuses (e.g., pooling of saliva, asymmetry, lesions)*
- *Examination by mirror of larynx including the condition of the epiglottis, false vocal cords, true vocal cords and mobility of larynx (Use of mirror not required in children)*
- *Examination by mirror of nasopharynx including appearance of the mucosa, adenoids, posterior choanae and eustachian tubes (Use of mirror not required in children)*

Neck
- *Examination of neck (e.g., masses, overall appearance, symmetry, tracheal position, crepitus)*
- *Examination of thyroid (e.g., enlargement, tenderness, mass)*

Respiratory
- *Inspection of chest including symmetry, expansion and/or assessment of respiratory effort (e.g., intercostal retractions, use of accessory muscles, diaphragmatic movement)*
- *Auscultation of lungs (e.g., breath sounds, adventitious sounds, rubs)*

Cardiovascular
- *Auscultation of heart with notation of abnormal sounds and murmurs*
- *Examination of peripheral vascular system by observation (e.g., swelling, varicosities) and palpation (e.g., pulses, temperature, edema, tenderness)*

Chest (Breasts)

Gastrointestinal (Abdomen)

125

Genitourinary

Lymphatic   • *Palpation of lymph nodes in neck, axillae, groin and/or other location*

Musculoskeletal

Extremities

Skin

Neurological/Psychiatric   • *Test cranial nerves with notation of any deficits*

Brief assessment of mental status including:

• *Orientation to time, place and person*

• *Mood and affect (e.g., depression, anxiety, agitation)*

CONTENT AND DOCUMENTATION REQUIREMENTS

Level of Exam	Perform and Document:
Problem Focused	One to five elements identified by a bullet.
Expanded Problem Focused	At least six elements identified by a bullet.
Detailed	At least twelve elements identified by a bullet.
Comprehensive	Perform all elements identified by a bullet; document every element in each box with a shaded border and at least one element in each box with an unshaded border.

EYE EXAMINATION

SYSTEM/BODY AREA   ELEMENTS OF EXAMINATION

Constitutional

Head and Face

Eyes

- Test visual acuity (Does not include determination of refractive error)

- Gross visual field testing by confrontation

- Test ocular motility including primary gaze alignment

- Inspection of bulbar and palpebral conjunctivae

- Examination of ocular adnexae including lids (e.g., ptosis or lagophthalmos), lacrimal glands, lacrimal drainage, orbits and preauricular lymph nodes

- Examination of pupils and irises including shape, direct and consensual reaction (afferent pupil), size (e.g., anisocoria) and morphology

- Slit lamp examination of the corneas including epithelium, stroma, endothelium, and tear film

- Slit lamp examination of the anterior chambers including depth, cells, and flare

- Slit lamp examination of the lenses including clarity, anterior and posterior capsule, cortex, and nucleus

- Measurement of intraocular pressures (except in children and patients with trauma or infectious disease)

- Ophthalmoscopic examination through dilated pupils (unless contraindicated) of

- Optic discs including size, C/D ratio, appearance (e.g., atrophy, cupping, tumor elevation) and nerve fiber layer

- Posterior segments including retina and vessels (e.g., exudates and hemorrhages)

127

Ears, Nose, Mouth and Throat

Neck

Respiratory

Cardiovascular

Chest (Breasts)

Gastrointestinal (Abdomen)

Genitourinary

Lymphatic

Musculoskeletal

Extremities

Skin

Neurological/Psychiatric   *Brief assessment of mental status including:*

- *Orientation to time, place and person*
- *Mood and affect (e.g., depression, anxiety, agitation)*

CONTENT AND DOCUMENTATION REQUIREMENTS

Level of Exam	Perform and Document:
Problem Focused	One to five elements identified by a bullet.
Expanded Problem Focused	At least six elements identified by a bullet.
Detailed	At least nine elements identified by a bullet.
Comprehensive	Perform all elements identified by a bullet; document every element in each box with a shaded border and at least one element in each box with an unshaded border.

GENITOURINARY EXAMINATION

SYSTEM/BODY AREA	ELEMENTS OF EXAMINATION
Constitutional	• *Measurement of any three of the following seven vital signs: 1) sitting or standing blood pressure, 2) supine blood pressure, 3) pulse rate and regularity, 4) respiration, 5) temperature, 6) height, 7) weight (May be measured and recorded by ancillary staff)* • *General appearance of patient (e.g., development, nutrition, body habitus, deformities, attention to grooming)*
Head and Face	
Eyes	
Ears, Nose, Mouth and Throat	
Neck	• *Examination of neck (e.g., masses, overall appearance, symmetry, tracheal position, crepitus)* • *Examination of thyroid (e.g., enlargement, tenderness, mass)*
Respiratory	• *Assessment of respiratory effort (e.g., intercostal retractions, use of accessory muscles, diaphragmatic movement)* • *Auscultation of lungs (e.g., breath sounds, adventitious sounds, rubs)*
Cardiovascular	• *Auscultation of heart with notation of abnormal sounds and murmurs* • *Examination of peripheral vascular system by observation (e.g., swelling, varicosities) and palpation (e.g., pulses, temperature, edema, tenderness)*
Chest (Breasts)	*[See genitourinary (female)]*

Gastrointestinal (Abdomen)	• *Examination of abdomen with notation of presence of masses or tenderness*
	• *Examination for presence or absence of hernia*
	• *Examination of liver and spleen*
	• *Obtain stool sample for occult blood test when indicated*
Genitourinary (male)	• *Inspection of anus and perineum*
	Examination (with or without specimen collection for smears and cultures) of genitalia including:
	• *Scrotum (e.g., lesions, cysts, rashes)*
	• *Epididymides (e.g., size, symmetry, masses)*
	• *Testes (e.g., size, symmetry, masses)*
	• *Urethral meatus (e.g., size, location, lesions, discharge)*
	• *Penis (e.g., lesions, presence or absence of foreskin, foreskin retractability, plaque, masses, scarring, deformities)*
	Digital rectal examination including:
	• *Prostate gland (e.g., size, symmetry, nodularity, tenderness)*
	• *Seminal vesicles (e.g., symmetry, tenderness, masses, enlargement)*
	• *Sphincter tone, presence of hemorrhoids, rectal masses*
Genitourinary (female)	*Includes at least seven of the following eleven elements identified by bullets:*
	• *Inspection and palpation of breasts (e.g., masses or lumps, tenderness, symmetry, nipple discharge)*
	• *Digital rectal examination including sphincter tone, presence of hemorrhoids, rectal masses*
	Pelvic examination (with or without specimen collection for smears and cultures) including:

- *External genitalia (e.g., general appearance, hair distribution, lesions)*

- *Urethral meatus (e.g., size, location, lesions, prolapse)*

- *Urethra (e.g., masses, tenderness, scarring)*

- *Bladder (e.g., fullness, masses, tenderness)*

- *Vagina (e.g., general appearance, estrogen effect, discharge, lesions, pelvic support, cystocele, rectocele)*

- *Cervix (e.g., general appearance, lesions, discharge)*

- *Uterus (e.g., size, contour, position, mobility, tenderness, consistency, descent or support)*

- *Adnexa/parametria (e.g., masses, tenderness, organomegaly, nodularity)*

- *Anus and perineum*

Lymphatic
- *Palpation of lymph nodes in neck, axillae, groin and/or other location*

Musculoskeletal

Extremities

Skin
- *Inspection and/or palpation of skin and subcutaneous tissue (e.g., rashes, lesions, ulcers)*

Neurological/Psychiatric
Brief assessment of mental status including:

- *Orientation (e.g., time, place and person) and*

- *Mood and affect (e.g., depression, anxiety, agitation)*

CONTENT AND DOCUMENTATION REQUIREMENTS

Level of Exam	*Perform and Document:*
Problem Focused	One to five elements identified by a bullet.
Expanded Problem Focused	At least six elements identified by a bullet.
Detailed	At least twelve elements identified by a bullet.
Comprehensive	Perform all elements identified by a bullet; document every element in each box with a shaded border and at least one element in each box with an unshaded border.

HEMATOLOGIC, LYMPHATIC, AND/OR IMMUNOLOGIC EXAMINATION

SYSTEM/BODY AREA	ELEMENTS OF EXAMINATION
Constitutional	• *Measurement of any three of the following seven vital signs: 1) sitting or standing blood pressure, 2) supine blood pressure, 3) pulse rate and regularity, 4) respiration, 5) temperature, 6) height, 7) weight (May be measured and recorded by ancillary staff)* • *General appearance of patient (e.g., development, nutrition, body habitus, deformities, attention to grooming)*
Head and Face	• *Palpation and/or percussion of face with notation of presence or absence of sinus tenderness*
Eyes	• *Inspection of conjunctivae and lids*
Ears, Nose, Mouth and Throat	• *Otoscopic examination of external auditory canals and tympanic membranes* • *Inspection of nasal mucosa, septum and turbinates* • *Inspection of teeth and gums* • *Examination of oropharynx (e.g., oral mucosa, hard and soft palates, tongue, tonsils, posterior pharynx)*
Neck	• *Examination of neck (e.g., masses, overall appearance, symmetry, tracheal position, crepitus)* • *Examination of thyroid (e.g., enlargement, tenderness, mass)*
Respiratory	• *Assessment of respiratory effort (e.g., intercostal retractions, use of accessory muscles, diaphragmatic movement)* • *Auscultation of lungs (e.g., breath sounds, adventitious sounds, rubs)*

| **Cardiovascular** | • Auscultation of heart with notation of abnormal sounds and murmurs

• Examination of peripheral vascular system by observation (e.g., swelling, varicosities) and palpation (e.g., pulses, temperature, edema, tenderness) |

Chest (Breasts)

| **Gastrointestinal (Abdomen)** | • Examination of abdomen with notation of presence of masses or tenderness

• Examination of liver and spleen |

Genitourinary

| **Lymphatic** | • Palpation of lymph nodes in neck, axillae, groin, and/or other location |

Musculoskeletal

| **Extremities** | • Inspection and palpation of digits and nails (e.g., clubbing, cyanosis, inflammation, petechiae, ischemia, infections, nodes) |

| **Skin** | • Inspection and/or palpation of skin and subcutaneous tissue (e.g., rashes, lesions, ulcers, ecchymoses, bruises) |

| **Neurological/Psychiatric** | Brief assessment of mental status including:

• Orientation to time, place and person

• Mood and affect (e.g., depression, anxiety, agitation) |

CONTENT AND DOCUMENTATION REQUIREMENTS

Level of Exam	Perform and Document:
Problem Focused	One to five elements identified by a bullet.
Expanded Problem Focused	At least six elements identified by a bullet.
Detailed	At least twelve elements identified by a bullet.
Comprehensive	Perform all elements identified by a bullet; document every element in each box with a shaded border and at least one element in each box with an unshaded border.

MUSCULOSKELETAL EXAMINATION

SYSTEM/BODY AREA	ELEMENTS OF EXAMINATION
Constitutional	• *Measurement of any three of the following seven vital signs: 1) sitting or standing blood pressure, 2) supine blood pressure, 3) pulse rate and regularity, 4) respiration, 5) temperature, 6) height, 7) weight (May be measured and recorded by ancillary staff)* • *General appearance of patient (e.g., development, nutrition, body habitus, deformities, attention to grooming)*
Head and Face	
Eyes	
Ears, Nose, Mouth and Throat	
Neck	
Respiratory	
Cardiovascular	• *Examination of peripheral vascular system by observation (e.g., swelling, varicosities) and palpation (e.g., pulses, temperature, edema, tenderness)*
Chest (Breasts)	
Gastrointestinal (Abdomen)	
Genitourinary	
Lymphatic	• *Palpation of lymph nodes in neck, axillae, groin and/or other location*

Musculoskeletal

- *Examination of gait and station*

- *Examination of joint(s), bone(s) and muscle(s)/ tendon(s) of four of the following six areas: 1) head and neck; 2) spine, ribs and pelvis; 3) right upper extremity; 4) left upper extremity; 5) right lower extremity; and 6) left lower extremity. The examination of a given area includes:*

- *Inspection, percussion and/or palpation with notation of any misalignment, asymmetry, crepitation, defects, tenderness, masses or effusions*

- *Assessment of range of motion with notation of any pain (e.g., straight leg raising), crepitation or contracture*

- *Assessment of stability with notation of any dislocation (luxation), subluxation or laxity*

- *Assessment of muscle strength and tone (e.g., flaccid, cog wheel, spastic) with notation of any atrophy or abnormal movements*

NOTE: For the comprehensive level of examination, all four of the elements identified by a bullet must be performed and documented for each of four anatomic areas. For the three lower levels of examination, each element is counted separately for each body area. For example, assessing range of motion in two extremities constitutes two elements.

Extremities

[See musculoskeletal and skin]

Skin

- *Inspection and/or palpation of skin and subcutaneous tissue (e.g., scars, rashes, lesions, cafe-au-lait spots, ulcers) in four of the following six areas: 1) head and neck; 2) trunk; 3) right upper extremity; 4) left upper extremity; 5) right lower extremity; and 6) left lower extremity.*

NOTE: For the comprehensive level, all four areas must be examined and documented. For the three lower levels, each body area is counted separately. For example, inspection and/or palpation of the skin and subcutaneous tissue of two extremities constitutes two elements.

137

Neurological/Psychiatric	• *Test coordination (e.g., finger/nose, heel/knee/shin, rapid alternating movements in the upper and lower extremities, evaluation of fine motor coordination in young children)*
	• *Examination of deep tendon reflexes and/or nerve stretch test with notation of pathological reflexes (e.g., Babinski)*
	• *Examination of sensation (e.g., by touch, pin, vibration, proprioception)*
	Brief assessment of mental status including
	• *Orientation to time, place and person*
	• *Mood and affect (e.g., depression, anxiety, agitation)*

CONTENT AND DOCUMENTATION REQUIREMENTS

Level of Exam	*Perform and Document:*
Problem Focused	*One to five elements identified by a bullet.*
Expanded Problem Focused	*At least six elements identified by a bullet.*
Detailed	*At least twelve elements identified by a bullet.*
Comprehensive	*Perform all elements identified by a bullet; document every element in each box with a shaded border and at least one element in each box with an unshaded border.*

NEUROLOGICAL EXAMINATION

SYSTEM/BODY AREA   ELEMENTS OF EXAMINATION

Constitutional
- *Measurement of any three of the following seven vital signs: 1) sitting or standing blood pressure, 2) supine blood pressure, 3) pulse rate and regularity, 4) respiration, 5) temperature, 6) height, 7) weight (May be measured and recorded by ancillary staff)*
- *General appearance of patient (e.g., development, nutrition, body habitus, deformities, attention to grooming)*

Head and Face

Eyes
- *Ophthalmoscopic examination of optic discs (e.g., size, C/D ratio, appearance) and posterior segments (e.g., vessel changes, exudates, hemorrhages)*

Ears, Nose, Mouth and Throat

Neck

Respiratory

Cardiovascular
- *Examination of carotid arteries (e.g., pulse amplitude, bruits)*
- *Auscultation of heart with notation of abnormal sounds and murmurs*
- *Examination of peripheral vascular system by observation (e.g., swelling, varicosities) and palpation (e.g., pulses, temperature, edema, tenderness)*

Chest (Breasts)

Gastrointestinal (Abdomen)

Genitourinary

Lymphatic

139

Musculoskeletal	• *Examination of gait and station*
	Assessment of motor function including:
	• *Muscle strength in upper and lower extremities*
	• *Muscle tone in upper and lower extremities (e.g., flaccid, cog wheel, spastic) with notation of any atrophy or abnormal movements (e.g., fasciculation, tardive dyskinesia)*
Extremities	*[See musculoskeletal]*

Skin

Neurological/Psychiatric	*Evaluation of higher integrative functions including:*
	• *Orientation to time, place and person*
	• *Recent and remote memory*
	• *Attention span and concentration*
	• *Language (e.g., naming objects, repeating phrases, spontaneous speech)*
	• *Fund of knowledge (e.g., awareness of current events, past history, vocabulary)*
	Test the following cranial nerves:
	• *2nd cranial nerve (e.g., visual acuity, visual fields, fundi)*
	• *3rd, 4th and 6th cranial nerves (e.g., pupils, eye movements)*
	• *5th cranial nerve (e.g., facial sensation, corneal reflexes)*
	• *7th cranial nerve (e.g., facial symmetry, strength)*
	• *8th cranial nerve (e.g., hearing with tuning fork, whispered voice and/or finger rub)*
	• *9th cranial nerve (e.g., spontaneous or reflex palate movement)*
	continued

- *11th cranial nerve (e.g., shoulder shrug strength)*

- *12th cranial nerve (e.g., tongue protrusion)*

- *Examination of sensation (e.g., by touch, pin, vibration, proprioception)*

- *Examination of deep tendon reflexes in upper and lower extremities with notation of pathological reflexes (e.g., Babinski)*

- *Test coordination (e.g., finger/nose, heel/knee/shin, rapid alternating movements in the upper and lower extremities, evaluation of fine motor coordination in young children)*

CONTENT AND DOCUMENTATION REQUIREMENTS

Level of Exam	Perform and Document:
Problem Focused	One to five elements identified by a bullet.
Expanded Problem Focused	At least six elements identified by a bullet.
Detailed	At least twelve elements identified by a bullet.
Comprehensive	Perform all elements identified by a bullet; document every element in each box with a shaded border and at least one element in each box with an unshaded border.

PSYCHIATRIC EXAMINATION

SYSTEM/BODY AREA	ELEMENTS OF EXAMINATION
Constitutional	• *Measurement of any three of the following seven vital signs: 1) sitting or standing blood pressure, 2) supine blood pressure, 3) pulse rate and regularity, 4) respiration, 5) temperature, 6) height, 7) weight (May be measured and recorded by ancillary staff)* • *General appearance of patient (e.g., development, nutrition, body habitus, deformities, attention to grooming)*
Head and Face	
Eyes	
Ears, Nose, Mouth and Throat	
Neck	
Respiratory	
Cardiovascular	
Chest (Breasts)	
Gastrointestinal (Abdomen)	
Genitourinary	
Lymphatic	
Musculoskeletal	• *Assessment of muscle strength and tone (e.g., flaccid, cog wheel, spastic) with notation of any atrophy and abnormal movements* • *Examination of gait and station*
Extremities	
Skin	

Neurological

| *Psychiatric* | • *Description of speech including: rate; volume; articulation; coherence; and spontaneity with notation of abnormalities (e.g., perseveration, paucity of language)* |

• *Description of thought processes including: rate of thoughts; content of thoughts (e.g., logical vs. illogical, tangential); abstract reasoning; and computation*

• *Description of associations (e.g., loose, tangential, circumstantial, intact)*

• *Description of abnormal or psychotic thoughts including: hallucinations; delusions; preoccupation with violence; homicidal or suicidal ideation; and obsessions*

• *Description of the patient's judgment (e.g., concerning everyday activities and social situations) and insight (e.g., concerning psychiatric condition)*

Complete mental status examination including:

• *Orientation to time, place and person*

• *Recent and remote memory*

• *Attention span and concentration*

• *Language (e.g., naming objects, repeating phrases)*

• *Fund of knowledge (e.g., awareness of current events, past history, vocabulary)*

• *Mood and affect (e.g., depression, anxiety, agitation, hypomania, lability)*

CONTENT AND DOCUMENTATION REQUIREMENTS

Level of Exam	Perform and Document:
Problem Focused	One to five elements identified by a bullet.
Expanded Problem Focused	At least six elements identified by a bullet.
Detailed	At least nine elements identified by a bullet.
Comprehensive	Perform all elements identified by a bullet; document every element in each box with a shaded border and at least one element in each box with an unshaded border.

RESPIRATORY EXAMINATION

SYSTEM/BODY AREA	ELEMENTS OF EXAMINATION
Constitutional	• Measurement of any three of the following seven vital signs: 1) sitting or standing blood pressure, 2) supine blood pressure, 3) pulse rate and regularity, 4) respiration, 5) temperature, 6) height, 7) weight (May be measured and recorded by ancillary staff) • General appearance of patient (e.g., development, nutrition, body habitus, deformities, attention to grooming)
Head and Face	
Eyes	
Ears, Nose, Mouth and Throat	• Inspection of nasal mucosa, septum and turbinates • Inspection of teeth and gums • Examination of oropharynx (e.g., oral mucosa, hard and soft palates, tongue, tonsils and posterior pharynx)
Neck	• Examination of neck (e.g., masses, overall appearance, symmetry, tracheal position, crepitus) • Examination of thyroid (e.g., enlargement, tenderness, mass) • Examination of jugular veins (e.g., distension; a, v or cannon a waves)
Respiratory	• Inspection of chest with notation of symmetry and expansion • Assessment of respiratory effort (e.g., intercostal retractions, use of accessory muscles, diaphragmatic movement) • Percussion of chest (e.g., dullness, flatness, hyperresonance) *continued*

145

- *Palpation of chest (e.g., tactile fremitus)*

- *Auscultation of lungs (e.g., breath sounds, adventitious sounds, rubs)*

Cardiovascular

- *Auscultation of heart including sounds, abnormal sounds and murmurs*

- *Examination of peripheral vascular system by observation (e.g., swelling, varicosities) and palpation (e.g., pulses, temperature, edema, tenderness)*

Chest (Breasts)

Gastrointestinal (Abdomen)

- *Examination of abdomen with notation of presence of masses or tenderness*

- *Examination of liver and spleen*

Genitourinary

Lymphatic

- *Palpation of lymph nodes in neck, axillae, groin and/or other location*

Musculoskeletal

- *Assessment of muscle strength and tone (e.g., flaccid, cog wheel, spastic) with notation of any atrophy and abnormal movements*

- *Examination of gait and station*

Extremities

- *Inspection and palpation of digits and nails (e.g., clubbing, cyanosis, inflammation, petechiae, ischemia, infections, nodes)*

Skin

- *Inspection and/or palpation of skin and subcutaneous tissue (e.g., rashes, lesions, ulcers)*

Neurological/Psychiatric

Brief assessment of mental status including:

- *Orientation to time, place and person*

- *Mood and affect (e.g., depression, anxiety, agitation)*

CONTENT AND DOCUMENTATION REQUIREMENTS

Level of Exam	Perform and Document:
Problem Focused	One to five elements identified by a bullet.
Expanded Problem Focused	At least six elements identified by a bullet.
Detailed	At least twelve elements identified by a bullet.
Comprehensive	Perform all elements identified by a bullet; document every element in each box with a shaded border and at least one element in each box with an unshaded border.

SKIN EXAMINATION

SYSTEM/BODY AREA	ELEMENTS OF EXAMINATION
Constitutional	• *Measurement of any three of the following seven vital signs: 1) sitting or standing blood pressure, 2) supine blood pressure, 3) pulse rate and regularity, 4) respiration, 5) temperature, 6) height, 7) weight (May be measured and recorded by ancillary staff)* • *General appearance of patient (e.g., development, nutrition, body habitus, deformities, attention to grooming)*
Head and Face	
Eyes	• *Inspection of conjunctivae and lids*
Ears, Nose, Mouth and Throat	• *Inspection of lips, teeth and gums* • *Examination of oropharynx (e.g., oral mucosa, hard and soft palates, tongue, tonsils, posterior pharynx)*
Neck	• *Examination of thyroid (e.g., enlargement, tenderness, mass)*
Respiratory	
Cardiovascular	• *Examination of peripheral vascular system by observation (e.g., swelling, varicosities) and palpation (e.g., pulses, temperature, edema, tenderness)*
Chest (Breasts)	
Gastrointestinal (Abdomen)	• *Examination of liver and spleen* • *Examination of anus for condyloma and other lesions*
Genitourinary	

Lymphatic

- *Palpation of lymph nodes in neck, axillae, groin and/or other location*

Musculoskeletal

Extremities

- *Inspection and palpation of digits and nails (e.g., clubbing, cyanosis, inflammation, petechiae, ischemia, infections, nodes)*

Skin

- *Palpation of scalp and inspection of hair of scalp, eyebrows, face, chest, pubic area (when indicated) and extremities*

  Inspection and/or palpation of skin and subcutaneous tissue (e.g., rashes, lesions, ulcers, susceptibility to and presence of photo damage) in eight of the following ten areas:

- *Head, including the face and*

- *Neck*

- *Chest, including breasts and axillae*

- *Abdomen*

- *Genitalia, groin, buttocks*

- *Back*

- *Right upper extremity*

- *Left upper extremity*

- *Right lower extremity*

- *Left lower extremity*

NOTE: For the comprehensive level, the examination of at least eight anatomic areas must be performed and documented. For the three lower levels of examination, each body area is counted separately. For example, inspection and/or palpation of the skin and subcutaneous tissue of the right upper extremity and the left upper extremity constitutes two elements.

- *Inspection of eccrine and apocrine glands of skin and subcutaneous tissue with identification and location of any hyperhidrosis, chromhidroses or bromhidrosis*

Neurological/Psychiatric	*Brief assessment of mental status including:*
	● *Orientation to time, place and person*
	● *Mood and affect (e.g., depression, anxiety, agitation)*

CONTENT AND DOCUMENTATION REQUIREMENTS

Level of Exam	*Perform and Document:*
Problem Focused	*One to five elements identified by a bullet.*
Expanded Problem Focused	*At least six elements identified by a bullet.*
Detailed	*At least twelve elements identified by a bullet.*
Comprehensive	*Perform all elements identified by a bullet; document every element in each box with a shaded border and at least one element in each box with an unshaded border.*

DOCUMENTATION OF THE COMPLEXITY OF MEDICAL DECISION MAKING

The levels of evaluation and management services recognize four types of medical decision making (straight-forward, low complexity, moderate complexity and high complexity). Medical decision making refers to the complexity of establishing a diagnosis and/or selecting a management option as measured by:

- the number of possible diagnoses and/or the number of management options that must be considered;

- the amount and/or complexity of medical records, diagnostic tests, and/or other information that must be obtained, reviewed and analyzed; and

- the risk of significant complications, morbidity and/or mortality, as well as comorbidities, associated with the patient's presenting problem(s), the diagnostic procedure(s) and/or the possible management options.

The following chart illustrates the progression of the elements required for each level of medical decision making. To qualify for a given type of decision making, two of the three elements in the table must be either met or exceeded.

NUMBER OF DIAGNOSES OR MANAGEMENT OPTIONS

The number of possible diagnoses and/or the number of management options that must be considered is based on the number and types of problems addressed during the encounter, the complexity of establishing a diagnosis and the management decisions that are made by the physician.

Generally, decision making with respect to a diagnosed problem is easier than that for an identified but undiagnosed problem. The number and type of diagnostic tests employed may be an indicator of the number of possible diagnoses. Problems which are improving or resolving are less complex than those which are worsening or failing to change as expected. The need to seek advice from others is another indicator of complexity of diagnostic or management problems.

- **●DG:** *For each encounter, an assessment, clinical impression, or diagnosis should be documented. It may be explicitly stated or implied in documented decisions regarding management plans and/or further evaluation.*

  - *For a presenting problem with an established diagnosis, the record should reflect whether the problem is: a) improved, well controlled, resolving or resolved; or, b) inadequately controlled, worsening, or failing to change as expected.*

  - *For a presenting problem without an established diagnosis, the assessment or clinical impression may be stated in the form of differential diagnoses or as a "possible", "probable", or "rule out" (R/O) diagnosis.*

151

Number of Diagnoses	Amount of Data to Review	Risk of Complication	Type of Decision Making
Minimal	Minimal or None	Minimal	**Straightforward**
Limited	Limited	Low	**Low Complexity**
Multiple	Moderate	Moderate	**Moderate Complexity**
Extensive	Extensive	High	**High Complexity**

Each of the elements of medical decision making is described below

●**DG:** *The initiation of, or changes in, treatment should be documented. Treatment includes a wide range of management options including patient instructions, nursing instructions, therapies, and medications.*

●**DG:** *If referrals are made, consultations requested or advice sought, the record should indicate to whom or where the referral or consultation is made or from whom the advice is requested.*

AMOUNT AND/OR COMPLEXITY OF DATA TO BE REVIEWED

The amount and complexity of data to be reviewed is based on the types of diagnostic testing ordered or reviewed. A decision to obtain and review old medical records and/or obtain history from sources other than the patient increases the amount and complexity of data to be reviewed.

Discussion of contradictory or unexpected test results with the physician who performed or interpreted the test is an indication of the complexity of data being reviewed. On occasion the physician who ordered a test may personally review the image, tracing or specimen to supplement information from the physician who prepared the test report or interpretation; this is another indication of the complexity of data being reviewed.

●**DG:** *If a diagnostic service (test or procedure) is ordered, planned, scheduled, or performed at the time of the evaluation and management encounter, the type of service, e.g., lab or x-ray, should be documented.*

●**DG:** *The review of lab, radiology and/or other diagnostic tests should be documented. A simple notation such as "WBC elevated" or "chest x-ray unremarkable" is acceptable. Alternatively, the review may be documented by initialing and dating the report containing the test results.*

●**DG:** *A decision to obtain old records or decision to obtain additional history from the family, caretaker or other source to supplement that obtained from the patient should be documented.*

●*DG:*   *Relevant findings from the review of old records, and/or the receipt of additional history from the family, caretaker or other source to supplement that obtained from the patient should be documented. If there is no relevant information beyond that already obtained, that fact should be documented. A notation of "Old records reviewed" or "additional history obtained from family" without elaboration is insufficient.*

●*DG:*   *The results of discussion of laboratory, radiology or other diagnostic tests with the physician who performed or interpreted the study should be documented.*

●*DG:*   *The direct visualization and independent interpretation of an image, tracing or specimen previously or subsequently interpreted by another physician should be documented.*

RISK OF SIGNIFICANT COMPLICATIONS, MORBIDITY AND/OR MORTALITY

The risk of significant complications, morbidity, and/or mortality is based on the risks associated with the presenting problem(s), the diagnostic procedure(s), and the possible management options.

●*DG:*   *Comorbidities/underlying diseases or other factors that increase the complexity of medical decision making by increasing the risk of complications, morbidity, and/or mortality should be documented.*

●*DG:*   *If a surgical or invasive diagnostic procedure is ordered, planned or scheduled at the time of the evaluation and management encounter, the type of procedure, e.g., laparoscopy, should be documented.*

●*DG:*   *If a surgical or invasive diagnostic procedure is performed at the time of the evaluation and management encounter, the specific procedure should be documented.*

●*DG:*   *The referral for or decision to perform a surgical or invasive diagnostic procedure on an urgent basis should be documented or implied.*

The Table of Risk on the following page may be used to help determine whether the risk of significant complications, morbidity, and/or mortality is minimal, low, moderate, or high. Because the determination of risk is complex and not readily quantifiable, the table includes common clinical examples rather than absolute measures of risk. The assessment of risk of the presenting problem(s) is based on the risk related to the disease process anticipated between the present encounter and the next one. The assessment of risk of selecting diagnostic procedures and management options is based on the risk during and immediately following any procedures or treatment. The highest level of risk in any one category (presenting problem(s), diagnostic procedure(s), or management options) determines the overall risk.

153

DOCUMENTATION OF AN ENCOUNTER DOMINATED BY COUNSELING OR COORDINATION OF CARE

In the case where counseling and/or coordination of care dominates (more than 50%) of the physician/patient and/or family encounter (face-to-face time in the office or other or outpatient setting, floor/unit time in the hospital or nursing facility), time is considered the key or controlling factor to qualify for a particular level of evaluation and management services.

●DG: *If the physician elects to report the level of service based on counseling and/or coordination of care, the total length of time of the encounter (face-to-face or floor time, as appropriate) should be documented and the record should describe the counseling and/or activities to coordinate care.*

TABLE OF RISK

LEVEL OF RISK	PRESENTING PROBLEM(S)	DIAGNOSTIC PROCEDURES	MANAGEMENT OPTIONS
Minimal	● One self-limited or minor problem, (eg, cold, insect bite, tinea corporis)	● Laboratory tests requiring venipuncture ● Chest x-rays ● EKG/EEG ● Urinalysis ● Ultrasound, (eg, echocardiography) ● KOH prep	● Rest ● Gargles ● Elastic bandages ● Superficial dressings
Low	● Two or more self-limited or minor problems ● One stable chronic illness, (eg, well controlled hypertension, non-insulin dependent diabetes, cataract, BPH) ● Acute uncomplicated illness or injury, (eg, cystitis, allergic rhinitis, simple sprain)	● Physiologic tests not under stress, (eg, pulmonary function tests) ● Non-cardiovascular imaging studies with contrast,(eg, barium enema) ● Superficial needle biopsies ● Clinical laboratory tests requiring arterial puncture ● Skin biopsies	● Over-the-counter drugs ● Minor surgery with no identified risk factors ● Physical therapy ● Occupational therapy ● IV fluids without additives

continued

TABLE OF RISK (continued)

LEVEL OF RISK	PRESENTING PROBLEM(S)	DIAGNOSTIC PROCEDURES	MANAGEMENT OPTIONS
Moderate	• One or more chronic illnesses with mild exacerbation, progression, or side effects of treatment • Two or more stable chronic illnesses • Undiagnosed new problem with uncertain prognosis, (eg, lump in breast) • Acute illness with systemic symptoms, (eg, pyelonephritis, pneumonitis, colitis) • Acute complicated injury, (eg, head injury with brief loss of consciousness)	• Physiologic tests under stress, (eg, cardiac stress test, fetal contraction stress test) • Diagnostic endoscopies with no identified risk factors • Deep needle or incisional biopsy • Cardiovascular imaging studies with contrast and no identified risk factors, (eg, arteriogram, cardiac catheterization) • Obtain fluid from body cavity, (eg, lumbar puncture, thoracentesis, culdocentesis)	• Minor surgery with identified risk factors • Elective major surgery (open, percutaneous or endoscopic) with no identified risk factors • Prescription drug management • Therapeutic nuclear medicine • IV fluids with additives • Closed treatment of fracture or dislocation without manipulation
High	• One or more chronic illnesses with severe exacerbation, progression, or side effects of treatment • Acute or chronic illnesses or injuries that pose a threat to life or bodily function, (eg, multiple trauma, acute MI, pulmonary embolus, severe respiratory distress, progressive severe rheumatoid arthritis, psychiatric illness with potential threat to self or others, peritonitis, acute renal failure) • An abrupt change in neurologic status, (eg, seizure, TIA, weakness, sensory loss)	• Cardiovascular imaging studies with contrast with identified risk factors • Cardiac electrophysiological tests • Diagnostic endoscopies with identified risk factors • Discography	• Elective major surgery (open, percutaneous or endoscopic) with identified risk factors • Emergency major surgery (open, percutaneous or endoscopic) • Parenteral controlled substances • Drug therapy requiring intensive monitoring for toxicity • Decision not to resuscitate or to de-escalate care because of poor prognosis

This page intentionally left blank.

EVALUATION AND MANAGEMENT

OFFICE OR OTHER OUTPATIENT SERVICES

Evaluation and management codes 99201-99215 are used to report services provided to new and established patients in the office or other outpatient facility, including the emergency department when the physician is not assigned to the emergency department. The key coding issues are the extent of history obtained, the extent of examination performed, and the complexity of medical decision making. Additional reporting issues include counseling and/or coordination of care, the nature of presenting problem(s), and the duration of face-to-face time spent with the patient and/or family.

CODING RULES

1.   *A patient is considered an outpatient until admitted as an inpatient to a health care facility.*

2.   *If outpatient evaluation and management services are provided in conjunction with, or result in, an inpatient admission, the service is reported using CPT codes for initial hospital care.*

3.   *CPT codes in this section may also be used to report the services provided by a physician to a patient in an observation area of a hospital.*

4.   *Laboratory tests, radiology services, and diagnostic or therapeutic procedures performed in conjunction with evaluation and management services are reported in addition to the basic evaluation and management service.*

5.   *Supplies and materials provided by the physician over and above those usually included with the evaluation and management or other services rendered may be listed separately. List all drugs, trays, supplies and materials provided.*

NEW PATIENT

99201   Office or other outpatient visit for the evaluation and management of a new patient, which requires these three key components:

- a problem focused history;

 Separate Procedure

 Unlisted Procedure

 CCI Comp. Code

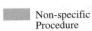 Non-specific Procedure

- a problem focused examination; and
- straightforward medical decision making.

Counseling and/or coordination of care with other providers or agencies are provided consistent with the nature of the problem(s) and the patient's and/or family's needs.

Usually, the presenting problems are self limited or minor. Physicians typically spend 10 minutes face-to-face with the patient and/or family.

99202 Office or other outpatient visit for the evaluation and management of a new patient, which requires these three key components:

- an expanded problem focused history;
- an expanded problem focused examination; and
- straightforward medical decision making.

Counseling and/or coordination of care with other providers or agencies are provided consistent with the nature of the problem(s) and the patient's and/or family's needs.

Usually, the presenting problem(s) are of low to moderate severity. Physicians typically spend 20 minutes face-to-face with the patient and/or family.

99203 Office or other outpatient visit for the evaluation and management of a new patient, which requires these three key components:

- a detailed history;
- a detailed examination; and
- medical decision making of low complexity.

Counseling and/or coordination of care with other providers or agencies are provided consistent with the nature of the problem(s) and the patient's and/or family's needs.

Usually, the presenting problem(s) are of moderate severity. Physicians typically spend 30 minutes face-to-face with the patient and/or family.

99204 Office or other outpatient visit for the evaluation and management of a new patient, which requires these three key components:

- a comprehensive history;

- a comprehensive examination; and
- medical decision making of moderate complexity.

Counseling and/or coordination of care with other providers or agencies are provided consistent with the nature of the problem(s) and the patient's and/or family's needs.

Usually, the presenting problem(s) are of moderate to high severity. Physicians typically spend 45 minutes face-to-face with the patient and/or family.

99205 Office or other outpatient visit for the evaluation and management of a new patient, which requires these three key components:

- a comprehensive history;
- a comprehensive examination; and
- medical decision making of high complexity.

Counseling and/or coordination of care with other providers or agencies are provided consistent with the nature of the problem(s) and the patient's and/or family's needs.

Usually, the presenting problem(s) are of moderate to high severity. Physicians typically spend 60 minutes face-to-face with the patient and/or family.

ESTABLISHED PATIENT

99211 Office or other outpatient visit for the evaluation and management of an established patient, that may not require the presence of a physician. Usually, the presenting problem(s) are minimal. Typically, 5 minutes are spent performing or supervising these services.

99212 Office or other outpatient visit for the evaluation and management of an established patient, which requires at least two of these three key components:

- a problem focused history;
- a problem focused examination;
- straightforward medical decision making.

Counseling and/or coordination of care with other providers or agencies are provided consistent with the nature of the problem(s) and the patient's and/or family's needs.

159

Usually, the presenting problem(s) are self limited or minor. Physicians typically 10 minutes face-to-face with the patient and/or family.

99213 Office or other outpatient visit for the evaluation and management of an established patient, which requires at least two of these three key components:

- an expanded problem focused history;
- an expanded problem focused examination;
- medical decision making of low complexity.

Counseling and coordination of care with other providers or agencies are provided consistent with the nature of the problem(s) and the patient's and/or family's needs.

Usually, the presenting problem(s) are of low to moderate severity. Physicians typically spend 15 minutes face-to-face with the patient and/or family.

99214 Office or other outpatient visit for the evaluation and management of an established patient, which requires at least two of these three key components:

- a detailed history;
- a detailed examination;
- medical decision making of moderate complexity.

Counseling and/or coordination of care with other providers or agencies are provided consistent with the nature of the problem(s) and the patient's and/or family's needs.

Usually, the presenting problem(s) are of moderate to high severity. Physicians typically spend 25 minutes face-to-face with the patient and/or family.

99215 Office or other outpatient visit for the evaluation and management of an established patient, which requires at least two of these three key components:

- a comprehensive history;
- a comprehensive examination;
- medical decision making of high complexity.

Counseling and/or coordination of care with other providers or agencies are provided consistent with the nature of the problem(s) and the patient's and/or family's needs.

● New Code   ▲ Revised Code   ✚ Add-On Code   ⊘ Modifier -51 Exempt

Usually, the presenting problem(s) are of moderate to high severity. Physicians typically spend 40 minutes face-to-face with the patient and/or family.

HOSPITAL OBSERVATION SERVICES

Occasionally a physician will watch or "observe" a patient in an area of an inpatient hospital designated as an "observation" area. This area is frequently located in or near the emergency room, and the observation typically after any acute care is rendered.

The purpose of the observation is to determine if the patient's condition requires inpatient hospitalization. Patients considered under observation status may be discharged from the observation area or admitted to the hospital as an inpatient.

All observation care services are "per day" and should be coded only once per date of service. CPT code 99217 is used to report all services provided on discharge from "observation status" if the discharge is on other than the initial date of "observation status."

OBSERVATION CARE DISCHARGE SERVICES

99217 Observation care discharge day management (This code is to be utilized by the physician to report all services provided to a patient on discharge from "observation status" if the discharge is on other than the initial date of "observation status." To report services to a patient designated as "observation status" or "inpatient status" and discharged on the same date, use codes for Observation or Inpatient Care Services [including Admission and Discharge Services, 99234-99236 as appropriate]).

INITIAL OBSERVATION CARE

NEW OR ESTABLISHED PATIENT

99218 Initial observation care, per day, for the evaluation and management of a patient which requires these three key components:

- a detailed or comprehensive history;

- a detailed or comprehensive examination; and

- medical decision making that is straightforward or of low complexity.

Counseling and/or coordination of care with other providers or agencies are provided consistent with the nature of the problem(s) and the patient's and/or family's needs.

 Separate Procedure   Unlisted Procedure   CCI Comp. Code 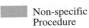 Non-specific Procedure

Usually, the problem(s) requiring admission to "observation status" are of low severity.

99219   Initial observation care, per day, for the evaluation and management of a patient, which requires these three key components:

- a comprehensive history;

- a comprehensive examination; and

- medical decision making of moderate complexity.

Counseling and/or coordination of care with other providers or agencies are provided consistent with the nature of the problem(s) and the patient's and/or family's needs.

Usually, the problem(s) requiring admission to "observation status" are of moderate severity.

99220   Initial observation care, per day, for the evaluation and management of a patient, which requires these three key components:

- a comprehensive history;

- a comprehensive examination; and

- medical decision making of high complexity.

Counseling and/or coordination of care with other providers or agencies are provided consistent with the nature of the problem(s) and the patient's and/or family's needs.

Usually, the problem(s) requiring admission to "observation status" are of high severity.

HOSPITAL INPATIENT SERVICES

Hospital inpatient services refer to hospital visits during the course of an inpatient hospital stay. The services may be provided by the patient's primary physician and/or other physicians in the event of multiple illnesses or injuries. Evaluation and management codes 99221-99239 are used to report services provided in the hospital. The key coding issues are the extent of history obtained, the extent of examination performed, and the complexity of medical decision making. Additional reporting issues include counseling and/or coordination of care, the nature of presenting problem(s), and the time spent at the bedside and on the patient's facility floor or unit.

● New Code	▲ Revised Code	+ Add-On Code	⊘ Modifier -51 Exempt

CODING RULES

1. *CPT codes defined as Initial Hospital Care are used to report the first hospital inpatient encounter with the patient by the admitting physician.*

2. *The admitting physician should report all service related to the admission provided in all other locations.*

3. *For observation care or inpatient hospital care services provided to patients who are admitted and discharged on the same date, report with CPT codes 99234-99236 from the Observation or Inpatient Care services subsections.*

INITIAL HOSPITAL CARE

NEW OR ESTABLISHED PATIENT

99221 Initial hospital care, per day, for the evaluation and management of a patient which requires these three key components:

- a detailed or comprehensive history;
- a detailed or comprehensive examination; and
- medical decision making that is straightforward or of low complexity.

Counseling and/or coordination of care with other providers or agencies are provided consistent with the nature of the problem(s) and the patient's and/or family's needs.

Usually, the problem(s) requiring admission are of low severity. Physicians typically spend 30 minutes at the bedside and on the patient's hospital floor or unit.

99222 Initial hospital care, per day, for the evaluation and management of a patient, which requires these three key components:

- a comprehensive history;
- a comprehensive examination; and
- medical decision making of moderate complexity.

Counseling and/or coordination of care with other providers or agencies are provided consistent with the nature of the problem(s) and the patient's and/or family's needs.

Usually, the problem(s) requiring admission are of moderate severity. Physicians typically spend 50 minutes at the bedside and on the patient's hospital floor or unit.

Separate Procedure   Unlisted Procedure   CCI Comp. Code   Non-specific Procedure

99223 Initial hospital care, per day, for the evaluation and management of a patient, which requires these three key components:

- a comprehensive history;
- a comprehensive examination; and
- medical decision making of high complexity.

Counseling and/or coordination of care with other providers or agencies are provided consistent with the nature of the problem(s) and the patient's and/or family's needs.

Usually, the problem(s) requiring admission are of high severity. Physicians typically spend 70 minutes at the bedside and on the patient's hospital floor or unit.

SUBSEQUENT HOSPITAL CARE

99231 Subsequent hospital care, per day, for the evaluation and management of a patient, which requires at least two of these three key components:

- a problem focused interval history;
- a problem focused examination;
- medical decision making that is straightforward or of low complexity.

Counseling and/or coordination of care with other providers or agencies are provided consistent with the nature of the problem(s) and the patient's and/or family's needs.

Usually, the patient is stable, recovering or improving. Physicians typically spend 15 minutes at the bedside and on the patient's hospital floor or unit.

99232 Subsequent hospital care, per day, for the evaluation and management of a patient, which requires at least two of these three key components:

- an expanded problem focused interval history;
- an expanded problem focused examination;
- medical decision making of moderate complexity.

Counseling and/or coordination of care with other providers or agencies are provided consistent with the nature of the problem(s) and the patient's and/or family's needs.

● New Code   ▲ Revised Code   + Add-On Code   ⊘ Modifier -51 Exempt

Usually, the patient is responding inadequately to therapy or has developed a minor complication. Physicians typically spend 25 minutes at the bedside and on the patient's hospital floor or unit.

99233 Subsequent hospital care, per day, for the evaluation and management of a patient, which requires at least two of these three key components:

- a detailed interval history;

- a detailed examination;

- medical decision making of high complexity.

Counseling and/or coordination of care with other providers or agencies are provided consistent with the nature of the problem(s) and the patient's and/or family's needs.

Usually, the patient is unstable or has developed a significant complication or a significant new problem. Physicians typically spend 35 minutes at the bedside and on the patient's hospital floor or unit.

OBSERVATION OR INPATIENT CARE SERVICES (INCLUDING ADMISSION AND DISCHARGE SERVICES)

99234 Observation or inpatient hospital care, for the evaluation and management of a patient including admission and discharge on the same date which requires these three key components:

- a detailed or comprehensive history;

- a detailed or comprehensive examination; and

- medical decision making that is straightforward or of low complexity.

Counseling and/or coordination of care with other providers or agencies are provided consistent with the nature of the problem(s) and the patient's and/or family's needs.

Usually the presenting problem(s) requiring admission are of low severity.

99235 Observation or inpatient hospital care, for the evaluation and management of a patient including admission and discharge on the same date which requires these three key components:

- a comprehensive history;

- a comprehensive examination; and

- medical decision making of moderate complexity.

165

 Separate Procedure   Unlisted Procedure   CCI Comp. Code   Non-specific Procedure

Counseling and/or coordination of care with other providers or agencies are provided consistent with the nature of the problem(s) and the patient's and/or family's needs.

Usually the presenting problem(s) requiring admission are of moderate severity.

99236 Observation or inpatient hospital care, for the evaluation and management of a patient including admission and discharge on the same date which requires these three key components:

- a comprehensive history;

- a comprehensive examination; and

- medical decision making of high complexity.

Counseling and/or coordination of care with other providers or agencies are provided consistent with the nature of the problem(s) and the patient's and/or family's needs.

Usually the presenting problem(s) requiring admission are of high severity.

HOSPITAL DISCHARGE SERVICES

99238 Hospital discharge day management; 30 minutes or less

99239 Hospital discharge day management; more than 30 minutes

(These codes are to be utilized by the physician to report all services provided to a patient on the date of discharge, if other than the initial date of inpatient status. To report services to a patient who is admitted as an inpatient, and discharged on the same date, see codes 99234-99236 for observation or inpatient hospital care including the admission and discharge of the patient on the same date. To report concurrent care services provided by a physician(s) other than the attending physician, use subsequent hospital care codes (99231-99233) on the day of discharge.)

(For Observation Care Discharge, use 99217)

(For observation or inpatient hospital care including the admission and discharge of the patient on the same date, see 99234-99236)

(For Nursing Facility Care Discharge, 99315, 99316)

(For discharge services provided to newborns admitted and discharged on the same date, use 99435)

● New Code	▲ Revised Code	+ Add-On Code	⊘ Modifier -51 Exempt

CONSULTATIONS

A consultation is the process of taking a history, performing a physical examination, and ordering and interpreting appropriate diagnostic tests, for the purpose of rendering an expert opinion about a patient's illness and/or injury.

A consultation may be requested by a patient's primary physician, by the patient or by a third party, such as a review organization.

The key coding issues are the location of the service, the extent of history obtained, the extent of examination performed, and the complexity of medical decision making. Additional reporting issues include counseling and/or coordination of care, the nature of presenting problem(s), and the time, depending on location, spent either face-to-face with the patient and/or family or at the bedside and on the patient's facility floor or unit.

CODING RULES

1. *The request for a consultation from the attending physician or other appropriate source, and the need for a consultation must be documented in the patient's medical record.*

2. *The consulting physician must document all services provided and the resulting opinion in the patient's medical record.*

3. *Modifier -32 must be added to the consulting service CPT code if a confirmatory consultation is required by a third party, such as a PRO.*

4. *If the consulting physician assumes responsibility for the continuing care of the patient, the service is no longer considered a consultation, and any subsequent visit services rendered are coded using evaluation and management codes.*

OFFICE OR OTHER OUTPATIENT CONSULTATIONS

NEW OR ESTABLISHED PATIENT

99241 Office consultation for a new or established patient, which requires these three key components:

- a problem focused history;
- a problem focused examination; and
- straightforward medical decision making.

Counseling and/or coordination of care with other providers or agencies are provided consistent with the nature of the problem(s) and the patient's and/or family's needs.

167

 Separate Procedure

Unlisted Procedure

 CCI Comp. Code

Non-specific Procedure

Usually, the presenting problem(s) are self limited or minor. Physicians typically spend 15 minutes face-to-face with the patient and/or family.

99242 Office consultation for a new or established patient, which requires these three key components:

- an expanded problem focused history;

- an expanded problem focused examination; and

- straightforward medical decision making.

Counseling and/or coordination of care with other providers or agencies are provided consistent with the nature of the problem(s) and the patient's and/or family's needs.

Usually, the presenting problem(s) are of low severity. Physicians typically spend 30 minutes face-to-face with the patient and/or family.

99243 Office consultation for a new or established patient, which requires these three key components:

- a detailed history;

- a detailed examination; and

- medical decision making of low complexity.

Counseling and/or coordination of care with other providers or agencies are provided consistent with the nature of the problem(s) and the patient's and/or family's needs.

Usually, the presenting problem(s) are of moderate severity. Physicians typically spend 40 minutes face-to-face with the patient and/or family.

99244 Office consultation for a new or established patient, which requires these three key components:

- a comprehensive history;

- a comprehensive examination; and

- medical decision making of moderate complexity.

Counseling and/or coordination of care with other providers or agencies are provided consistent with the nature of the problem(s) and the patient's and/or family's needs.

Usually, the presenting problem(s) are of moderate to high severity. Physicians typically spend 60 minutes face-to-face with the patient and/or family.

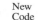

168 ● New Code   ▲ Revised Code   + Add-On Code   ⊘ Modifier -51 Exempt

99245 Office consultation for a new or established patient, which requires these three key components:

- a comprehensive history;

- a comprehensive examination; and

- medical decision making of high complexity.

Counseling and/or coordination of care with other providers or agencies are provided consistent with the nature of the problem(s) and the patient's and/or family's needs.

Usually, the presenting problem(s) are of moderate to high severity. Physicians typically spend 80 minutes face-to-face with the patient and/or family.

INITIAL INPATIENT CONSULTATIONS

NEW OR ESTABLISHED PATIENT

The following CPT codes are used to report physician consultations provided to hospital inpatients, residents of nursing facilities, or patients in a partial hospital setting. Only one initial consultation should be reported by the consultant per admission.

99251 Initial inpatient consultation for a new or established patient, which requires these three key components:

- a problem focused history;

- a problem focused examination; and

- straightforward medical decision making.

Counseling and/or coordination of care with other providers or agencies are provided consistent with the nature of the problem(s) and the patient's and/or family's needs.

Usually, the presenting problem(s) are self limited or minor. Physicians typically spend 20 minutes at the bedside and on the patient's hospital floor or unit.

99252 Initial inpatient consultation for a new or established patient, which requires these three key components:

- an expanded problem focused history;

- an expanded problem focused examination; and

- straightforward medical decision making.

Counseling and/or coordination of care with other providers or agencies are provided consistent with the nature of the problem(s) and the patient's and/or family's needs.

169

 Separate Procedure

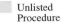 Unlisted Procedure

 CCI Comp. Code

 Non-specific Procedure

Usually, the presenting problem(s) are of low severity. Physicians typically spend 40 minutes at the bedside and on the patient's hospital floor or unit.

99253   Initial inpatient consultation for a new or established patient, which requires these three key components:

- a detailed history;

- a detailed examination; and

- medical decision making of low complexity.

Counseling and/or coordination of care with other providers or agencies are provided consistent with the nature of the problem(s) and the patient's and/or family's needs.

Usually, the presenting problem(s) are of moderate severity. Physicians typically spend 55 minutes at the bedside and on the patient's hospital floor or unit.

99254   Initial inpatient consultation for a new or established patient, which requires three key components:

- a comprehensive history;

- a comprehensive examination; and

- medical decision making of moderate complexity.

Counseling and/or coordination of care with other providers or agencies are provided consistent with the nature of the problem(s) and the patient's and/or family's needs.

Usually, the presenting problem(s) are of moderate to high severity. Physicians typically spend 80 minutes at the bedside and on the patient's hospital floor or unit.

99255   Initial inpatient consultation for a new or established patient, which requires these three key components:

- a comprehensive history;

- a comprehensive examination; and

- medical decision making of high complexity.

Counseling and/or coordination of care with other providers or agencies are provided consistent with the nature of the problem(s) and the patient's and/or family's needs.

Usually, the presenting problem(s) are of moderate to high severity. Physicians typically spend 110 minutes at the bedside and on the patient's hospital floor or unit.

● New Code   ▲ Revised Code   + Add-On Code   ⊘ Modifier -51 Exempt

FOLLOW-UP INPATIENT CONSULTATIONS

ESTABLISHED PATIENT

Follow-up consultations are visits to complete the initial consultation or subsequent consultative visits requested by the attending physician. A follow-up consultation includes monitoring progress, recommending management modifications or advising on a new plan of care in response to changes in the patient's status.

If the physician consultant has initiated treatment at the initial consultation, and participates thereafter in the patient's management, the codes for subsequent hospital care should be used (99231-99233).

99261 Follow-up inpatient consultation for an established patient, which requires at least two of these three key components:

- a problem focused interval history;

- a problem focused examination;

- medical decision making that is straightforward or of low complexity.

Counseling and/or coordination of care with other providers or agencies are provided consistent with nature of the problem(s) and the patient's and/or family's needs.

Usually, the patient is stable, recovering or improving. Physicians typically 10 minutes at the bedside and on the patient's hospital floor or unit.

99262 Follow-up inpatient consultation for an established patient which requires at least two of these three key components:

- an expanded problem focused interval history;

- an expanded problem focused examination;

- medical decision making of moderate complexity.

Counseling and/or coordination of care with other providers or agencies are provided consistent with the nature of the problem(s) and the patient's and/or family's needs.

Usually, the patient is responding inadequately to therapy or has developed a minor complication. Physicians typically spend 20 minutes at the bedside and on the patient's hospital floor or unit.

99263 Follow-up inpatient consultation for an established patient which requires at least two of these three key components:

- a detailed interval history;

Separate Procedure	Unlisted Procedure	CCI Comp. Code	Non-specific Procedure

- a detailed examination;

- medical decision making of high complexity.

Counseling and/or coordination of care with other providers or agencies are provided consistent with the nature of the problem(s) and the patient's and/or family's needs.

Usually, the patient is unstable or has developed a significant complication or a significant new problem. Physicians typically spend 30 minutes at the bedside and on the patient's hospital floor or unit.

CONFIRMATORY CONSULTATIONS

NEW OR ESTABLISHED PATIENT

Confirmatory consultation codes are used when the consultation is requested by the patient, or other agency. Typically the consultation will involve a second or third opinion on the necessity or appropriateness of a medical treatment or surgical procedure recommended by another physician.

Note that there are special modifiers in the CPT coding system which are used to modify these codes. Use the following guidelines when adding modifiers to mandated consultations.

- *If the second opinion is mandated by a professional review organization, use CPT modifier -32 if the patient IS NOT a Medicare patient and HCPCS Level II modifier -SF if the patient IS a Medicare patient.*

- *Many Medicare intermediaries have assigned HCPCS Level III modifiers for second opinions requested by the patient. Check with the local Medicare intermediary before reporting these services.*

99271 Confirmatory consultation for a new or established patient, which requires these three key components:

- a problem focused history;

- a problem focused examination; and

- straightforward medical decision making.

Counseling and/or coordination of care with other providers or agencies are provided consistent with the nature of the problem(s) and the patient's and/or family's needs.

Usually, the presenting problem(s) are self limited or minor.

99272 Confirmatory consultation for a new or established patient, which requires these three key components:

- an expanded problem focused history;

172

- New
Code

▲ Revised
Code

+ Add-On
Code

⊘ Modifier -51
Exempt

- an expanded problem focused examination; and
- straightforward medical decision making.

Counseling and/or coordination of care with other providers or agencies are provided consistent with the nature of the problem(s) and the patient's and/or family's needs.

Usually, the presenting problem(s) are of low severity.

99273 Confirmatory consultation for a new or established patient, which requires these three key components:

- a detailed history;
- a detailed examination; and
- medical decision making of low complexity.

Counseling and/or coordination of care with other providers or agencies are provided consistent with the nature of the problem(s) and the patient's and/or family's needs.

Usually, the presenting problem(s) are of moderate severity.

99274 Confirmatory consultation for a new or established patient, which requires these three key components:

- a comprehensive history;
- a comprehensive examination; and
- medical decision making of moderate complexity.

Counseling and/or coordination of care with other providers or agencies are provided consistent with the nature of the problem(s) and the patient's and/or family's needs.

Usually, the presenting problem(s) are of moderate to high severity.

99275 Confirmatory consultation for a new or established patient, which requires these three key components:

- a comprehensive history;
- a comprehensive examination; and
- medical decision making of high complexity.

Counseling and/or coordination of care with other providers or agencies are provided consistent with the nature of the problem(s) and the patient's and/or family's needs.

Usually, the presenting problem(s) are of moderate to high severity.

173

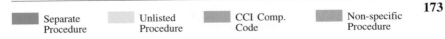

| Separate Procedure | Unlisted Procedure | CCI Comp. Code | Non-specific Procedure |

EMERGENCY DEPARTMENT SERVICES

Evaluation and management codes 99281-99288 are used to report services provided to new or established patients in the emergency department. The emergency department is defined as a facility for the treatment of patients with emergent conditions. The emergency department must be attached to a hospital and operate on a 24/7 basis.

The key coding issues for evaluation and management emergency services are the extent of history obtained, the extent of examination performed, and the complexity of medical decision making. Additional reporting issues include counseling and/or coordination of care, and the nature of presenting problem(s).

Time is not a descriptive component for evaluation and management services provided in the emergency department. These services are typically provided on a variable intensity basis, often involving multiple encounters with several patients over an extended period of time. Therefore, it is difficult for physicians to provide accurate estimates of the time spent face-to-face with the patient in the emergency department.

CODING RULES

1. No distinction is made between new and established patients in the emergency department.

2. If the emergency department is used for observation or inpatient care services, report using codes from the Observation Care services subsection of the CPT coding system.

3. For critical care services provided in the emergency department, use the appropriate codes from the Critical Care subsection of the CPT coding system.

EMERGENCY DEPARTMENT SERVICES

NEW OR ESTABLISHED PATIENT

99281 Emergency department visit for the evaluation and management of a patient, which requires these three key components:

- a problem focused history;
- a problem focused examination; and
- straightforward medical decision making.

Counseling and/or coordination of care with other providers or agencies are provided consistent with the nature of the problem(s) and the patient's and/or family's needs.

Usually, the presenting problem(s) are self limited or minor.

| ● New Code | ▲ Revised Code | + Add-On Code | ⊘ Modifier -51 Exempt |

99282 Emergency department visit for the evaluation and management of a patient, which requires these three key components:

- an expanded problem focused history;

- an expanded problem focused examination; and

- medical decision making of low complexity.

Counseling and/or coordination of care with other providers or agencies are provided consistent with the nature of the problem(s) and the patient's and/or family's needs.

Usually, the presenting problem(s) are of low to moderate severity.

99283 Emergency department visit for the evaluation and management of a patient, which requires these three key components:

- an expanded problem focused history;

- an expanded problem focused examination; and

- medical decision making of moderate complexity.

Counseling and/or coordination of care with other providers or agencies are provided consistent with the nature of the problem(s) and the patient's and/or family's needs.

Usually, the presenting problem(s) are of moderate severity.

99284 Emergency department visit for the evaluation and management of a patient, which requires these three key components:

- a detailed history;

- a detailed examination; and

- medical decision making of moderate complexity.

Counseling and/or coordination of care with other providers or agencies are provided consistent with the nature of the problem(s) and the patient's and/or family's needs.

Usually, the presenting problem(s) are of high severity, and require urgent evaluation by the physician but do not pose an immediate significant threat to life or physiologic function.

99285 Emergency department visit for the evaluation and management of a patient, which requires these three key components within the constraints imposed by the urgency of the patient's clinical condition and/or mental status:

- a comprehensive history;

- a comprehensive examination; and

175

 Separate Procedure   Unlisted Procedure   CCI Comp. Code   Non-specific Procedure

- medical decision making of high complexity.

Counseling and/or coordination of care with other providers or agencies are provided consistent with the nature of the problem(s) and the patient's and/or family's needs.

Usually, the presenting problem(s) are of high severity and pose an immediate significant threat to life or physiologic function.

OTHER EMERGENCY SERVICES

99288 Physician direction of emergency medical systems (EMS) emergency care, advanced life support

PEDIATRIC CRITICAL CARE PATIENT TRANSPORT

The following codes 99289 and 99290 are used to report the physical attendance and direct fact-to-face care by a physician during the interfacility transport of a critically ill or critically injured pediatric patient.

99289 Critical care services delivered by a physician, face-to-face, during an interfacility transport of critically ill or critically injured pediatric patient, 24 months of age or less; first 30-74 minutes of hands on care during transport

+ 99290   each additional 30 minutes (List separately in addition to code for primary service)

(Use 99290 in conjunction with 99289)

(Critical care of less than 30 minutes total duration should be reported with the appropriate E/M code)

CRITICAL CARE SERVICES

Critical care includes the care of critically ill patients in a variety of medical emergencies that requires the constant attention of the physician. Cardiac arrest, shock, bleeding, respiratory failure, postoperative complications, or a critically ill neonate are examples of medical emergencies defined in CPT. Critical care is usually, but not always, given in a critical area, such as the coronary care unit, intensive care unit, respiratory care unit, or the emergency care facility.

CPT codes listed in this section are intended to include cardiopulmonary resuscitation (CPR) and the variety of services commonly employed with this procedure as well as other acute emergency situations. Other services, such as catheter placement, cardiac output measurement, dialysis management, control of

176 ● New Code ▲ Revised Code ＋ Add-On Code ⊘ Modifier -51 Exempt

gastrointestinal hemorrhage, cardioversion, etc. are considered to be included when reporting critical care services under these time-based CPT codes.

Evaluation and management codes 99291-99292 are used to report services for specific conditions (usually) provided in a critical care area. Key coding issues include the condition of the patient (supported by diagnostic coding), the service(s) provided, and the amount of time spent. Follow-up critical care services may be reported using either evaluation and management codes from this section or hospital evaluation and management codes from the series 99231-99233.

CODING RULES

1. *The critical care CPT codes are used to report the total duration of time spent by a physician providing constant attention to a critically ill patient.*

2. *Critical care code 99291 is used to report the first hour of critical care on a given day. It may be reported only once per day even if the time spent is not continuous on that day.*

3. *Critical care 99292 is used to report each additional 30 minutes beyond the first hour.*

4. *Other procedures which are not considered included in the critical care services, for example, suturing of lacerations, setting of fractures, reduction of joint dislocations, lumbar puncture, peritoneal lavage and bladder tap, are reported separately.*

CORRECT CODING CHART FOR CRITICAL CARE SERVICES

DURATION OF CRITICAL CARE	CODE(S) TO REPORT
less than 30 minutes	appropriate E/M codes
30- 74 minutes	99291 once
75-104 minutes	99291 once and 99292 once
105-134 minutes	99291 once and 99292 twice
135-164 minutes	99291 once and 99292 three times
165-194 minutes	99291 once and 99292 four times
194 minutes or longer	99291 and 99292 as appropriate (see illustrated reporting examples above)

CRITICAL CARE SERVICES

99291   Critical care, evaluation and management of the critically ill or critically injured patient; first 30-74 minutes

---

Separate Procedure	Unlisted Procedure	CCI Comp. Code	Non-specific Procedure

177

+ 99292   each additional 30 minutes (List separately in addition to code for primary service)

(Use 99292 in conjunction with 99291)

INPATIENT NEONATAL AND PEDIATRIC CRITICAL CARE SERVICES

Neonatal intensive care refers to services, including management, monitoring and treatment, provided to a critically ill newborn or infant, usually in the neonatal intensive care unit (NICU). Counseling of parents, case management services and personal direct supervision of the NICU team are bundled into these codes.

CODING RULES

1. *Neonatal intensive care services start with the date of admission and are coded only once per day, per patient.*

2. *Once the neonate is no longer considered to be critically ill, report with CPT codes for subsequent hospital care instead of neonatal intensive care.*

3. *Neonatal intensive care CPT codes are coded in addition to physician stand-by code 99360 or newborn resuscitation code 99440 when the physician is present for the delivery and newborn resuscitation is required.*

4. *Procedures which are routinely performed as part of NICU care are included in the bundled NICU codes. These routine procedures include: venous/arterial catheterization, bladder catheterization, intubation, lumbar puncture, mechanical ventilation/CPAP, IV and/or blood transfusions, and monitoring.*

INPATIENT PEDIATRIC CRITICAL CARE

▲ **99293**   Initial inpatient pediatric critical care, 31 days up through 24 months of age, per day, for the evaluation and management of a critically ill infant or young child.

▲ **99294**   Subsequent inpatient pediatric critical care, 31 days up through 24 months of age, per day, for the evaluation and management of a critically ill infant or young child.

INPATIENT NEONATAL CRITICAL CARE

▲ **99295**   Initial inpatient neonatal critical care, per day, for the evaluation and management of a critically ill neonate 30 days of age or less.

● New Code   ▲ Revised Code   + Add-On Code   ⊘ Modifier -51 Exempt

This code is reserved for the date of admission for neonates who are critically ill. Critically ill neonates require cardiac and/or respiratory support (including ventilator or nasal CPAP when indicated), continuous or frequent vital sign monitoring, laboratory and blood gas interpretations, follow-up physician reevaluations, and constant observation by the health care team under direct physician supervision. Immediate preoperative evaluation and stabilization of neonates with life threatening surgical or cardiac conditions are included under this code. Neonates with life threatening surgical or cardiac conditions are included under this code.

Care for neonates who require an intensive care setting but who are not critically ill is reported using the initial hospital care codes (99221-99223).

▲ **99296** Subsequent inpatient neonatal critical care, per day, for the evaluation and management of a critically ill neonate 30 days of age or less.

A critically ill and unstable neonate will require cardiac and/or respiratory support (including ventilator or nasal CPAP when indicated), continuous or frequent vital sign monitoring, laboratory and blood gas interpretations, follow-up physician re-evaluations throughout a 24-hour period, and constant observation by the health care team under direct physician supervision. In addition, most will require frequent ventilator changes, intravenous fluid alterations, and/or early initiation of parenteral nutrition. Neonates in the immediate post-operative period or those who become critically ill and unstable during the hospital stay will commonly qualify for this level of care.

(99297   deleted 2003 edition. To report, use 99296)

INTENSIVE (NON-CRITICAL) LOW BIRTH WEIGHT SERVICES

99298 Subsequent intensive care, per day, for the evaluation and management of the recovering very low birth weight infant (present body weight less than 1500 grams).

Infants with present body weight less than 1500 grams who are no longer critically ill continue to require intensive cardiac and respiratory monitoring, continuous and/or frequent vital sign monitoring, heat maintenance, enteral and/or parenteral nutritional adjustments, laboratory and oxygen monitoring and constant observation by the health care team under direct physician supervision.

179

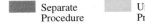 Separate Procedure   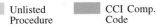 Unlisted Procedure   CCI Comp. Code   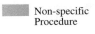 Non-specific Procedure

99299 Subsequent intensive care, per day, for the evaluation and management of the recovering low birth weight infant (present body weight of 1500-2500 grams).

Infants with present body weight of 1500-2500 grams who are no longer critically ill continue to require intensive cardiac and respiratory monitoring, continuous and/or frequent vital sign monitoring, heat maintenance, enteral and/or parenteral nutritional adjustments, laboratory and oxygen monitoring, and constant observation by the health care team under direct physician supervision.

NURSING FACILITY SERVICES

A patient may be transferred from an inpatient hospital to a nursing facility for supervised care when the patient no longer requires the skill levels of the inpatient hospital. Evaluation and management service codes 99301-99313 are used to report services provided in nursing facilities. The key coding issues are the extent of history obtained, the extent of examination performed, and the complexity of medical decision making. Additional reporting issues include counseling and/or coordination of care, the nature of presenting problem(s), and the time spent at the bedside and on the patient's facility floor or unit.

These CPT codes are also used to report evaluation and management services provided to a patient in a psychiatric residential treatment center. If procedures such as medical psychotherapy are provided in addition to evaluation and management services, these are coded in addition to the evaluation and management services.

CPT codes in this section apply to Comprehensive Nursing Facility Assessments and Subsequent Nursing Facility care. Both subcategories apply to new and established patients. Comprehensive Assessments may be performed at one or more sites during the assessment process; including the hospital, the office, a nursing facility, a domiciliary facility and/or the patient's home.

CODING RULES

1. *If a patient is admitted to the nursing facility after receiving services in the physician's office or hospital emergency department, all evaluation and management services are considered inclusive in the initial nursing facility care.*

2. *With the exception of hospital discharge services, evaluation and management service on the same date provided in locations other than the nursing facility that are related to the admission should not be coded separately.*

● New Code ▲ Revised Code + Add-On Code ⊘ Modifier -51 Exempt

3.   *When reporting these CPT codes to Medicare include the HCPCS Level II modifier -SP or -MP, or HCPCS Level III modifier if specified by the local Medicare carrier.*

COMPREHENSIVE NURSING FACILITY ASSESSMENTS

NEW OR ESTABLISHED PATIENT

99301   Evaluation and management of a new or established patient involving an annual nursing facility assessment which requires these three key components:

- a detailed interval history;

- a comprehensive examination; and

- medical decision making that is straightforward or of low complexity.

Counseling and/or coordination of care with other providers or agencies are provided consistent with the nature of the problem(s) and the patient's and/or family's needs.

Usually, the patient is stable, recovering or improving. The review and affirmation of the medical plan of care is required. Physicians typically spend 30 minutes at the bedside and on the patient's facility floor or unit.

99302   Evaluation and management of a new or established patient involving a nursing facility assessment which requires these three key components:

- a detailed interval history;

- a comprehensive examination; and

- medical decision making of moderate to high complexity.

Counseling and/or coordination of care with other providers or agencies are provided consistent with the nature of the problem(s) and the patient's and/or family's needs.

Usually, the patient has developed a significant complication or a significant new problem and has had a major permanent change in status.

The creation of a new medical plan of care is required. Physicians typically spend 40 minutes at the bedside and on the patient's facility floor or unit.

Separate Procedure   Unlisted Procedure   CCI Comp. Code   Non-specific Procedure

99303 Evaluation and management of a new or established patient involving a nursing facility assessment at the time of initial admission or readmission to the facility, which requires these three key components:

- a comprehensive history;

- a comprehensive examination; and

- medical decision making of moderate to high complexity.

Counseling and/or coordination of care with other providers or agencies are provided consistent with the nature of the problem(s) and the patient's and/or family's needs.

The creation of a medical plan of care is required. Physicians typically spend 50 minutes at the bedside and on the patient's facility floor or unit.

SUBSEQUENT NURSING FACILITY CARE

NEW OR ESTABLISHED PATIENT

99311 Subsequent nursing facility care, per day, for the evaluation and management of a new or established patient, which requires at least two of these three key components:

- a problem focused interval history;

- a problem focused examination;

- medical decision making that is straightforward or of low complexity.

Counseling and/or coordination of care with other providers or agencies are provided consistent with the nature of the problem(s) and the patient's and/or family's needs.

Usually, the patient is stable, recovering or improving. Physicians typically spend 15 minutes at the bedside and on the patient's facility floor or unit.

99312 Subsequent nursing facility care, per day, for the evaluation and management of a new or established patient, which requires at least two of these three key components:

- an expanded problem focused interval history;

- an expanded problem focused examination;

- medical decision making of moderate complexity.

Counseling and/or coordination of care with other providers or agencies are provided consistent with the nature of the problem(s) and the patient's and/or family's needs.

●	New Code	▲	Revised Code	+	Add-On Code	⊘	Modifier -51 Exempt

Usually, the patient is responding inadequately to therapy or has developed a minor complication. Physicians typically spend 25 minutes at the bedside and on the patient's facility floor or unit.

99313 Subsequent nursing facility care, per day, for the evaluation and management of a new or established patient, which requires at least two of these three key components:

- a detailed interval history;
- a detailed examination;
- medical decision making of moderate to high complexity.

Counseling and/or coordination of care with other providers or agencies are provided consistent with the nature of the problem(s) and the patient's and/or family's needs.

Usually, the patient has developed a significant complication or a significant new problem. Physicians typically spend 35 minutes at the bedside and on the patient's facility floor or unit.

NURSING FACILITY DISCHARGE SERVICES

99315 Nursing facility discharge day management; 30 minutes or less

99316 more than 30 minutes

DOMICILIARY, REST HOME (eg, BOARDING HOME), OR CUSTODIAL CARE SERVICES

Evaluation and management service codes 99321-99333 are used to report services provided to new and established patients in domiciliary, rest home or custodial care facilities. The key coding issues are the extent of history obtained, the extent of examination performed, and the complexity of medical decision making. Additional reporting issues include counseling and/or coordination of care, the nature of presenting problem(s).

When reporting these CPT codes to Medicare include HCPCS modifier -SP or -MP to indicate single or multiple patients seen during the visit. Consult the local Medicare intermediary before using these modifiers.

NEW PATIENT

99321 Domiciliary or rest home visit for the evaluation and management of a new patient which requires these three key components:

- a problem focused history;

183

	Separate Procedure		Unlisted Procedure		CCI Comp. Code		Non-specific Procedure

- a problem focused examination; and

- medical decision making that is straightforward or of low complexity.

Counseling and/or coordination of care with other providers or agencies are provided consistent with the nature of the problem(s) and the patient's and/or family's needs.

Usually, the presenting problem(s) are of low severity.

99322 Domiciliary or rest home visit for the evaluation and management of a new patient, which requires these three key components:

- an expanded problem focused history;

- an expanded problem focused examination; and

- medical decision making of moderate complexity.

Counseling and/or coordination of care with other providers or agencies are provided consistent with the nature of the problem(s) and the patient's and/or family's needs.

Usually, the presenting problem(s) are of moderate severity.

99323 Domiciliary or rest home visit for the evaluation and management of a new patient, which requires these three key components:

- a detailed history;

- a detailed examination; and

- medical decision making of high complexity.

Counseling and/or coordination of care with other providers or agencies are provided consistent with the nature of the problem(s) and the patient's and/or family's needs.

Usually, the presenting problem(s) are of high complexity.

ESTABLISHED PATIENT

99331 Domiciliary or rest home visit for the evaluation and management of an established patient, which requires at least two of these three key components:

- a problem focused interval history;

- a problem focused examination;

- medical decision making that is straightforward or of low complexity.

● New Code   ▲ Revised Code   + Add-On Code   ⊘ Modifier -51 Exempt

Counseling and/or coordination of care with other providers or agencies are provided consistent with the nature of the problem(s) and the patient's and/or family's needs.

Usually, the patient is stable, recovering or improving.

99332 Domiciliary or rest home visit for the evaluation and management of an established patient, which requires at least two of these three key components:

- an expanded problem focused interval history;
- an expanded problem focused examination;
- medical decision making of moderate complexity.

Counseling and/or coordination of care with other providers or agencies are provided consistent with the nature of the problem(s) and the patient's and/or family's needs.

Usually, the patient is responding inadequately to therapy or has developed a minor complication.

99333 Domiciliary or rest home visit for the evaluation and management of an established patient, which requires at least two of these three key components:

- a detailed interval history;
- a detailed examination;
- medical decision making of high complexity.

Counseling and/or coordination of care with other providers or agencies are provided consistent with the nature of the problem(s) and the patient's and/or family's needs.

Usually, the patient is unstable or has developed a significant complication or a significant new problem.

HOME SERVICES

Evaluation and management codes 99341-99350 are used to report services provided to new and established patients in the patient's home. The key coding issues are the extent of history obtained, the extent of examination performed, and the complexity of medical decision making. Additional reporting issues include counseling and/or coordination of care, and the nature of presenting problem(s).

| Separate Procedure | Unlisted Procedure | CCI Comp. Code | Non-specific Procedure |

NEW PATIENT

99341 Home visit for the evaluation and management of a new patient, which requires these three key components:

- a problem focused history;
- a problem focused examination; and
- straightforward medical decision making.

Counseling and/or coordination of care with other providers or agencies are provided consistent with the nature of the problem(s) and the patient's and/or family's needs.

Usually, the presenting problem(s) are of low severity. Physicians typically spend 20 minutes face-to-face with the patient and/or family.

99342 Home visit for the evaluation and management of a new patient, which requires these three key components:

- an expanded problem focused history;
- an expanded problem focused examination; and
- medical decision making of low complexity.

Counseling and/or coordination of care with other providers or agencies are provided consistent with the nature of the problem(s) and the patient's and/or family's needs.

Usually, the presenting problem(s) are of moderate severity. Physicians typically spend 30 minutes face-to-face with the patient and/or family.

99343 Home visit for the evaluation and management of a new patient, which requires these three key components:

- a detailed history;
- a detailed examination; and
- medical decision making of moderate complexity.

Counseling and/or coordination of care with other providers or agencies are provided consistent with the nature of the problem(s) and the patient's and/or family's needs.

Usually, the presenting problem(s) are of moderate to high severity. Physicians typically spend 45 minutes face-to-face with the patient and/or family.

99344 Home visit for the evaluation and management of a new patient, which requires these three components:

- a comprehensive history;

- a comprehensive examination; and

- medical decision making of moderate complexity.

Counseling and/or coordination of care with other providers or agencies are provided consistent with the nature of the problem(s) and the patient's and/or family's needs.

Usually, the presenting problem(s) are of high severity. Physicians typically spend 60 minutes face-to-face with the patient and/or family.

99345 Home visit for the evaluation and management of a new patient, which requires these three key components:

- a comprehensive history;

- a comprehensive examination; and

- medical decision making of high complexity.

Counseling and/or coordination of care with other providers or agencies are provided consistent with the nature of the problem(s) and the patient's and/or family's needs.

Usually, the patient is unstable or has developed a significant new problem requiring immediate physician attention. Physicians typically spend 75 minutes face-to-face with the patient and/or family.

ESTABLISHED PATIENT

99347 Home visit for the evaluation and management of an established patient, which requires at least two of these three key components:

- a problem focused interval history;

- a problem focused examination;

- straightforward medical decision making.

Counseling and/or coordination of care with other providers or agencies are provided consistent with the nature of the problem(s) and the patient's and/or family's needs.

Usually, the presenting problem(s) are self-limited or minor. Physicians typically spend 15 minutes face-to-face with the patient and/or family.

187

| | Separate Procedure | | Unlisted Procedure | | CCI Comp. Code | | Non-specific Procedure |

99348 Home visit for the evaluation and management of an established patient, which requires at least two of these three key components:

- an expanded problem focused interval history;
- an expanded problem focused examination;
- medical decision making of low complexity.

Counseling and/or coordination of care with other providers or agencies are provided consistent with the nature of the problem(s) and the patient's and/or family's needs.

Usually, the presenting problem(s) are of low to moderate severity. Physicians typically spend 25 minutes face-to-face with the patient and/or family.

99349 Home visit for the evaluation and management of an established patient, which requires at least two of these three key components:

- a detailed interval history;
- a detailed examination;
- medical decision making of moderate complexity.

Counseling and/or coordination of care with other providers or agencies are provided consistent with the nature of the problem(s) and the patient's and/or family's needs.

Usually, the presenting problem(s) are moderate to high severity. Physicians typically spend 40 minutes face-to-face with the patient and/or family.

99350 Home visit for the evaluation and management of an established patient, which requires at least two of these three key components:

- a comprehensive interval history;
- a comprehensive examination;
- medical decision making of moderate to high complexity.

Counseling and/or coordination of care with other providers or agencies are provided consistent with the nature of the problem(s) and the patient's and/or family's needs.

Usually, the presenting problem(s) are of moderate to high severity. The patient may be unstable or may have developed a significant new problem requiring immediate physician attention. Physicians typically spend 60 minutes face-to-face with the patient and/or family.

● New Code   ▲ Revised Code   **+** Add-On Code   ⃠ Modifier -51 Exempt

PROLONGED SERVICES

Evaluation and management service CPT codes -99360 are used to report inpatient or outpatient services which include prolonged service or physician standby service that is beyond the usual service. The key coding issues are the location of the service, whether the service is direct (face-to-face) or not direct, and the total duration of the prolonged service.

CODING RULES

1. *Prolonged services are reported in addition to other physician services.*

2. *Prolonged services involving direct (face-to-face) time are reported as cumulative time on a given date, even if the time is not continuous.*

3. *If the total duration of prolonged services is less than 30 minutes, the prolonged service is not reported.*

CORRECT CODING CHART FOR PROLONGED SERVICES

DURATION OF PROLONGED SERVICE	CODE(S) TO REPORT
less than 30 minutes	not reported separately
30- 74 minutes	99354 once
75-104 minutes	99354 once and 99355 once
105-134 minutes	99354 once and 99355 twice
135-164 minutes	99354 once and 99355 three times
165-194 minutes	99354 once and 99355 four times

PROLONGED PHYSICIAN SERVICE WITH DIRECT (FACE-TO-FACE) PATIENT CONTACT

+ **99354** Prolonged physician service in the office or other outpatient setting requiring direct (face-to-face) patient contact beyond the usual service (eg, prolonged care and treatment of an acute asthmatic patient in an outpatient setting); first hour (List separately in addition to code for office or other outpatient Evaluation and Management service)

(Use in conjunction with codes 99201-99215, 99241-99245, 99301-99350)

+ **99355** each additional 30 minutes (List separately in addition to code for prolonged physician service)

(Use 99355 in conjunction with codes)

189

	Separate Procedure		Unlisted Procedure		CCI Comp. Code		Non-specific Procedure

+ 99356 Prolonged physician service in the inpatient setting, requiring direct (face-to-face) patient contact beyond the usual service (eg, maternal fetal monitoring for high risk delivery or other physiological monitoring, prolonged care of an acutely ill inpatient); first hour (List separately in addition to code for inpatient Evaluation and Management service)

(Use 99356 in conjunction with codes 99221-99233, 99251-99255, 99261-99263)

+ 99357 each additional 30 minutes (List separately in addition to code for prolonged physician service)

(Use 99357 in conjunction with code 99356)

PROLONGED PHYSICIAN SERVICE WITHOUT DIRECT (FACE-TO-FACE) PATIENT CONTACT

+ 99358 Prolonged evaluation and management service before and/or after direct (face-to-face) patient care (eg, review of extensive records and tests, communication with other professionals and/or the patient/family); first hour (List separately in addition to code(s) for other physician service(s) and/or inpatient or outpatient Evaluation and Management service)

+ 99359 each additional 30 minutes (List separately in addition to code for prolonged physician service)

(Use 99359 in conjunction with code 99358)

(To report telephone calls, see 99371-99373)

PHYSICIAN STANDBY SERVICE

99360 Physician standby service, requiring prolonged physician attendance, each 30 minutes (eg, operative standby, standby for frozen section, for cesarean/high risk delivery, for monitoring EEG)

(For hospital mandated on call services, see 99026, 99027)

(99360 may be reported in addition to 99431, 99440 as appropriate)

(99360 may not be reported in addition to 99436)

190

| ● New Code | ▲ Revised Code | + Add-On Code | ⃠ Modifier -51 Exempt |

CASE MANAGEMENT SERVICES

Case management is a process wherein a physician is responsible for direct care of the patient and has the additional responsibility of coordinating all other services provided to the patient. Case management services may be provided during medical conferences, or by telephone. The key coding issues are the type of service, the amount of time spent, and the level of service provided.

TEAM CONFERENCES

99361   Medical conference by a physician with interdisciplinary team of health professionals or representatives of community agencies to coordinate activities of patient care (patient not present); approximately 30 minutes

99362   approximately 60 minutes

TELEPHONE CALLS

99371   Telephone call by a physician to patient or for consultation or medical management or for coordinating medical management with other health care professionals (eg, nurses, therapists, social workers, nutritionists, physicians, pharmacists); simple or brief (eg, to report on tests and/or laboratory results, to clarify or alter previous instructions, to integrate new information from other health professionals into the medical treatment plan, or to adjust therapy)

99372   intermediate (eg, to provide advice to an established patient on a new problem, to initiate therapy that can be handled by telephone, to discuss test results in detail, to coordinate medical management of a new problem in an established patient, to discuss and evaluate new information and details, or to initiate new plan of care)

99373   complex or lengthy (eg, lengthy counseling session with anxious or distraught patient, detailed or prolonged discussion with family members regarding seriously ill patient, lengthy communication necessary to coordinate complex services of several different health professionals working on different aspects of the total patient care plan)

191

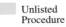 Separate Procedure   Unlisted Procedure   CCI Comp. Code   Non-specific Procedure

CARE PLAN OVERSIGHT SERVICES

Care plans prepared and/or reviewed by a physician are frequently required for patients under the care of home health agencies, hospices, or residing in nursing facilities. Evaluation and management service codes 99374-99380 are used to report care plan oversight services. The key coding issues are the location of service, the complexity of the plan, and the amount of physician time provided within a 30-day period.

CODING RULES

1. *Evaluation and management services are not inclusive of care plan oversight services. Care plan oversight is coded separately.*

2. *Care plan oversight services may be coded only by a single physician for each patient during a specific period of time.*

99374 Physician supervision of a patient under care of home health agency (patient not present) in home, domiciliary or equivalent environment (eg, Alzheimer's facility) requiring complex and multidisciplinary care modalities involving regular physician development and/or revision of care plans, review of subsequent reports of patient status, review of related laboratory and other studies, communication (including telephone calls) for purposes of assessment or care decisions with health care professional(s), family member(s), surrogate decision maker(s) (eg., legal guardian) and/or key caregiver(s) involved in patient's care, integration of new information into the medical treatment plan and/or adjustment of medical therapy, within a calendar month; 15-29 minutes

99375 30 minutes or more

99377 Physician supervision of a hospice patient (patient not present) requiring complex and multidisciplinary care modalities involving regular physician development and/or revision of care plans, review of subsequent reports of patient status, review of related laboratory and other studies, communication (including telephone calls) for purposes of assessment or care decisions with health care professional(s), family member(s), surrogate decision maker(s) (eg, legal guardian) and/or key caregiver(s) involved in patient's care, integration of new information into the medical treatment plan and/or adjustment of medical therapy, within a calendar month; 15-29 minutes

99378 30 minutes or more

● New Code ▲ Revised Code + Add-On Code ⃠ Modifier -51 Exempt

99379   Physician supervision of a nursing facility patient (patient not present) requiring complex and multidisciplinary care modalities involving regular physician development and/or revision of care plans, review of subsequent reports of patient status, review of related laboratory and other studies, communication (including telephone calls) for purposes of assessment or care decisions with health care professional(s), family member(s), surrogate decision maker(s) (eg, legal guardian) and/or key caregiver(s) involved in patient's care, integration of new information into the medical treatment plan and/or adjustment of medical therapy, within a calendar month; 15-29 minutes

99380   30 minutes or more

PREVENTIVE MEDICINE SERVICES

Preventive medicine services codes are used to report routine evaluation and management of adults and children in the absence of patient complaints or counseling and/or risk factor reduction intervention services to healthy individuals. The key coding issues are whether the patient is a new patient or established patient, the age of the patient, the circumstances of the examination, and the nature of any abnormalities encountered, and for counseling services, whether the service was provided to an individual or to a group and the amount of time spent counseling.

CODING RULES

1.   *The selection of Preventive Medicine codes is mostly dependent upon the age of the patient.*

2.   *Preventive medicine codes are coded only in the absence of illness. If illness, injury is discovered during provision of a preventive medicine service, office/outpatient evaluation and management codes are coded.*

3.   *Immunizations and diagnostic studies involving laboratory or radiology, or other procedures are not included in the preventive medicine service and should be coded separately.*

NEW PATIENT

99381   Initial comprehensive preventive medicine evaluation and management of an individual including an age and gender appropriate history, examination, counseling/anticipatory guidance/risk factor reduction interventions, and the ordering of appropriate immunization(s), laboratory/diagnostic procedures, new patient; infant (age under 1 year)

193

 Separate Procedure   Unlisted Procedure   CCI Comp. Code   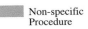 Non-specific Procedure

99382   early childhood (age 1 through 4 years)

99383   late childhood (age 5 through 11 years)

99384   adolescent (age 12 through 17 years)

99385   18-39 years

99386   40-64 years

99387   65 years and over

ESTABLISHED PATIENT

99391   Periodic comprehensive preventive medicine reevaluation and management of an individual including an age and gender appropriate history, examination, counseling/anticipatory guidance/risk factor reduction interventions, and the ordering of appropriate immunization(s), laboratory/diagnostic procedures, established patient; infant (age under 1 year)

99392   early childhood (age 1 through 4 years)

99393   late childhood (age 5 through 11 years)

99394   adolescent (age 12 through 17 years)

99395   18-39 years

99396   40-64 years

99397   65 years and over

COUNSELING AND/OR RISK FACTOR REDUCTION INTERVENTION

NEW OR ESTABLISHED PATIENT

Preventive Medicine, Individual Counseling

99401   Preventive medicine counseling and/or risk factor reduction intervention(s) provided to an individual (separate procedure); approximately 15 minutes

99402   approximately 30 minutes

● New Code   ▲ Revised Code   ✛ Add-On Code   ⊘ Modifier -51 Exempt

99403   approximately 45 minutes

99404   approximately 60 minutes

Preventive Medicine, Group Counseling

99411   Preventive medicine counseling and/or risk factor reduction intervention(s) provided to individuals in a group setting (separate procedure); approximately 30 minutes

99412   approximately 60 minutes

Other Preventive Medicine Services

99420   Administration and interpretation of health risk assessment instrument (eg, health hazard appraisal)

99429   Unlisted preventive medicine service

NEWBORN CARE SERVICES

99431   History and examination of the normal newborn infant, initiation of diagnostic and treatment programs and preparation of hospital records. (This code should also be used for birthing room deliveries.)

99432   Normal newborn care in other than hospital or birthing room setting, including physical examination of baby and conference(s) with parent(s)

99433   Subsequent hospital care, for the evaluation and management of a normal newborn, per day

99435   History and examination of the normal newborn infant, including the preparation of medical records. (This code should only be used for newborns assessed and discharged from the hospital or birthing room on the same date.)

99436   Attendance at delivery (when requested by delivering physician) and initial stabilization of newborn

(99436 may be reported in addition to 99431)

(99436 may not be reported in addition to 99440)

195

	Separate Procedure		Unlisted Procedure		CCI Comp. Code		Non-specific Procedure

99440 Newborn resuscitation: provision of positive pressure ventilation and/or chest compressions in the presence of acute inadequate ventilation and/or cardiac output

SPECIAL EVALUATION AND MANAGEMENT SERVICES

BASIC LIFE AND/OR DISABILITY EVALUATION SERVICES

99450 Basic life and/or disability examination that includes:
- measurement of height, weight and blood pressure;
- completion of a medical history following a life insurance pro forma;
- collection of blood sample and/or urinalysis complying with "chain of custody" protocols; and
- completion of necessary documentation/certificates.

WORK RELATED OR MEDICAL DISABILITY EVALUATION SERVICES

99455 Work related or medical disability examination by the treating physician that includes:
- completion of a medical history commensurate with the patient's condition;
- performance of an examination commensurate with the patient's condition;
- formulation of a diagnosis, assessment of capabilities and stability, and calculation of impairment;
- development of future medical treatment plan; and
- completion of necessary documentation/certificates and report.

99456 Work related or medical disability examination by other than the treating physician that includes:
- completion of a medical history commensurate with the patient's condition;
- performance of an examination commensurate with the patient's condition;

● New Code ▲ Revised Code + Add-On Code ⊘ Modifier -51 Exempt

- formulation of a diagnosis, assessment of capabilities and stability, and calculation of impairment;

- development of future medical treatment plan; and

- completion of necessary documentation/certificates and report.

(Do not report 99455, 99456 with 99080 for the completion of Workman's Compensation forms)

OTHER EVALUATION AND MANAGEMENT SERVICES

99499   Unlisted evaluation and management service

Separate Procedure   Unlisted Procedure   CCI Comp. Code   Non-specific Procedure

This page intentionally left blank.

● New
Code

▲ Revised
Code

✚ Add-On
Code

⊘ Modifier -51
Exempt

ANESTHESIA

ANESTHESIA OVERVIEW

The second section of the CPT coding system is the anesthesia section, which includes service codes for the delivery of anesthesia. Within each subsection, the CPT codes are arranged by anatomical site.

The Anesthesiologist provides pain relief and maintenance, or restoration, of a stable condition during and immediately following an operation, an obstetric or diagnostic procedure. The Anesthesiologist assesses the risk of the patient undergoing surgery and optimizes the patient's condition prior to, during, and after surgery.

Reporting of anesthesia services is dependent on the third party payer involved. Anesthesia services covered by Medicare are coded using codes from the ANESTHESIA section of the CPT coding system. For most other third party payers, anesthesia services are coded using codes from the SURGERY section of the CPT coding system to describe the major surgical procedure.

Anesthesia services may be coded by anesthesiologists or anesthetists working under the supervision of the anesthesiologist. Anesthesia services include pre- and post-op visits, anesthesia delivery, giving fluids and/or blood needed during a procedure, and monitoring. Anesthesia delivery includes general, regional, supplementing local anesthesia, and other supportive services.

KEY POINTS ABOUT ANESTHESIA CODING

1. *Time recording for anesthesia services starts with patient preparation for anesthesia induction and ends when the anesthesiologist or anesthetist has completed his/her services and transfers responsibility for postoperative supervision.*

2. *Consultations and/or other evaluation and management services which are not included in the administration or supervising the administration of anesthesia, regardless of location provided, are reporting using CPT codes from the evaluation and management section of the CPT book.*

3. *Any supplies and/or materials provided by the anesthesiologist or anesthetist which are not considered to be included in the standard service may be coded separately.*

4. *Multiple procedures provided on the same date of service should be coded separately.*

199

 Separate Procedure   Unlisted Procedure   CCI Comp. Code   Non-specific Procedure

5. *Any service which may be considered rare, unusual, variable or not defined should be supported with a special report which clearly defines the need for the unusual service. These services are generally coded with an unlisted CPT code or by adding modifier -22 to the CPT code which defines the procedure.*

ANESTHESIA SERVICE MODIFIERS

A physical status modifier must be added to all CPT codes when reporting anesthesia services. The physical status modifier defines the physical condition of the patient and ranges from a normal health patient to a declared brain-dead patient whose organs are being harvested for a transplant.

PHYSICAL STATUS MODIFIERS

-P1   A normal healthy patient.

-P2   A patient with a mild systemic disease.

-P3   A patient with severe systemic disease.

-P4   A patient with severe systemic disease that is a constant threat to life.

-P5   A moribund patient who is not expected to survive without the operation.

-P6   A declared brain-dead patient whose organs are being removed for donor purposes.

OTHER ANESTHESIA SERVICE MODIFIERS

Under certain circumstances, medical services and procedures may need to be further modified. Other CPT coding system modifiers commonly used with ANESTHESIA services include:

-22   Unusual services

-23   Anesthesia

-32   Mandated services

-51   Multiple procedures

● New Code   ▲ Revised Code   + Add-On Code   ⊘ Modifier -51 Exempt

QUALIFYING CIRCUMSTANCES FOR ANESTHESIA

In the case of difficult and/or extraordinary circumstances such as extreme youth or age, extraordinary condition of the patient, and/or unusual risk factors it may be appropriate to report one or more of the following qualifying circumstances in addition to the anesthesia services.

+ **99100**   Anesthesia for patient of extreme age, under one year and over seventy

   (For procedure performed on infants less than 1 year of age at time of surgery, see 00833, 00834)

+ **99116**   Anesthesia complicated by utilization of total body hypothermia

+ **99135**   Anesthesia complicated by utilization of controlled hypotension

+ **99140**   Anesthesia complicated by emergency conditions (specify) (List separately in addition to code for primary anesthesia procedure)

   (An emergency is defined as existing when delay in treatment of the patient would lead to a significant increase in the threat to life or body part.)

201

 Separate Procedure   Unlisted Procedure   CCI Comp. Code   Non-specific Procedure

This page intentionally left blank.

● New Code   ▲ Revised Code   ✚ Add-On Code   ⊘ Modifier -51 Exempt

ANESTHESIA CODES

HEAD

00100 Anesthesia for procedures on salivary glands, including biopsy

00102 Anesthesia for procedures on plastic repair of cleft lip

00103 Anesthesia for reconstructive procedures of eyelid (eg, blepharoplasty, ptosis surgery)

00104 Anesthesia for electroconvulsive therapy

00120 Anesthesia for procedures on external, middle, and inner ear including biopsy; not otherwise specified

00124 otoscopy

00126 tympanotomy

00140 Anesthesia for procedures on eye; not otherwise specified

00142 lens surgery

00144 corneal transplant

00145 vitreoretinal surgery

00147 iridectomy

00148 ophthalmoscopy

00160 Anesthesia for procedures on nose and accessory sinuses; not otherwise specified

00162 radical surgery

00164 biopsy, soft tissue

00170 Anesthesia for intraoral procedures, including biopsy; not otherwise specified

00172 repair of cleft palate

203

 Separate Procedure   Unlisted Procedure   CCI Comp. Code   Non-specific Procedure

00174   excision of retropharyngeal tumor

00176   radical surgery

00190   Anesthesia for procedures on facial bones or skull; not otherwise specified

00192   radical surgery (including prognathism)

00210   Anesthesia for intracranial procedures; not otherwise specified

00212   subdural taps

00214   burr holes, including ventriculography

00215   cranioplasty or elevation of depressed skull fracture, extradural (simple or compound)

00216   vascular procedures

00218   procedures in sitting position

00220   cerebrospinal fluid shunting procedures

00222   electrocoagulation of intracranial nerve

NECK

00300   Anesthesia for all procedures on the integumentary system, muscles and nerves of head, neck, and posterior trunk, not otherwise specified

00320   Anesthesia for all procedures on esophagus, thyroid, larynx, trachea and lymphatic system of neck; not otherwise specified, age 1 year or older

00322   needle biopsy of thyroid

(For procedures on cervical spine and cord, see 00600, 00604, 00670)

00326   Anesthesia for all procedures on the larynx and trachea in children less than 1 year of age

(Do not report 00326 in conjunction with code 99100)

● New Code   ▲ Revised Code   + Add-On Code   ⊘ Modifier -51 Exempt

00350 Anesthesia for procedures on major vessels of neck; not otherwise specified

00352 simple ligation

(For arteriography, use 01916)

THORAX (CHEST WALL AND SHOULDER GIRDLE)

00400 Anesthesia for procedures on the integumentary system on the extremities, anterior trunk and perineum; not otherwise specified

00402 reconstructive procedures on breast (eg, reduction or augmentation mammoplasty, muscle flaps)

00404 radical or modified radical procedures on breast

00406 radical or modified radical procedures on breast with internal mammary node dissection

00410 electrical conversion of arrhythmias

00450 Anesthesia for procedures on clavicle and scapula; not otherwise specified

00452 radical surgery

00454 biopsy of clavicle

00470 Anesthesia for partial rib resection; not otherwise specified

00472 thoracoplasty (any type)

00474 radical procedures (eg, pectus excavatum)

INTRATHORACIC

00500 Anesthesia for all procedures on esophagus

00520 Anesthesia for closed chest procedures; (including bronchoscopy) not otherwise specified

00522 needle biopsy of pleura

205

	Separate Procedure		Unlisted Procedure		CCI Comp. Code		Non-specific Procedure

00524   pneumocentesis

▲ **00528**   mediastinoscopy and diagnostic thoracoscopy not utilizing one lung ventilation

(For tracheobronchial reconstruction, use 00539)

● **00529**   mediastinoscopy and diagnostic thoracoscopy utilizing one lung ventilation

00530   Anesthesia for permanent transvenous pacemaker insertion

00532   Anesthesia for access to central venous circulation

00534   Anesthesia for transvenous insertion or replacement of pacing cardioverter/defibrillator

(For transthoracic approach, use 00560)

00537   Anesthesia for cardiac electrophysiologic procedures including radiofrequency ablation

00539   Anesthesia for tracheobronchial reconstruction

00540   Anesthesia for thoracotomy procedures involving lungs, pleura, diaphragm, and mediastinum (including surgical thoracoscopy); not otherwise specified

00541   utilizing one lung ventilation

00542   decortication

(**00544**   deleted 2004 edition. To report, use 00542)

00546   pulmonary resection with thoracoplasty

00548   intrathoracic procedures on the trachea and bronchi

00550   Anesthesia for sternal debridement

00560   Anesthesia for procedures on heart, pericardial sac, and great vessels of chest; without pump oxygenator

00562   with pump oxygenator

00563   with pump oxygenator with hypothermic circulatory arrest

206

| ● | New Code | ▲ | Revised Code | + | Add-On Code | ⊘ | Modifier -51 Exempt |

00566 Anesthesia for direct coronary artery bypass grafting without pump oxygenator

00580 Anesthesia for heart transplant or heart/lung transplant

SPINE AND SPINAL CORD

00600 Anesthesia for procedures on cervical spine and cord; not otherwise specified

(For myelography and diskography, see radiological procedures 01905)

00604 procedures with patient in the sitting position

00620 Anesthesia for procedures on thoracic spine and cord; not otherwise specified

00622 thoracolumbar sympathectomy

00630 Anesthesia for procedures in lumbar region; not otherwise specified

00632 lumbar sympathectomy

00634 chemonucleolysis

00635 diagnostic or therapeutic lumbar puncture

00640 Anesthesia for manipulation of the spine or for closed procedures on the cervical, thoracic or lumbar spine

00670 Anesthesia for extensive spine and spinal cord procedures (eg, spinal instrumentation or vascular procedures)

UPPER ABDOMEN

00700 Anesthesia for procedures on upper anterior abdominal wall; not otherwise specified

00702 percutaneous liver biopsy

00730 Anesthesia for procedures on upper posterior abdominal wall

---

207

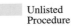 Separate Procedure   Unlisted Procedure    CCI Comp. Code   Non-specific Procedure

00740 Anesthesia for upper gastrointestinal endoscopic procedures, endoscope introduced proximal to duodenum

00750 Anesthesia for hernia repairs in upper abdomen; not otherwise specified

00752 lumbar and ventral (incisional) hernias and/or wound dehiscence

00754 omphalocele

00756 transabdominal repair of diaphragmatic hernia

00770 Anesthesia for all procedures on major abdominal blood vessels

00790 Anesthesia for intraperitoneal procedures in upper abdomen including laparoscopy; not otherwise specified

00792 partial hepatectomy or management of liver hemorrhage (excluding liver biopsy)

00794 pancreatectomy, partial or total (eg, Whipple procedure)

00796 liver transplant (recipient)

(For harvesting of liver, use 01990)

00797 gastric restrictive procedure for morbid obesity

LOWER ABDOMEN

00800 Anesthesia for procedures on lower anterior abdominal wall; not otherwise specified

00802 panniculectomy

00810 Anesthesia for lower intestinal endoscopic procedures, endoscope introduced distal to duodenum

00820 Anesthesia for procedures on lower posterior abdominal wall

00830 Anesthesia for hernia repairs in lower abdomen; not otherwise specified

00832 ventral and incisional hernias

● New Code ▲ Revised Code + Add-On Code ⊘ Modifier -51 Exempt

(For hernia repairs in the infant 1 year of age or younger, see 00834, 00836)

00834 Anesthesia for hernia repairs in the lower abdomen not otherwise specified, under 1 year of age

(Do not report 00834 in conjunction with code 99100)

00836 Anesthesia for hernia repairs in the lower abdomen not otherwise specified, infants less than 37 weeks gestational age at birth and less than 50 weeks gestational age at time of surgery

(Do not report 00836 in conjunction with code 99100)

00840 Anesthesia for intraperitoneal procedures in lower abdomen including laparoscopy; not otherwise specified

00842 amniocentesis

00844 abdominoperineal resection

00846 radical hysterectomy

00848 pelvic exenteration

(00850 deleted 2002 edition. To report, use 01961)

00851 tubal ligation/transection

(00855 deleted 2002 edition. To report, use 01963)

(00857 deleted 2002 edition. To report, use 01968, 01969)

00860 Anesthesia for extraperitoneal procedures in lower abdomen, including urinary tract; not otherwise specified

00862 renal procedures, including upper 1/3 of ureter, or donor nephrectomy

00864 total cystectomy

00865 radical prostatectomy (suprapubic, retropubic)

00866 adrenalectomy

00868 renal transplant (recipient)

Separate Procedure	Unlisted Procedure	CCI Comp. Code	Non-specific Procedure

(For donor nephrectomy, use 00862)

(For harvesting kidney from brain-dead patient, use 01990)

(00869   deleted 2003 edition. To report, use 00921)

00870   cystolithotomy

00872   Anesthesia for lithotripsy, extracorporeal shock wave; with water bath

00873   without water bath

00880   Anesthesia for procedures on major lower abdominal vessels; not otherwise specified

00882   inferior vena cava ligation

(00884   deleted 2002 edition. To report, use 01930)

PERINEUM

00902   Anesthesia for; anorectal procedure

00904   radical perineal procedure

00906   vulvectomy

00908   perineal prostatectomy

00910   Anesthesia for transurethral procedures (including urethrocystoscopy); not otherwise specified

00912   transurethral resection of bladder tumor(s)

00914   transurethral resection of prostate

00916   post-transurethral resection bleeding

00918   with fragmentation, manipulation and/or removal of ureteral calculus

00920   Anesthesia for procedures on male genitalia (including open urethral procedures); not otherwise specified

● New Code   ▲ Revised Code   + Add-On Code   ⊘ Modifier -51 Exempt

00921   vasectomy, unilateral/bilateral

00922   seminal vesicles

00924   undescended testis, unilateral or bilateral

00926   radical orchiectomy, inguinal

00928   radical orchiectomy, abdominal

00930   orchiopexy, unilateral or bilateral

00932   complete amputation of penis

00934   radical amputation of penis with bilateral inguinal lymphadenectomy

00936   radical amputation of penis with bilateral inguinal and iliac lymphadenectomy

00938   insertion of penile prosthesis (perineal approach)

00940   Anesthesia for vaginal procedures (including biopsy of labia, vagina, cervix or endometrium); not otherwise specified

00942   colpotomy, vaginectomy, colporrhaphy and open urethral procedures

00944   vaginal hysterectomy

(00946   deleted 2002 edition. To report, use 01960)

00948   cervical cerclage

00950   culdoscopy

00952   hysteroscopy and/or hysterosalpingography

(00955   deleted 2002 edition. To report, use 01967)

211

 Separate Procedure   Unlisted Procedure   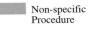 CCI Comp. Code   Non-specific Procedure

PELVIS (EXCEPT HIP)

01112 Anesthesia for bone marrow aspiration and/or biopsy, anterior or posterior iliac crest

01120 Anesthesia for procedures on bony pelvis

01130 Anesthesia for body cast application or revision

01140 Anesthesia for interpelviabdominal (hindquarter) amputation

01150 Anesthesia for radical procedures for tumor of pelvis, except hindquarter amputation

01160 Anesthesia for closed procedures involving symphysis pubis or sacroiliac joint

01170 Anesthesia for open procedures involving symphysis pubis or sacroiliac joint

● **01173** Anesthesia for open repair of fracture disruption of pelvis or column fracture involving acetabulum

01180 Anesthesia for obturator neurectomy; extrapelvic

01190 intrapelvic

UPPER LEG (EXCEPT KNEE)

01200 Anesthesia for all closed procedures involving hip joint

01202 Anesthesia for arthroscopic procedures of hip joint

01210 Anesthesia for open procedures involving hip joint; not otherwise specified

01212 hip disarticulation

01214 total hip arthroplasty

01215 revision of total hip arthroplasty

01220 Anesthesia for all closed procedures involving upper 2/3 of femur

---

● New Code	▲ Revised Code	✛ Add-On Code	⊘ Modifier -51 Exempt

01230 Anesthesia for open procedures involving upper 2/3 of femur; not otherwise specified

01232 amputation

01234 radical resection

01250 Anesthesia for all procedures on nerves, muscles, tendons, fascia, and bursae of upper leg

01260 Anesthesia for all procedures involving veins of upper leg, including exploration

01270 Anesthesia for procedures involving arteries of upper leg, including bypass graft; not otherwise specified

01272 femoral artery ligation

01274 femoral artery embolectomy

KNEE AND POPLITEAL AREA

(Surgical endoscopy/arthroscopy always includes a diagnostic endoscopy/arthroscopy.)

01320 Anesthesia for all procedures on nerves, muscles, tendons, fascia, and bursae of knee and/or popliteal area

01340 Anesthesia for all closed procedures on lower 1/3 of femur

01360 Anesthesia for all open procedures on lower 1/3 of femur

01380 Anesthesia for all closed procedures on knee joint

01382 Anesthesia for diagnostic arthroscopic procedures of knee joint

01390 Anesthesia for all closed procedures on upper ends of tibia, fibula, and/or patella

01392 Anesthesia for all open procedures on upper ends of tibia, fibula, and/or patella

01400 Anesthesia for open or surgical arthroscopic procedures on knee joint; not otherwise specified

01402 total knee arthroplasty

213

| | Separate Procedure | | Unlisted Procedure | | CCI Comp. Code | | Non-specific Procedure |

01404   disarticulation at knee

01420   Anesthesia for all cast applications, removal, or repair involving knee joint

01430   Anesthesia for procedures on veins of knee and popliteal area; not otherwise specified

01432   arteriovenous fistula

01440   Anesthesia for procedures on arteries of knee and popliteal area; not otherwise specified

01442   popliteal thromboendarterectomy, with or without patch graft

01444   popliteal excision and graft or repair for occlusion or aneurysm

LOWER LEG (BELOW KNEE, INCLUDES ANKLE AND FOOT)

(Surgical endoscopy/arthroscopy always includes a diagnostic endoscopy/arthroscopy.)

01462   Anesthesia for all closed procedures on lower leg, ankle, and foot

01464   Anesthesia for arthroscopic procedures of ankle and/or foot

01470   Anesthesia for procedures on nerves, muscles, tendons, and fascia of lower leg, ankle, and foot; not otherwise specified

01472   repair of ruptured Achilles tendon, with or without graft

01474   gastrocnemius recession (eg, Strayer procedure)

01480   Anesthesia for open procedures on bones of lower leg, ankle, and foot; not otherwise specified

01482   radical resection (including below knee amputation)

01484   osteotomy or osteoplasty of tibia and/or fibula

01486   total ankle replacement

214

| ● New Code | ▲ Revised Code | + Add-On Code | ⊘ Modifier -51 Exempt |

01490	Anesthesia for lower leg cast application, removal, or repair
01500	Anesthesia for procedures on arteries of lower leg, including bypass graft; not otherwise specified
01502	embolectomy, direct or with catheter
01520	Anesthesia for procedures on veins of lower leg; not otherwise specified
01522	venous thrombectomy, direct or with catheter

SHOULDER AND AXILLA

(Surgical endoscopy/arthroscopy always includes a diagnostic endoscopy/arthroscopy.)

(Includes humeral head and neck, sternoclavicular joint, acromioclavicular joint, and shoulder joint)

01610	Anesthesia for all procedures on nerves, muscles, tendons, fascia, and bursae of shoulder and axilla
01620	Anesthesia for all closed procedures on humeral head and neck, sternoclavicular joint, acromioclavicular joint, and shoulder joint
01622	Anesthesia for diagnostic arthroscopic procedures of shoulder joint
01630	Anesthesia for open or surgical arthroscopic procedures on humeral head and neck, sternoclavicular joint, acromioclavicular joint, and shoulder joint; not otherwise specified
01632	radical resection
01634	shoulder disarticulation
01636	interthoracoscapular (forequarter) amputation
01638	total shoulder replacement
01650	Anesthesia for procedures on arteries of shoulder and axilla; not otherwise specified
01652	axillary-brachial aneurysm

215

 Separate Procedure   Unlisted Procedure   CCI Comp. Code   Non-specific Procedure

| 01654 | bypass graft |

| 01656 | axillary-femoral bypass graft |

| 01670 | Anesthesia for all procedures on veins of shoulder and axilla |

| 01680 | Anesthesia for shoulder cast application, removal or repair; not otherwise specified |

| 01682 | shoulder spica |

UPPER ARM AND ELBOW

(Surgical endoscopy/arthroscopy always includes a diagnostic endoscopy/arthroscopy.)

| 01710 | Anesthesia for procedures on nerves, muscles, tendons, fascia, and bursae of upper arm and elbow; not otherwise specified |

| 01712 | tenotomy, elbow to shoulder, open |

| 01714 | tenoplasty, elbow to shoulder |

| 01716 | tenodesis, rupture of long tendon of biceps |

| 01730 | Anesthesia for all closed procedures on humerus and elbow |

| 01732 | Anesthesia for diagnostic arthroscopic procedures of elbow joint |

| 01740 | Anesthesia for open or surgical arthroscopic procedures of the elbow; not otherwise specified |

| 01742 | osteotomy of humerus |

| 01744 | repair of nonunion or malunion of humerus |

| 01756 | radical procedures |

| 01758 | excision of cyst or tumor of humerus |

| 01760 | total elbow replacement |

| 01770 | Anesthesia for procedures on arteries of upper arm and elbow; not otherwise specified |

● New Code   ▲ Revised Code   + Add-On Code   ⊘ Modifier -51 Exempt

01772   embolectomy

01780   Anesthesia for procedures on veins of upper arm and elbow; not otherwise specified

01782   phleborrhaphy

FOREARM, WRIST, AND HAND

01810   Anesthesia for all procedures on nerves, muscles, tendons, fascia, and bursae of forearm, wrist, and hand

01820   Anesthesia for all closed procedures on radius, ulna, wrist, or hand bones

01829   Anesthesia for diagnostic arthroscopic procedures on the wrist

01830   Anesthesia for open or surgical arthroscopic/endoscopic procedures on distal radius, distal ulna, wrist, or hand joints; not otherwise specified

01832   total wrist replacement

01840   Anesthesia for procedures on arteries of forearm, wrist, and hand; not otherwise specified

01842   embolectomy

01844   Anesthesia for vascular shunt, or shunt revision, any type (eg, dialysis)

01850   Anesthesia for procedures on veins of forearm, wrist, and hand; not otherwise specified

01852   phleborrhaphy

01860   Anesthesia for forearm, wrist, or hand cast application, removal, or repair

217

 Separate Procedure   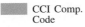 Unlisted Procedure   CCI Comp. Code   Non-specific Procedure

RADIOLOGICAL PROCEDURES

(01904   deleted 2002 edition. To report, use 01905)

01905   Anesthesia for myelography, diskography, vertebroplasty

(01906   deleted 2002 edition. To report, use 01905)

(01908   deleted 2002 edition. To report, use 01905)

(01910   deleted 2002 edition. To report, use 01905)

(01912   deleted 2002 edition. To report, use 01905)

(01914   deleted 2002 edition. To report, use 01905)

01916   Anesthesia for diagnostic arteriography/venography

(Do not report 01916 in conjunction with therapeutic codes 01924-01926, 01930-01933)

(01918   deleted 2002 edition. To report, use 01916)

01920   Anesthesia for cardiac catheterization including coronary angiography and ventriculography (not to include Swan-Ganz catheter)

(01921   deleted 2002 edition. To report, see 01924-01926)

01922   Anesthesia for non-invasive imaging or radiation therapy

01924   Anesthesia for therapeutic interventional radiologic procedures involving the arterial system; not otherwise specified

01925   carotid or coronary

01926   intracranial, intracardiac, or aortic

01930   Anesthesia for therapeutic interventional radiologic procedures involving the venous/lymphatic system (not to include access to the central circulation); not otherwise specified

01931   intrahepatic or portal circulation (eg, transcutaneous porto-caval shunt (TIPS))

● New Code   ▲ Revised Code   + Add-On Code   ⊘ Modifier -51 Exempt

01932   intrathoracic or jugular

01933   intracranial

BURN EXCISIONS OR DEBRIDEMENT

01951   Anesthesia for second and third degree burn excision or debridement with or without skin grafting, any site, for total body surface area (TBSA) treated during anesthesia and surgery; less than four percent total body surface area

01952   between four and nine percent of total body surface area

+ 01953   each additional nine percent total body surface area or part thereof (List separately in addition to code for primary procedure)

(Use 01953 in conjunction with code 01952)

OBSTETRIC

● **01958**   Anesthesia for external cephalic version procedure

01960   Anesthesia for vaginal delivery only

01961   Anesthesia for cesarean delivery only

01962   Anesthesia for urgent hysterectomy following delivery

01963   Anesthesia for cesarean hysterectomy without any labor analgesia/anesthesia care

01964   Anesthesia for abortion procedures

01967   Neuraxial labor analgesia/anesthesia for planned vaginal delivery (this includes any repeat subarachnoid needle placement and drug injection and/or any necessary replacement of an epidural catheter during labor)

+ 01968   Anesthesia for cesarean delivery following neuraxial labor analgesia/anesthesia (List separately in addition to code for primary procedure)

(Use 01968 in conjunction with code 01967)

 Separate Procedure   Unlisted Procedure   CCI Comp. Code   Non-specific Procedure

+ 01969 Anesthesia for cesarean hysterectomy following neuraxial labor analgesia/anesthesia (List separately in addition to code for primary procedure)

(Use 01969 in conjunction with code 01967)

OTHER PROCEDURES

01990 Physiological support for harvesting of organ(s) from brain-dead patient

01991 Anesthesia for diagnostic or therapeutic nerve blocks and injections (when block or injection is performed by a different provider); other than the prone position

01992 prone position

(Do not report code 01991 or 01992 in conjunction with 99141)

01995 Regional intravenous administration of local anesthetic agent or other medication (upper or lower extremity)

(For intra-arterial or intravenous therapy for pain management, see 90783, 90784)

01996 Daily hospital management of epidural or subarachnoid continuous drug administration

(Report code 01996 for daily hospital management of continuous epidural or subarachnoid drug administration performed after insertion of an epidural or subarachnoid catheter placed primarily for anesthesia administration during an operative session, but retained for post-operative pain management)

01999 Unlisted anesthesia procedure(s)

● New Code ▲ Revised Code + Add-On Code ⊘ Modifier -51 Exempt

SURGERY

SURGERY SECTION OVERVIEW

The third section of the CPT coding system is the surgery section, and it includes surgical procedure codes for all body areas. Within each subsection, the CPT codes are arranged by anatomical site.

It is essential to understand the organization of the CPT surgery section in order to locate the correct procedure code. Understanding other or alternative terms which may apply to a procedure, injury, illness or condition may also make the location of the appropriate procedure easier and faster.

All procedures listed in the surgery section of the CPT book include local, metacarpal/digital block or topical anesthesia if used, the surgical procedure, and normal uncomplicated follow-up care. For diagnostic surgical procedures, follow-up care includes only the care related to recovery from the diagnostic procedure. For therapeutic surgical procedures, follow-up care includes only the care which would usually be included in the surgical service. Any complications resulting in additional services are not considered to be included and should be coded separately.

KEY POINTS ABOUT SURGERY SERVICES

- *Evaluation and management services provided by surgeons in the office, home or hospital, plus consultations and other medical services are coded using evaluation and management service codes.*

- *Any supplies and/or materials provided by the surgeon which are not considered to be included in the standard service may be coded separately.*

GLOBAL SURGICAL PACKAGE

Third-party payers differ in their definition of a surgical or global surgical package concept. Medicare defines the global surgical package as follows:

- *The surgeon's initial evaluation or consultation will be paid separately.*

- *There is a one day preoperative period covered under the global surgical package.*

- *Included in the package are all intraoperative services that are considered to be usual and necessary. Separate billing of these services would be considered unbundling.*

- *Any treatment of complications by the surgeon not requiring a return to the operating room is included in the package.*

221

 Separate Procedure   Unlisted Procedure   CCI Comp. Code   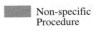 Non-specific Procedure

- *The surgical package contains a standard 90-day postoperative period which includes all visits to the physician during that time unless the visit is for a totally different reason than that for the surgery.*

- *In cases of organ transplant, immunosuppressive therapy is not included in the global package.*

- *Minor surgical procedures are those with a 0 or 10-day postoperative period, and are excluded from the surgical package definition.*

SPECIAL REPORT

Surgical procedures which are new, unusual or vary significantly from the standard definition may require a special report. When preparing reports to accompany health insurance claim forms the provider should include a description of the nature, extent, and need for the procedure, and the time, effort, and equipment necessary to provides the service. Try to keep these reports as brief and simple as possible. Additional items which may be needed are:

- *complexity of symptoms*

- *final diagnosis*

- *pertinent physical findings*

- *diagnostic and therapeutic procedures*

- *concurrent problems*

- *follow-up care*

MULTIPLE SURGICAL PROCEDURES

It is common for several surgical procedures to be performed at the same operative session. When multiple procedures are performed on the same day or at the same session, the "major" procedure or service is listed first followed by secondary, additional, or "lessor" procedures or services. CPT modifier -51 is added to all procedures following the first one.

Reporting multiple procedures incorrectly may have a serious impact on reimbursement from health insurance payers. An inexperienced health insurance biller may simply list the procedures on the health insurance claim form in the order dictated or described in the operative report.

There are two critical decisions related to reporting multiple surgical procedures correctly; namely: 1) The order in which the procedures are listed on the health insurance claim form, and 2) whether or not to list the additional procedures with full or reduced fees.

● New Code   ▲ Revised Code   + Add-On Code   ⊘ Modifier -51 Exempt

ORDER OF LISTING MULTIPLE PROCEDURES

The first procedure to be listed when reporting services under the multiple procedure rule is the procedure with the highest fee. Additional procedures should be listed in descending order by fee. Modifier -51 should be added to each additional procedure.

All third party payers will reduce the allowance for the additional procedures, typically by 50 percent for the second procedure, and 50 to 75 percent for the third and subsequent procedures. Listing the procedures in descending order by fee minimizes the possibility of an incorrect reduction.

21. DIAGNOSIS OR NATURE OF ILLNESS OR INJURY. (RELATE ITEMS 1,2,3 OR 4 TO ITEM 24E BY LINE)						
1. 952 . 10				3.		
2.				4.		

24 A DATE(S) OF SERVICE FROM MM DD YY — FROM MM DD YY	B Place of Service	C Type of Service	D PROCEDURES, SERVICES, OR SUPPLIES (Explain Unusual Circumstances) CPT/HCPCS MODIFIER	E DIAGNOSIS CODE
1 06 15 04	21		63046	
2 06 15 04	21		62223 51	
3				
4				

BILLING FULL VERSUS REDUCED FEES

The full fee should be listed for each procedure coded on the health insurance claim form as part of multiple surgical procedures. Third party payers will automatically reduce the allowances for the additional procedures by a specific formula. Listing all multiple procedures with full fees in descending fee order (the procedure with the highest fee first, the procedure with the next highest fee second, et cetera) will result in the maximum total allowable reimbursement for the provider or the insured.

After the maximum benefit has been paid by the health insurance company, the balance remaining, less any patient co-insurance or deductible requirements, should be written off. Note that billing practices vary in different areas of the country. Providers should continue to use the method that is customary or required by third party payers in the provider's practice location.

223

Separate Procedure   Unlisted Procedure   CCI Comp. Code   Non-specific Procedure

SEPARATE PROCEDURE

Some surgical procedures are considered to be an integral part of a more extensive surgical procedure. In this circumstance, the integral procedure is not coded. When the integral procedure is performed independently and is unrelated to other services, it should be listed as a "separate procedure."

SURGERY SUBSECTIONS

The SURGERY section of the CPT coding system is divided into 17 subsections:

Integumentary System	10040-19499
Musculoskeletal System	20000-29999
Respiratory System	30000-32999
Cardiovascular System	33010-37799
Hemic and Lymphatic Systems	38100-38999
Mediastinum and Diaphragm	39000-39599
Digestive System	40490-49999
Urinary System	50010-53899
Male Genital System	54000-55899
Intersex Surgery	55970-55980
Female Genital Surgery	56400-58999
Maternity Care and Delivery	59000-59899
Endocrine System	60000-60699
Nervous System	61000-64999
Eye and Ocular Adnexa	65091-68899
Auditory System	69000-69979
Operating Microscope	69990

Each sub-section of the SURGERY section of the CPT coding system is divided into organs then into procedures involving anatomic sites. Each anatomic site is further separated into surgical processes such as incision, excision, repair, removal, amputation, etc.

SURGERY SECTION MODIFIERS

Due to various circumstances, surgical procedures may be considered to be modified in comparison to the full or complete procedure. Modified procedures are identified by reporting a two-digit modifier to the CPT procedure code(s). The following CPT modifiers may be coded with surgical procedures:

-22   Unusual Procedural Services

-26   Professional Component

-32   Mandated Services

-47   Anesthesia by Surgeon

224

● New Code   ▲ Revised Code   + Add-On Code   ⊘ Modifier -51 Exempt

-50   Bilateral Procedure

-51   Multiple Procedures

-52   Reduced Services

-54   Surgical Care Only

-55   Postoperative Management Only

-56   Preoperative Management Only

-57   Decision for Surgery

-58   Staged or Related Procedure or Service by the Same Physician During the Postoperative Period

-62   Two Surgeons

-66   Surgical Team

-76   Repeat Procedure by Same Physician

-77   Repeat Procedure by Another Physician

-78   Return to the Operating Room for a Related Procedure During the Postoperative Period

-79   Unrelated Procedure or Service by the Same Physician During the Postoperative Period

-80   Assistant Surgeon

-81   Minimum Assistant Surgeon

-82   Assistant Surgeon (when qualified resident surgeon not available)

-90   Reference (Outside) Laboratory

-99   Multiple modifiers

 Separate Procedure   Unlisted Procedure    CCI Comp. Code   Non-specific Procedure

ADD-ON CODES

Many surgical procedures are performed secondary to primary surgical procedures. These procedures are classified as "additional" or "supplemental" procedures and are designated as "add-on" codes in the CPT coding system. "Add-on" CPT codes are identified in the CPT code book by a black plus sign "+" placed to the left of the code number.

Many of the CPT "Add-on" codes are further identified by phrases included within the descriptions of the definition of the CPT code or include the phrase "(List separately in addition to primary procedure)" following the definition. Examples of CPT codes identified as "add-on" codes in CPT 2003 include:

+11001 Debridement of extensive eczematous or infected skin; each additional 10% of the body surface (List separately in addition to code for primary procedure)

+33530 Reoperation, coronary artery bypass procedure or valve procedure, more than one month after original operation (List separately in addition to code for primary procedure)

STARRED PROCEDURES

CPT used to define minor surgical procedures by placing a star (*) after the procedure code number. This designation was removed in CPT 2004.

MEDICAL AND SURGICAL SUPPLIES

HCPCS Level II codes for medical and surgical supplies, A4000-A4999, may be used to report supplies and materials provided to Medicare patients if the supplies and materials are not considered to be included with or part of the basic service(s) or procedure(s).

226

● New Code   ▲ Revised Code   **+** Add-On Code   ⊘ Modifier -51 Exempt

SURGERY CODES

GENERAL

(10000-10020 have been deleted. To report, see 10060, 10061)

10021   Fine needle aspiration; without imaging guidance

10022   with imaging guidance

(For radiological supervision and interpretation, see 76003, 76360, 76393, 76942)

(For percutaneous needle biopsy other than fine needle aspiration, see 20206 for muscle, 32400 for pleura, 32405 for lung or mediastinum, 42400 for salivary gland, 47000, 47001 for liver, 48102 for pancreas, 49180 for abdominal or retroperitoneal mass, 60100 for thyroid, 62269 for spinal cord)

(For evaluation of fine needle aspirate, see 88172, 88173)

 Separate Procedure   Unlisted Procedure   CCI Comp. Code   Non-specific Procedure

This page intentionally left blank.

INTEGUMENTARY SYSTEM

SKIN, SUBCUTANEOUS AND ACCESSORY STRUCTURES

INCISION AND DRAINAGE

(For excision, see 11400, et seq)

10040 Acne surgery (eg, marsupialization, opening or removal of multiple milia, comedones, cysts, pustules)

10060 Incision and drainage of abscess (eg, carbuncle, suppurative hidradenitis, cutaneous or subcutaneous abscess, cyst, furuncle, or paronychia); simple or single

10061 complicated or multiple

10080 Incision and drainage of pilonidal cyst; simple

10081 complicated

(For excision of pilonidal cyst, see 11770-11772)

10120 Incision and removal of foreign body, subcutaneous tissues; simple

10121 complicated

(To report wound exploration due to penetrating trauma without laparotomy or thoracotomy, see 20100-20103, as appropriate)

(To report debridement associated with open fracture(s) and/or dislocation(s), use 11010-11012, as appropriate)

10140 Incision and drainage of hematoma, seroma or fluid collection

(If imaging guidance is performed, see 76360, 76393, 76942)

10160 Puncture aspiration of abscess, hematoma, bulla, or cyst

(If imaging guidance is performed, see 76360, 76393, 76942)

10180 Incision and drainage, complex, postoperative wound infection

(For secondary closure of surgical wound, see 12020, 12021, 13160)

229

 Separate Procedure   Unlisted Procedure   CCI Comp. Code   Non-specific Procedure

EXCISION-DEBRIDEMENT

(For dermabrasions, see 15780-15783)

(For nail debridement, see 11720-11721)

(For burn(s), see 16000-16035)

11000   Debridement of extensive eczematous or infected skin; up to 10% of body surface

+ 11001   each additional 10% of the body surface (List separately in addition to code for primary procedure)

(Use 11001 in conjunction with code 11000)

11010   Debridement including removal of foreign material associated with open fracture(s) and/or dislocation(s); skin and subcutaneous tissues

11011   skin, subcutaneous tissue, muscle fascia, and muscle

11012   skin, subcutaneous tissue, muscle fascia, muscle, and bone

11040   Debridement; skin, partial thickness

11041   skin, full thickness

11042   skin, and subcutaneous tissue

11043   skin, subcutaneous tissue, and muscle

11044   skin, subcutaneous tissue, muscle, and bone

(Do not report 11040-11044 in addition to 97601, 97602)

PARING OR CUTTING

11055   Paring or cutting of benign hyperkeratotic lesion (eg, corn or callus); single lesion

11056   two to four lesions

11057   more than four lesions

   ● New Code   ▲ Revised Code   + Add-On Code   ⊘ Modifier -51 Exempt

BIOPSY

(For biopsy of conjunctiva, use 68100; eyelid, use 67810)

▲ **11100** Biopsy of skin, subcutaneous tissue and/or mucous membrane (including simple closure), unless otherwise listed; single lesion

+ **11101** each separate/additional lesion (List separately in addition to code for primary procedure)

(Use 11101 in conjunction with code 11100)

REMOVAL OF SKIN TAGS

11200 Removal of skin tags, multiple fibrocutaneous tags, any area; up to and including 15 lesions

+ **11201** each additional ten lesions (List separately in addition to code for primary procedure)

(Use 11201 in conjunction with code 11200)

SHAVING OF EPIDERMAL OR DERMAL LESIONS

Many of the procedure codes listed in the integumentary system subsection of the CPT manual are designated in centimeters or square centimeters. Many physicians document sizes using inches or millimeters. Make sure to verify, and convert if necessary, measurements before assigning a code.

To be able to code lesion removal appropriately, the site, size in centimeters, method of removal and morphology must be documented in the medical record. Always code morphology from the pathology report.

Excision of lesion codes are determined by the diameter of the actual lesion, not the specimen sent to pathology. However, the size of the specimen can be used when the size of the lesion cannot be located in the operative report or elsewhere in the medical record.

When more than one dimension of a lesion is provided in the documentation, select the code based on the largest size. For example, if the dimensions indicated are 3 cm x 2 cm x 1.5 cm, the lesion should be coded as 3 cm. Excision of benign and malignant lesions includes anesthesia and simple repair of the defect site.

11300 Shaving of epidermal or dermal lesion, single lesion, trunk, arms or legs; lesion diameter 0.5 cm or less

11301 lesion diameter 0.6 to 1.0 cm

11302 lesion diameter 1.1 to 2.0 cm

231

| | Separate Procedure | | Unlisted Procedure | | CCI Comp. Code | | Non-specific Procedure |

11303   lesion diameter over 2.0 cm

11305   Shaving of epidermal or dermal lesion, single lesion, scalp, neck, hands, feet, genitalia; lesion diameter 0.5 cm or less

11306   lesion diameter 0.6 to 1.0 cm

11307   lesion diameter 1.1 to 2.0 cm

11308   lesion diameter over 2.0 cm

11310   Shaving of epidermal or dermal lesion, single lesion, face, ears, eyelids, nose, lips, mucous membrane; lesion diameter 0.5 cm or less

11311   lesion diameter 0.6 to 1.0 cm

11312   lesion diameter 1.1 to 2.0 cm

11313   lesion diameter over 2.0 cm

EXCISION OF BENIGN LESIONS

(For excision of benign lesions requiring more than simple closure, ie, requiring intermediate or complex closure, report 11400-11466 in addition to appropriate intermediate (12031-12057) or complex closure (13100-13153) codes. For reconstructive closure, see 11400-14300, 15000-15261, 15570-15770)

(For shave removal, see 11300 et seq., and for electrosurgical and other methods, see 17000 et seq.)

11400   Excision, benign lesion including margins, except skin tag (unless listed elsewhere), trunk, arms or legs; excised diameter 0.5 cm or less

11401   excised diameter 0.6 to 1.0 cm

11402   excised diameter 1.1 to 2.0 cm

11403   excised diameter 2.1 to 3.0 cm

11404   excised diameter 3.1 to 4.0 cm

11406   excised diameter over 4.0 cm

● New Code   ▲ Revised Code   + Add-On Code   ⊘ Modifier -51 Exempt

(For unusual or complicated excision, add modifier -22)

11420   Excision, benign lesion including margins, except skin tag (unless listed elsewhere), scalp, neck, hands, feet, genitalia; excised diameter 0.5 cm or less

11421   excised diameter 0.6 to 1.0 cm

11422   excised diameter 1.1 to 2.0 cm

11423   excised diameter 2.1 to 3.0 cm

11424   excised diameter 3.1 to 4.0 cm

11426   excised diameter over 4.0 cm

(For unusual or complicated excision, add modifier -22)

11440   Excision, other benign lesion including margins (unless listed elsewhere), face, ears, eyelids, nose, lips, mucous membrane; excised diameter 0.5 cm or less

11441   excised diameter 0.6 to 1.0 cm

11442   excised diameter 1.1 to 2.0 cm

11443   excised diameter 2.1 to 3.0 cm

11444   excised diameter 3.1 to 4.0 cm

11446   excised diameter over 4.0 cm

(For unusual or complicated excision, add modifier -22)

(For eyelids involving more than skin, see also 67800 et seq.)

11450   Excision of skin and subcutaneous tissue for hidradenitis, axillary; with simple or intermediate repair

11451   with complex repair

11462   Excision of skin and subcutaneous tissue for hidradenitis, inguinal; with simple or intermediate repair

11463   with complex repair

 Separate Procedure   Unlisted Procedure   CCI Comp. Code   Non-specific Procedure

| 11470 | Excision of skin and subcutaneous tissue for hidradenitis, perianal, perineal, or umbilical; with simple or intermediate repair |

| 11471 | with complex repair |

(When skin graft or flap is used for closure, use appropriate procedure code in addition)

(For bilateral procedure, add modifier -50)

EXCISION OF MALIGNANT LESIONS

(For excision of malignant lesions requiring more than simple closure, i.e., requiring intermediate or complex closure, report 11600-11646 in addition to appropriate intermediate (12031-12057) or complex closure (13100-13153) codes. For reconstructive closure, see 14000-14300, 15000-15261, 15570-15770)

| 11600 | Excision, malignant lesion including margins, trunk, arms, or legs; excised diameter 0.5 cm or less |

| 11601 | excised diameter 0.6 to 1.0 cm |

| 11602 | excised diameter 1.1 to 2.0 cm |

| 11603 | excised diameter 2.1 to 3.0 cm |

| 11604 | excised diameter 3.1 to 4.0 cm |

| 11606 | excised diameter over 4.0 cm |

| 11620 | Excision, malignant lesion including margins, scalp, neck, hands, feet, genitalia; excised diameter 0.5 cm or less |

| 11621 | excised diameter 0.6 to 1.0 cm |

| 11622 | excised diameter 1.1 to 2.0 cm |

| 11623 | excised diameter 2.1 to 3.0 cm |

| 11624 | excised diameter 3.1 to 4.0 cm |

| 11626 | excised diameter over 4.0 cm |

● New Code   ▲ Revised Code   + Add-On Code   ⊘ Modifier -51 Exempt

11640 Excision, malignant lesion including margins, face, ears, eyelids, nose, lips; excised diameter 0.5 cm or less

11641 excised diameter 0.6 to 1.0 cm

11642 excised diameter 1.1 to 2.0 cm

11643 excised diameter 2.1 to 3.0 cm

11644 excised diameter 3.1 to 4.0 cm

11646 excised diameter over 4.0 cm

(For eyelids involving more than skin, see also 67800 et seq)

NAILS

(For drainage of paronychia or onychia, see 10060, 10061)

11719 Trimming of nondystrophic nails, any number

11720 Debridement of nail(s) by any method(s); one to five

11721 six or more

11730 Avulsion of nail plate, partial or complete, simple; single

+ 11732 each additional nail plate (List separately in addition to code for primary procedure)

(Use 11732 in conjunction with code 11730)

11740 Evacuation of subungual hematoma

11750 Excision of nail and nail matrix, partial or complete, (eg, ingrown or deformed nail) for permanent removal;

11752 with amputation of tuft of distal phalanx

(For skin graft, if used, use 15050)

11755 Biopsy of nail unit (eg, plate, bed, matrix, hyponychium, proximal and lateral nail folds) (separate procedure)

11760 Repair of nail bed

11762 Reconstruction of nail bed with graft

	Separate Procedure		Unlisted Procedure		CCI Comp. Code		Non-specific Procedure

235

| 11765 | Wedge excision of skin of nail fold (eg, for ingrown toenail) |

PILONIDAL CYST

| 11770 | Excision of pilonidal cyst or sinus; simple |

| 11771 | extensive |

| 11772 | complicated |

(For incision of pilonidal cyst, see 10080, 10081)

INTRODUCTION

| 11900 | Injection, intralesional; up to and including seven lesions |

| 11901 | more than seven lesions |

(11900, 11901 are not to be used for preoperative local anesthetic injection)

(For veins, see 36470, 36471)

(For intralesional chemotherapy administration, see 96405, 96406)

| 11920 | Tattooing, intradermal introduction of insoluble opaque pigments to correct color defects of skin, including micropigmentation; 6.0 sq cm or less |

| 11921 | 6.1 to 20.0 sq cm |

+ 11922   each additional 20.0 sq cm (List separately in addition to code for primary procedure)

(Use 11922 in conjunction with code 11921)

| 11950 | Subcutaneous injection of filling material (eg, collagen); 1 cc or less |

| 11951 | 1.1 to 5.0 cc |

| 11952 | 5.1 to 10.0 cc |

| 11954 | over 10.0 cc |

| 11960 | Insertion of tissue expander(s) for other than breast, including subsequent expansion |

● New Code   ▲ Revised Code   + Add-On Code   ⊘ Modifier -51 Exempt

(For breast reconstruction with tissue expander(s), use 19357)

11970 Replacement of tissue expander with permanent prosthesis

11971 Removal of tissue expander(s) without insertion of prosthesis

11975 Insertion, implantable contraceptive capsules

11976 Removal, implantable contraceptive capsules

11977 Removal with reinsertion, implantable contraceptive capsules

11980 Subcutaneous hormone pellet implantation (implantation of estradiol and/or testosterone pellets beneath the skin)

11981 Insertion, non-biodegradable drug delivery implant

11982 Removal, non-biodegradable drug delivery implant

11983 Removal with reinsertion, non-biodegradable drug delivery implant

REPAIR (CLOSURE)

To be able to code wound repair appropriately, the site, length of wound in centimeters and type of repair must be documented in the medical record. Review the definitions of simple, intermediate and complex repair in the current CPT coding system.

Multiple wound repairs from the same body site (category of codes) that were repaired using the same type of closure (simple, intermediate, or complex) should be coded as one wound. Add the measurements of each wound and assign a single code for the repair.

Simple exploration of nerves, blood vessels or tendons exposed in an open wound are integral part of the wound repair treatment and should not be coded separately. If the wound requires enlargement, extension of dissection, debridement, removal of foreign body, ligation or coagulation of minor subcutaneous and/or muscular blood vessel(s), of the subcutaneous tissue, muscle fascia, and/or muscle, not requiring thoracotomy or laparotomy, use wound exploration codes (20100-20103), as appropriate.

REPAIR — SIMPLE

12001 Simple repair of superficial wounds of scalp, neck, axillae, external genitalia, trunk and/or extremities (including hands and feet); 2.5 cm or less

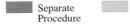 Separate Procedure    Unlisted Procedure   CCI Comp. Code   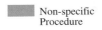 Non-specific Procedure

12002   2.6 cm to 7.5 cm

12004   7.6 cm to 12.5 cm

12005   12.6 cm to 20.0 cm

12006   20.1 cm to 30.0 cm

12007   over 30.0 cm

12011   Simple repair of superficial wounds of face, ears, eyelids, nose, lips and/or mucous membranes; 2.5 cm or less

12013   2.6 cm to 5.0 cm

12014   5.1 cm to 7.5 cm

12015   7.6 cm to 12.5 cm

12016   12.6 cm to 20.0 cm

12017   20.1 cm to 30.0 cm

12018   over 30.0 cm

12020   Treatment of superficial wound dehiscence; simple closure

12021   with packing

(For extensive or complicated secondary wound closure, use 13160)

REPAIR — INTERMEDIATE

12031   Layer closure of wounds of scalp, axillae, trunk and/or extremities (excluding hands and feet); 2.5 cm or less

12032   2.6 cm to 7.5 cm

12034   7.6 cm to 12.5 cm

12035   12.6 cm to 20.0 cm

12036   20.1 cm to 30.0 cm

12037   over 30.0 cm

● New Code   ▲ Revised Code   ✛ Add-On Code   ⊘ Modifier -51 Exempt

| 12041 | Layer closure of wounds of neck, hands, feet and/or external genitalia; 2.5 cm or less |

| 12042 | 2.6 cm to 7.5 cm |

| 12044 | 7.6 cm to 12.5 cm |

| 12045 | 12.6 cm to 20.0 cm |

| 12046 | 20.1 cm to 30.0 cm |

| 12047 | over 30.0 cm |

| 12051 | Layer closure of wounds of face, ears, eyelids, nose, lips and/or mucous membranes; 2.5 cm or less |

| 12052 | 2.6 cm to 5.0 cm |

| 12053 | 5.1 cm to 7.5 cm |

| 12054 | 7.6 cm to 12.5 cm |

| 12055 | 12.6 cm to 20.0 cm |

| 12056 | 20.1 cm to 30.0 cm |

| 12057 | over 30.0 cm |

REPAIR — COMPLEX

(For full thickness repair of lip or eyelid, see respective anatomical subsections)

| 13100 | Repair, complex, trunk; 1.1 cm to 2.5 cm |

(For 1.0 cm or less, see simple or intermediate repairs)

| 13101 | 2.6 cm to 7.5 cm |

| + 13102 | each additional 5 cm or less (List separately in addition to code for primary procedure) |

(Use 13102 in conjunction with code 13101)

| 13120 | Repair, complex, scalp, arms, and/or legs; 1.1 cm to 2.5 cm |

(For 1.0 cm or less, see simple or intermediate repairs)

239

 Separate Procedure   Unlisted Procedure   CCI Comp. Code   Non-specific Procedure

13121 2.6 cm to 7.5 cm

+ **13122** each additional 5 cm or less (List separately in addition to code for primary procedure)

(Use 13122 in conjunction with 13121)

13131 Repair, complex, forehead, cheeks, chin, mouth, neck, axillae, genitalia, hands and/or feet; 1.1 cm to 2.5 cm

(For 1.0 cm or less, see simple or intermediate repairs)

13132 2.6 cm to 7.5 cm

+ **13133** each additional 5 cm or less (List separately in addition to code for primary procedure)

(Use 13133 in conjunction with 13132)

13150 Repair, complex, eyelids, nose, ears and/or lips; 1.0 cm or less

(See also 40650-40654, 67961-67975)

13151 1.1 cm to 2.5 cm

13152 2.6 cm to 7.5 cm

+ **13153** each additional 5 cm or less (List separately in addition to code for primary procedure)

(Use 13153 in conjunction with code 13152)

13160 Secondary closure of surgical wound or dehiscence, extensive or complicated

(For packing or simple secondary wound closure, see 12020, 12021)

ADJACENT TISSUE TRANSFER OR REARRANGEMENT

Codes for adjacent tissue transfer or rearrangement (14000-14350) are determined by the size and location of the defect site. Excision of lesions performed prior to an adjacent tissue transfer or rearrangement are included in codes 14000 to 14350.

14000 Adjacent tissue transfer or rearrangement, trunk; defect 10 sq cm or less

14001 defect 10.1 sq cm to 30.0 sq cm

---

240 ● New Code ▲ Revised Code + Add-On Code ⊘ Modifier -51 Exempt

14020 Adjacent tissue transfer or rearrangement, scalp, arms and/or legs; defect 10 sq cm or less

14021   defect 10.1 sq cm to 30.0 sq cm

14040 Adjacent tissue transfer or rearrangement, forehead, cheeks, chin, mouth, neck, axillae, genitalia, hands and/or feet; defect 10 sq cm or less

14041   defect 10.1 sq cm to 30.0 sq cm

14060 Adjacent tissue transfer or rearrangement, eyelids, nose, ears and/or lips; defect 10 sq cm or less

14061   defect 10.1 sq cm to 30.0 sq cm

(For eyelid, full thickness, see 67961 et seq)

14300 Adjacent tissue transfer or rearrangement, more than 30 sq cm, unusual or complicated, any area

14350 Filleted finger or toe flap, including preparation of recipient site

FREE SKIN GRAFTS

When coding free skin grafts, the choice of CPT codes is based on the size and location of the defect (recipient area) and the type of graft to be used. The graft CPT codes include simple debridement of granulations or recent avulsion.

When a primary procedure such as orbitectomy, radical mastectomy or deep tumor removal requires skin graft for definite closure, use CPT codes from the appropriate anatomical subsection for the primary procedure and CPT codes from the series 15000-15416 for the skin graft. Note that the repair of a donor site requiring skin graft or local flaps should be coded as an additional procedure. HCPCS Level II codes for medical and surgical supplies, A4000-A4999, may be used to report supplies and materials provided to Medicare patients if the supplies and materials are not considered to be included with or part of the basic service(s) or procedure(s).

(Use 15000 for initial wound preparation)

(Use 15100-15261 for autogenous skin grafts)

(For microvascular flaps, see 15756-15758)

15000 Surgical preparation or creation of recipient site by excision of open wounds, burn eschar, or scar (including subcutaneous tissues); first 100 sq cm or one percent of body area of infants and children

241

 Separate Procedure    Unlisted Procedure   CCI Comp. Code   Non-specific Procedure

(For appropriate skin grafts, see 15050-15261; list the free graft separately by its procedure number when the graft, immediate or delayed, is applied)

+ 15001   each additional 100 sq cm or each additional one percent of body area of infants and children (List separately in addition to code for primary procedure)

(Use code 15001 in conjunction with code 15000)

(For excision of benign lesions, see 11400-11471)

(For excision of malignant lesions, see 11600-11646)

(For excision with alloplastic dressing, use 15000 only)

(For excision with immediate skin grafting use 15050-15261 in addition to 15000)

(For excision with immediate allograft placement use 15350 in addition to 15000)

(For excision with immediate xenograft placement use 15400 in addition to 15000)

15050   Pinch graft, single or multiple, to cover small ulcer, tip of digit, or other minimal open area (except on face), up to defect size 2 cm diameter

15100   Split graft, trunk, arms, legs; first 100 sq cm or less, or one percent of body area of infants and children (except 15050)

+ 15101   each additional 100 sq cm, or each additional one percent of body area of infants and children, or part thereof (List separately in addition to code for primary procedure)

(Use 15101 in conjunction with code 15100)

15120   Split graft, face, scalp, eyelids, mouth, neck, ears, orbits, genitalia, hands, feet and/or multiple digits; first 100 sq cm or less, or one percent of body area of infants and children (except 15050)

+ 15121   each additional 100 sq cm, or each additional one percent of body area of infants and children, or part thereof (List separately in addition to code for primary procedure)

(Use 15121 in conjunction with code 15120)

(For eyelids, see also 67961 et seq)

● New Code   ▲ Revised Code   + Add-On Code   ⊘ Modifier -51 Exempt

15200   Full thickness graft, free, including direct closure of donor site, trunk; 20 sq cm or less

+ 15201   each additional 20 sq cm (List separately in addition to code for primary procedure)

(Use 15201 in conjunction with 15200)

15220   Full thickness graft, free, including direct closure of donor site, scalp, arms, and/or legs; 20 sq cm or less

+ 15221   each additional 20 sq cm (List separately in addition to code for primary procedure)

(Use 15221 in conjunction with 15220)

15240   Full thickness graft, free, including direct closure of donor site, forehead, cheeks, chin, mouth, neck, axillae, genitalia, hands, and/or feet; 20 sq cm or less

(For finger tip graft, use 15050)

(For repair of syndactyly, fingers, see 26560-26562)

+ 15241   each additional 20 sq cm (List separately in addition to code for primary procedure)

(Use 15241 in conjunction with code 15240)

15260   Full thickness graft, free, including direct closure of donor site, nose, ears, eyelids, and/or lips; 20 sq cm or less

+ 15261   each additional 20 sq cm (List separately in addition to code for primary procedure)

(Use 15261 in conjunction with code 15260)

(For eyelids, see also 67961 et seq)

(Repair of donor site requiring skin graft or local flaps, to be added as additional separate procedure)

15342   Application of bilaminate skin substitute/neodermis; 25 sq cm

+ 15343   each additional 25 sq cm (List separately in addition to code for primary procedure)

(Use 15343 in conjunction with code 15342)

15350   Application of allograft, skin; 100 sq cm or less

243

 Separate Procedure   Unlisted Procedure   CCI Comp. Code   Non-specific Procedure

(For staged tissue graft implantation, use modifier -58)

+ 15351   each additional 100 sq cm (List separately in addition to code for primary procedure)

(Use 15351 in conjunction with code 15350)

15400   Application of xenograft, skin; 100 sq cm or less

+ 15401   each additional 100 sq cm (List separately in addition to code for primary procedure)

(Use 15401 in conjunction with code 15400)

FLAPS (SKIN AND/OR DEEP TISSUES)

(For microvascular flaps, see 15756-15758)

15570   Formation of direct or tubed pedicle, with or without transfer; trunk

15572   scalp, arms, or legs

15574   forehead, cheeks, chin, mouth, neck, axillae, genitalia, hands or feet

15576   eyelids, nose, ears, lips, or intraoral

15600   Delay of flap or sectioning of flap (division and inset); at trunk

15610   at scalp, arms, or legs

15620   at forehead, cheeks, chin, neck, axillae, genitalia, hands, or feet

15630   at eyelids, nose, ears, or lips

15650   Transfer, intermediate, of any pedicle flap (eg, abdomen to wrist, Walking tube), any location

(For eyelids, nose, ears, or lips, see also anatomical area)

(For revision, defatting or rearranging of transferred pedicle flap or skin graft, see 13100-14300)

(Procedures 15732-15738 are described by donor site of the muscle, myocutaneous, or fasciocutaneous flap)

15732 Muscle, myocutaneous, or fasciocutaneous flap; head and neck (eg, temporalis, masseter muscle, sternocleidomastoid, levator scapulae)

15734 trunk

15736 upper extremity

15738 lower extremity

OTHER FLAPS AND GRAFTS

15740 Flap; island pedicle

15750 neurovascular pedicle

15756 Free muscle or myocutaneous flap with microvascular anastomosis

(Do not report code 69990 in addition to code 15756)

15757 Free skin flap with microvascular anastomosis

(Do not report code 69990 in addition to code 15757)

15758 Free fascial flap with microvascular anastomosis

(Do not report code 69990 in addition to code 15758)

15760 Graft; composite (eg, full thickness of external ear or nasal ala), including primary closure, donor area

15770 derma-fat-fascia

15775 Punch graft for hair transplant; 1 to 15 punch grafts

15776 more than 15 punch grafts

(For strip transplant, use 15220)

OTHER PROCEDURES

15780 Dermabrasion; total face (eg, for acne scarring, fine wrinkling, rhytids, general keratosis)

15781 segmental, face

15782 regional, other than face

245

Separate   Unlisted   CCI Comp.   Non-specific
Procedure   Procedure   Code   Procedure

| 15783 | superficial, any site, (eg, tattoo removal) |

| 15786 | Abrasion; single lesion (eg, keratosis, scar) |

+ 15787   each additional four lesions or less (List separately in addition to code for primary procedure)

(Use 15787 in conjunction with code 15786)

| 15788 | Chemical peel, facial; epidermal |

| 15789 | dermal |

| 15792 | Chemical peel, nonfacial; epidermal |

| 15793 | dermal |

| 15810 | Salabrasion; 20 sq cm or less |

| 15811 | over 20 sq cm |

| 15819 | Cervicoplasty |

| 15820 | Blepharoplasty, lower eyelid; |

| 15821 | with extensive herniated fat pad |

| 15822 | Blepharoplasty, upper eyelid; |

| 15823 | with excessive skin weighting down lid |

(For bilateral blepharoplasty, add modifier -50)

| 15824 | Rhytidectomy; forehead |

(For repair of brow ptosis, use 67900)

| 15825 | neck with platysmal tightening (platysmal flap, P-flap) |

| 15826 | glabellar frown lines |

| 15828 | cheek, chin, and neck |

| 15829 | superficial musculoaponeurotic system (SMAS) flap |

(For bilateral rhytidectomy, add modifier -50)

● New Code   ▲ Revised Code   + Add-On Code   ⦸ Modifier -51 Exempt

15831 Excision, excessive skin and subcutaneous tissue (including lipectomy); abdomen (abdominoplasty)

15832 thigh

15833 leg

15834 hip

15835 buttock

15836 arm

15837 forearm or hand

15838 submental fat pad

15839 other area

(For bilateral procedure, add modifier -50)

15840 Graft for facial nerve paralysis; free fascia graft (including obtaining fascia)

(For bilateral procedure, add modifier -50)

15841 free muscle graft (including obtaining graft)

15842 free muscle flap by microsurgical technique

(Do not report code 69990 in addition to code 15842)

15845 regional muscle transfer

(For intravenous fluorescein examination of blood flow in graft or flap, use 15860)

(For nerve transfers, decompression, or repair, see 64831-64876, 64905, 64907, 69720, 69725, 69740, 69745, 69955)

15850 Removal of sutures under anesthesia (other than local), same surgeon

15851 Removal of sutures under anesthesia (other than local), other surgeon

15852 Dressing change (for other than burns) under anesthesia (other than local)

| Separate Procedure | Unlisted Procedure | CCI Comp. Code | Non-specific Procedure |

247

15860 Intravenous injection of agent (eg, fluorescein) to test vascular flow in flap or graft

15876 Suction assisted lipectomy; head and neck

15877 trunk

15878 upper extremity

15879 lower extremity

PRESSURE ULCERS (DECUBITUS ULCERS)

15920 Excision, coccygeal pressure ulcer, with coccygectomy; with primary suture

15922 with flap closure

15931 Excision, sacral pressure ulcer, with primary suture;

15933 with ostectomy

15934 Excision, sacral pressure ulcer, with skin flap closure;

15935 with ostectomy

15936 Excision, sacral pressure ulcer, in preparation for muscle or myocutaneous flap or skin graft closure;

15937 with ostectomy

(For repair of defect using muscle or myocutaneous flap, use code(s) 15734 and/or 15738 in addition to 15936, 15937. For repair of defect using split skin graft, use codes 15100 and/or 15101 in addition to 15936, 15937)

15940 Excision, ischial pressure ulcer, with primary suture;

15941 with ostectomy (ischiectomy)

15944 Excision, ischial pressure ulcer, with skin flap closure;

15945 with ostectomy

15946 Excision, ischial pressure ulcer, with ostectomy, in preparation for muscle or myocutaneous flap or skin graft closure

(For repair of defect using muscle or myocutaneous flap, use code(s) 15734 and/or 15738 in addition to 15946. For repair of defect using split skin graft, use codes 15100 and/or 15101 in addition to 15946)

15950 Excision, trochanteric pressure ulcer, with primary suture;

15951 with ostectomy

15952 Excision, trochanteric pressure ulcer, with skin flap closure;

15953 with ostectomy

15956 Excision, trochanteric pressure ulcer, in preparation for muscle or myocutaneous flap or skin graft closure;

15958 with ostectomy

(For repair of defect using muscle or myocutaneous flap, use code(s) 15734 and/or 15738 in addition to 15956, 15958. For repair of defect using split skin graft, use codes 15100 and/or 15101 in addition to 15956, 15958)

15999 Unlisted procedure, excision pressure ulcer

(For free skin graft to close ulcer or donor site, see 15000 et seq)

BURNS, LOCAL TREATMENT

(For skin graft, see 15100-15650)

16000 Initial treatment, first degree burn, when no more than local treatment is required

16010 Dressings and/or debridement, initial or subsequent; under anesthesia, small

16015 under anesthesia, medium or large, or with major debridement

16020 without anesthesia, office or hospital, small

16025 without anesthesia, medium (eg, whole face or whole extremity)

16030 without anesthesia, large (eg, more than one extremity)

16035   Escharotomy; initial incision

+ **16036**   each additional incision (List separately in addition to code for primary procedure)

(Use 16036 in conjunction with code 16035)

(For debridement, curettement of burn wound, see 16010-16030)

DESTRUCTION

(For destruction of lesion(s) in specific anatomic sites, see 40820, 46900-46917, 46924, 54050-54057, 54065, 56501, 56515, 57061, 57065, 67850, 68135)

(For paring or cutting of benign hyperkeratotic lesions (eg, corns or calluses), see 11055-11057)

(For sharp removal or electrosurgical destruction of skin tags and fibrocutaneous tags, see 11200, 11201)

(For cryotherapy of acne, use 17340)

(For initiation or follow-up care of topical chemotherapy (eg, 5-FU or similar agents), see appropriate office visits)

(For shaving of epidermal or dermal lesions, see 11300-11313)

DESTRUCTION, BENIGN OR PREMALIGNANT LESIONS

17000   Destruction (eg, laser surgery, electrosurgery, cryosurgery, chemosurgery, surgical curettement), all benign or premalignant lesions (eg, actinic keratoses) other than skin tags or cutaneous vascular proliferative lesions; first lesion

+ **17003**   second through 14 lesions, each (List separately in addition to code for first lesion)

(Use 17003 in conjunction with 17000)

⊘ 17004   Destruction (eg, laser surgey, electrosurgery, cryosurgery, chemosurgery, surgical curettement), all benign or premalignant lesions (eg, actinic keratoses) other than skin tags or cutaneous vascular proliferative lesions; 15 or more lesions

(Do not report 17004 in conjunction with codes 17000-17003)

17106   Destruction of cutaneous vascular proliferative lesions (eg, laser technique); less than 10 sq cm

17107   10.0 to 50.0 sq cm

250

● New Code	▲ Revised Code	+ Add-On Code	⊘ Modifier -51 Exempt

17108   over 50.0 sq cm

17110   Destruction (eg, laser surgery, electrosurgery, cryosurgery, chemosurgery, surgical curettement), of flat warts, molluscum contagiosum, or milia; up to 14 lesions

17111   15 or more lesions

(For destruction of common or plantar warts, see 17000, 17003, 17004)

17250   Chemical cauterization of granulation tissue (proud flesh, sinus or fistula)

(17250 is not to be used with removal or excision codes for the same lesion)

DESTRUCTION, MALIGNANT LESIONS, ANY METHOD

17260   Destruction, malignant lesion (eg, laser surgery, electrosurgery, cryosurgery, chemosurgery, surgical curettement), trunk, arms or legs; lesion diameter 0.5 cm or less

17261   lesion diameter 0.6 to 1.0 cm

17262   lesion diameter 1.1 to 2.0 cm

17263   lesion diameter 2.1 to 3.0 cm

17264   lesion diameter 3.1 to 4.0 cm

17266   lesion diameter over 4.0 cm

17270   Destruction, malignant lesion (eg, laser surgery, electrosurgery, cryosurgery, chemosurgery, surgical curettement), scalp, neck, hands, feet, genitalia; lesion diameter 0.5 cm or less

17271   lesion diameter 0.6 to 1.0 cm

17272   lesion diameter 1.1 to 2.0 cm

17273   lesion diameter 2.1 to 3.0 cm

17274   lesion diameter 3.1 to 4.0 cm

17276   lesion diameter over 4.0 cm

251

 Separate Procedure    Unlisted Procedure   CCI Comp. Code   Non-specific Procedure

17280	Destruction, malignant lesion, (eg, laser surgery, electrosurgery, cryosurgery, chemosurgery, surgical curettement), face, ears, eyelids, nose, lips, mucous membrane; lesion diameter 0.5 cm or less
17281	lesion diameter 0.6 to 1.0 cm
17282	lesion diameter 1.1 to 2.0 cm
17283	lesion diameter 2.1 to 3.0 cm
17284	lesion diameter 3.1 to 4.0 cm
17286	lesion diameter over 4.0 cm

MOHS MICROGRAPHIC SURGERY

⊘ **17304** Chemosurgery (Mohs micrographic technique), including removal of all gross tumor, surgical excision of tissue specimens, mapping, color coding of specimens, microscopic examination of specimens by the surgeon, and complete histopathologic preparation including the first routine stain (eg, hematoxylin and eosin, toluidine blue); first stage, fresh tissue technique, up to 5 specimens

(If additional special pathology procedures, stains or immunostains are required, use 88311-88314, 88342)

⊘ **17305** second stage, fixed or fresh tissue, up to 5 specimens

⊘ **17306** third stage, fixed or fresh tissue, up to 5 specimens

⊘ **17307** additional stage(s), up to 5 specimens, each stage

+ **17310** each additional specimen, after the first 5 specimens, fixed or fresh tissue, any stage (List separately in addition to code for primary procedure)

(Use 17310 in conjunction with codes 17304-17307)

OTHER PROCEDURES

17340	Cryotherapy (CO_2 slush, liquid N_2) for acne
17360	Chemical exfoliation for acne (eg, acne paste, acid)
17380	Electrolysis epilation, each 1/2 hour

252 ● New Code ▲ Revised Code + Add-On Code ⊘ Modifier -51 Exempt

(For actinotherapy, use 96900)

17999 Unlisted procedure, skin, mucous membrane and subcutaneous tissue

BREAST

INCISION

19000 Puncture aspiration of cyst of breast;

+ 19001 each additional cyst (List separately in addition to code for primary procedure)

(Use 19001 in conjunction with code 19000)

(If imaging guidance is performed, see 76095, 76096, 76393, 76942)

19020 Mastotomy with exploration or drainage of abscess, deep

19030 Injection procedure only for mammary ductogram or galactogram

(For radiological supervision and interpretation, see 76086, 76088)

(For catheter lavage of mammary ducts for collection of cytology specimens, use Category III codes 0046T, 0047T)

EXCISION

(All codes for bilateral procedures have been deleted. To report, add modifier -50)

19100 Biopsy of breast; percutaneous, needle core, not using imaging guidance (separate procedure)

(For fine needle aspiration, use 10021)

(For image guided breast biopsy, see 19102, 19103, 10022)

19101 open, incisional

19102 percutaneous, needle core, using imaging guidance

(For placement of percutaneous localization clip, use 19295)

19103 percutaneous, automated vacuum assisted or rotating biopsy device, using imaging guidance

							253
	Separate Procedure		Unlisted Procedure		CCI Comp. Code		Non-specific Procedure

(For imaging guidance performed in conjunction with 19102, 19103, see 76095, 76096, 76360, 76393, 76942)

(For placement of percutaneous localization clip, use 19295)

19110 Nipple exploration, with or without excision of a solitary lactiferous duct or a papilloma lactiferous duct

19112 Excision of lactiferous duct fistula

19120 Excision of cyst, fibroadenoma, or other benign or malignant tumor, aberrant breast tissue, duct lesion, nipple or areolar lesion (except 19140), open, male or female, one or more lesions

19125 Excision of breast lesion identified by preoperative placement of radiological marker, open; single lesion

+ 19126 each additional lesion separately identified by a preoperative radiological marker (List separately in addition to code for primary procedure)

(Use 19126 in conjunction with code 19125)

19140 Mastectomy for gynecomastia

19160 Mastectomy, partial;

19162 with axillary lymphadenectomy

19180 Mastectomy, simple, complete

(For immediate or delayed insertion of implant, use 19340 or 19342)

(For gynecomastia, use 19140)

19182 Mastectomy, subcutaneous

19200 Mastectomy, radical, including pectoral muscles, axillary lymph nodes

19220 Mastectomy, radical, including pectoral muscles, axillary and internal mammary lymph nodes (Urban type operation)

19240 Mastectomy, modified radical, including axillary lymph nodes, with or without pectoralis minor muscle, but excluding pectoralis major muscle

● New Code   ▲ Revised Code   + Add-On Code   ⊘ Modifier -51 Exempt

SURGERY

19260   Excision of chest wall tumor including ribs

19271   Excision of chest wall tumor involving ribs, with plastic reconstruction; without mediastinal lymphadenectomy

19272   with mediastinal lymphadenectomy

INTRODUCTION

19290   Preoperative placement of needle localization wire, breast;

+ **19291**   each additional lesion (List separately in addition to code for primary procedure)

(Use 19291 in conjunction with code 19290)

(For radiological supervision and interpretation see 76095, 76096, 76942)

+ **19295**   Image guided placement, metallic localization clip, percutaneous, during breast biopsy (List separately in addition to code for primary procedure)

(Use 19295 in conjunction with codes 19102, 19103)

REPAIR AND/OR RECONSTRUCTION

19316   Mastopexy

19318   Reduction mammaplasty

19324   Mammaplasty, augmentation; without prosthetic implant

19325   with prosthetic implant

(For flap or graft, use also appropriate number)

19328   Removal of intact mammary implant

19330   Removal of mammary implant material

19340   Immediate insertion of breast prosthesis following mastopexy, mastectomy or in reconstruction

19342   Delayed insertion of breast prosthesis following mastopexy, mastectomy or in reconstruction

(For supply of implant, use 99070)

255

 Separate Procedure   Unlisted Procedure   CCI Comp. Code   Non-specific Procedure

(For preparation of custom breast implant, use 19396)

19350 Nipple/areola reconstruction

19355 Correction of inverted nipples

19357 Breast reconstruction, immediate or delayed, with tissue expander, including subsequent expansion

19361 Breast reconstruction with latissimus dorsi flap, with or without prosthetic implant

19364 Breast reconstruction with free flap

(Do not report code 69990 in addition to code 19364)

(19364 includes harvesting of the flap, microvascular transfer, closure of the donor site, and inset shaping the flap into a breast)

19366 Breast reconstruction with other technique

(For operating microscope, use 69990)

(For insertion of prosthesis, use also 19340 or 19342)

19367 Breast reconstruction with transverse rectus abdominis myocutaneous flap (TRAM), single pedicle, including closure of donor site;

19368 with microvascular anastomosis (supercharging)

(Do not report code 69990 in addition to code 19368)

19369 Breast reconstruction with transverse rectus abdominis myocutaneous flap (TRAM), double pedicle, including closure of donor site

19370 Open periprosthetic capsulotomy, breast

19371 Periprosthetic capsulectomy, breast

19380 Revision of reconstructed breast

19396 Preparation of moulage for custom breast implant

● New Code ▲ Revised Code + Add-On Code ⊘ Modifier -51 Exempt

OTHER PROCEDURES

(For microwave thermotherapy of the breast, use Category III code 0061T)

19499   Unlisted procedure, breast

| | Separate Procedure | | Unlisted Procedure | | CCI Comp. Code | | Non-specific Procedure |

This page intentionally left blank.

● New
Code
▲ Revised
Code
✚ Add-On
Code
⊘ Modifier -51
Exempt

MUSCULOSKELETAL SYSTEM

Musculoskeletal procedure codes include the application and removal of the initial cast or traction device. Use codes in range 29000 to 29799 to report subsequent cast or traction-device applications. Review the instructional notes under the "Application of Casts and Strapping" to identify other uses for these codes.

The procedures and services listed in this section of the CPT coding system include the application and removal of the first cast or traction device only. Subsequent replacement of the cast and/or traction device may be coded using the cast and strapping procedure CPT codes appearing at the end of the section.

MISCELLANEOUS CODING RULES

Most bone, cartilage and fascia graft procedures include obtaining of the graft by the operating surgeon. When a surgical associate obtains the graft for the operating surgeon, the additional service should be coded and coded separately using CPT codes from the 20900-20926 range. In addition, a surgical modifier for assistant surgeon or co-surgeon should be included when reporting the associates services.

CPT codes 20100-20103 relate to treatment of wounds resulting from penetrating trauma (e.g., gunshot, stab wound). Use these codes for wound explorations only if the procedure does not require a thoracotomy or laparotomy and/or repairs to major structure(s) or major blood vessels.

The term "complicated" appears in some narratives in the musculoskeletal subsection. This term implies that an infection occurred, treatment was delayed, or the surgery took longer than usual to perform. Send supporting documentation when the codes containing this descriptor are assigned.

MUSC-
SKEL
29000

An intermediate repair associated with a musculoskeletal surgery is an integral portion of the surgery and should not be coded separately.

Code the injection codes according to the location of the joint injected or aspirated. Example: small joint = fingers, toes; intermediate joint = wrist, elbow; and major joint = shoulder, hip, or knee.

When removing a foreign body or performing soft tissue biopsy, determine the site and whether or not the foreign body/biopsy is superficial or deep.

FRACTURES

Remember to differentiate between the type of fracture and the type of treatment when coding fractures. Review the meanings of open and closed treatment of fractures. Dislocations must also be coded with emphasis on whether the treatment is open or closed.

259

 Separate Procedure   Unlisted Procedure   CCI Comp. Code   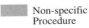 Non-specific Procedure

When coding the re-reduction of a fracture and/or dislocation performed by the primary physician, add modifier -76 to the procedure code. If the re-reduction were performed by another physician, then modifier -77 would be added to the procedure code.

GENERAL

INCISION

20000 Incision of soft tissue abscess (eg, secondary to osteomyelitis); superficial

20005 deep or complicated

WOUND EXPLORATION—TRAUMA (EG, PENETRATING GUNSHOT, STAB WOUND)

20100 Exploration of penetrating wound (separate procedure); neck

20101 chest

20102 abdomen/flank/back

20103 extremity

EXCISION

20150 Excision of epiphyseal bar, with or without autogenous soft tissue graft obtained through same fascial incision

(For aspiration of bone marrow, use 38220)

20200 Biopsy, muscle; superficial

20205 deep

20206 Biopsy, muscle, percutaneous needle

(If imaging guidance is performed, see 76360, 76393, 76942)

(For fine needle aspiration, use 10021 or 10022)

(For evaluation of fine needle aspirate, see 88172-88173)

(For excision of muscle tumor, deep, see specific anatomic section)

● New Code ▲ Revised Code + Add-On Code ⊘ Modifier -51 Exempt

20220 Biopsy, bone, trocar, or needle; superficial (eg, ilium, sternum, spinous process, ribs)

20225 deep (eg, vertebral body, femur)

(For bone marrow biopsy, use 38221)

(For radiologic supervision and interpretation, see 76003, 76360, 76393)

▲ **20240** Biopsy, bone, open; superficial (eg, ilium, sternum, spinous process, ribs, trochanter of femur)

20245 deep (eg, humerus, ischium, femur)

20250 Biopsy, vertebral body, open; thoracic

20251 lumbar or cervical

(For sequestrectomy, osteomyelitis or drainage of bone abscess, see anatomical area)

INTRODUCTION OR REMOVAL

(For injection procedure for arthrography, see anatomical area)

20500 Injection of sinus tract; therapeutic (separate procedure)

20501 diagnostic (sinogram)

(For radiological supervision and interpretation, use 76080)

20520 Removal of foreign body in muscle or tendon sheath; simple

20525 deep or complicated

20526 Injection, therapeutic (eg, local anesthetic, corticosteroid), carpal tunnel

20550 Injection(s); single tendon sheath, or ligament, aponeurosis (eg, plantar "fascia")

▲ **20551** single tendon origin/insertion

▲ **20552** Injection(s); single or multiple trigger point(s), one or two muscle(s)

261

 Separate Procedure

 Unlisted Procedure

 CCI Comp. Code

 Non-specific Procedure

20553   single or multiple trigger point(s), three or more muscle(s)

(If imaging guidance is performed, see 76003, 76393, 76942)

20600 Arthrocentesis, aspiration and/or injection; small joint or bursa (eg, fingers, toes)

20605   intermediate joint or bursa (eg, temporomandibular, acromioclavicular, wrist, elbow or ankle, olecranon bursa)

20610   major joint or bursa (eg, shoulder, hip, knee joint, subacromial bursa)

(If imaging guidance is performed, see 76003, 76360, 76393, 76942)

20612 Aspiration and/or injection of ganglion cyst(s) any location

(To report multiple ganglion cyst aspirations/injections, use 20612 and append modifier '-59')

20615 Aspiration and injection for treatment of bone cyst

20650 Insertion of wire or pin with application of skeletal traction, including removal (separate procedure)

⊘ **20660** Application of cranial tongs, caliper, or stereotactic frame, including removal (separate procedure)

20661 Application of halo, including removal; cranial

20662   pelvic

20663   femoral

20664 Application of halo, including removal, cranial, 6 or more pins placed, for thin skull osteology (eg, pediatric patients, hydrocephalus, osteogenesis imperfecta), requiring general anesthesia

20665 Removal of tongs or halo applied by another physician

20670 Removal of implant; superficial, (eg, buried wire, pin or rod) (separate procedure)

20680   deep (eg, buried wire, pin, screw, metal band, nail,rod or plate)

● New Code   ▲ Revised Code   + Add-On Code   ⊘ Modifier -51 Exempt

⊘ **20690** Application of a uniplane (pins or wires in one plane), unilateral, external fixation system

⊘ **20692** Application of a multiplane (pins or wires in more than one plane), unilateral, external fixation system (eg, Ilizarov, Monticelli type)

20693 Adjustment or revision of external fixation system requiring anesthesia (eg, new pin(s) or wire(s) and/or new ring(s) or bar(s))

20694 Removal, under anesthesia, of external fixation system

REPLANTATION

20802 Replantation, arm (includes surgical neck of humerus through elbow joint), complete amputation

20805 Replantation, forearm (includes radius and ulna to radial carpal joint), complete amputation

20808 Replantation, hand (includes hand through metacarpophalangeal joints), complete amputation

20816 Replantation, digit, excluding thumb (includes metacarpophalangeal joint to insertion of flexor sublimis tendon), complete amputation

20822 Replantation, digit, excluding thumb (includes distal tip to sublimis tendon insertion), complete amputation

20824 Replantation, thumb (includes carpometacarpal joint to MP joint), complete amputation

20827 Replantation, thumb (includes distal tip to MP joint), complete amputation

20838 Replantation, foot, complete amputation

GRAFTS (OR IMPLANTS)

(For spinal surgery bone graft(s) see codes 20930-20938)

⊘ **20900** Bone graft, any donor area; minor or small (eg, dowel or button)

⊘ **20902** major or large

 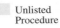

⊘ **20910** Cartilage graft; costochondral

⊘ **20912** nasal septum

(For ear cartilage, use 21235)

⊘ **20920** Fascia lata graft; by stripper

⊘ **20922** by incision and area exposure, complex or sheet

⊘ **20924** Tendon graft, from a distance (eg, palmaris, toe extensor, plantaris)

⊘ **20926** Tissue grafts, other (eg, paratenon, fat, dermis)

(Codes 20930-20938 are reported in addition to codes for the definitive procedure(s) without modifier -51)

⊘ **20930** Allograft for spine surgery only; morselized

⊘ **20931** structural

⊘ **20936** Autograft for spine surgery only (includes harvesting the graft); local (eg, ribs, spinous process, or laminar fragments) obtained from same incision

⊘ **20937** morselized (through separate skin or fascial incision)

⊘ **20938** structural, bicortical or tricortical (through separate skin or fascial incision)

(For needle aspiration of bone marrow for the purpose of bone grafting, use 38220)

OTHER PROCEDURES

20950 Monitoring of interstitial fluid pressure (includes insertion of device,eg, wick catheter technique, needle manometer technique) in detection of muscle compartment syndrome

20955 Bone graft with microvascular anastomosis; fibula

20956 iliac crest

20957 metatarsal

20962 other than fibula, iliac crest, or metatarsal

264

● New Code   ▲ Revised Code   ✚ Add-On Code   ⊘ Modifier -51 Exempt

(Do not report code 69990 in addition to codes 20955-20962)

20969   Free osteocutaneous flap with microvascular anastomosis; other than iliac crest, metatarsal, or great toe

20970   iliac crest

20972   metatarsal

20973   great toe with web space

(Do not report code 69990 in addition to codes 20969-20973)

(For great toe, wrap-around procedure, use 26551)

⊘ **20974**   Electrical stimulation to aid bone healing; noninvasive (nonoperative)

⊘ **20975**   invasive (operative)

20979   Low intensity ultrasound stimulation to aid bone healing, noninvasive (nonoperative)

● **20982**   Ablation, bone tumor(s) (eg, osteoid osteoma, metastasis) radiofrequency, percutaneous, including computed tomographic guidance

20999   Unlisted procedure, musculoskeletal system, general

HEAD

INCISION

(For drainage of superficial abscess and hematoma, use 20000)

(For removal of embedded foreign body from dentoalveolar structure, see 41805, 41806)

21010   Arthrotomy, temporomandibular joint

EXCISION

(For biopsy, see 20220, 20240)

21015   Radical resection of tumor (eg, malignant neoplasm), soft tissue of face or scalp

21025   Excision of bone (eg, for osteomyelitis or bone abscess); mandible

265

| Separate Procedure | Unlisted Procedure | CCI Comp. Code | Non-specific Procedure |

21026　　　facial bone(s)

21029　Removal by contouring of benign tumor of facial bone (eg, fibrous dysplasia)

21030　Excision of benign tumor or cyst of maxilla or zygoma by enucleation and curettage

21031　Excision of torus mandibularis

21032　Excision of maxillary torus palatinus

21034　Excision of malignant tumor of maxilla or zygoma

21040　Excision of benign tumor or cyst of mandible, by enucleation and/or curettage

(21041　deleted 2003 edition. For enucleation and/or curettage of benign cysts or tumors of mandible not requiring osteotomy, use 21040)

(For excision of benign tumor or cyst of mandible requiring osteotomy, see 21046-21047)

21044　Excision of malignant tumor of mandible;

21045　　　radical resection

(For bone graft, use 21215)

21046　Excision of benign tumor or cyst of mandible; requiring intra-oral osteotomy (eg, locally aggressive or destructive lesion(s))

21047　　　requiring extra-oral osteotomy and partial mandibulectomy (eg, locally aggressive or destructive lesion(s))

21048　Excision of benign tumor or cyst of maxilla; requiring intra-oral osteotomy (eg, locally aggressive or destructive lesion(s))

21049　　　requiring extra-oral osteotomy and partial maxillectomy (eg, locally aggressive or destructive lesion(s))

21050　Condylectomy, temporomandibular joint (separate procedure)

21060　Meniscectomy, partial or complete, temporomandibular joint (separate procedure)

266　● New Code　　▲ Revised Code　　＋ Add-On Code　　⊘ Modifier -51 Exempt

21070   Coronoidectomy (separate procedure)

INTRODUCTION OR REMOVAL

21076   Impression and custom preparation; surgical obturator prosthesis

21077   orbital prosthesis

21079   interim obturator prosthesis

21080   definitive obturator prosthesis

21081   mandibular resection prosthesis

21082   palatal augmentation prosthesis

21083   palatal lift prosthesis

21084   speech aid prosthesis

21085   oral surgical splint

21086   auricular prosthesis

21087   nasal prosthesis

21088   facial prosthesis

21089   Unlisted maxillofacial prosthetic procedure

21100   Application of halo type appliance for maxillofacial fixation, includes removal (separate procedure)

21110   Application of interdental fixation device for conditions other than fracture or dislocation, includes removal

(For removal of interdental fixation by another physician, see 20670-20680)

21116   Injection procedure for temporomandibular joint arthrography

(For radiological supervision and interpretation, use 70332. Do not report 76003 in addition to 70332)

| | Separate Procedure | | Unlisted Procedure | | CCI Comp. Code | | Non-specific Procedure |

REPAIR, REVISION AND/OR RECONSTRUCTION

(For cranioplasty, see 21179, 21180 and 62116, 62120, 62140-62147)

21120   Genioplasty; augmentation (autograft, allograft, prosthetic material)

21121   sliding osteotomy, single piece

21122   sliding osteotomies, two or more osteotomies (eg, wedge excision or bone wedge reversal for asymmetrical chin)

21123   sliding, augmentation with interpositional bone grafts (includes obtaining autografts)

21125   Augmentation, mandibular body or angle; prosthetic material

21127   with bone graft, onlay or interpositional (includes obtaining autograft)

21137   Reduction forehead; contouring only

21138   contouring and application of prosthetic material or bone graft (includes obtaining autograft)

21139   contouring and setback of anterior frontal sinus wall

21141   Reconstruction midface, LeFort I; single piece, segment movement in any direction (eg, for Long Face Syndrome), without bone graft

21142   two pieces, segment movement in any direction, without bone graft

21143   three or more pieces, segment movement in any direction, without bone graft

21145   single piece, segment movement in any direction, requiring bone grafts (includes obtaining autografts)

21146   two pieces, segment movement in any direction, requiring bone grafts (includes obtaining autografts) (eg, ungrafted unilateral alveolar cleft)

268

● New Code   ▲ Revised Code   + Add-On Code   ⊘ Modifier -51 Exempt

21147   three or more pieces, segment movement in any direction, requiring bone grafts (includes obtaining autografts) (eg, ungrafted bilateral alveolar cleft or multiple osteotomies)

21150   Reconstruction midface, LeFort II; anterior intrusion (eg, Treacher-Collins Syndrome)

21151   any direction, requiring bone grafts (includes obtaining autografts)

21154   Reconstruction midface, LeFort III (extracranial), any type, requiring bone grafts (includes obtaining autografts); without LeFort I

21155   with LeFort I

21159   Reconstruction midface, LeFort III (extra and intracranial) with forehead advancement (eg, mono bloc), requiring bone grafts (includes obtaining autografts); without LeFort I

21160   with LeFort I

21172   Reconstruction superior-lateral orbital rim and lower forehead, advancement or alteration, with or without grafts (includes obtaining autografts)

(For frontal or parietal craniotomy performed for craniosynostosis, use 61556)

21175   Reconstruction, bifrontal, superior-lateral orbital rims and lower forehead, advancement or alteration (eg, plagiocephaly, trigonocephaly, brachycephaly), with or without grafts (includes obtaining autografts)

(For bifrontal craniotomy performed for craniosynostosis, use 61557)

21179   Reconstruction, entire or majority of forehead and/or supraorbital rims; with grafts (allograft or prosthetic material)

21180   with autograft (includes obtaining grafts)

(For extensive craniectomy for multiple suture craniosynostosis, use only 61558 or 61559)

21181   Reconstruction by contouring of benign tumor of cranial bones (eg, fibrous dysplasia), extracranial

---

269

 Separate Procedure   Unlisted Procedure   CCI Comp. Code   Non-specific Procedure

21182 Reconstruction of orbital walls, rims, forehead, nasoethmoid complex following intra- and extracranial excision of benign tumor of cranial bone (eg, fibrous dysplasia), with multiple autografts (includes obtaining grafts); total area of bone grafting less than 40 sq cm

21183 total area of bone grafting greater than 40 sq cm but less than 80 sq cm

21184 total area of bone grafting greater than 80 sq cm

(For excision of benign tumor of cranial bones, see 61563, 61564)

21188 Reconstruction midface, osteotomies (other than LeFort type) and bone grafts (includes obtaining autografts)

21193 Reconstruction of mandibular rami, horizontal, vertical, C, or L osteotomy; without bone graft

21194 with bone graft (includes obtaining graft)

21195 Reconstruction of mandibular rami and/or body, sagittal split; without internal rigid fixation

21196 with internal rigid fixation

21198 Osteotomy, mandible, segmental;

21199 with genioglossus advancement

21206 Osteotomy, maxilla, segmental (eg, Wassmund or Schuchard)

21208 Osteoplasty, facial bones; augmentation (autograft, allograft, or prosthetic implant)

21209 reduction

21210 Graft, bone; nasal, maxillary or malar areas (includes obtaining graft)

(For cleft palate repair, see 42200-42225)

21215 mandible (includes obtaining graft)

21230 Graft; rib cartilage, autogenous, to face, chin, nose or ear (includes obtaining graft)

● New Code ▲ Revised Code + Add-On Code ⊘ Modifier -51 Exempt

21235   ear cartilage, autogenous, to nose or ear (includes obtaining graft)

21240   Arthroplasty, temporomandibular joint, with or without autograft (includes obtaining graft)

21242   Arthroplasty, temporomandibular joint, with allograft

21243   Arthroplasty, temporomandibular joint, with prosthetic joint replacement

21244   Reconstruction of mandible, extraoral, with transosteal bone plate (eg, mandibular staple bone plate)

21245   Reconstruction of mandible or maxilla, subperiosteal implant; partial

21246   complete

21247   Reconstruction of mandibular condyle with bone and cartilage autografts (includes obtaining grafts) (eg, for hemifacial microsomia)

21248   Reconstruction of mandible or maxilla, endosteal implant (eg, blade, cylinder); partial

21249   complete

21255   Reconstruction of zygomatic arch and glenoid fossa with bone and cartilage (includes obtaining autografts)

21256   Reconstruction of orbit with osteotomies (extracranial) and with bone grafts (includes obtaining autografts) (eg, micro-ophthalmia)

21260   Periorbital osteotomies for orbital hypertelorism, with bone grafts; extracranial approach

21261   combined intra- and extracranial approach

21263   with forehead advancement

21267   Orbital repositioning, periorbital osteotomies, unilateral, with bone grafts; extracranial approach

21268   combined intra- and extracranial approach

Separate Procedure · Unlisted Procedure · CCI Comp. Code · Non-specific Procedure

21270 Malar augmentation, prosthetic material

(For malar augmentation with bone graft, use 21210)

21275 Secondary revision of orbitocraniofacial reconstruction

21280 Medial canthopexy (separate procedure)

(For medial canthoplasty, use 67950)

21282 Lateral canthopexy

21295 Reduction of masseter muscle and bone (eg, for treatment of benign masseteric hypertrophy); extraoral approach

21296   intraoral approach

OTHER PROCEDURES

21299 Unlisted craniofacial and maxillofacial procedure

FRACTURE AND/OR DISLOCATION

21300 Closed treatment of skull fracture without operation

(For operative repair, see 62000-62010)

21310 Closed treatment of nasal bone fracture without manipulation

21315 Closed treatment of nasal bone fracture; without stabilization

21320   with stabilization

21325 Open treatment of nasal fracture; uncomplicated

21330   complicated, with internal and/or external skeletal fixation

21335   with concomitant open treatment of fractured septum

21336 Open treatment of nasal septal fracture, with or without stabilization

21337 Closed treatment of nasal septal fracture, with or without stabilization

21338 Open treatment of nasoethmoid fracture; without external fixation

● New Code   ▲ Revised Code   + Add-On Code   ⊘ Modifier -51 Exempt

21339   with external fixation

21340   Percutaneous treatment of nasoethmoid complex fracture, with splint, wire or headcap fixation, including repair of canthal ligaments and/or the nasolacrimal apparatus

21343   Open treatment of depressed frontal sinus fracture

21344   Open treatment of complicated (eg, comminuted or involving posterior wall) frontal sinus fracture, via coronal or multiple approaches

21345   Closed treatment of nasomaxillary complex fracture (LeFort II type), with interdental wire fixation or fixation of denture or splint

21346   Open treatment of nasomaxillary complex fracture (LeFort II type); with wiring and/or local fixation

21347   requiring multiple open approaches

21348   with bone grafting (includes obtaining graft)

21355   Percutaneous treatment of fracture of malar area, including zygomatic arch and malar tripod, with manipulation

21356   Open treatment of depressed zygomatic arch fracture (eg, Gillies approach)

21360   Open treatment of depressed malar fracture, including zygomatic arch and malar tripod

21365   Open treatment of complicated (eg, comminuted or involving cranial nerve foramina) fracture(s) of malar area, including zygomatic arch and malar tripod; with internal fixation and multiple surgical approaches

21366   with bone grafting (includes obtaining graft)

21385   Open treatment of orbital floor blowout fracture; transantral approach (Caldwell-Luc type operation)

21386   periorbital approach

21387   combined approach

| Separate Procedure | Unlisted Procedure | CCI Comp. Code | Non-specific Procedure |

21390   periorbital approach, with alloplastic or other implant

21395   periorbital approach with bone graft (includes obtaining graft)

21400   Closed treatment of fracture of orbit, except blowout; without manipulation

21401   with manipulation

21406   Open treatment of fracture of orbit, except blowout; without implant

21407   with implant

21408   with bone grafting (includes obtaining graft)

21421   Closed treatment of palatal or maxillary fracture (LeFort I type), with interdental wire fixation or fixation of denture or splint

21422   Open treatment of palatal or maxillary fracture (LeFort I type);

21423   complicated (comminuted or involving cranial nerve foramina), multiple approaches

21431   Closed treatment of craniofacial separation (LeFort III type) using interdental wire fixation of denture or splint

21432   Open treatment of craniofacial separation (LeFort III type); with wiring and/or internal fixation

21433   complicated (eg, comminuted or involving cranial nerve foramina), multiple surgical approaches

21435   complicated, utilizing internal and/or external fixation techniques (eg, head cap, halo device, and/or intermaxillary fixation)

(For removal of internal or external fixation device, use 20670)

21436   complicated, multiple surgical approaches, internal fixation, with bone grafting (includes obtaining graft)

21440   Closed treatment of mandibular or maxillary alveolar ridge fracture (separate procedure)

● New Code   ▲ Revised Code   + Add-On Code   ⊘ Modifier -51 Exempt

21445 Open treatment of mandibular or maxillary alveolar ridge fracture (separate procedure)

21450 Closed treatment of mandibular fracture; without manipulation

21451   with manipulation

21452 Percutaneous treatment of mandibular fracture, with external fixation

21453 Closed treatment of mandibular fracture with interdental fixation

21454 Open treatment of mandibular fracture with external fixation

21461 Open treatment of mandibular fracture; without interdental fixation

21462   with interdental fixation

21465 Open treatment of mandibular condylar fracture

21470 Open treatment of complicated mandibular fracture by multiple surgical approaches including internal fixation, interdental fixation, and/or wiring of dentures or splints

21480 Closed treatment of temporomandibular dislocation; initial or subsequent

21485   complicated (eg, recurrent requiring intermaxillary fixation or splinting), initial or subsequent

21490 Open treatment of temporomandibular dislocation

(For interdental wire fixation, use 21497)

21493 Closed treatment of hyoid fracture; without manipulation

21494   with manipulation

21495 Open treatment of hyoid fracture

(For treatment of fracture of larynx, see 31584-31586)

21497 Interdental wiring, for condition other than fracture

275

 Separate Procedure   Unlisted Procedure   CCI Comp. Code   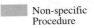 Non-specific Procedure

OTHER PROCEDURES

21499 Unlisted musculoskeletal procedure, head

(For unlisted craniofacial or maxillofacial procedure, use 21299)

NECK (SOFT TISSUES) AND THORAX

(For cervical spine and back, see 21920 et seq)

(For injection of fracture site or trigger point, use 20550)

INCISION

(For incision and drainage of abscess or hematoma, superficial, see 10060, 10140)

21501 Incision and drainage, deep abscess or hematoma, soft tissues of neck or thorax;

21502 with partial rib ostectomy

21510 Incision, deep, with opening of bone cortex (eg, for osteomyelitis or bone abscess), thorax

EXCISION

(For bone biopsy, see 20220-20251)

21550 Biopsy, soft tissue of neck or thorax

(For needle biopsy of soft tissue, use 20206)

21555 Excision tumor, soft tissue of neck or thorax; subcutaneous

21556 deep, subfascial, intramuscular

21557 Radical resection of tumor (eg, malignant neoplasm), soft tissue of neck or thorax

21600 Excision of rib, partial

(For radical resection of chest wall and rib cage for tumor, use 19260)

(For radical debridement of chest wall and rib cage for injury, see 11040-11044)

21610 Costotransversectomy (separate procedure)

276

● New Code ▲ Revised Code ✚ Add-On Code ⊘ Modifier -51 Exempt

21615	Excision first and/or cervical rib;
21616	with sympathectomy
21620	Ostectomy of sternum, partial
21627	Sternal debridement

(For debridement and closure, use 21750)

21630	Radical resection of sternum;
21632	with mediastinal lymphadenectomy

REPAIR, REVISION, AND/OR RECONSTRUCTION

(For superficial wound, see Integumentary System section under Repair, Simple)

● **21685**   Hyoid myotomy and suspension

21700	Division of scalenus anticus; without resection of cervical rib
21705	with resection of cervical rib
21720	Division of sternocleidomastoid for torticollis, open operation; without cast application

(For transection of spinal accessory and cervical nerves, see 63191, 64722)

21725	with cast application
21740	Reconstructive repair of pectus excavatum or carinatum; open
21742	minimally invasive approach (Nuss procedure), without thoracoscopy
21743	minimally invasive approach (Nuss procedure), with thoracoscopy
21750	Closure of median sternotomy separation with or without debridement (separate procedure)

FRACTURE AND/OR DISLOCATION

21800	Closed treatment of rib fracture, uncomplicated, each

277

Separate Procedure   Unlisted Procedure   CCI Comp. Code   Non-specific Procedure

21805 Open treatment of rib fracture without fixation, each

21810 Treatment of rib fracture requiring external fixation (flail chest)

21820 Closed treatment of sternum fracture

21825 Open treatment of sternum fracture with or without skeletal fixation

(For sternoclavicular dislocation, see 23520-23532)

OTHER PROCEDURES

21899 Unlisted procedure, neck or thorax

BACK AND FLANK

EXCISION

21920 Biopsy, soft tissue of back or flank; superficial

21925   deep

(For needle biopsy of soft tissue, use 20206)

21930 Excision, tumor, soft tissue of back or flank

21935 Radical resection of tumor (eg, malignant neoplasm), soft tissue of back or flank

SPINE (VERTEBRAL COLUMN)

(Do not append modifier -62 to bone graft code 20931)

(For injection procedure for myelography, use 62284)

(For injection procedure for diskography, see 62290, 62291)

(For injection procedure, chemonucleolysis, single or multiple leveles, use 62292)

(For injection procedure for facet joints, see 64470-64476, 64622-64627)

(For needle or trocar biopsy, see 20220-20225)

● New Code ▲ Revised Code + Add-On Code ⊘ Modifier -51 Exempt

EXCISION

(For bone biopsy, see 20220-20251)

22100 Partial excision of posterior vertebral component (eg, spinous process, lamina or facet) for intrinsic bony lesion, single vertebral segment; cervical

22101 thoracic

22102 lumbar

+ **22103** each additional segment (List separately in addition to code for primary procedure)

(Use 22103 in conjunction with codes 22100, 22101, 22102)

22110 Partial excision of vertebral body, for intrinsic bony lesion, without decompression of spinal cord or nerve root(s), single vertebral segment; cervical

22112 thoracic

22114 lumbar

+ **22116** each additional vertebral segment (List separately in addition to code for primary procedure)

(Use 22116 in conjunction with codes 22110, 22112, 22114)

OSTEOTOMY

22210 Osteotomy of spine, posterior or posterolateral approach, one vertebral segment; cervical

22212 thoracic

22214 lumbar

+ **22216** each additional vertebral segment (List separately in addition to primary procedure)

(Use 22216 in conjunction with codes 22210, 22212, 22214)

22220 Osteotomy of spine, including diskectomy, anterior approach, single vertebral segment; cervical

22222 thoracic

279

 Separate Procedure   Unlisted Procedure   CCI Comp. Code   Non-specific Procedure

| 22224 | lumbar |

+ 22226 each additional vertebral segment (List separately in addition to code for primary procedure)

(Use 22226 in conjunction with codes 22220, 22222, 22224)

FRACTURE AND/OR DISLOCATION

22305 Closed treatment of vertebral process fracture(s)

22310 Closed treatment of vertebral body fracture(s), without manipulation, requiring and including casting or bracing

22315 Closed treatment of vertebral fracture(s) and/or dislocation(s) requiring casting or bracing, with and including casting and/or bracing, with or without anesthesia, by manipulation or traction

(For spinal subluxation, use 97140)

22318 Open treatment and/or reduction of odontoid fracture(s) and or dislocation(s) (including os odontoideum), anterior approach, including placement of internal fixation; without grafting

22319 with grafting

22325 Open treatment and/or reduction of vertebral fracture(s) and/or dislocation(s), posterior approach, one fractured vertebrae or dislocated segment; lumbar

22326 cervical

22327 thoracic

+ 22328 each additional fractured vertebrae or dislocated segment (List separately in addition to code for primary procedure)

(Use 22328 in conjunction with codes 22325, 22326, 22327)

(For treatment of vertebral fracture by the anterior approach, see corpectomy 63081-63091, and appropriate arthrodesis, bone graft and instrument codes)

MANIPULATION

22505 Manipulation of spine requiring anesthesia, any region

● New Code   ▲ Revised Code   + Add-On Code   ⊘ Modifier -51 Exempt

VERTEBRAL BODY, EMBOLIZATION OR INJECTION

22520   Percutaneous vertebroplasty, one vertebral body, unilateral or bilateral injection; thoracic

22521   lumbar

+ 22522   each additional thoracic or lumbar body (List separately in addition to code for primary procedure)

(Use 22522 in conjunction with codes 22520, 22521 as appropriate)

(For radiological supervision and interpretation, see 76012, 76013)

LATERAL EXTRACAVITARY APPROACH TECHNIQUE

● **22532**   Arthrodesis, lateral extracavitary technique, including minimal diskectomy to prepare interspace (other than for decompression); thoracic

● **22533**   lumbar

●+**22534**   thoracic or lumbar, each additional vertebral segment (List separately in addition to code for primary procedure)

(Use 22534 in conjunction with 22532 and 22533)

ARTHRODESIS

Anterior or Anterolateral Approach Technique

22548   Arthrodesis, anterior transoral or extraoral technique, clivus-C1-C2 (atlas-axis), with or without excision of odontoid process

22554   Arthrodesis, anterior interbody technique, including minimal diskectomy to prepare interspace (other than for decompression); cervical below C2

22556   thoracic

22558   lumbar

+ 22585   each additional interspace (List separately in addition to code for primary procedure)

(Use 22585 in conjunction with codes 22554, 22556, 22558)

281

 Separate Procedure   Unlisted Procedure   CCI Comp. Code   Non-specific Procedure

Posterior, Posterolateral or Lateral Transverse Process Technique

22590 Arthrodesis, posterior technique, craniocervical (occiput-C2)

22595 Arthrodesis, posterior technique, atlas-axis (C1-C2)

22600 Arthrodesis, posterior or posterolateral technique, single level; cervical below C2 segment

22610 thoracic (with or without lateral transverse technique)

22612 lumbar (with or without lateral transverse technique)

+ **22614** each additional vertebral segment (List separately in addition to code for primary procedure)

(Use 22614 in conjunction with codes 22600, 22610, 22612)

22630 Arthrodesis, posterior interbody technique, including laminectomy and/or diskectomy to prepare interspace (other than for decompression), single interspace; lumbar

+ **22632** each additional interspace (List separately in addition to code for primary procedure)

(Use 22632 in conjunction with code 22630)

SPINE DEFORMITY (eg, SCOLIOSIS, KYPHOSIS)

22800 Arthrodesis, posterior, for spinal deformity, with or without cast; up to 6 vertebral segments

22802 7 to 12 vertebral segments

22804 13 or more vertebral segments

22808 Arthrodesis, anterior, for spinal deformity, with or without cast; 2 to 3 vertebral segments

22810 4 to 7 vertebral segments

22812 8 or more vertebral segments

22818 Kyphectomy, circumferential exposure of spine and resection of vertebral segment(s) (including body and posterior elements); single or 2 segments

● New Code ▲ Revised Code + Add-On Code ⃠ Modifier -51 Exempt

| 22819 | 3 or more segments |

(To report arthrodesis, see 22800-22804 and add modifier -51)

EXPLORATION

| 22830 | Exploration of spinal fusion |

SPINAL INSTRUMENTATION

(List codes 22840-22848, 22851 separately, in addition to code for fracture, dislocation, or arthrodesis of the spine, 22325, 22326, 22327, 22548-22812)

⊘ **22840** Posterior non-segmental instrumentation (eg, Harrington rod technique, pedicle fixation across one interspace, atlantoaxial transarticular screw fixation, sublaminar wiring at C1, facet screw fixation)

⊘ **22841** Internal spinal fixation by wiring of spinous processes

⊘ **22842** Posterior segmental instrumentation (eg, pedicle fixation, dual rods with multiple hooks and sublaminar wires); 3 to 6 vertebral segments

⊘ **22843** 7 to 12 vertebral segments

⊘ **22844** 13 or more vertebral segments

⊘ **22845** Anterior instrumentation; 2 to 3 vertebral segments

⊘ **22846** 4 to 7 vertebral segments

⊘ **22847** 8 or more vertebral segments

⊘ **22848** Pelvic fixation (attachment of caudal end of instrumentation to pelvic bony structures) other than sacrum

| 22849 | Reinsertion of spinal fixation device |

| 22850 | Removal of posterior nonsegmental instrumentation (eg, Harrington rod) |

⊘ **22851** Application of intervertebral biomechanical device(s) (eg, synthetic cage(s), threaded bone dowel(s), methylmethacrylate) to vertebral defector interspace

| 22852 | Removal of posterior segmental instrumentation |

22855   Removal of anterior instrumentation

OTHER PROCEDURES

22899   Unlisted procedure, spine

ABDOMEN

EXCISION

22900   Excision, abdominal wall tumor, subfascial (eg, desmoid)

OTHER PROCEDURES

22999   Unlisted procedure, abdomen, musculoskeletal system

SHOULDER

INCISION

23000   Removal of subdeltoid calcareous deposits, open

(For arthroscopic removal of bursal deposits, use 29999)

23020   Capsular contracture release (eg, Sever type procedure)

(For incision and drainage procedures, superficial, see 10040-10160)

23030   Incision and drainage, shoulder area; deep abscess or hematoma

23031   infected bursa

23035   Incision, bone cortex (eg, osteomyelitis or bone abscess), shoulder area

23040   Arthrotomy, glenohumeral joint, including exploration, drainage, or removal of foreign body

23044   Arthrotomy, acromioclavicular, sternoclavicular joint, including exploration, drainage, or removal of foreign body

EXCISION

23065   Biopsy, soft tissue of shoulder area; superficial

| ● | New Code | ▲ | Revised Code | + | Add-On Code | ⊘ | Modifier -51 Exempt |

23066	deep

(For needle biopsy of soft tissue, use 20206)

23075	Excision, soft tissue tumor, shoulder area; subcutaneous
23076	deep, subfascial, or intramuscular
23077	Radical resection of tumor (eg, malignant neoplasm), soft tissue of shoulder area
23100	Arthrotomy, glenohumeral joint, including biopsy
23101	Arthrotomy, acromioclavicular joint or sternoclavicular joint, including biopsy and/or excision of torn cartilage
23105	Arthrotomy; glenohumeral joint, with synovectomy, with or without biopsy
23106	sternoclavicular joint, with synovectomy, with or without biopsy
23107	Arthrotomy, glenohumeral joint, with joint exploration, with or without removal of loose or foreign body
23120	Claviculectomy; partial

(For arthroscopic procedure, use 29824)

23125	total
23130	Acromioplasty or acromionectomy, partial, with or without coracoacromial ligament release
23140	Excision or curettage of bone cyst or benign tumor of clavicle or scapula;
23145	with autograft (includes obtaining graft)
23146	with allograft
23150	Excision or curettage of bone cyst or benign tumor of proximal humerus;
23155	with autograft (includes obtaining graft)
23156	with allograft

285

Separate Procedure	Unlisted Procedure	CCI Comp. Code	Non-specific Procedure

23170	Sequestrectomy (eg, for osteomyelitis or bone abscess), clavicle
23172	Sequestrectomy (eg, for osteomyelitis or bone abscess), scapula
23174	Sequestrectomy (eg, for osteomyelitis or bone abscess), humeral head to surgical neck
23180	Partial excision (craterization, saucerization, or diaphysectomy) bone (eg, osteomyelitis), clavicle
23182	Partial excision (craterization, saucerization, or diaphysectomy) bone (eg, osteomyelitis), scapula
23184	Partial excision (craterization, saucerization, or diaphysectomy) bone (eg, osteomyelitis), proximal humerus
23190	Ostectomy of scapula, partial (eg, superior medial angle)
23195	Resection, humeral head

(For replacement with implant, use 23470)

23200	Radical resection for tumor; clavicle
23210	scapula
23220	Radical resection of bone tumor, proximal humerus;
23221	with autograft (includes obtaining graft)
23222	with prosthetic replacement

INTRODUCTION OR REMOVAL

(For arthrocentesis or needling of bursa, use 20610)

(For K-wire or pin insertion or removal, see 20650, 20670, 20680)

23330	Removal of foreign body, shoulder; subcutaneous
23331	deep (eg, Neer hemiarthroplasty removal)
23332	complicated (eg, total shoulder)
23350	Injection procedure for shoulder arthrography or enhanced CT/MRI shoulder arthrography

286

| ● | New Code | ▲ | Revised Code | + | Add-On Code | ⊘ | Modifier -51 Exempt |

(For radiographic arthrography, radiological supervision and interpretation, use 73040. Fluoroscopy (76003) is inclusive of radiographic arthrography)

(When fluoroscopic guided injection is performed for enhanced CT arthrography, use codes 23350, 76003, and 73201 or 73202)

(When fluoroscopic guided injection is performed for enhanced MR arthrography, use codes 23350, 76003, and 73222 or 73223)

(For enhanced CT or enhanced MRI arthrography, use 76003 and either 73201, 73202, 73222 or 73223)

REPAIR, REVISION AND/OR RECONSTRUCTION

23395 Muscle transfer, any type, shoulder or upper arm; single

23397   multiple

23400 Scapulopexy (eg, Sprengels deformity or for paralysis)

23405 Tenotomy, shoulder area; single tendon

23406   multiple tendons through same incision

23410 Repair of ruptured musculotendinous cuff (eg, rotator cuff) open; acute

23412   chronic

(For arthroscopic procedure, use 29827)

23415 Coracoacromial ligament release, with or without acromioplasty

(For arthroscopic procedure, use 29826)

23420 Reconstruction of complete shoulder (rotator) cuff avulsion, chronic (includes acromioplasty)

23430 Tenodesis of long tendon of biceps

23440 Resection or transplantation of long tendon of biceps

23450 Capsulorrhaphy, anterior; Putti-Platt procedure or Magnuson type operation

(To report arthroscopic thermal capsulorrhaphy, use 29999)

287

| | Separate Procedure | | Unlisted Procedure | CCI Comp. Code | Non-specific Procedure |

23455   with labral repair (eg, Bankart procedure)

(For arthroscopic procedure, use 29806)

23460   Capsulorrhaphy, anterior, any type; with bone block

23462   with coracoid process transfer

(To report open thermal capsulorrhaphy, use 23929)

23465   Capsulorrhaphy, glenohumeral joint, posterior, with or without bone block

(For sternoclavicular and acromioclavicular reconstruction, see 23530, 23550)

23466   Capsulorrhaphy, glenohumeral joint, any type multi-directional instability

23470   Arthroplasty, glenohumeral joint; hemiarthroplasty

23472   total shoulder (glenoid and proximal humeral replacement (eg, total shoulder))

(For removal of total shoulder implants, see 23331, 23332)

(For osteotomy, proximal humerus, use 24400)

23480   Osteotomy, clavicle, with or without internal fixation;

23485   with bone graft for nonunion or malunion (includes obtaining graft and/or necessary fixation)

23490   Prophylactic treatment (nailing, pinning, plating or wiring) with or without methylmethacrylate; clavicle

23491   proximal humerus

FRACTURE AND/OR DISLOCATION

23500   Closed treatment of clavicular fracture; without manipulation

23505   with manipulation

23515   Open treatment of clavicular fracture, with or without internal or external fixation

● New
Code

▲ Revised
Code

+ Add-On
Code

⊘ Modifier -51
Exempt

23520 Closed treatment of sternoclavicular dislocation; without manipulation

23525 with manipulation

23530 Open treatment of sternoclavicular dislocation, acute or chronic;

23532 with fascial graft (includes obtaining graft)

23540 Closed treatment of acromioclavicular dislocation; without manipulation

23545 with manipulation

23550 Open treatment of acromioclavicular dislocation, acute or chronic;

23552 with fascial graft (includes obtaining graft)

23570 Closed treatment of scapular fracture; without manipulation

23575 with manipulation, with or without skeletal traction (with or without shoulder joint involvement)

23585 Open treatment of scapular fracture (body, glenoid or acromion) with or without internal fixation

23600 Closed treatment of proximal humeral (surgical or anatomical neck) fracture; without manipulation

23605 with manipulation, with or without skeletal traction

23615 Open treatment of proximal humeral (surgical or anatomical neck) fracture, with or without internal or external fixation, with or without repair of tuberosity(-ies);

23616 with proximal humeral prosthetic replacement

23620 Closed treatment of greater humeral tuberosity fracture; without manipulation

23625 with manipulation

23630 Open treatment of greater humeral tuberosity fracture, with or without internal or external fixation

289

| | Separate Procedure | | Unlisted Procedure | | CCI Comp. Code | | Non-specific Procedure |

23650   Closed treatment of shoulder dislocation, with manipulation; without anesthesia

23655   requiring anesthesia

23660   Open treatment of acute shoulder dislocation

        (Repairs for recurrent dislocations, see 23450-23466)

23665   Closed treatment of shoulder dislocation, with fracture of greater humeral tuberosity, with manipulation

23670   Open treatment of shoulder dislocation, with fracture of greater humeral tuberosity, with or without internal or external fixation

23675   Closed treatment of shoulder dislocation, with surgical or anatomical neck fracture, with manipulation

23680   Open treatment of shoulder dislocation, with surgical or anatomical neck fracture, with or without internal or external fixation

MANIPULATION

23700   Manipulation under anesthesia, shoulder joint, including application of fixation apparatus (dislocation excluded)

ARTHRODESIS

23800   Arthrodesis, glenohumeral joint;

23802   with autogenous graft (includes obtaining graft)

AMPUTATION

23900   Interthoracoscapular amputation (forequarter)

23920   Disarticulation of shoulder;

23921   secondary closure or scar revision

OTHER PROCEDURES

23929   Unlisted procedure, shoulder

●   New Code   ▲   Revised Code   ✚   Add-On Code   ⊘   Modifier -51 Exempt

HUMERUS (UPPER ARM) AND ELBOW

INCISION

(For incision and drainage procedures, superficial, see 10040-10160)

23930 Incision and drainage, upper arm or elbow area; deep abscess or hematoma

23931 bursa

23935 Incision, deep, with opening of bone cortex (eg, for osteomyelitis or bone abscess), humerus or elbow

24000 Arthrotomy, elbow, including exploration, drainage, or removal of foreign body

24006 Arthrotomy of the elbow, with capsular excision for capsular release (separate procedure)

EXCISION

24065 Biopsy, soft tissue of upper arm or elbow area; superficial

24066 deep (subfascial or intramuscular)

(For needle biopsy of soft tissue, use 20206)

24075 Excision, tumor, soft tissue of upper arm or elbow area; subcutaneous

24076 deep (subfascial or intramuscular)

24077 Radical resection of tumor (eg, malignant neoplasm), soft tissue of upper arm or elbow area

24100 Arthrotomy, elbow; with synovial biopsy only

24101 with joint exploration, with or without biopsy, with or without removal of loose or foreign body

24102 with synovectomy

24105 Excision, olecranon bursa

24110 Excision or curettage of bone cyst or benign tumor, humerus;

291

 Separate Procedure   Unlisted Procedure   CCI Comp. Code   Non-specific Procedure

24115 with autograft (includes obtaining graft)

24116 with allograft

24120 Excision or curettage of bone cyst or benign tumor of head or neck of radius or olecranon process;

24125 with autograft (includes obtaining graft)

24126 with allograft

24130 Excision, radial head

(For replacement with implant, use 24366)

24134 Sequestrectomy (eg, for osteomyelitis or bone abscess), shaft or distal humerus

24136 Sequestrectomy (eg, for osteomyelitis or bone abscess), radial head or neck

24138 Sequestrectomy (eg, for osteomyelitis or bone abscess), olecranon process

24140 Partial excision (craterization, saucerization, or diaphysectomy) bone (eg, osteomyelitis), humerus

24145 Partial excision (craterization, saucerization, or diaphysectomy) bone (eg, osteomyelitis), radial head or neck

24147 Partial excision (craterization, saucerization, or diaphysectomy) bone (eg, osteomyelitis), olecranon process

24149 Radical resection of capsule, soft tissue, and heterotopic bone, elbow, with contracture release (separate procedure)

(For capsular and soft tissue release only, use 24006)

24150 Radical resection for tumor, shaft or distal humerus;

24151 with autograft (includes obtaining graft)

24152 Radical resection for tumor, radial head or neck;

24153 with autograft (includes obtaining graft)

24155 Resection of elbow joint (arthrectomy)

292　● New Code　▲ Revised Code　+ Add-On Code　⊘ Modifier -51 Exempt

INTRODUCTION OR REMOVAL

(For K-wire or pin insertion or removal, see 20650, 20670, 20680)

(For arthrocentesis or needling of bursa or joint, use 20605)

24160 Implant removal; elbow joint

24164 radial head

24200 Removal of foreign body, upper arm or elbow area; subcutaneous

24201 deep (subfascial or intramuscular)

24220 Injection procedure for elbow arthrography

(For radiological supervision and interpretation, use 73085. Do not report 76003 in addition to 73085)

(For injection of tennis elbow, use 20550)

REPAIR, REVISION, AND/OR RECONSTRUCTION

24300 Manipulation, elbow, under anesthesia

(For application of external fixation, see 20690 or 20692)

24301 Muscle or tendon transfer, any type, upper arm or elbow, single (excluding 24320-24331)

24305 Tendon lengthening, upper arm or elbow, each tendon

24310 Tenotomy, open, elbow to shoulder, each tendon

24320 Tenoplasty, with muscle transfer, with or without free graft, elbow to shoulder, single (Seddon-Brookes type procedure)

24330 Flexor-plasty, elbow (eg, Steindler type advancement);

24331 with extensor advancement

24332 Tenolysis, triceps

24340 Tenodesis of biceps tendon at elbow (separate procedure)

293

 Separate Procedure

 Unlisted Procedure

 CCI Comp. Code

 Non-specific Procedure

24341 Repair, tendon or muscle, upper arm or elbow, each tendon or muscle, primary or secondary (excludes rotator cuff)

24342 Reinsertion of ruptured biceps or triceps tendon, distal, with or without tendon graft

24343 Repair lateral collateral ligament, elbow, with local tissue

24344 Reconstruction lateral collateral ligament, elbow, with tendon graft (includes harvesting of graft)

24345 Repair medial collateral ligament, elbow, with local tissue

24346 Reconstruction medial collateral ligament, elbow, with tendon graft (includes harvesting of graft)

24350 Fasciotomy, lateral or medial (eg, tennis elbow or epicondylitis);

24351 with extensor origin detachment

24352 with annular ligament resection

24354 with stripping

24356 with partial ostectomy

24360 Arthroplasty, elbow; with membrane (eg, fascial)

24361 with distal humeral prosthetic replacement

24362 with implant and fascia lata ligament reconstruction

24363 with distal humerus and proximal ulnar prosthetic replacement (eg, total elbow)

24365 Arthroplasty, radial head;

24366 with implant

24400 Osteotomy, humerus, with or without internal fixation

24410 Multiple osteotomies with realignment on intramedullary rod, humeral shaft (Sofield type procedure)

24420 Osteoplasty, humerus (eg, shortening or lengthening) (excluding 64876)

● New Code ▲ Revised Code + Add-On Code ⊘ Modifier -51 Exempt

24430 Repair of nonunion or malunion, humerus; without graft (eg, compression technique)

24435 with iliac or other autograft (includes obtaining graft)

(For proximal radius and/or ulna, see 25400-25420)

24470 Hemiepiphyseal arrest (eg, cubitus varus or valgus, distal humerus)

24495 Decompression fasciotomy, forearm, with brachial artery exploration

24498 Prophylactic treatment (nailing, pinning, plating or wiring), with or without methylmethacrylate, humeral shaft

FRACTURE AND/OR DISLOCATION

24500 Closed treatment of humeral shaft fracture; without manipulation

24505 with manipulation, with or without skeletal traction

24515 Open treatment of humeral shaft fracture with plate/screws, with or without cerclage

24516 Treatment of humeral shaft fracture, with insertion of intramedullary implant, with or without cerclage and/or locking screws

24530 Closed treatment of supracondylar or transcondylar humeral fracture, with or without intercondylar extension; without manipulation

24535 with manipulation, with or without skin or skeletal traction

24538 Percutaneous skeletal fixation of supracondylar or transcondylar humeral fracture, with or without intercondylar extension

24545 Open treatment of humeral supracondylar or transcondylar fracture, with or without internal or external fixation; without intercondylar extension

24546 with intercondylar extension

24560 Closed treatment of humeral epicondylar fracture, medial or lateral; without manipulation

24565   with manipulation

24566   Percutaneous skeletal fixation of humeral epicondylar fracture, medial or lateral, with manipulation

24575   Open treatment of humeral epicondylar fracture, medial or lateral, with or without internal or external fixation

24576   Closed treatment of humeral condylar fracture, medial or lateral; without manipulation

24577   with manipulation

24579   Open treatment of humeral condylar fracture, medial or lateral, with or without internal or external fixation

24582   Percutaneous skeletal fixation of humeral condylar fracture, medial or lateral, with manipulation

24586   Open treatment of periarticular fracture and/or dislocation of the elbow (fracture distal humerus and proximal ulna and/or proximal radius);

24587   with implant arthroplasty

(See also 24361)

24600   Treatment of closed elbow dislocation; without anesthesia

24605   requiring anesthesia

24615   Open treatment of acute or chronic elbow dislocation

24620   Closed treatment of Monteggia type of fracture dislocation at elbow (fracture proximal end of ulna with dislocation of radial head), with manipulation

24635   Open treatment of Monteggia type of fracture dislocation at elbow (fracture proximal end of ulna with dislocation of radial head), with or without internal or external fixation

24640   Closed treatment of radial head subluxation in child, nursemaid elbow, with manipulation

24650   Closed treatment of radial head or neck fracture; without manipulation

296

● New Code   ▲ Revised Code   + Add-On Code   ⊘ Modifier -51 Exempt

24655   with manipulation

24665   Open treatment of radial head or neck fracture, with or without internal fixation or radial head excision;

24666   with radial head prosthetic replacement

24670   Closed treatment of ulnar fracture, proximal end (olecranon process); without manipulation

24675   with manipulation

24685   Open treatment of ulnar fracture proximal end (olecranon process), with or without internal or external fixation

ARTHRODESIS

24800   Arthrodesis, elbow joint; local

24802   with autogenous graft (includes obtaining graft)

AMPUTATION

24900   Amputation, arm through humerus; with primary closure

24920   open, circular (guillotine)

24925   secondary closure or scar revision

24930   re-amputation

24931   with implant

24935   Stump elongation, upper extremity

24940   Cineplasty, upper extremity, complete procedure

OTHER PROCEDURES

24999   Unlisted procedure, humerus or elbow

FOREARM AND WRIST

INCISION

25000   Incision, extensor tendon sheath, wrist (eg, deQuervains disease)

297

 Separate Procedure   Unlisted Procedure   CCI Comp. Code   Non-specific Procedure

(For decompression median nerve or for carpal tunnel syndrome, use 64721)

25001   Incision, flexor tendon sheath, wrist (eg, flexor carpi radialis)

25020   Decompression fasciotomy, forearm and/or wrist, flexor OR extensor compartment; without debridement of nonviable muscle and/or nerve

25023   with debridement of nonviable muscle and/or nerve

(For decompression fasciotomy with brachial artery exploration, use 24495)

(For incision and drainage procedures, superficial, see 10040-10160)

(For debridement, see also 11000-11044)

25024   Decompression fasciotomy, forearm and/or wrist, flexor AND extensor compartment; without debridement of nonviable muscle and/or nerve

25025   with debridement of nonviable muscle and/or nerve

25028   Incision and drainage, forearm and/or wrist; deep abscess or hematoma

25031   bursa

25035   Incision, deep, bone cortex, forearm and/or wrist (eg, osteomyelitis or bone abscess)

25040   Arthrotomy, radiocarpal or midcarpal joint, with exploration, drainage, or removal of foreign body

EXCISION

25065   Biopsy, soft tissue of forearm and/or wrist; superficial

25066   deep (subfascial or intramuscular)

(For needle biopsy of soft tissue, use 20206)

25075   Excision, tumor, soft tissue of forearm and/or wrist area; subcutaneous

25076   deep (subfascial or intramuscular)

298

| ● | New Code | ▲ | Revised Code | + | Add-On Code | ⃠ | Modifier -51 Exempt |

25077 Radical resection of tumor (eg, malignant neoplasm), soft tissue of forearm and/or wrist area

25085 Capsulotomy, wrist (eg, contracture)

25100 Arthrotomy, wrist joint; with biopsy

25101 with joint exploration, with or without biopsy, with or without removal of loose or foreign body

25105 with synovectomy

25107 Arthrotomy, distal radioulnar joint including repair of triangular cartilage, complex

25110 Excision, lesion of tendon sheath, forearm and/or wrist

25111 Excision of ganglion, wrist (dorsal or volar); primary

25112 recurrent

(For hand or finger, use 26160)

25115 Radical excision of bursa, synovia of wrist, or forearm tendon sheaths (eg, tenosynovitis, fungus, Tbc, or other granulomas, rheumatoid arthritis); flexors

25116 extensors, with or without transposition of dorsal retinaculum

(For finger synovectomies, use 26145)

25118 Synovectomy, extensor tendon sheath, wrist, single compartment;

25119 with resection of distal ulna

25120 Excision or curettage of bone cyst or benign tumor of radius or ulna (excluding head or neck of radius and olecranon process);

(For head or neck of radius or olecranon process, see 24120-24126)

25125 with autograft (includes obtaining graft)

25126 with allograft

299

 Separate Procedure

 Unlisted Procedure

 CCI Comp. Code

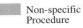 Non-specific Procedure

25130 Excision or curettage of bone cyst or benign tumor of carpal bones;

25135 with autograft (includes obtaining graft)

25136 with allograft

25145 Sequestrectomy (eg, for osteomyelitis or bone abscess), forearm and/or wrist

25150 Partial excision (craterization, saucerization, or diaphysectomy) of bone (eg, for osteomyelitis); ulna

25151 radius

(For head or neck of radius or olecranon process, see 24145, 24147)

25170 Radical resection for tumor, radius or ulna

25210 Carpectomy; one bone

(For carpectomy with implant, see 25441-25445)

25215 all bones of proximal row

25230 Radial styloidectomy (separate procedure)

25240 Excision distal ulna partial or complete (eg, Darrach type or matched resection)

(For implant replacement, distal ulna, use 25442)

(For obtaining fascia for interposition, see 20920, 20922)

INTRODUCTION OR REMOVAL

(For K-wire, pin or rod insertion or removal, see 20650, 20670, 20680)

25246 Injection procedure for wrist arthrography

(For radiological supervision and interpretation, use 73115. Do not report 76003 in addition to 73115)

(For foreign body removal, superficial use 20520)

25248 Exploration with removal of deep foreign body, forearm or wrist

● New Code ▲ Revised Code + Add-On Code ○ Modifier -51 Exempt

25250 Removal of wrist prosthesis; (separate procedure)

25251 complicated, including total wrist

25259 Manipulation, wrist, under anesthesia

(For application of external fixation, see 20690 or 20692)

REPAIR, REVISION, AND/OR RECONSTRUCTION

25260 Repair, tendon or muscle, flexor, forearm and/or wrist; primary, single, each tendon or muscle

25263 secondary, single, each tendon or muscle

25265 secondary, with free graft (includes obtaining graft), each tendon or muscle

25270 Repair, tendon or muscle, extensor, forearm and/or wrist; primary, single, each tendon or muscle

25272 secondary, single, each tendon or muscle

25274 secondary, with free graft (includes obtaining graft), each tendon or muscle

25275 Repair, tendon sheath, extensor, forearm and/or wrist, with free graft (includes obtaining graft) (eg, for extensor carpi ulnaris subluxation)

25280 Lengthening or shortening of flexor or extensor tendon, forearm and/or wrist, single, each tendon

25290 Tenotomy, open, flexor or extensor tendon, forearm and/or wrist, single, each tendon

25295 Tenolysis, flexor or extensor tendon, forearm and/or wrist, single, each tendon

25300 Tenodesis at wrist; flexors of fingers

25301 extensors of fingers

25310 Tendon transplantation or transfer, flexor or extensor, forearm and/or wrist, single; each tendon

25312 with tendon graft(s) (includes obtaining graft), each tendon

301

| | Separate Procedure | | Unlisted Procedure | | CCI Comp. Code | | Non-specific Procedure |

25315 Flexor origin slide (eg, for cerebral palsy, Volkmann contracture), forearm and/or wrist;

25316 with tendon(s) transfer

25320 Capsulorrhaphy or reconstruction, wrist, open (eg, capsulodesis, ligament repair, tendon transfer or graft) (includes synovectomy, capsulotomy and open reduction) for carpal instability

25332 Arthroplasty, wrist, with or without interposition, with or without external or internal fixation

(For obtaining fascia for interposition, see 20920, 20922)

(For prosthetic replacement arthroplasty, see 25441-25446)

25335 Centralization of wrist on ulna (eg, radial club hand)

25337 Reconstruction for stabilization of unstable distal ulna or distal radioulnar joint, secondary by soft tissue stabilization (eg, tendon transfer, tendon graft or weave, or tenodesis) with or without open reduction of distal radioulnar joint

(For harvesting of fascia lata graft, see 20920, 20922)

25350 Osteotomy, radius; distal third

25355 middle or proximal third

25360 Osteotomy; ulna

25365 radius AND ulna

25370 Multiple osteotomies, with realignment on intramedullary rod (Sofield type procedure); radius OR ulna

25375 radius AND ulna

25390 Osteoplasty, radius OR ulna; shortening

25391 lengthening with autograft

25392 Osteoplasty, radius AND ulna; shortening (excluding 64876)

25393 lengthening with autograft

25394 Osteoplasty, carpal bone, shortening

● New Code ▲ Revised Code + Add-On Code ⃠ Modifier -51 Exempt

25400 Repair of nonunion or malunion, radius OR ulna; without graft (eg, compression technique)

25405 with autograft (includes obtaining graft)

25415 Repair of nonunion or malunion, radius AND ulna; without graft (eg, compression technique)

25420 with autograft (includes obtaining graft)

25425 Repair of defect with autograft; radius OR ulna

25426 radius AND ulna

25430 Insertion of vascular pedicle into carpal bone (eg, Hori procedure)

25431 Repair of nonunion of carpal bone (excluding carpal scaphoid (navicular) (includes obtaining graft and necessary fixation), each bone

25440 Repair of nonunion, scaphoid carpal (navicular) bone, with or without radial styloidectomy (includes obtaining graft and necessary fixation)

25441 Arthroplasty with prosthetic replacement; distal radius

25442 distal ulna

25443 scaphoid carpal (navicular)

25444 lunate

25445 trapezium

25446 distal radius and partial or entire carpus (total wrist)

25447 Arthroplasty, interposition, intercarpal or carpometacarpal joints

(For wrist arthroplasty, use 25332)

25449 Revision of arthroplasty, including removal of implant, wrist joint

25450 Epiphyseal arrest by epiphysiodesis or stapling; distal radius OR ulna

303

Separate Procedure   Unlisted Procedure   CCI Comp. Code   Non-specific Procedure

25455   distal radius AND ulna

25490   Prophylactic treatment (nailing, pinning, plating or wiring) with or without methylmethacrylate; radius

25491   ulna

25492   radius AND ulna

FRACTURE AND/OR DISLOCATION

25500   Closed treatment of radial shaft fracture; without manipulation

25505   with manipulation

25515   Open treatment of radial shaft fracture, with or without internal or external fixation

25520   Closed treatment of radial shaft fracture and closed treatment of dislocation of distal radioulnar joint (Galeazzi fracture/dislocation)

25525   Open treatment of radial shaft fracture, with internal and/or external fixation and closed treatment of dislocation of distal radioulnar joint (Galeazzi fracture/dislocation), with or without percutaneous skeletal fixation

25526   Open treatment of radial shaft fracture, with internal and/or external fixation and open treatment, with or without internal or external fixation of distal radioulnar joint (Galeazzi fracture/dislocation), includes repair of triangular fibrocartilage complex

25530   Closed treatment of ulnar shaft fracture; without manipulation

25535   with manipulation

25545   Open treatment of ulnar shaft fracture, with or without internal or external fixation

25560   Closed treatment of radial and ulnar shaft fractures; without manipulation

25565   with manipulation

25574   Open treatment of radial AND ulnar shaft fractures, with internal or external fixation; of radius OR ulna

● New Code   ▲ Revised Code   + Add-On Code   ⊘ Modifier -51 Exempt

25575   of radius AND ulna

25600   Closed treatment of distal radial fracture (eg, Colles or Smith type) or epiphyseal separation, with or without fracture of ulnar styloid; without manipulation

25605   with manipulation

25611   Percutaneous skeletal fixation of distal radial fracture (eg, Colles or Smith type) or epiphyseal separation, with or without fracture of ulnar styloid, requiring manipulation, with or without external fixation

25620   Open treatment of distal radial fracture (eg, Colles or Smith type) or epiphyseal separation, with or without fracture of ulnar styloid, with or without internal or external fixation

25622   Closed treatment of carpal scaphoid (navicular) fracture; without manipulation

25624   with manipulation

25628   Open treatment of carpal scaphoid (navicular) fracture, with or without internal or external fixation

25630   Closed treatment of carpal bone fracture (excluding carpal scaphoid (navicular)); without manipulation, each bone

25635   with manipulation, each bone

25645   Open treatment of carpal bone fracture (other than carpal scaphoid (navicular)), each bone

25650   Closed treatment of ulnar styloid fracture

25651   Percutaneous skeletal fixation of ulnar styloid fracture

25652   Open treatment of ulnar styloid fracture

25660   Closed treatment of radiocarpal or intercarpal dislocation, one or more bones, with manipulation

25670   Open treatment of radiocarpal or intercarpal dislocation, one or more bones

25671   Percutaneous skeletal fixation of distal radioulnar dislocation

305

	Separate Procedure		Unlisted Procedure		CCI Comp. Code		Non-specific Procedure

25675 Closed treatment of distal radioulnar dislocation with manipulation

25676 Open treatment of distal radioulnar dislocation, acute or chronic

25680 Closed treatment of trans-scaphoperilunar type of fracture dislocation, with manipulation

25685 Open treatment of trans-scaphoperilunar type of fracture dislocation

25690 Closed treatment of lunate dislocation, with manipulation

25695 Open treatment of lunate dislocation

ARTHRODESIS

25800 Arthrodesis, wrist; complete, without bone graft (includes radiocarpal and/or intercarpal and/or carpometacarpal joints)

25805   with sliding graft

25810   with iliac or other autograft (includes obtaining graft)

25820 Arthrodesis, wrist; limited, without bone graft (eg, intercarpal or radiocarpal)

25825   with autograft (includes obtaining graft)

25830 Arthrodesis, distal radioulnar joint with segmental resection of ulna, with or without bone graft (eg, Sauve-Kapandji procedure)

AMPUTATION

25900 Amputation, forearm, through radius and ulna;

25905   open, circular (guillotine)

25907   secondary closure or scar revision

25909   re-amputation

25915 Krukenberg procedure

25920 Disarticulation through wrist;

25922 secondary closure or scar revision

25924 re-amputation

25927 Transmetacarpal amputation;

25929 secondary closure or scar revision

25931 re-amputation

OTHER PROCEDURES

25999 Unlisted procedure, forearm or wrist

HAND AND FINGERS

INCISION

26010 Drainage of finger abscess; simple

26011 complicated (eg, felon)

26020 Drainage of tendon sheath, digit and/or palm, each

26025 Drainage of palmar bursa; single, bursa

26030 multiple bursa

26034 Incision, bone cortex, hand or finger (eg, osteomyelitis or bone abscess)

26035 Decompression fingers and/or hand, injection injury (eg, grease gun)

26037 Decompressive fasciotomy, hand (excludes 26035)

(For injection injury, use 26035)

26040 Fasciotomy, palmar (eg, Dupuytren's contracture); percutaneous

26045 open, partial

(For fasciectomy, see 26121-26125)

26055 Tendon sheath incision (eg, for trigger finger)

307

 Separate Procedure   Unlisted Procedure   CCI Comp. Code 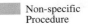 Non-specific Procedure

26060   Tenotomy, percutaneous, single, each digit

26070   Arthrotomy, with exploration, drainage, or removal of loose or foreign body; carpometacarpal joint

26075   metacarpophalangeal joint, each

26080   interphalangeal joint, each

EXCISION

26100   Arthrotomy with biopsy; carpometacarpal joint, each

26105   metacarpophalangeal joint, each

26110   interphalangeal joint, each

26115   Excision, tumor or vascular malformation, soft tissue of hand or finger; subcutaneous

26116   deep (subfascial or intramuscular)

26117   Radical resection of tumor (eg, malignant neoplasm), soft tissue of hand or finger

26121   Fasciectomy, palm only, with or without Z-plasty, other local tissue rearrangement, or skin grafting (includes obtaining graft)

26123   Fasciectomy, partial palmar with release of single digit including proximal interphalangeal joint, with or without Z-plasty, other local tissue rearrangement, or skin grafting (includes obtaining graft);

+ 26125   each additional digit (List separately in addition to code for primary procedure)

(Use 26125 in conjunction with code 26123)

(For fasciotomy, see 26040, 26045)

26130   Synovectomy, carpometacarpal joint

26135   Synovectomy, metacarpophalangeal joint including intrinsic release and extensor hood reconstruction, each digit

26140   Synovectomy, proximal interphalangeal joint, including extensor reconstruction, each interphalangeal joint

| ● | New Code | ▲ | Revised Code | + | Add-On Code | ⊘ | Modifier -51 Exempt |

26145 Synovectomy, tendon sheath, radical (tenosynovectomy), flexor tendon, palm and/or finger, each tendon

(For tendon sheath synovectomies at wrist, see 25115, 25116)

26160 Excision of lesion of tendon sheath or joint capsule (eg, cyst, mucous cyst, or ganglion), hand or finger

(For wrist ganglion, see 25111, 25112)

(For trigger digit, use 26055)

26170 Excision of tendon, palm, flexor, single (separate procedure), each

26180 Excision of tendon, finger, flexor (separate procedure), each tendon

26185 Sesamoidectomy, thumb or finger (separate procedure)

26200 Excision or curettage of bone cyst or benign tumor of metacarpal;

26205 with autograft (includes obtaining graft)

26210 Excision or curettage of bone cyst or benign tumor of proximal, middle, or distal phalanx of finger;

26215 with autograft (includes obtaining graft)

26230 Partial excision (craterization, saucerization, or diaphysectomy) bone (eg, osteomyelitis); metacarpal

26235 proximal or middle phalanx of finger

26236 distal phalanx of finger

26250 Radical resection, metacarpal (eg, tumor);

26255 with autograft (includes obtaining graft)

26260 Radical resection, proximal or middle phalanx of finger (eg, tumor);

26261 with autograft (includes obtaining graft)

26262 Radical resection, distal phalanx of finger (eg, tumor)

309

| | Separate Procedure | | Unlisted Procedure | | CCI Comp. Code | | Non-specific Procedure |

INTRODUCTION OR REMOVAL

26320   Removal of implant from finger or hand

(For removal of foreign body in hand or finger, see 20520, 20525)

REPAIR, REVISION, AND/OR RECONSTRUCTION

26340   Manipulation, finger joint, under anesthesia, each joint

(For application of external fixation, see 20690 or 20692)

26350   Repair or advancement, flexor tendon, not in zone 2 digital flexor tendon sheath (eg, no man's land); primary or secondary without free graft, each tendon

26352   secondary with free graft (includes obtaining graft), each tendon

▲ **26356**   Repair or advancement, flexor tendon, in zone 2 digital flexor tendon sheath (eg, no man's land); primary, without free graft, each tendon

▲ **26357**   secondary, without free graft, each tendon

26358   secondary with free graft (includes obtaining graft), each tendon

26370   Repair or advancement of profundus tendon, with intact superficialis tendon; primary, each tendon

26372   secondary with free graft (includes obtaining graft), each tendon

26373   secondary without free graft, each tendon

26390   Excision flexor tendon, with implantation of synthetic rod for delayed tendon graft, hand or finger, each rod

26392   Removal of synthetic rod and insertion of flexor tendon graft, hand or finger (includes obtaining graft), each rod

26410   Repair, extensor tendon, hand, primary or secondary; without free graft, each tendon

26412   with free graft (includes obtaining graft), each tendon

310

● New Code	▲ Revised Code	✛ Add-On Code	⊘ Modifier -51 Exempt

26415 Excision of extensor tendon, with implantation of synthetic rod for delayed tendon graft, hand or finger, each rod

26416 Removal of synthetic rod and insertion of extensor tendon graft (includes obtaining graft), hand or finger, each rod

26418 Repair, extensor tendon, finger, primary or secondary; without free graft, each tendon

26420 with free graft (includes obtaining graft) each tendon

26426 Repair of extensor tendon, central slip, secondary (eg, boutonniere deformity); using local tissue(s), including lateral band(s), each finger

26428 with free graft (includes obtaining graft), each finger

26432 Closed treatment of distal extensor tendon insertion, with or without percutaneous pinning (eg, mallet finger)

26433 Repair of extensor tendon, distal insertion, primary or secondary; without graft (eg, mallet finger)

26434 with free graft (includes obtaining graft)

(for tenovaginotomy for trigger finger, use 26055)

26437 Realignment of extensor tendon, hand, each tendon

26440 Tenolysis, flexor tendon; palm OR finger, each tendon

26442 palm AND finger, each tendon

26445 Tenolysis, extensor tendon, hand OR finger; each tendon

26449 Tenolysis, complex, extensor tendon, finger, including forearm, each tendon

26450 Tenotomy, flexor, palm, open, each tendon

26455 Tenotomy, flexor, finger, open, each tendon

26460 Tenotomy, extensor, hand or finger, open, each tendon

26471 Tenodesis; of proximal interphalangeal joint, each joint

---

311

 Separate Procedure    Unlisted Procedure   CCI Comp. Code   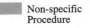 Non-specific Procedure

26474   of distal joint, each joint

26476   Lengthening of tendon, extensor, hand or finger, each tendon

26477   Shortening of tendon, extensor, hand or finger, each tendon

26478   Lengthening of tendon, flexor, hand or finger, each tendon

26479   Shortening of tendon, flexor, hand or finger, each tendon

26480   Transfer or transplant of tendon, carpometacarpal area or dorsum of hand; without free graft, each tendon

26483   with free tendon graft (includes obtaining graft), each tendon

26485   Transfer or transplant of tendon, palmar; without free tendon graft, each tendon

26489   with free tendon graft (includes obtaining graft), each tendon

26490   Opponensplasty; superficialis tendon transfer type, each tendon

26492   tendon transfer with graft (includes obtaining graft), each tendon

26494   hypothenar muscle transfer

26496   other methods

        (For thumb fusion in opposition, use 26820)

26497   Transfer of tendon to restore intrinsic function; ring and small finger

26498   all four fingers

26499   Correction claw finger, other methods

26500   Reconstruction of tendon pulley, each tendon; with local tissues (separate procedure)

26502   with tendon or fascial graft (includes obtaining graft) (separate procedure)

---

312   ● New   ▲ Revised   + Add-On   ⊘ Modifier -51
         Code   Code   Code   Exempt

26504 with tendon prosthesis (separate procedure)

26508 Release of thenar muscle(s) (eg, thumb contracture)

26510 Cross intrinsic transfer, each tendon

26516 Capsulodesis, metacarpophalangeal joint; single digit

26517 two digits

26518 three or four digits

26520 Capsulectomy or capsulotomy; metacarpophalangeal joint, each joint

26525 interphalangeal joint, each joint

26530 Arthroplasty, metacarpophalangeal joint; each joint

26531 with prosthetic implant, each joint

26535 Arthroplasty, interphalangeal joint; each joint

26536 with prosthetic implant, each joint

26540 Repair of collateral ligament, metacarpophalangeal or interphalangeal joint

26541 Reconstruction, collateral ligament, metacarpophalangeal joint, single; with tendon or fascial graft (includes obtaining graft)

26542 with local tissue (eg, adductor advancement)

26545 Reconstruction, collateral ligament, interphalangeal joint, single, including graft, each joint

26546 Repair non-union, metacarpal or phalanx, (includes obtaining bone graft with or without external or internal fixation)

26548 Repair and reconstruction, finger, volar plate, interphalangeal joint

26550 Pollicization of a digit

313

 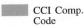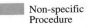

26551 Transfer, toe-to-hand with microvascular anastomosis; great toe wrap-around with bone graft

(For great toe with web space, use 20973)

26553 other than great toe, single

26554 other than great toe, double

(Do not report code 69990 in addition to codes 26551-26554)

26555 Transfer, finger to another position without microvascular anastomosis

26556 Transfer, free toe joint, with microvascular anastomosis

(Do not report code 69990 in addition to code 26556)

26560 Repair of syndactyly (web finger) each web space; with skin flaps

26561 with skin flaps and grafts

26562 complex (eg, involving bone, nails)

26565 Osteotomy; metacarpal, each

26567 phalanx of finger, each

26568 Osteoplasty, lengthening, metacarpal or phalanx

26580 Repair cleft hand

(26585 deleted 2002 edition. To report, use 26587)

26587 Reconstruction of polydactylous digit, soft tissue and bone

(For excision of polydactylous digit, soft tissue only, use 11200)

26590 Repair macrodactylia, each digit

26591 Repair, intrinsic muscles of hand, each muscle

26593 Release, intrinsic muscles of hand, each muscle

● New Code ▲ Revised Code + Add-On Code ⊘ Modifier -51 Exempt

26596 Excision of constricting ring of finger, with multiple Z-plasties

(26597 deleted 2002 edition. To report, see 11041-11042, 14040-14041, or 15120, 15240)

FRACTURE AND/OR DISLOCATION

26600 Closed treatment of metacarpal fracture, single; without manipulation, each bone

26605 with manipulation, each bone

26607 Closed treatment of metacarpal fracture, with manipulation, with external fixation, each bone

26608 Percutaneous skeletal fixation of metacarpal fracture, each bone

26615 Open treatment of metacarpal fracture, single, with or without internal or external fixation, each bone

26641 Closed treatment of carpometacarpal dislocation, thumb, with manipulation

26645 Closed treatment of carpometacarpal fracture dislocation, thumb (Bennett fracture), with manipulation

26650 Percutaneous skeletal fixation of carpometacarpal fracture dislocation, thumb (Bennett fracture), with manipulation, with or without external fixation

26665 Open treatment of carpometacarpal fracture dislocation, thumb (Bennett fracture), with or without internal or external fixation

26670 Closed treatment of carpometacarpal dislocation, other than thumb, with manipulation, each joint; without anesthesia

26675 requiring anesthesia

26676 Percutaneous skeletal fixation of carpometacarpal dislocation, other than thumb, with manipulation, each joint

26685 Open treatment of carpometacarpal dislocation, other than thumb; with or without internal or external fixation, each joint

26686 complex, multiple or delayed reduction

315

 Separate Procedure  Unlisted Procedure CCI Comp. Code 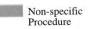 Non-specific Procedure

26700 Closed treatment of metacarpophalangeal dislocation, single, with manipulation; without anesthesia

26705 requiring anesthesia

26706 Percutaneous skeletal fixation of metacarpophalangeal dislocation, single, with manipulation

26715 Open treatment of metacarpophalangeal dislocation, single, with or without internal or external fixation

26720 Closed treatment of phalangeal shaft fracture, proximal or middle phalanx, finger or thumb; without manipulation, each

26725 with manipulation, with or without skin or skeletal traction, each

26727 Percutaneous skeletal fixation of unstable phalangeal shaft fracture, proximal or middle phalanx, finger or thumb, with manipulation, each

26735 Open treatment of phalangeal shaft fracture, proximal or middle phalanx, finger or thumb, with or without internal or external fixation, each

26740 Closed treatment of articular fracture, involving metacarpophalangeal or interphalangeal joint; without manipulation, each

26742 with manipulation, each

26746 Open treatment of articular fracture, involving metacarpophalangeal or interphalangeal joint, with or without internal or external fixation, each

26750 Closed treatment of distal phalangeal fracture, finger or thumb; without manipulation, each

26755 with manipulation, each

26756 Percutaneous skeletal fixation of distal phalangeal fracture, finger or thumb, each

26765 Open treatment of distal phalangeal fracture, finger or thumb, with or without internal or external fixation, each

26770 Closed treatment of interphalangeal joint dislocation, single, with manipulation; without anesthesia

26775 requiring anesthesia

26776 Percutaneous skeletal fixation of interphalangeal joint dislocation, single, with manipulation

26785 Open treatment of interphalangeal joint dislocation, with or without internal or external fixation, single

ARTHRODESIS

26820 Fusion in opposition, thumb, with autogenous graft (includes obtaining graft)

26841 Arthrodesis, carpometacarpal joint, thumb, with or without internal fixation;

26842 with autograft (includes obtaining graft)

26843 Arthrodesis, carpometacarpal joint, digit, other than thumb, each;

26844 with autograft (includes obtaining graft)

26850 Arthrodesis, metacarpophalangeal joint, with or without internal fixation;

26852 with autograft (includes obtaining graft)

26860 Arthrodesis, interphalangeal joint, with or without internal fixation;

+ 26861 each additional interphalangeal joint (List separately in addition to code for primary procedure)

(Use 26861 in conjunction with code 26860)

26862 with autograft (includes obtaining graft)

+ 26863 with autograft (includes obtaining graft), each additional joint (List separately in addition to code for primary procedure)

(Use 26863 in conjunction with code 26862)

317

 Separate Procedure   Unlisted Procedure   CCI Comp. Code   Non-specific Procedure

AMPUTATION

(For hand through metacarpal bones, use 25927)

26910 Amputation, metacarpal, with finger or thumb (ray amputation), single, with or without interosseous transfer

(For repositioning see 26550, 26555)

26951 Amputation, finger or thumb, primary or secondary, any joint or phalanx, single, including neurectomies; with direct closure

26952 with local advancement flaps (V-Y, hood)

(For repair of soft tissue defect requiring split or full thickness graft or other pedicle flaps, see 15050-15758)

OTHER PROCEDURES

26989 Unlisted procedure, hands or fingers

PELVIS AND HIP JOINT

INCISION

(For incision and drainage procedures, superficial, see 10040-10160)

26990 Incision and drainage, pelvis or hip joint area; deep abscess or hematoma

26991 infected bursa

26992 Incision, bone cortex, pelvis and/or hip joint (eg, osteomyelitis or bone abscess)

27000 Tenotomy, adductor of hip, percutaneous (separate procedure)

27001 Tenotomy, adductor of hip, open

27003 Tenotomy, adductor, subcutaneous, open, with obturator neurectomy

27005 Tenotomy, hip flexor(s), open (separate procedure)

27006 Tenotomy, abductors and/or extensor(s) of hip, open (separate procedure)

27025 Fasciotomy, hip or thigh, any type

27030 Arthrotomy, hip, with drainage (eg, infection)

27033 Arthrotomy, hip, including exploration or removal of loose or foreign body

27035 Denervation, hip joint, intrapelvic or extrapelvic intra-articular branches of sciatic, femoral, or obturator nerves

(For obturator neurectomy, see 64763, 64766)

27036 Capsulectomy or capsulotomy, hip, with or without excision of heterotopic bone, with release of hip flexor muscles (ie, gluteus medius, gluteus minimus, tensor fascia latae, rectus femoris, sartorius, iliopsoas)

EXCISION

27040 Biopsy, soft tissue of pelvis and hip area; superficial

27041 deep, subfascial or intramuscular

(For needle biopsy of soft tissue, use 20206)

27047 Excision, tumor, pelvis and hip area; subcutaneous tissue

27048 deep, subfascial, intramuscular

27049 Radical resection of tumor, soft tissue of pelvis and hip area (eg, malignant neoplasm)

27050 Arthrotomy, with biopsy; sacroiliac joint

27052 hip joint

27054 Arthrotomy with synovectomy, hip joint

27060 Excision; ischial bursa

27062 trochanteric bursa or calcification

(For arthrocentesis or needling of bursa, use 20610)

27065 Excision of bone cyst or benign tumor; superficial (wing of ilium, symphysis pubis, or greater trochanter of femur) with or without autograft

319

 Separate Procedure

Unlisted Procedure

 CCI Comp. Code

 Non-specific Procedure

27066   deep, with or without autograft

27067   with autograft requiring separate incision

27070 Partial excision (craterization, saucerization) (eg, osteomyelitis or bone abscess); superficial (eg, wing of ilium, symphysis pubis, or greater trochanter of femur)

27071   deep (subfascial or intramuscular)

27075 Radical resection of tumor or infection; wing of ilium, one pubic or ischial ramus or symphysis pubis

27076   ilium, including acetabulum, both pubic rami, or ischium and acetabulum

27077   innominate bone, total

27078   ischial tuberosity and greater trochanter of femur

27079   ischial tuberosity and greater trochanter of femur, with skin flaps

27080 Coccygectomy, primary

(For pressure (decubitus) ulcer, see 15920, 15922 and 15931-15958)

INTRODUCTION OR REMOVAL

27086 Removal of foreign body, pelvis or hip; subcutaneous tissue

27087   deep (subfascial or intramuscular)

27090 Removal of hip prosthesis; (separate procedure)

27091   complicated, including total hip prosthesis, methylmethacrylate with or without insertion of spacer

27093 Injection procedure for hip arthrography; without anesthesia

(For radiological supervision and interpretation, use 73525. Do not report 76003 in addition to 73525)

27095   with anesthesia

---

320   ● New Code   ▲ Revised Code   + Add-On Code   ⊘ Modifier -51 Exempt

(For radiological supervision and interpretation, use 73525. Do not report 76003 in addition to 73525)

27096 Injection procedure for sacroiliac joint, arthrography and/or anesthetic/steroid

(27096 is to be used only with imaging confirmation of intra-articular needle positioning)

(For radiological supervision and interpretation of sacroiliac joint arthrography, use 73542)

(For fluoroscopic guidance without formal arthrography, use 76005)

(Code 27096 is a unilateral procedure. For bilateral procedure, use modifier -50)

REPAIR, REVISION, AND/OR RECONSTRUCTION

27097 Release or recession, hamstring, proximal

27098 Transfer, adductor to ischium

27100 Transfer external oblique muscle to greater trochanter including fascial or tendon extension (graft)

27105 Transfer paraspinal muscle to hip (includes fascial or tendon extension graft)

27110 Transfer iliopsoas; to greater trochanter of femur

27111 to femoral neck

27120 Acetabuloplasty; (eg, Whitman, Colonna, Haygroves, or cup type)

27122 resection, femoral head (eg, Girdlestone procedure)

27125 Hemiarthroplasty, hip, partial (eg, femoral stem prosthesis, bipolar arthroplasty)

(For prosthetic replacement following fracture of the hip, use 27236)

27130 Arthroplasty, acetabular and proximal femoral prosthetic replacement (total hip arthroplasty), with or without autograft or allograft

321

27132 Conversion of previous hip surgery to total hip arthroplasty, with or without autograft or allograft

27134 Revision of total hip arthroplasty; both components, with or without autograft or allograft

27137 acetabular component only, with or without autograft or allograft

27138 femoral component only, with or without allograft

27140 Osteotomy and transfer of greater trochanter of femur (separate procedure)

27146 Osteotomy, iliac, acetabular or innominate bone;

27147 with open reduction of hip

27151 with femoral osteotomy

27156 with femoral osteotomy and with open reduction of hip

27158 Osteotomy, pelvis, bilateral (eg, congenital malformation)

27161 Osteotomy, femoral neck (separate procedure)

27165 Osteotomy, intertrochanteric or subtrochanteric including internal or external fixation and/or cast

27170 Bone graft, femoral head, neck, intertrochanteric or subtrochanteric area (includes obtaining bone graft)

27175 Treatment of slipped femoral epiphysis; by traction, without reduction

27176 by single or multiple pinning, in situ

27177 Open treatment of slipped femoral epiphysis; single or multiple pinning or bone graft (includes obtaining graft)

27178 closed manipulation with single or multiple pinning

27179 osteoplasty of femoral neck (Heyman type procedure)

27181 osteotomy and internal fixation

● New Code ▲ Revised Code + Add-On Code ⃠ Modifier -51 Exempt

27185 Epiphyseal arrest by epiphysiodesis or stapling, greater trochanter of femur

27187 Prophylactic treatment (nailing, pinning, plating or wiring) with or without methylmethacrylate, femoral neck and proximal femur

FRACTURE AND/OR DISLOCATION

27193 Closed treatment of pelvic ring fracture, dislocation, diastasis or subluxation; without manipulation

27194   with manipulation, requiring more than local anesthesia

27200 Closed treatment of coccygeal fracture

27202 Open treatment of coccygeal fracture

27215 Open treatment of iliac spine(s), tuberosity avulsion, or iliac wing fracture(s) (eg, pelvic fracture(s) which do not disrupt the pelvic ring), with internal fixation

27216 Percutaneous skeletal fixation of posterior pelvic ring fracture and/or dislocation (includes ilium, sacroiliac joint and/or sacrum)

27217 Open treatment of anterior ring fracture and/or dislocation with internal fixation (includes pubic symphysis and/or rami)

27218 Open treatment of posterior ring fracture and/or dislocation with internal fixation (includes ilium, sacroiliac joint and/or sacrum)

27220 Closed treatment of acetabulum (hip socket) fracture(s); without manipulation

27222   with manipulation, with or without skeletal traction

27226 Open treatment of posterior or anterior acetabular wall fracture, with internal fixation

27227 Open treatment of acetabular fracture(s) involving anterior or posterior (one) column, or a fracture running transversely across the acetabulum, with internal fixation

323

 Separate Procedure   Unlisted Procedure   CCI Comp. Code   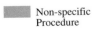 Non-specific Procedure

27228 Open treatment of acetabular fracture(s) involving anterior and posterior (two) columns, includes T-fracture and both column fracture with complete articular detachment, or single column or transverse fracture with associated acetabular wall fracture, with internal fixation

27230 Closed treatment of femoral fracture, proximal end, neck; without manipulation

27232 with manipulation, with or without skeletal traction

27235 Percutaneous skeletal fixation of femoral fracture, proximal end, neck

27236 Open treatment of femoral fracture, proximal end, neck, internal fixation or prosthetic replacement

27238 Closed treatment of intertrochanteric, pertrochanteric, or subtrochanteric femoral fracture; without manipulation

27240 with manipulation, with or without skin or skeletal traction

27244 Treatment of intertrochanteric, pertrochanteric or subtrochanteric femoral fracture; with plate/screw type implant, with or without cerclage

27245 with intramedullary implant, with or without interlocking screws and/or cerclage

27246 Closed treatment of greater trochanteric fracture, without manipulation

27248 Open treatment of greater trochanteric fracture, with or without internal or external fixation

27250 Closed treatment of hip dislocation, traumatic; without anesthesia

27252 requiring anesthesia

27253 Open treatment of hip dislocation, traumatic, without internal fixation

27254 Open treatment of hip dislocation, traumatic, with acetabular wall and femoral head fracture, with or without internal or external fixation

● New Code ▲ Revised Code + Add-On Code ⊘ Modifier -51 Exempt

27256 Treatment of spontaneous hip dislocation (developmental, including congenital or pathological), by abduction, splint or traction; without anesthesia, without manipulation

27257   with manipulation, requiring anesthesia

27258 Open treatment of spontaneous hip dislocation (developmental, including congenital or pathological), replacement of femoral head in acetabulum (including tenotomy, etc);

27259   with femoral shaft shortening

27265 Closed treatment of post hip arthroplasty dislocation; without anesthesia

27266   requiring regional or general anesthesia

MANIPULATION

27275 Manipulation, hip joint, requiring general anesthesia

ARTHRODESIS

27280 Arthrodesis, sacroiliac joint (including obtaining graft)

27282 Arthrodesis, symphysis pubis (including obtaining graft)

27284 Arthrodesis, hip joint (including obtaining graft);

27286   with subtrochanteric osteotomy

AMPUTATION

27290 Interpelviabdominal amputation (hindquarter amputation)

27295 Disarticulation of hip

OTHER PROCEDURES

27299 Unlisted procedure, pelvis or hip joint

325

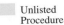 Separate Procedure   Unlisted Procedure   CCI Comp. Code   Non-specific Procedure

FEMUR (THIGH REGION) AND KNEE JOINT

INCISION

(For incision and drainage of abscess or hematoma, superficial, see 10040-10160)

27301 Incision and drainage, deep abscess, bursa, or hematoma, thigh or knee region

27303 Incision, deep, with opening of bone cortex, femur or knee (eg, osteomyelitis or bone abscess)

27305 Fasciotomy, iliotibial (tenotomy), open

(For combined Ober-Yount fasciotomy, use 27025)

27306 Tenotomy, percutaneous, adductor or hamstring; single tendon (separate procedure)

27307 multiple tendons

27310 Arthrotomy, knee, with exploration, drainage, or removal of foreign body(eg, infection)

27315 Neurectomy, hamstring muscle

27320 Neurectomy, popliteal (gastrocnemius)

EXCISION

27323 Biopsy, soft tissue of thigh or knee area; superficial

27324 deep (subfascial or intramuscular)

(For needle biopsy of soft tissue, use 20206)

27327 Excision, tumor, thigh or knee area; subcutaneous

27328 deep, subfascial, or intramuscular

27329 Radical resection of tumor (eg, malignant neoplasm), soft tissue of thigh or knee area

27330 Arthrotomy, knee; with synovial biopsy only

326

● New Code   ▲ Revised Code   ✛ Add-On Code   ⊘ Modifier -51 Exempt

27331   including joint exploration, biopsy, or removal of loose or foreign bodies

27332 Arthrotomy, with excision of semilunar cartilage (meniscectomy) knee; medial OR lateral

27333   medial AND lateral

27334 Arthrotomy, with synovectomy, knee; anterior OR posterior

27335   anterior AND posterior including popliteal area

27340 Excision, prepatellar bursa

27345 Excision of synovial cyst of popliteal space (eg, Baker's cyst)

27347 Excision of lesion of meniscus or capsule (eg, cyst, ganglion), knee

27350 Patellectomy or hemipatellectomy

27355 Excision or curettage of bone cyst or benign tumor of femur;

27356   with allograft

27357   with autograft (includes obtaining graft)

+ **27358**   with internal fixation (List in addition to code for primary procedure)

(Use 27358 in conjunction with codes 27355, 27356 or 27357)

27360 Partial excision (craterization, saucerization, or diaphysectomy) bone, femur, proximal tibia and/or fibula (eg, osteomyelitis or bone abscess)

27365 Radical resection of tumor, bone, femur or knee

(For radical resection of tumor, soft tissue, use 27329)

INTRODUCTION OR REMOVAL

27370 Injection procedure for knee arthrography

(For radiological supervision and interpretation, use 73580. Do not report 76003 in addition to 73580)

 Separate Procedure   Unlisted Procedure   CCI Comp. Code   Non-specific Procedure

27372   Removal of foreign body, deep, thigh region or knee area

(For removal of knee prosthesis including "total knee," use 27488)

REPAIR, REVISION, AND/OR RECONSTRUCTION

27380   Suture of infrapatellar tendon; primary

27381   secondary reconstruction, including fascial or tendon graft

27385   Suture of quadriceps or hamstring muscle rupture; primary

27386   secondary reconstruction, including fascial or tendon graft

27390   Tenotomy, open, hamstring, knee to hip; single tendon

27391   multiple tendons, one leg

27392   multiple tendons, bilateral

27393   Lengthening of hamstring tendon; single tendon

27394   multiple tendons, one leg

27395   multiple tendons, bilateral

27396   Transplant, hamstring tendon to patella; single tendon

27397   multiple tendons

27400   Transfer, tendon or muscle, hamstrings to femur (eg, Egger's type procedure)

27403   Arthrotomy with meniscus repair, knee

(For arthroscopic repair, use 29882)

27405   Repair, primary, torn ligament and/or capsule, knee; collateral

27407   cruciate

27409   collateral and cruciate ligaments

27418   Anterior tibial tubercleplasty (eg, Maquet type procedure)

328

●   New Code   ▲   Revised Code   ✛   Add-On Code   ⊘   Modifier -51 Exempt

27420 Reconstruction of dislocating patella; (eg, Hauser type procedure)

27422 with extensor realignment and/or muscle advancement or release (eg, Campbell, Goldwaite type procedure)

27424 with patellectomy

27425 Lateral retinacular release open

(For arthroscopic lateral release, use 29873)

27427 Ligamentous reconstruction (augmentation), knee; extra-articular

27428 intra-articular (open)

27429 intra-articular (open) and extra-articular

(For primary repair of ligament(s) performed in addition to reconstruction, report 27405, 27407 or 27409 in addition to code 27427, 27428 or 27429)

27430 Quadricepsplasty (eg, Bennett or Thompson type)

27435 Capsulotomy, posterior capsular release, knee

27437 Arthroplasty, patella; without prosthesis

27438 with prosthesis

27440 Arthroplasty, knee, tibial plateau;

27441 with debridement and partial synovectomy

27442 Arthroplasty, femoral condyles or tibial plateau(s), knee;

27443 with debridement and partial synovectomy

27445 Arthroplasty, knee, hinge prosthesis (eg, Walldius type)

27446 Arthroplasty, knee, condyle and plateau; medial OR lateral compartment

27447 medial AND lateral compartments with or without patella resurfacing (total knee arthroplasty)

329

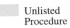 Separate Procedure
 Unlisted Procedure
 CCI Comp. Code
Non-specific Procedure

(For revision of total knee arthroplasty, use 27487)

(For removal of total knee prosthesis, use 27488)

27448 Osteotomy, femur, shaft or supracondylar; without fixation

27450 with fixation

27454 Osteotomy, multiple, with realignment on intramedullary rod, femoral shaft (eg, Sofield type procedure)

27455 Osteotomy, proximal tibia, including fibular excision or osteotomy (includes correction of genu varus (bowleg) or genu valgus (knock-knee)); before epiphyseal closure

27457 after epiphyseal closure

27465 Osteoplasty, femur; shortening (excluding 64876)

27466 lengthening

27468 combined, lengthening and shortening with femoral segment transfer

27470 Repair, nonunion or malunion, femur, distal to head and neck; without graft (eg, compression technique)

27472 with iliac or other autogenous bone graft (includes obtaining graft)

27475 Arrest, epiphyseal, any method (eg, epiphysiodesis); distal femur

27477 tibia and fibula, proximal

27479 combined distal femur, proximal tibia and fibula

27485 Arrest, hemiepiphyseal, distal femur or proximal tibia or fibula (eg, genu varus or valgus)

27486 Revision of total knee arthroplasty, with or without allograft; one component

27487 femoral and entire tibial component

27488 Removal of prosthesis, including total knee prosthesis, methylmethacrylate with or without insertion of spacer, knee

27495 Prophylactic treatment (nailing, pinning, plating or wiring) with or without methylmethacrylate, femur

27496 Decompression fasciotomy, thigh and/or knee, one compartment (flexor or extensor or adductor);

27497   with debridement of nonviable muscle and/or nerve

27498 Decompression fasciotomy, thigh and/or knee, multiple compartments;

27499   with debridement of nonviable muscle and/or nerve

FRACTURE AND/OR DISLOCATION

(For arthroscopic treatment of intercondylar spine(s) and tuberosity fracture(s) of the knee, see 29850, 29851)

(For arthroscopic treatment of tibial fracture, see 29855, 29856)

27500 Closed treatment of femoral shaft fracture, without manipulation

27501 Closed treatment of supracondylar or transcondylar femoral fracture with or without intercondylar extension, without manipulation

27502 Closed treatment of femoral shaft fracture, with manipulation, with or without skin or skeletal traction

27503 Closed treatment of supracondylar or transcondylar femoral fracture with or without intercondylar extension, with manipulation, with or without skin or skeletal traction

27506 Open treatment of femoral shaft fracture, with or without external fixation, with insertion of intramedullary implant, with or without cerclage and/or locking screws

27507 Open treatment of femoral shaft fracture with plate/screws, with or without cerclage

27508 Closed treatment of femoral fracture, distal end, medial or lateral condyle, without manipulation

27509 Percutaneous skeletal fixation of femoral fracture, distal end, medial or lateral condyle, or supracondylar or transcondylar, with or without intercondylar extension, or distal femoral epiphyseal separation

331

Separate Procedure   Unlisted Procedure   CCI Comp. Code   Non-specific Procedure

27510 Closed treatment of femoral fracture, distal end, medial or lateral condyle, with manipulation

27511 Open treatment of femoral supracondylar or transcondylar fracture without intercondylar extension, with or without internal or external fixation

27513 Open treatment of femoral supracondylar or transcondylar fracture with intercondylar extension, with or without internal or external fixation

27514 Open treatment of femoral fracture, distal end, medial or lateral condyle, with or without internal or external fixation

27516 Closed treatment of distal femoral epiphyseal separation; without manipulation

27517 with manipulation, with or without skin or skeletal traction

27519 Open treatment of distal femoral epiphyseal separation, with or without internal or external fixation

27520 Closed treatment of patellar fracture, without manipulation

27524 Open treatment of patellar fracture, with internal fixation and/or partial or complete patellectomy and soft tissue repair

27530 Closed treatment of tibial fracture, proximal (plateau); without manipulation

27532 with or without manipulation, with skeletal traction

(For arthroscopic treatment, see 29855, 29856)

27535 Open treatment of tibial fracture, proximal (plateau); unicondylar, with or without internal or external fixation

27536 bicondylar, with or without internal fixation

(For arthroscopic treatment, see 29855, 29856)

27538 Closed treatment of intercondylar spine(s) and/or tuberosity fracture(s) of knee, with or without manipulation

(For arthroscopic treatment, see 29850, 29851)

● New Code   ▲ Revised Code   + Add-On Code   ⊘ Modifier -51 Exempt

27540   Open treatment of intercondylar spine(s) and/or tuberosity fracture(s) of the knee, with or without internal or external fixation

27550   Closed treatment of knee dislocation; without anesthesia

27552   requiring anesthesia

27556   Open treatment of knee dislocation, with or without internal or external fixation; without primary ligamentous repair or augmentation/reconstruction

27557   with primary ligamentous repair

27558   with primary ligamentous repair, with augmentation/reconstruction

27560   Closed treatment of patellar dislocation; without anesthesia

(For recurrent dislocation, see 27420-27424)

27562   requiring anesthesia

27566   Open treatment of patellar dislocation, with or without partial or total patellectomy

MANIPULATION

27570   Manipulation of knee joint under general anesthesia (includes application of traction or other fixation devices)

ARTHRODESIS

27580   Arthrodesis, knee, any technique

AMPUTATION

27590   Amputation, thigh, through femur, any level;

27591   immediate fitting technique including first cast

27592   open, circular (guillotine)

27594   secondary closure or scar revision

27596   re-amputation

333

 Separate Procedure   Unlisted Procedure   CCI Comp. Code   Non-specific Procedure

| 27598 | Disarticulation at knee |

OTHER PROCEDURES

| 27599 | Unlisted procedure, femur or knee |

LEG (TIBIA AND FIBULA) AND ANKLE JOINT

INCISION

| 27600 | Decompression fasciotomy, leg; anterior and/or lateral compartments only |

| 27601 | posterior compartment(s) only |

| 27602 | anterior and/or lateral, and posterior compartment(s) |

(For incision and drainage procedures, superficial, see 10040-10160)

(For decompression fasciotomy with debridement, see 27892-27894)

| 27603 | Incision and drainage, leg or ankle; deep abscess or hematoma |

| 27604 | infected bursa |

| 27605 | Tenotomy, percutaneous, Achilles tendon (separate procedure); local anesthesia |

| 27606 | general anesthesia |

| 27607 | Incision (eg, osteomyelitis or bone abscess), leg or ankle |

| 27610 | Arthrotomy, ankle, including exploration, drainage, or removal of foreign body |

| 27612 | Arthrotomy, posterior capsular release, ankle, with or without Achilles tendon lengthening |

(See also 27685)

EXCISION

| 27613 | Biopsy, soft tissue of leg or ankle area; superficial |

| 27614 | deep (subfascial or intramuscular) |

● New Code   ▲ Revised Code   + Add-On Code   ⊘ Modifier -51 Exempt

(For needle biopsy of soft tissue, use 20206)

27615 Radical resection of tumor (eg, malignant neoplasm), soft tissue of leg or ankle area

27618 Excision, tumor, leg or ankle area; subcutaneous tissue

27619 deep (subfascial or intramuscular)

27620 Arthrotomy, ankle, with joint exploration, with or without biopsy, with or without removal of loose or foreign body

27625 Arthrotomy, with synovectomy, ankle;

27626 including tenosynovectomy

27630 Excision of lesion of tendon sheath or capsule (eg, cyst or ganglion), leg and/or ankle

27635 Excision or curettage of bone cyst or benign tumor, tibia or fibula;

27637 with autograft (includes obtaining graft)

27638 with allograft

27640 Partial excision (craterization, saucerization, or diaphysectomy) bone (eg, osteomyelitis or exostosis); tibia

27641 fibula

27645 Radical resection of tumor, bone; tibia

27646 fibula

27647 talus or calcaneus

INTRODUCTION OR REMOVAL

27648 Injection procedure for ankle arthrography

(For radiological supervision and interpretation use 73615. Do not report 76003 in addition to 73615)

(For ankle arthroscopy, see 29894-29898)

335

 Separate Procedure

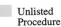 Unlisted Procedure

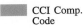 CCI Comp. Code

 Non-specific Procedure

REPAIR, REVISION, AND/OR RECONSTRUCTION

27650 Repair, primary, open or percutaneous, ruptured Achilles tendon;

27652 with graft (includes obtaining graft)

27654 Repair, secondary, Achilles tendon, with or without graft

27656 Repair, fascial defect of leg

27658 Repair, flexor tendon, leg; primary, without graft, each tendon

27659 secondary, with or without graft, each tendon

27664 Repair, extensor tendon, leg; primary, without graft, each tendon

27665 secondary, with or without graft, each tendon

27675 Repair, dislocating peroneal tendons; without fibular osteotomy

27676 with fibular osteotomy

27680 Tenolysis, flexor or extensor tendon, leg and/or ankle; single, each tendon

27681 multiple tendons (through separate incision(s))

27685 Lengthening or shortening of tendon, leg or ankle; single tendon (separate procedure)

27686 multiple tendons (through same incision), each

27687 Gastrocnemius recession (eg, Strayer procedure)

(Toe extensors are considered as a group to be single tendon when transplanted into midfoot)

27690 Transfer or transplant of single tendon (with muscle redirection or rerouting); superficial (eg, anterior tibial extensors into midfoot)

27691 deep (eg, anterior tibial or posterior tibial through interosseous space, flexor digitorum longus, flexor hallucis longus, or peroneal tendon to midfoot or hind foot)

● New Code   ▲ Revised Code   + Add-On Code   ⊘ Modifier -51 Exempt

+ 27692   each additional tendon (List separately in addition to code for primary procedure)

(Use 27692 in conjunction with codes 27690, 27691)

27695   Repair, primary, disrupted ligament, ankle; collateral

27696   both collateral ligaments

27698   Repair, secondary disrupted ligament, ankle, collateral (eg, Watson-Jones procedure)

27700   Arthroplasty, ankle;

27702   with implant (total ankle)

27703   revision, total ankle

27704   Removal of ankle implant

27705   Osteotomy; tibia

27707   fibula

27709   tibia and fibula

27712   multiple, with realignment on intramedullary rod (eg, Sofield type procedure)

(For osteotomy to correct genu varus (bowleg) or genu valgus (knock-knee), see 27455-27457)

27715   Osteoplasty, tibia and fibula, lengthening or shortening

27720   Repair of nonunion or malunion, tibia; without graft, (eg, compression technique)

27722   with sliding graft

27724   with iliac or other autograft (includes obtaining graft)

27725   by synostosis, with fibula, any method

27727   Repair of congenital pseudarthrosis, tibia

337

| ■ Separate Procedure | ▨ Unlisted Procedure | ▨ CCI Comp. Code | ▨ Non-specific Procedure |

27730 Arrest, epiphyseal (epiphysiodesis), open; distal tibia

27732 distal fibula

27734 distal tibia and fibula

27740 Arrest, epiphyseal (epiphysiodesis), any method, combined, proximal and distal tibia and fibula;

27742 and distal femur

(For epiphyseal arrest of proximal tibia and fibula, use 27477)

27745 Prophylactic treatment (nailing, pinning, plating or wiring) with or without methylmethacrylate, tibia

FRACTURE AND/OR DISLOCATION

27750 Closed treatment of tibial shaft fracture (with or without fibular fracture); without manipulation

27752 with manipulation, with or without skeletal traction

27756 Percutaneous skeletal fixation of tibial shaft fracture (with or without fibular fracture) (eg, pins or screws)

27758 Open treatment of tibial shaft fracture, (with or without fibular fracture) with plate/screws, with or without cerclage

27759 Treatment of tibial shaft fracture (with or without fibular fracture) by intramedullary implant, with or without interlocking screws and/or cerclage

27760 Closed treatment of medial malleolus fracture; without manipulation

27762 with manipulation, with or without skin or skeletal traction

27766 Open treatment of medial malleolus fracture, with or without internal or external fixation

27780 Closed treatment of proximal fibula or shaft fracture; without manipulation

27781 with manipulation

● New
Code

▲ Revised
Code

✚ Add-On
Code

⊘ Modifier -51
Exempt

27784 Open treatment of proximal fibula or shaft fracture, with or without internal or external fixation

27786 Closed treatment of distal fibular fracture (lateral malleolus); without manipulation

27788 with manipulation

27792 Open treatment of distal fibular fracture (lateral malleolus), with or without internal or external fixation

27808 Closed treatment of bimalleolar ankle fracture, (including Potts); without manipulation

27810 with manipulation

27814 Open treatment of bimalleolar ankle fracture, with or without internal or external fixation

27816 Closed treatment of trimalleolar ankle fracture; without manipulation

27818 with manipulation

27822 Open treatment of trimalleolar ankle fracture, with or without internal or external fixation, medial and/or lateral malleolus; without fixation of posterior lip

27823 with fixation of posterior lip

27824 Closed treatment of fracture of weight bearing articular portion of distal tibia (eg, pilon or tibial plafond), with or without anesthesia; without manipulation

27825 with skeletal traction and/or requiring manipulation

27826 Open treatment of fracture of weight bearing articular surface/portion of distal tibia (eg, pilon or tibial plafond), with internal or external fixation; of fibula only

27827 of tibia only

27828 of both tibia and fibula

27829 Open treatment of distal tibiofibular joint (syndesmosis) disruption, with or without internal or external fixation

339

| | Separate Procedure | | Unlisted Procedure | | CCI Comp. Code | | Non-specific Procedure |

27830 Closed treatment of proximal tibiofibular joint dislocation; without anesthesia

27831 requiring anesthesia

27832 Open treatment of proximal tibiofibular joint dislocation, with or without internal or external fixation, or with excision of proximal fibula

27840 Closed treatment of ankle dislocation; without anesthesia

27842 requiring anesthesia, with or without percutaneous skeletal fixation

27846 Open treatment of ankle dislocation, with or without percutaneous skeletal fixation; without repair or internal fixation

27848 with repair or internal or external fixation

MANIPULATION

27860 Manipulation of ankle under general anesthesia (includes application of traction or other fixation apparatus)

ARTHRODESIS

27870 Arthrodesis, ankle, open

(For arthroscopic ankle arthrodesis, use 29899)

27871 Arthrodesis, tibiofibular joint, proximal or distal

AMPUTATION

27880 Amputation, leg, through tibia and fibula;

27881 with immediate fitting technique including application of first cast

27882 open, circular (guillotine)

27884 secondary closure or scar revision

27886 re-amputation

27888   Amputation, ankle, through malleoli of tibia and fibula (eg, Syme, Pirogoff type procedures), with plastic closure and resection of nerves

27889   Ankle disarticulation

OTHER PROCEDURES

27892   Decompression fasciotomy, leg; anterior and/or lateral compartments only, with debridement of nonviable muscle and/or nerve

(For decompression fasciotomy of the leg without debridement, use 27600)

27893   posterior compartment(s) only, with debridement of nonviable muscle and/or nerve

(For decompession fasciotomy of the leg without debridement, use 27601)

27894   anterior and/or lateral, and posterior compartment(s), with debridement of nonviable muscle and/or nerve

(For decompression fasciotomy of the leg without debridement, use 27602)

27899   Unlisted procedure, leg or ankle

FOOT AND TOES

INCISION

(For incision and drainage procedures, superficial, see 10040-10160)

28001   Incision and drainage, bursa, foot

28002   Incision and drainage below fascia, with or without tendon sheath involvement, foot; single bursal space

28003   multiple areas

28005   Incision, bone cortex (eg, osteomyelitis or bone abscess), foot

28008   Fasciotomy, foot and/or toe

(See also 28060, 28062, 28250)

341

28010 Tenotomy, percutaneous, toe; single tendon

28011   multiple tendons

    (For open tenotomy, see 28230-28234)

28020 Arthrotomy, including exploration, drainage, or removal of loose or foreign body; intertarsal or tarsometatarsal joint

28022   metatarsophalangeal joint

28024   interphalangeal joint

28030 Neurectomy, intrinsic musculature of foot

28035 Release, tarsal tunnel (posterior tibial nerve decompression)

    (For other nerve entrapments, see 64704, 64722)

EXCISION

28043 Excision, tumor, foot; subcutaneous tissue

28045   deep, subfascial, intramuscular

28046 Radical resection of tumor (eg, malignant neoplasm), soft tissue of foot

28050 Arthrotomy with biopsy; intertarsal or tarsometatarsal joint

28052   metatarsophalangeal joint

28054   interphalangeal joint

28060 Fasciectomy, plantar fascia; partial (separate procedure)

28062   radical (separate procedure)

    (For plantar fasciotomy, see 28008, 28250)

28070 Synovectomy; intertarsal or tarsometatarsal joint, each

28072   metatarsophalangeal joint, each

28080 Excision, interdigital (Morton) neuroma, single, each

28086 Synovectomy, tendon sheath, foot; flexor

● New Code   ▲ Revised Code   + Add-On Code   ⊘ Modifier -51 Exempt

28088   extensor

28090   Excision of lesion, tendon, tendon sheath, or capsule (including synovectomy) (eg, cyst or ganglion); foot

28092   toe(s), each

28100   Excision or curettage of bone cyst or benign tumor, talus or calcaneus;

28102   with iliac or other autograft (includes obtaining graft)

28103   with allograft

28104   Excision or curettage of bone cyst or benign tumor, tarsal or metatarsal, except talus or calcaneus;

28106   with iliac or other autograft (includes obtaining graft)

28107   with allograft

28108   Excision or curettage of bone cyst or benign tumor, phalanges of foot

(For ostectomy, partial (eg, hallux valgus, Silver type procedure), use 28290)

28110   Ostectomy, partial excision, fifth metatarsal head (bunionette) (separate procedure)

28111   Ostectomy, complete excision; first metatarsal head

28112   other metatarsal head (second, third or fourth)

28113   fifth metatarsal head

28114   all metatarsal heads, with partial proximal phalangectomy, excluding first metatarsal (eg, Clayton type procedure)

28116   Ostectomy, excision of tarsal coalition

28118   Ostectomy, calcaneus;

28119   for spur, with or without plantar fascial release

343

 Separate Procedure   Unlisted Procedure   CCI Comp. Code   Non-specific Procedure

| 28120 | Partial excision (craterization, saucerization, sequestrectomy, or diaphysectomy) bone (eg, osteomyelitis or bossing); talus or calcaneus |

| 28122 | tarsal or metatarsal bone, except talus or calcaneus |

(For partial excision of talus or calcaneus, use 28120)

(For cheilectomy for hallux rigidus, use 28289)

| 28124 | phalanx of toe |

| 28126 | Resection, partial or complete, phalangeal base, each toe |

| 28130 | Talectomy (astragalectomy) |

| 28140 | Metatarsectomy |

| 28150 | Phalangectomy, toe, each toe |

| 28153 | Resection, condyle(s), distal end of phalanx, each toe |

| 28160 | Hemiphalangectomy or interphalangeal joint excision, toe, proximal end of phalanx, each |

| 28171 | Radical resection of tumor, bone; tarsal (except talus or calcaneus) |

| 28173 | metatarsal |

| 28175 | phalanx of toe |

(For talus or calcaneus, use 27647)

INTRODUCTION OR REMOVAL

| 28190 | Removal of foreign body, foot; subcutaneous |

| 28192 | deep |

| 28193 | complicated |

REPAIR, REVISION, AND/OR RECONSTRUCTION

| 28200 | Repair, tendon, flexor, foot; primary or secondary, without free graft, each tendon |

344

| ● | New Code | ▲ | Revised Code | + | Add-On Code | ⊘ | Modifier -51 Exempt |

28202   secondary with free graft, each tendon (includes obtaining graft)

28208   Repair, tendon, extensor, foot; primary or secondary, each tendon

28210   secondary with free graft, each tendon (includes obtaining graft)

28220   Tenolysis, flexor, foot; single tendon

28222   multiple tendons

28225   Tenolysis, extensor, foot; single tendon

28226   multiple tendons

28230   Tenotomy, open, tendon flexor; foot, single or multiple tendon(s) (separate procedure)

28232   toe, single tendon (separate procedure)

28234   Tenotomy, open, extensor, foot or toe, each tendon

28238   Reconstruction (advancement), posterior tibial tendon with excision of accessory tarsal navicular bone (eg, Kidner type procedure)

(For subcutaneous tenotomy, see 28010, 28011)

(For transfer or transplant of tendon with muscle redirection or rerouting, see 27690-27692)

(For extensor hallucis longus transfer with great toe IP fusion (Jones procedure), use 28760)

28240   Tenotomy, lengthening, or release, abductor hallucis muscle

28250   Division of plantar fascia and muscle (eg, Steindler stripping) (separate procedure)

28260   Capsulotomy, midfoot; medial release only (separate procedure)

28261   with tendon lengthening

28262   extensive, including posterior talotibial capsulotomy and tendon(s) lengthening (eg, resistant clubfoot deformity)

345

Separate Procedure   Unlisted Procedure   CCI Comp. Code   Non-specific Procedure

28264 Capsulotomy, midtarsal (eg, Heyman type procedure)

28270 Capsulotomy; metatarsophalangeal joint, with or without tenorrhaphy, each joint (separate procedure)

28272 interphalangeal joint, each joint (separate procedure)

28280 Syndactylization, toes (eg, webbing or Kelikian type procedure)

28285 Correction, hammertoe (eg, interphalangeal fusion, partial or total phalangectomy)

28286 Correction, cock-up fifth toe, with plastic skin closure (eg, Ruiz-Mora type procedure)

28288 Ostectomy, partial, exostectomy or condylectomy, metatarsal head, each metatarsal head

28289 Hallux rigidus correction with cheilectomy, debridement and capsular release of the first metatarsophalangeal joint

28290 Correction, hallux valgus (bunion), with or without sesamoidectomy; simple exostectomy (eg, Silver type procedure)

28292 Keller, McBride, or Mayo type procedure

28293 resection of joint with implant

28294 with tendon transplants (eg, Joplin type procedure)

28296 with metatarsal osteotomy (eg, Mitchell, Chevron, or concentric type procedures)

28297 Lapidus type procedure

28298 by phalanx osteotomy

28299 by double osteotomy

28300 Osteotomy; calcaneus (eg, Dwyer or Chambers type procedure), with or without internal fixation

28302 talus

28304 Osteotomy, tarsal bones, other than calcaneus or talus;

346

| | New Code | ▲ Revised Code | + Add-On Code | ⊘ Modifier -51 Exempt |

28305   with autograft (includes obtaining graft) (eg, Fowler type)

28306 Osteotomy, with or without lengthening, shortening or angular correction, metatarsal; first metatarsal

28307   first metatarsal with autograft (other than first toe)

28308   other than first metatarsal, each

28309   multiple (eg, Swanson type cavus foot procedure)

28310 Osteotomy, shortening, angular or rotational correction; proximal phalanx, first toe (separate procedure)

28312   other phalanges, any toe

28313 Reconstruction, angular deformity of toe, soft tissue procedures only (eg, overlapping second toe, fifth toe, curly toes)

28315 Sesamoidectomy, first toe (separate procedure)

28320 Repair, nonunion or malunion; tarsal bones

28322   metatarsal, with or without bone graft (includes obtaining graft)

28340 Reconstruction, toe, macrodactyly; soft tissue resection

28341   requiring bone resection

28344 Reconstruction, toe(s); polydactyly

28345   syndactyly, with or without skin graft(s), each web

28360 Reconstruction, cleft foot

FRACTURE AND/OR DISLOCATION

28400 Closed treatment of calcaneal fracture; without manipulation

28405   with manipulation

28406 Percutaneous skeletal fixation of calcaneal fracture, with manipulation

347

 Separate Procedure   Unlisted Procedure    CCI Comp. Code   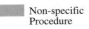 Non-specific Procedure

28415 Open treatment of calcaneal fracture, with or without internal or external fixation;

28420 with primary iliac or other autogenous bone graft (includes obtaining graft)

28430 Closed treatment of talus fracture; without manipulation

28435 with manipulation

28436 Percutaneous skeletal fixation of talus fracture, with manipulation

28445 Open treatment of talus fracture, with or without internal or external fixation

28450 Treatment of tarsal bone fracture (except talus and calcaneus); without manipulation, each

28455 with manipulation, each

28456 Percutaneous skeletal fixation of tarsal bone fracture (except talus and calcaneus), with manipulation, each

28465 Open treatment of tarsal bone fracture (except talus and calcaneus), with or without internal or external fixation, each

28470 Closed treatment of metatarsal fracture; without manipulation, each

28475 with manipulation, each

28476 Percutaneous skeletal fixation of metatarsal fracture, with manipulation, each

28485 Open treatment of metatarsal fracture, with or without internal or external fixation, each

28490 Closed treatment of fracture great toe, phalanx or phalanges; without manipulation

28495 with manipulation

28496 Percutaneous skeletal fixation of fracture great toe, phalanx or phalanges, with manipulation

● New Code   ▲ Revised Code   + Add-On Code   ⊘ Modifier -51 Exempt

28505 Open treatment of fracture great toe, phalanx or phalanges, with or without internal or external fixation

28510 Closed treatment of fracture, phalanx or phalanges, other than great toe; without manipulation, each

28515 with manipulation, each

28525 Open treatment of fracture, phalanx or phalanges, other than great toe, with or without internal or external fixation, each

28530 Closed treatment of sesamoid fracture

28531 Open treatment of sesamoid fracture, with or without internal fixation

28540 Closed treatment of tarsal bone dislocation, other than talotarsal; without anesthesia

28545 requiring anesthesia

28546 Percutaneous skeletal fixation of tarsal bone dislocation, other than talotarsal, with manipulation

28555 Open treatment of tarsal bone dislocation, with or without internal or external fixation

28570 Closed treatment of talotarsal joint dislocation; without anesthesia

28575 requiring anesthesia

28576 Percutaneous skeletal fixation of talotarsal joint dislocation, with manipulation

28585 Open treatment of talotarsal joint dislocation, with or without internal or external fixation

28600 Closed treatment of tarsometatarsal joint dislocation; without anesthesia

28605 requiring anesthesia

28606 Percutaneous skeletal fixation of tarsometatarsal joint dislocation, with manipulation

349

 Separate Procedure   Unlisted Procedure   CCI Comp. Code   Non-specific Procedure

28615	Open treatment of tarsometatarsal joint dislocation, with or without internal or external fixation
28630	Closed treatment of metatarsophalangeal joint dislocation; without anesthesia
28635	requiring anesthesia
28636	Percutaneous skeletal fixation of metatarsophalangeal joint dislocation, with manipulation
28645	Open treatment of metatarsophalangeal joint dislocation, with or without internal or external fixation
28660	Closed treatment of interphalangeal joint dislocation; without anesthesia
28665	requiring anesthesia
28666	Percutaneous skeletal fixation of interphalangeal joint dislocation, with manipulation
28675	Open treatment of interphalangeal joint dislocation, with or without internal or external fixation

ARTHRODESIS

28705	Arthrodesis; pantalar
28715	triple
28725	subtalar
28730	Arthrodesis, midtarsal or tarsometatarsal, multiple or transverse;
28735	with osteotomy (eg, flatfoot correction)
28737	Arthrodesis, with tendon lengthening and advancement, midtarsal, tarsal navicular-cuneiform (eg, Miller type procedure)
28740	Arthrodesis, midtarsal or tarsometatarsal, single joint
28750	Arthrodesis, great toe; metatarsophalangeal joint
28755	interphalangeal joint

● New Code ▲ Revised Code + Add-On Code ⊘ Modifier -51 Exempt

28760 Arthrodesis, with extensor hallucis longus transfer to first metatarsal neck, great toe, interphalangeal joint (eg, Jones type procedure)

(For hammertoe operation or interphalangeal fusion, use 28285)

AMPUTATION

28800 Amputation, foot; midtarsal (eg, Chopart type procedure)

28805 transmetatarsal

28810 Amputation, metatarsal, with toe, single

28820 Amputation, toe; metatarsophalangeal joint

28825 interphalangeal joint

(For amputation of tuft of distal phalanx, use 11752)

OTHER PROCEDURES

(For extracorporeal shock wave therapy involving musculoskeletal system, or plantar fascia, see Category III codes 0019T, 0020T)

28899 Unlisted procedure, foot or toes

APPLICATION OF CASTS AND STRAPPING

CPT codes in this section are used only when the cast application or strapping is a replacement procedure performed during or after the period of follow-up care. An additional evaluation and management service code, dependent on location, is reportable only if significant identifiable other services are provided at the time of the cast application or strapping.

For coding cast or strap application in situations not involving surgery, for example, casting of a sprained ankle or knee, use the appropriate level of evaluation and management services code plus code 99070 or equivalent HCPCS Level II code to report casting materials.

(For orthotics fitting and training, use 97504)

BODY AND UPPER EXTREMITY

Casts

29000 Application of halo type body cast (see 20661-20663 for insertion)

351

| | Separate Procedure | | Unlisted Procedure | | CCI Comp. Code | | Non-specific Procedure |

29010   Application of Risser jacket, localizer, body; only

29015   including head

29020   Application of turnbuckle jacket, body; only

29025   including head

29035   Application of body cast, shoulder to hips;

29040   including head, Minerva type

29044   including one thigh

29046   including both thighs

29049   Application, cast; figure-of-eight

29055   shoulder spica

29058   plaster Velpeau

29065   shoulder to hand (long arm)

29075   elbow to finger (short arm)

29085   hand and lower forearm (gauntlet)

29086   finger (eg, contracture)

Splints

29105   Application of long arm splint (shoulder to hand)

29125   Application of short arm splint (forearm to hand); static

29126   dynamic

29130   Application of finger splint; static

29131   dynamic

Strapping - Any Age

29200   Strapping; thorax

● New Code   ▲ Revised Code   + Add-On Code   ⊘ Modifier -51 Exempt

29220   low back

29240   shoulder (eg, Velpeau)

29260   elbow or wrist

29280   hand or finger

LOWER EXTREMITY

Casts

29305   Application of hip spica cast; one leg

29325   one and one-half spica or both legs

(For hip spica (body) cast, including thighs only, use 29046)

29345   Application of long leg cast (thigh to toes);

29355   walker or ambulatory type

29358   Application of long leg cast brace

29365   Application of cylinder cast (thigh to ankle)

29405   Application of short leg cast (below knee to toes);

29425   walking or ambulatory type

29435   Application of patellar tendon bearing (PTB) cast

29440   Adding walker to previously applied cast

29445   Application of rigid total contact leg cast

29450   Application of clubfoot cast with molding or manipulation, long or short leg

Splints

29505   Application of long leg splint (thigh to ankle or toes)

29515   Application of short leg splint (calf to foot)

353

■ Separate Procedure   ■ Unlisted Procedure   ■ CCI Comp. Code   ■ Non-specific Procedure

Strapping - Any Age

29520 Strapping; hip

29530 knee

29540 ankle and/or foot

29550 toes

29580 Unna boot

29590 Denis-Browne splint strapping

REMOVAL OR REPAIR

29700 Removal or bivalving; gauntlet, boot or body cast

29705 full arm or full leg cast

29710 shoulder or hip spica, Minerva, or Risser jacket, etc.

29715 turnbuckle jacket

29720 Repair of spica, body cast or jacket

29730 Windowing of cast

29740 Wedging of cast (except clubfoot casts)

29750 Wedging of clubfoot cast

OTHER PROCEDURES

29799 Unlisted procedure, casting or strapping

ENDOSCOPY/ARTHROSCOPY

Surgical arthroscopy always includes a diagnostic arthroscopy and is therefore never reported in addition to the surgical procedure. However, there are several arthroscopy procedures defined as separate procedures, indicating that the codes may be reported if the diagnostic arthroscopy is the only procedure performed.

29800 Arthroscopy, temporomandibular joint, diagnostic, with or without synovial biopsy (separate procedure)

● New Code   ▲ Revised Code   + Add-On Code   ⊘ Modifier -51 Exempt

29804 Arthroscopy, temporomandibular joint, surgical

(For open procedure, use 21010)

29805 Arthroscopy, shoulder, diagnostic, with or without synovial biopsy (separate procedure)

(For open procedure, see 23065-23066, 23100-23101)

29806 Arthroscopy, shoulder, surgical; capsulorrhaphy

(For open procedure, see 23450-23466)

(To report thermal capsulorrhaphy, use 29999)

29807 repair of slap lesion

(29815 deleted 2002 edition. To report, use 29805)

29819 Arthroscopy, shoulder, surgical; with removal of loose body or foreign body

(For open procedure, see 23040-23044, 23107)

29820 synovectomy, partial

(For open procedure, see 23105)

29821 synovectomy, complete

(For open procedure, see 23105)

29822 debridement, limited

(For open procedure, see specific open shoulder procedure performed)

29823 debridement, extensive

(For open procedure, see specific open shoulder procedure performed)

29824 distal claviculectomy including distal articular surface (Mumford procedure)

(For open procedure, use 23120)

 Separate Procedure    Unlisted Procedure   CCI Comp. Code   Non-specific Procedure

29825   with lysis and resection of adhesions, with or without manipulation

(For open procedure, see specific open shoulder procedure performed)

29826   decompression of subacromial space with partial acromioplasty, with or without coracoacromial release

(For open procedure, use 23130 or 23415)

29827   with rotator cuff repair

(For open or mini-open rotator cuff repair, use 23412)

(When arthroscopic subacromial decompression is performed at the same setting, use 29826 and append modifier '-51')

(When arthroscopic distal clavicle resection is performed at the same setting, use 29824 and append modifier '-51')

29830   Arthroscopy, elbow, diagnostic, with or without synovial biopsy (separate procedure)

29834   Arthroscopy, elbow, surgical; with removal of loose body or foreign body

29835   synovectomy, partial

29836   synovectomy, complete

29837   debridement, limited

29838   debridement, extensive

29840   Arthroscopy, wrist, diagnostic, with or without synovial biopsy (separate procedure)

29843   Arthroscopy, wrist, surgical; for infection, lavage and drainage

29844   synovectomy, partial

29845   synovectomy, complete

29846   excision and/or repair of triangular fibrocartilage and/or joint debridement

29847   internal fixation for fracture or instability

356

● New Code   ▲ Revised Code   + Add-On Code   ⊘ Modifier -51 Exempt

29848 Endoscopy, wrist, surgical, with release of transverse carpal ligament

(For open procedure, use 64721)

29850 Arthroscopically aided treatment of intercondylar spine(s) and/or tuberosity fracture(s) of the knee, with or without manipulation; without internal or external fixation (includes arthroscopy)

29851 with internal or external fixation (includes arthroscopy)

(For bone graft, use 20900, 20902)

29855 Arthroscopically aided treatment of tibial fracture, proximal (plateau); nicondylar, with or without internal or external fixation (includes arthroscopy)

29856 bicondylar, with or without internal or external fixation (includes arthroscopy)

(For bone graft, use 20900, 20902)

29860 Arthroscopy, hip, diagnostic with or without synovial biopsy (separate procedure)

29861 Arthroscopy, hip, surgical; with removal of loose body or foreign body

29862 with debridement/shaving of articular cartilage (chondroplasty), abrasion arthroplasty, and/or resection of labrum

29863 with synovectomy

29870 Arthroscopy, knee, diagnostic, with or without synovial biopsy (separate procedure)

(For surgical arthroscopy of the knee with implantation of osteochondral graft for treatment of articular surface defect, see Category III codes 0012T, 0013T)

(For meniscal transplantation, medial or lateral, knee, use Category III code 0014T)

29871 Arthroscopy, knee, surgical; for infection, lavage and drainage

29873 with lateral release

(For open lateral release, use 27425)

Separate Procedure · Unlisted Procedure · CCI Comp. Code · Non-specific Procedure

29874 for removal of loose body or foreign body (eg, osteochondritis dissecans fragmentation, chondral fragmentation)

29875 synovectomy, limited (eg, plica or shelf resection) (separate procedure)

29876 synovectomy, major, two or more compartments (eg, medial or lateral)

29877 debridement/shaving of articular cartilage (chondroplasty)

29879 abrasion arthroplasty (includes chondroplasty where necessary) or multiple drilling or microfracture

29880 with meniscectomy (medial AND lateral, including any meniscal shaving)

29881 with meniscectomy (medial OR lateral, including any meniscal shaving)

29882 with meniscus repair (medial OR lateral)

29883 with meniscus repair (medial AND lateral)

29884 with lysis of adhesions, with or without manipulation (separate procedure)

29885 drilling for osteochondritis dissecans with bone grafting, with or without internal fixation (including debridement of base of lesion)

29886 drilling for intact osteochondritis dissecans lesion

29887 drilling for intact osteochondritis dissecans lesion with internal fixation

29888 Arthroscopically aided anterior cruciate ligament repair/augmentation or reconstruction

29889 Arthroscopically aided posterior cruciate ligament repair/augmentation or reconstruction

(Procedures 29888 and 29889 should not be used with reconstruction procedures 27427-27429)

358 ● New Code ▲ Revised Code + Add-On Code ⊘ Modifier -51 Exempt

29891 Arthroscopy, ankle, surgical; excision of osteochondral defect of talus and/or tibia, including drilling of the defect

29892 Arthroscopically aided repair of large osteochondritis dissecans lesion, talar dome fracture, or tibial plafond fracture, with or without internal fixation (includes arthroscopy)

29893 Endoscopic plantar fasciotomy

29894 Arthroscopy, ankle (tibiotalar and fibulotalar joints), surgical; with removal of loose body or foreign body

29895 synovectomy, partial

29897 debridement, limited

29898 debridement, extensive

29899 with ankle arthrodesis

(For open ankle arthrodesis, use 27870)

29900 Arthroscopy, metacarpophalangeal joint, diagnostic, includes synovial biopsy

(Do not report 29900 with 29901, 29902)

29901 Arthroscopy, metacarpophalangeal joint, surgical; with debridement

29902 with reduction of displaced ulnar collateral ligament (eg, Stenar lesion)

(29909 deleted 2002 edition. To report, use 29999)

29999 Unlisted procedure, arthroscopy

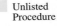 Separate Procedure

 Unlisted Procedure

 CCI Comp. Code

Non-specific Procedure

RESPIRATORY SYSTEM

CPT codes from this section of the CPT coding system are used to report invasive and surgical procedures performed on the nose, sinuses, larynx, trachea and bronchi, and the lungs and pleura.

MISCELLANEOUS CODING RULES

Functional Endoscopic Sinus Surgery (FESS) codes are coded based on the procedures described in the operative report or on the nasal sinus endoscopy report. Each FESS code represents a unilateral procedure. To express that a procedure was performed bilaterally requires the application of the modifier -50, bilateral procedure.

Indirect laryngoscopy involves the visualization of the larynx using a warm laryngeal mirror positioned at the back of the throat. Direct laryngoscopy involves the visualization using a rigid or fiberoptic endoscope. Operative direct laryngoscopy involves an endoscopic examination under general anesthesia.

To code nasal hemorrhages appropriately, documentation needs to substantiate whether the hemorrhage is anterior or posterior and how the hemorrhage is controlled. Control of anterior nasal hemorrhage typically involves the insertion of gauze packing, or anterior packing or performance of cauterization. Control of posterior nasal hemorrhage most likely requires the insertion of nasal stents, tampons, balloon catheters, or posterior packing.

NOSE

INCISION

30000 Drainage abscess or hematoma, nasal, internal approach

(For external approach, see 10060, 10140)

30020 Drainage abscess or hematoma, nasal septum

(For lateral rhinotomy, see specific application (eg, 30118, 30320))

EXCISION

30100 Biopsy, intranasal

(For biopsy skin of nose, see 11100, 11101)

30110 Excision, nasal polyp(s), simple

360
● New Code   ▲ Revised Code   + Add-On Code   ⊘ Modifier -51 Exempt

(30110 would normally be completed in an office setting)

30115 Excision, nasal polyp(s), extensive

(30115 would normally require the facilities available in a hospital setting)

30117 Excision or destruction (eg, laser), intranasal lesion; internal approach

30118   external approach (lateral rhinotomy)

30120 Excision or surgical planing of skin of nose for rhinophyma

30124 Excision dermoid cyst, nose; simple, skin, subcutaneous

30125   complex, under bone or cartilage

30130 Excision turbinate, partial or complete, any method

30140 Submucous resection turbinate, partial or complete, any method

(For submucous resection of nasal septum, use 30520)

(For reduction of turbinates, use 30140 with modifier -52)

30150 Rhinectomy; partial

30160   total

(For closure and/or reconstruction, primary or delayed, see Integumentary System, 13150-13160, 14060-14300, 15120, 15121, 15260, 15261, 15760, 20900-20912)

INTRODUCTION

30200 Injection into turbinate(s), therapeutic

30210 Displacement therapy (Proetz type)

30220 Insertion, nasal septal prosthesis (button)

REMOVAL OF FOREIGN BODY

30300 Removal foreign body, intranasal; office type procedure

30310   requiring general anesthesia

RESP
CVS
30000

361

 Separate Procedure   Unlisted Procedure   CCI Comp. Code   Non-specific Procedure

30320   by lateral rhinotomy

REPAIR

(For obtaining tissues for graft, see 20900-20926, 21210)

30400   Rhinoplasty, primary; lateral and alar cartilages and/or elevation of nasal tip

(For columellar reconstruction, see 13150 et seq)

30410   complete, external parts including bony pyramid, lateral and alar cartilages, and/or elevation of nasal tip

30420   including major septal repair

30430   Rhinoplasty, secondary; minor revision (small amount of nasal tip work)

30435   intermediate revision (bony work with osteotomies)

30450   major revision (nasal tip work and osteotomies)

30460   Rhinoplasty for nasal deformity secondary to congenital cleft lip and/or palate, including columellar lengthening; tip only

30462   tip, septum, osteotomies

30465   Repair of nasal vestibular stenosis (eg, spreader grafting, lateral nasal wall reconstruction)

(30465 excludes obtaining graft. For graft procedure, see 20900-20926, 21210)

(30465 is used to report a bilateral procedure. For unilateral procedure, use modifier -52)

30520   Septoplasty or submucous resection, with or without cartilage scoring, contouring or replacement with graft

(For submucous resection of turbinates, use 30140)

30540   Repair choanal atresia; intranasal

30545   transpalatine

(Do not report modifier '-63' in conjunction with 30540, 30545)

---

362   ● New Code   ▲ Revised Code   + Add-On Code   ⊘ Modifier -51 Exempt

30560 Lysis intranasal synechia

30580 Repair fistula; oromaxillary (combine with 31030 if antrotomy is included)

30600 oronasal

30620 Septal or other intranasal dermatoplasty (does not include obtaining graft)

30630 Repair nasal septal perforations

DESTRUCTION

30801 Cautery and/or ablation, mucosa of turbinates, unilateral or bilateral, any method, (separate procedure); superficial

30802 intramural

OTHER PROCEDURES

30901 Control nasal hemorrhage, anterior, simple (limited cautery and/or packing) any method

30903 Control nasal hemorrhage, anterior, complex (extensive cautery and/or packing) any method

30905 Control nasal hemorrhage, posterior, with posterior nasal packs and/or cautery, any method; initial

30906 subsequent

30915 Ligation arteries; ethmoidal

30920 internal maxillary artery, transantral

(For ligation external carotid artery, use 37600)

30930 Fracture nasal turbinate(s), therapeutic

30999 Unlisted procedure, nose

363

Separate Procedure	Unlisted Procedure	CCI Comp. Code	Non-specific Procedure

ACCESSORY SINUSES

INCISION

31000 Lavage by cannulation; maxillary sinus (antrum puncture or natural ostium)

31002   sphenoid sinus

31020 Sinusotomy, maxillary (antrotomy); intranasal

31030   radical (Caldwell-Luc) without removal of antrochoanal polyps

31032   radical (Caldwell-Luc) with removal of antrochoanal polyps

31040 Pterygomaxillary fossa surgery, any approach

(For transantral ligation of internal maxillary artery, use 30920)

31050 Sinusotomy, sphenoid, with or without biopsy;

31051   with mucosal stripping or removal of polyp(s)

31070 Sinusotomy frontal; external, simple (trephine operation)

31075   transorbital, unilateral (for mucocele or osteoma, Lynch type)

31080   obliterative without osteoplastic flap, brow incision (includes ablation)

31081   obliterative, without osteoplastic flap, coronal incision (includes ablation)

31084   obliterative, with osteoplastic flap, brow incision

31085   obliterative, with osteoplastic flap, coronal incision

31086   nonobliterative, with osteoplastic flap, brow incision

31087   nonobliterative, with osteoplastic flap, coronal incision

31090 Sinusotomy, unilateral, three or more paranasal sinuses (frontal, maxillary, ethmoid, sphenoid)

● New Code   ▲ Revised Code   + Add-On Code   ⊘ Modifier -51 Exempt

EXCISION

31200 Ethmoidectomy; intranasal, anterior

31201   intranasal, total

31205   extranasal, total

31225 Maxillectomy; without orbital exenteration

31230   with orbital exenteration (en bloc)

    (For orbital exenteration only, see 65110 et seq)

    (For skin graft, see 15120 et seq)

ENDOSCOPY

31231 Nasal endoscopy, diagnostic, unilateral or bilateral (separate procedure)

31233 Nasal/sinus endoscopy, diagnostic with maxillary sinusoscopy (via inferior meatus or canine fossa puncture)

31235 Nasal/sinus endoscopy, diagnostic with sphenoid sinusoscopy (via puncture of sphenoidal face or cannulation of ostium)

31237 Nasal/sinus endoscopy, surgical; with biopsy, polypectomy or debridement (separate procedure)

31238   with control of nasal hemorrhage

31239   with dacryocystorhinostomy

31240   with concha bullosa resection

31254   with ethmoidectomy, partial (anterior)

31255   with ethmoidectomy, total (anterior andposterior)

31256 Nasal/sinus endoscopy, surgical, with maxillary antrostomy;

31267   with removal of tissue from maxillary sinus

31276 Nasal/sinus endoscopy, surgical with frontal sinus exploration, with or without removal of tissue from frontal sinus

 Separate Procedure   Unlisted Procedure   CCI Comp. Code   Non-specific Procedure

365

31287 Nasal/sinus endoscopy, surgical, with sphenoidotomy;

31288 with removal of tissue from the sphenoid sinus

31290 Nasal/sinus endoscopy, surgical, with repair of cerebrospinal fluid leak; ethmoid region

31291 sphenoid region

31292 Nasal/sinus endoscopy, surgical; with medial or inferior orbital wall decompression

31293 with medial orbital wall and inferior orbital wall decompression

31294 with optic nerve decompression

OTHER PROCEDURES

(For hypophysectomy, transantral or transeptal approach, use 61548)

(For transcranial hypophysectomy, use 61546)

31299 Unlisted procedure, accessory sinuses

LARYNX

EXCISION

31300 Laryngotomy (thyrotomy, laryngofissure); with removal of tumor or laryngocele, cordectomy

31320 diagnostic

31360 Laryngectomy; total, without radical neck dissection

31365 total, with radical neck dissection

31367 subtotal supraglottic, without radical neck dissection

31368 subtotal supraglottic, with radical neck dissection

31370 Partial laryngectomy (hemilaryngectomy); horizontal

31375 laterovertical

● New Code ▲ Revised Code + Add-On Code ⊘ Modifier -51 Exempt

31380 anterovertical

31382 antero-latero-vertical

31390 Pharyngolaryngectomy, with radical neck dissection; without reconstruction

31395 with reconstruction

31400 Arytenoidectomy or arytenoidopexy, external approach

(For endoscopic arytenoidecomy, use 31560)

31420 Epiglottidectomy

INTRODUCTION

⊘ **31500** Intubation, endotracheal, emergency procedure

(For injection procedure for bronchography, see 31656, 31708, 31710)

31502 Tracheotomy tube change prior to establishment of fistula tract

ENDOSCOPY

31505 Laryngoscopy, indirect; diagnostic (separate procedure)

31510 with biopsy

31511 with removal of foreign body

31512 with removal of lesion

31513 with vocal cord injection

31515 Laryngoscopy direct, with or without tracheoscopy; for aspiration

31520 diagnostic, newborn

(Do not report modifier '-63' in conjunction with 31520)

31525 diagnostic, except newborn

31526 diagnostic, with operating microscope

367

 Separate Procedure   Unlisted Procedure    CCI Comp. Code   Non-specific Procedure

(Do not report code 69990 in addition to code 31526)

31527   with insertion of obturator

31528   with dilation, initial

31529   with dilation, subsequent

31530 Laryngoscopy, direct, operative, with foreign body removal;

31531   with operating microscope

(Do not report code 69990 in addition to code 31531)

31535 Laryngoscopy, direct, operative, with biopsy;

31536   with operating microscope

(Do not report code 69990 in addition to code 31536)

31540 Laryngoscopy, direct, operative, with excision of tumor and/or stripping of vocal cords or epiglottis;

31541   with operating microscope

(Do not report code 69990 in addition to code 31541)

31560 Laryngoscopy, direct, operative, with arytenoidectomy;

31561   with operating microscope

(Do not report code 69990 in addition to code 31561)

31570 Laryngoscopy, direct, with injection into vocal cord(s), therapeutic;

31571   with operating microscope

(Do not report code 69990 in addition to code 31571)

31575 Laryngoscopy, flexible fiberoptic; diagnostic

31576   with biopsy

31577   with removal of foreign body

31578   with removal of lesion

368   ● New Code   ▲ Revised Code   + Add-On Code   ⊘ Modifier -51 Exempt

(To report flexible fiberoptic endoscopic evaluation of swallowing, see 92612-92613)

(To report flexible fiberoptic endoscopic evaluation with sensory testing, see 92614-92615)

(To report flexible fiberoptic endoscopic evaluation of swallowing with sensory testing, see 92616-92617)

(For flexible fiberoptic laryngoscopy as part of flexible fiberoptic endoscopic evaluation of swallowing and/or laryngeal sensory testing by cine or video recording, see 92612-92617)

31579 Laryngoscopy, flexible or rigid fiberoptic, with stroboscopy

REPAIR

31580 Laryngoplasty; for laryngeal web, two stage, with keel insertion and removal

31582 for laryngeal stenosis, with graft or core mold, including tracheotomy

31584 with open reduction of fracture

31585 Treatment of closed laryngeal fracture; without manipulation

31586 with closed manipulative reduction

31587 Laryngoplasty, cricoid split

31588 Laryngoplasty, not otherwise specified (eg, for burns, reconstruction after partial laryngectomy)

31590 Laryngeal reinnervation by neuromuscular pedicle

DESTRUCTION

31595 Section recurrent laryngeal nerve, therapeutic (separate procedure), unilateral

OTHER PROCEDURES

31599 Unlisted procedure, larynx

369

 Separate Procedure   Unlisted Procedure   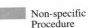 CCI Comp. Code   Non-specific Procedure

TRACHEA AND BRONCHI

INCISION

31600   Tracheostomy, planned (separate procedure);

31601   under two years

31603   Tracheostomy, emergency procedure; transtracheal

31605   cricothyroid membrane

31610   Tracheostomy, fenestration procedure with skin flaps

(For endotracheal intubation, use 31500)

(For tracheal aspiration under direct vision, use 31515)

31611   Construction of tracheoesophageal fistula and subsequent insertion of an alaryngeal speech prosthesis (eg, voice button, Blom-Singer prosthesis)

31612   Tracheal puncture, percutaneous with transtracheal aspiration and/or injection

31613   Tracheostoma revision; simple, without flap rotation

31614   complex, with flap rotation

ENDOSCOPY

(For tracheoscopy, see laryngoscopy codes 31515-31578)

31615   Tracheobronchoscopy through established tracheostomy incision

▲ **31622**   Bronchoscopy, rigid or flexible, with or without fluoroscopic guidance; diagnostic, with or without cell washing (separate procedure)

31623   with brushing or protected brushings

31624   with bronchial alveolar lavage

▲ **31625**   with bronchial or endobronchial biopsy(s), single or multiple sites

▲ **31628**   with transbronchial lung biopsy(s), single lobe

● New Code   ▲ Revised Code   + Add-On Code   ⊘ Modifier -51 Exempt

(31628 should be reported only once regardless of how many transbronchial lung biopsies are performed in a lobe)

(To report transbronchial lung biopsies performed on additional lobe(s), use 31632)

▲ **31629** with transbronchial needle aspiration biopsy(s), trachea, main stem and/or lobar bronchus(i)

(31629 should be reported only once for upper airway biopsies regardless of how many transbronchial needle aspiration biopsies are performed in the upper airway or in a lobe)

(To report transbronchial needle aspiration biopsies performed on additional lobe(s), use 31633)

31630 with tracheal or bronchial dilation or closed reduction of fracture

31631 with tracheal dilation and placement of tracheal stent

●+**31632** with transbronchial lung biopsy(s), each additional lobe (List separately in addition to code for primary procedure)

(Use 31632 in conjunction with 31628)

(31632 should be reported only once regardless of how many transbronchial lung biopsies are performed in a lobe)

●+**31633** with transbronchial needle aspiration biopsy(s), each additional lobe (List separately in addition to code for primary procedure)

(Use 31633 in conjunction with 31629)

(31633 should be reported only once regardless of how many transbronchial needle aspiration biopsies are performed in the trachea or the additional lobe)

31635 with removal of foreign body

31640 with excision of tumor

31641 Bronchoscopy, (rigid or flexible); with destruction of tumor or relief of stenosis by any method other than excision (eg, laser therapy, cryotherapy)

(For bronchoscopic photodynamic therapy, report 31641 in addition to 96570, 96571 as appropriate)

371

 Separate Procedure   Unlisted Procedure    CCI Comp. Code   Non-specific Procedure

31643   with placement of catheter(s) for intracavitary radioelement application

(For intracavitary radioelement application, see 77761-77763, 77781-77784)

31645   with therapeutic aspiration of tracheobronchial tree, initial (eg, drainage of lung abscess)

31646   with therapeutic aspiration of tracheobronchial tree, subsequent

(For catheter aspiration of tracheobronchial tree at bedside, use 31725)

31656   with injection of contrast material for segmental bronchography (fiberscope only)

(For radiological supervision and interpretation, see 71040, 71060)

INTRODUCTION

(For endotracheal intubation, use 31500)

(For tracheal aspiration under direct vision, see 31515)

31700   Catheterization, transglottic (separate procedure)

31708   Instillation of contrast material for laryngography or bronchography, without catheterization

(For radiological supervision and interpretation, see 70373, 71040, 71060)

31710   Catheterization for bronchography, with or without instillation of contrast material

(For bronchoscopic catheterization for bronchography, fiberscope only, use 31656)

(For radiological supervision and interpretation, see 71040, 71060)

31715   Transtracheal injection for bronchography

(For radiological supervision and interpretation, see 71040, 71060)

(For prolonged services, see 99354-99360)

| ● New Code | ▲ Revised Code | + Add-On Code | ⊘ Modifier -51 Exempt |

31717 Catheterization with bronchial brush biopsy

31720 Catheter aspiration (separate procedure); nasotracheal

31725 tracheobronchial with fiberscope, bedside

31730 Transtracheal (percutaneous) introduction of needle wire dilator/stent or indwelling tube for oxygen therapy

REPAIR

31750 Tracheoplasty; cervical

31755 tracheopharyngeal fistulization, each stage

31760 intrathoracic

31766 Carinal reconstruction

31770 Bronchoplasty; graft repair

31775 excision stenosis and anastomosis

(For lobectomy and bronchoplasty, use 32501)

31780 Excision tracheal stenosis and anastomosis; cervical

31781 cervicothoracic

31785 Excision of tracheal tumor or carcinoma; cervical

31786 thoracic

31800 Suture of tracheal wound or injury; cervical

31805 intrathoracic

31820 Surgical closure tracheostomy or fistula; without plastic repair

31825 with plastic repair

(For repair tracheoesophageal fistula, see 43305, 43312)

31830 Revision of tracheostomy scar

 Separate Procedure

 Unlisted Procedure

 CCI Comp. Code

 Non-specific Procedure

OTHER PROCEDURES

31899 Unlisted procedure, trachea, bronchi

LUNGS AND PLEURA

INCISION

⊘ **32000** Thoracentesis, puncture of pleural cavity for aspiration, initial or subsequent

(If imaging guidance is performed, see 76003, 76360, 76942)

⊘ **32002** Thoracentesis with insertion of tube with or without water seal (eg, for pneumothorax) (separate procedure)

(If imaging guidance is performed, see 76003, 76360, 76942)

32005 Chemical pleurodesis (eg, for recurrent or persistent pneumothorax)

⊘ **32020** Tube thoracostomy with or without water seal (eg, for abscess, hemothorax, empyema) (separate procedure)

(If imaging guidance is performed, use 75989)

32035 Thoracostomy; with rib resection for empyema

32036   with open flap drainage for empyema

32095 Thoracotomy, limited, for biopsy of lung or pleura

(To report wound exploration due to penetrating trauma without thoractomy, use 20102)

32100 Thoracotomy, major; with exploration and biopsy

32110   with control of traumatic hemorrhage and/or repair of lung tear

32120   for postoperative complications

32124   with open intrapleural pneumonolysis

32140   with cyst(s) removal, with or without a pleural procedure

32141   with excision-plication of bullae, with or without any pleural procedure

● New Code ▲ Revised Code + Add-On Code ⊘ Modifier -51 Exempt

(For lung volume reduction, use 32491)

32150 with removal of intrapleural foreign body or fibrin deposit

32151 with removal of intrapulmonary foreign body

32160 with cardiac massage

(For segmental or other resections of lung, see 32480-32525)

32200 Pneumonostomy; with open drainage of abscess or cyst

32201 with percutaneous drainage of abscess or cyst

(For radiological supervision and interpretation, use 75989)

32215 Pleural scarification for repeat pneumothorax

32220 Decortication, pulmonary (separate procedure); total

32225 partial

EXCISION

32310 Pleurectomy, parietal (separate procedure)

32320 Decortication and parietal pleurectomy

32400 Biopsy, pleura; percutaneous needle

(If imaging guidance is performed, see 76003, 76360, 76393, 76942)

(For fine needle aspiration, use 10021 or 10022)

(For evaluation of fine needle aspirate, see 88172, 88173)

32402 open

32405 Biopsy, lung or mediastinum, percutaneous needle

(For radiological supervision and interpretation, see 76003, 76360, 76393, 76942)

(For fine needle aspiration, use 10022)

(For evaluation of fine needle aspirate, see 88172, 88173)

32420 Pneumocentesis, puncture of lung for aspiration

| Separate Procedure | Unlisted Procedure | CCI Comp. Code | Non-specific Procedure |

375

32440 Removal of lung, total pneumonectomy;

32442 with resection of segment of trachea followed by broncho-tracheal anastomosis (sleeve pneumonectomy)

32445 extrapleural

32480 Removal of lung, other than total pneumonectomy; single lobe (lobectomy)

32482 two lobes (bilobectomy)

32484 single segment (segmentectomy)

32486 with circumferential resection of segment of bronchus followed by broncho-bronchial anastomosis (sleeve lobectomy)

32488 all remaining lung following previous removal of a portion of lung (completion pneumonectomy)

32491 excision-plication of emphysematous lung(s) (bullous or non-bullous) for lung volume reduction, sternal split or transthoracic approach, with or without any pleural procedure

32500 wedge resection, single or multiple

+ 32501 Resection and repair of portion of bronchus (bronchoplasty) when performed at time of lobectomy or segmentectomy (List separately in addition to code for primary procedure)

(Use 32501 in conjunction with codes 32480, 32482, 32484)

(32501 is to be used when a portion of the bronchus to preserved lung is removed and requires plastic closure to preserve function of that preserved lung. It is not to be used for closure for the proximal end of a resected bronchus.)

32520 Resection of lung; with resection of chest wall

32522 with reconstruction of chest wall, without prosthesis

32525 with major reconstruction of chest wall, with prosthesis

32540 Extrapleural enucleation of empyema (empyemectomy)

● New Code   ▲ Revised Code   + Add-On Code   ⊘ Modifier -51 Exempt

ENDOSCOPY

32601 Thoracoscopy, diagnostic (separate procedure); lungs and pleural space, without biopsy

32602 lungs and pleural space, with biopsy

32603 pericardial sac, without biopsy

32604 pericardial sac, with biopsy

32605 mediastinal space, without biopsy

32606 mediastinal space, with biopsy

(Surgical thoracoscopy always includes diagnostic thoracoscopy)

32650 Thoracoscopy, surgical; with pleurodesis (eg, mechanical or chemical)

32651 with partial pulmonary decortication

32652 with total pulmonary decortication, including intrapleural pneumonolysis

32653 with removal of intrapleural foreign body or fibrin deposit

32654 with control of traumatic hemorrhage

32655 with excision-plication of bullae, including any pleural procedure

32656 with parietal pleurectomy

32657 with wedge resection of lung, single or multiple

32658 with removal of clot or foreign body from pericardial sac

32659 with creation of pericardial window or partial resection of pericardial sac for drainage

32660 with total pericardiectomy

32661 with excision of pericardial cyst, tumor, or mass

32662 with excision of mediastinal cyst, tumor, or mass

Separate Procedure	Unlisted Procedure	CCI Comp. Code	Non-specific Procedure

377

32663	with lobectomy, total or segmental
32664	with thoracic sympathectomy
32665	with esophagomyotomy (Heller type)

REPAIR

32800	Repair lung hernia through chest wall
32810	Closure of chest wall following open flap drainage for empyema (Clagett type procedure)
32815	Open closure of major bronchial fistula
32820	Major reconstruction, chest wall (posttraumatic)

LUNG TRANSPLANTATION

32850	Donor pneumonectomy(ies) with preparation and maintenance of allograft (cadaver)
32851	Lung transplant, single; without cardiopulmonary bypass
32852	with cardiopulmonary bypass
32853	Lung transplant, double (bilateral sequential or en bloc); without cardiopulmonary bypass
32854	with cardiopulmonary bypass

SURGICAL COLLAPSE THERAPY; THORACOPLASTY

(See also 32520-32525)

32900	Resection of ribs, extrapleural, all stages
32905	Thoracoplasty, Schede type or extrapleural (all stages);
32906	with closure of bronchopleural fistula

(For open closure of major bronchial fistula, use 32815)

(For resection of first rib for thoracic outlet compression, see 21615, 21616)

| ● | New Code | ▲ | Revised Code | + | Add-On Code | ⊘ | Modifier -51 Exempt |

32940 Pneumonolysis, extraperiosteal, including filling or packing procedures

32960 Pneumothorax, therapeutic, intrapleural injection of air

OTHER PROCEDURES

32997 Total lung lavage (unilateral)

(For bronchoscopic bronchial alveolar lavage, use 31624)

32999 Unlisted procedure, lungs and pleura

 Separate Procedure   Unlisted Procedure   CCI Comp. Code    Non-specific Procedure

CARDIOVASCULAR SYSTEM

CPT codes from this section of the CPT coding system are used to report invasive and surgical procedures performed on the heart and pericardium, including pacemakers or defibrillators; cardiac valves; coronary arteries; aorta; and arteries and veins.

For coding services such as monitoring, operation of pump and other non-surgical services performed during cardiovascular surgery, see the Special Services CPT codes 99150, 99151, 99160-99162 or CPT codes 99291-99292 and 99190-99192 from the evaluation and management section of the CPT coding system.

MISCELLANEOUS CODING RULES

A pacemaker system includes a pulse generator containing electronics, a battery, and one or more electrodes (leads) inserted one of several ways. Pulse generators may be placed in a subcutaneous "pocket" created in either a subclavicular or intra-abdominal site. Electrodes may be inserted through a vein (transvenous) or on the surface of the heart (epicardial). A single chamber system includes a pulse generator, one electrode inserted into either the atrium or ventricle. A dual chamber system includes a pulse generator, one electrode inserted in the atrium, and one electrode inserted in the ventricle.

Assign two CPT codes when a pacemaker or cardioverter-defibrillator "battery"/pulse generator is replaced. One code should describe the removal of the old pulse generator and the other should describe the insertion of the new pulse generator.

Cardiac catheterization codes are classified in the Medicine Section of the CPT coding system. Insertion of a dilator into a vein prior to the placement of a catheter should not be separately coded.

(For monitoring, operation of pump and other nonsurgical services, see 99190-99192, 99291, 99292, 99354-99360)

(For other medical or laboratory related services, see appropriate section)

(For radiological supervision and interpretation, see 75600-75978)

HEART AND PERICARDIUM

PERICARDIUM

33010 Pericardiocentesis; initial

380

● New Code

▲ Revised Code

+ Add-On Code

⊘ Modifier -51 Exempt

(For radiological supervision and interpretation, use 76930)

33011   subsequent

(For radiological supervision and interpretation, use 76930)

33015 Tube pericardiostomy

33020 Pericardiotomy for removal of clot or foreign body (primary procedure)

33025 Creation of pericardial window or partial resection for drainage

33030 Pericardiectomy, subtotal or complete; without cardiopulmonary bypass

33031   with cardiopulmonary bypass

33050 Excision of pericardial cyst or tumor

CARDIAC TUMOR

33120 Excision of intracardiac tumor, resection with cardiopulmonary bypass

33130 Resection of external cardiac tumor

TRANSMYOCARDIAL REVASCULARIZATION

33140 Transmyocardial laser revascularization, by thoracotomy (separate procedure)

+ 33141   performed at the time of other open cardiac procedure(s) (List separately in addition to code for primary procedure)

(Use 33141 in conjunction with codes 33400-33496, 33510-33536)

PACEMAKER OR PACING CARDIOVERTER-DEFIBRILLATOR

(For electronic, telephonic analysis of internal pacemaker system, see 93731-93736)

(For radiological supervision and interpretation with insertion of pacemaker, use 71090)

33200 Insertion of permanent pacemaker with epicardial electrode(s); by thoracotomy

381

 Separate Procedure   Unlisted Procedure   CCI Comp. Code   Non-specific Procedure

33201   by xiphoid approach

33206 Insertion or replacement of permanent pacemaker with transvenous electrode(s); atrial

33207   ventricular

33208   atrial and ventricular

(Codes 33206-33208 include subcutaneous insertion of the pulse generator and transvenous placement of electrode(s))

33210 Insertion or replacement of temporary transvenous single chamber cardiac electrode or pacemaker catheter (separate procedure)

33211 Insertion or replacement of temporary transvenous dual chamber pacing electrodes (separate procedure)

33212 Insertion or replacement of pacemaker pulse generator only; single chamber, atrial or ventricular

33213   dual chamber

33214 Upgrade of implanted pacemaker system, conversion of single chamber system to dual chamber system (includes removal of previously placed pulse generator, testing of existing lead, insertion of new lead, insertion of new pulse generator)

33215 Repositioning of previously implanted transvenous pacemaker or pacing cardioverter-defibillator (right atrial or right ventricular) electrode

33216 Insertion of a transvenous electrode (15 days or more after initial insertion); single chamber (one electrode) permanent pacemaker or single chamber pacing cardioverter-defibrillator

33217   dual chamber (two electrodes) permanent pacemaker or dual chamber pacing cardioverter-defibrillator

(Do not report 33216-33217 in conjunction with code 33214)

33218 Repair of single transvenous electrode for a single chamber, permanent pacemaker or single chamber pacing cardioverter-defibrillator

● New Code   ▲ Revised Code   + Add-On Code   ⊘ Modifier -51 Exempt

33220 Repair of two transvenous electrodes for a dual chamber permanent pacemaker or dual chamber pacing cardioverter-defibrillator

33222 Revision or relocation of skin pocket for pacemaker

33223 Revision of skin pocket for single or dual chamber pacing cardioverter-defibrillator

33224 Insertion of pacing electrode, cardiac venous system, for left ventricular pacing, with attachment to previously placed pacemaker or pacing cardioverter-defibrillator pulse generator (including revision of pocket, removal, insertion and/or replacement of generator)

+ **33225** Insertion of pacing electrode, cardiac venous system, for left ventricular pacing, at time of insertion of pacing cardioverter-defibrillator or pacemaker pulse generator (including upgrade to dual chamber system) (List separately in addition to code for primary procedure)

(Use 33225 in conjunction with 33206, 33207, 33208, 33212, 33213, 33214, 33216, 33217, 33222, 33233, 33234, 33235, 33240, 33249)

33226 Repositioning of previously implanted cardiac venous system (left ventricular) electrode (including removal, insertion and/or replacement of generator)

33233 Removal of permanent pacemaker pulse generator

33234 Removal of transvenous pacemaker electrode(s); single lead system, atrial or ventricular

33235 dual lead system

33236 Removal of permanent epicardial pacemaker and electrodes by thoracotomy; single lead system, atrial or ventricular

33237 dual lead system

33238 Removal of permanent transvenous electrode(s) by thoracotomy

33240 Insertion of single or dual chamber pacing cardioverter-defibrillator pulse generator

 Separate Procedure   Unlisted Procedure   CCI Comp. Code   Non-specific Procedure

33241 Subcutaneous removal of single or dual chamber pacing cardioverter-defibrillator pulse generator

(For removal of electrode(s) by thoracotomy, use 33243 in conjunction with code 33241)

(For removal of electrode(s) by transvenous extraction, use 33244 in conjunction with code 33241)

(For removal and reinsertion of a pacing cardioverter-defibrillator system (pulse generator and electrodes), report 33241 and 33243 or 33244 and 33249)

(33242 has been deleted. To report, see 33218, 33220)

33243 Removal of single or dual chamber pacing cardioverter-defibrillator electrode(s); by thoracotomy

33244   by transvenous extraction

(For subcutaneous removal of the pulse generator, use 33241 in conjunction with code 33243 or 33244)

33245 Insertion of epicardial single or dual chamber pacing cardioverter-defibrillator electrodes by thoracotomy;

33246   with insertion of pulse generator

33249 Insertion or repositioning of electrode lead(s) for single or dual chamber pacing cardioverter-defibrillator and insertion of pulse generator

(For removal and reinsertion of a pacing cardioverter-defibrillator system (pulse generator and electrodes), report 33241 and 33243 or 33244 and 33249)

ELECTROPHYSIOLOGIC OPERATIVE PROCEDURES

33250 Operative ablation of supraventricular arrhythmogenic focus or pathway (eg, Wolff-Parkinson-White, atrioventricular node re-entry), tract(s) and/or focus (foci); without cardiopulmonary bypass

33251   with cardiopulmonary bypass

33253 Operative incisions and reconstruction of atria for treatment of atrial fibrillation or atrial flutter (eg, maze procedure)

● New Code   ▲ Revised Code   + Add-On Code   ⊘ Modifier -51 Exempt

33261 Operative ablation of ventricular arrhythmogenic focus with cardiopulmonary bypass

PATIENT-ACTIVATED EVENT RECORDER

33282 Implantation of patient-activated cardiac event recorder

(Initial implantation includes programming. For subsequent electronic analysis and/or reprogramming, use 93727)

33284 Removal of an implantable, patient-activated cardiac event recorder

WOUNDS OF THE HEART AND GREAT VESSELS

33300 Repair of cardiac wound; without bypass

33305   with cardiopulmonary bypass

▲ **33310** Cardiotomy, exploratory (includes removal of foreign body, atrial or ventricular thrombus); without bypass

33315   with cardiopulmonary bypass

(Do not report removal of thrombus (33310-33315) in conjunction with other cardiac procedures unless a separate incision in the heart is required to remove the atrial or ventricular thrombus)

(If removal of thrombus with coronary bypass (33315) is reported in conjunction with 33120, 33130, 33420-33430, 33460-33468, 33496, 33542, 33545, 33641-33647, 33670, 33681, 33975-33980 which requires a separate heart incision, report 33315 with modifier '-59')

33320 Suture repair of aorta or great vessels; without shunt or cardiopulmonary bypass

33321   with shunt bypass

33322   with cardiopulmonary bypass

33330 Insertion of graft, aorta or great vessels; without shunt, or cardiopulmonary bypass

33332   with shunt bypass

33335   with cardiopulmonary bypass

385

 Separate Procedure   Unlisted Procedure   CCI Comp. Code   Non-specific Procedure

CARDIAC VALVES

Aortic Valve

33400 Valvuloplasty, aortic valve; open, with cardiopulmonary bypass

33401 open, with inflow occlusion

33403 using transventricular dilation, with cardiopulmonary bypass

(Do not report modifier '-63' in conjunction with 33401, 33403)

33404 Construction of apical-aortic conduit

33405 Replacement, aortic valve, with cardiopulmonary bypass; with prosthetic valve other than homograft or stentless valve

33406 with allograft valve (freehand)

33410 with stentless tissue valve

33411 Replacement, aortic valve; with aortic annulus enlargement, noncoronary cusp

33412 with transventricular aortic annulus enlargement (Konno procedure)

33413 by translocation of autologous pulmonary valve with allograft replacement of pulmonary valve (Ross procedure)

33414 Repair of left ventricular outflow tract obstruction by patch enlargement of the outflow tract

33415 Resection or incision of subvalvular tissue for discrete subvalvular aortic stenosis

33416 Ventriculomyotomy (-myectomy) for idiopathic hypertrophic subaortic stenosis (eg, asymmetric septal hypertrophy)

33417 Aortoplasty (gusset) for supravalvular stenosis

Mitral Valve

33420 Valvotomy, mitral valve; closed heart

33422 open heart, with cardiopulmonary bypass

386

● New Code   ▲ Revised Code   + Add-On Code   ⊘ Modifier -51 Exempt

33425	Valvuloplasty, mitral valve, with cardiopulmonary bypass;
33426	with prosthetic ring
33427	radical reconstruction, with or without ring
33430	Replacement, mitral valve, with cardiopulmonary bypass

Tricuspid Valve

33460	Valvectomy, tricuspid valve, with cardiopulmonary bypass
33463	Valvuloplasty, tricuspid valve; without ring insertion
33464	with ring insertion
33465	Replacement, tricuspid valve, with cardiopulmonary bypass
33468	Tricuspid valve repositioning and plication for Ebstein anomaly

Pulmonary Valve

33470	Valvotomy, pulmonary valve, closed heart; transventricular

(Do not report modifier '-63' in conjunction with 33470)

33471	via pulmonary artery

(To report percutaneous valvuloplasty of pulmonary valve, use 92990)

33472	Valvotomy, pulmonary valve, open heart; with inflow occlusion

(Do not report modifier '-63' in conjunction with 33472)

33474	with cardiopulmonary bypass
33475	Replacement, pulmonary valve
33476	Right ventricular resection for infundibular stenosis, with or without commissurotomy
33478	Outflow tract augmentation (gusset), with or without commissurotomy or infundibular resection

387

 Separate Procedure    Unlisted Procedure   CCI Comp. Code   Non-specific Procedure

OTHER VALVULAR PROCEDURES

33496 Repair of non-structural prosthetic valve dysfunction with cardiopulmonary bypass (separate procedure)

(For reoperation, use 33530 in addition to 33496)

CORONARY ARTERY ANOMALIES

33500 Repair of coronary arteriovenous or arteriocardiac chamber fistula; with cardiopulmonary bypass

33501 without cardiopulmonary bypass

33502 Repair of anomalous coronary artery; by ligation

33503 by graft, without cardiopulmonary bypass

(Do not report modifier '-63' in conjunction with 33502, 33503)

33504 by graft, with cardiopulmonary bypass

33505 with construction of intrapulmonary artery tunnel (Takeuchi procedure)

33506 by translocation from pulmonary artery to aorta

(Do not report modifier '-63' in conjunction with 33505, 33506)

ENDOSCOPY

(Surgical vascular endoscopy always includes diagnostic endoscopy)

+ 33508 Endoscopy, surgical, including video-assisted harvest of vein(s) for coronary artery bypass procedure (List separately in addition to code for primary procedure)

(Use 33508 in conjunction with code 33510-33523)

(For open harvest of upper extremity vein procedure, use 35500)

VENOUS GRAFTING ONLY FOR CORONARY ARTERY BYPASS

33510 Coronary artery bypass, vein only; single coronary venous graft

33511 two coronary venous grafts

---

388 ● New Code ▲ Revised Code + Add-On Code ⊘ Modifier -51 Exempt

33512   three coronary venous grafts

33513   four coronary venous grafts

33514   five coronary venous grafts

33516   six or more coronary venous grafts

COMBINED ARTERIAL-VENOUS GRAFTING FOR CORONARY BYPASS

⊘ **33517**   Coronary artery bypass, using venous graft(s) and arterial graft(s); single vein graft (List separately in addition to code for arterial graft)

⊘ **33518**   two venous grafts (List separately in addition to code for arterial graft)

⊘ **33519**   three venous grafts (List separately in addition to code for arterial graft)

⊘ **33521**   four venous grafts (List separately in addition to code for arterial graft)

⊘ **33522**   five venous grafts (List separately in addition to code for arterial graft)

⊘ **33523**   six or more venous grafts (List separately in addition to code for arterial graft)

+ **33530**   Reoperation, coronary artery bypass procedure or valve procedure, more than one month after original operation (List separately in addition to code for primary procedure)

       (Use 33530 in conjunction with codes 33400-33496; 33510-33536, 33863)

ARTERIAL GRAFTING FOR CORONARY ARTERY BYPASS

33533   Coronary artery bypass, using arterial graft(s); single arterial graft

33534   two coronary arterial grafts

33535   three coronary arterial grafts

33536   four or more coronary arterial grafts

389

| Separate Procedure | Unlisted Procedure | CCI Comp. Code | Non-specific Procedure |

33542 Myocardial resection (eg, ventricular aneurysmectomy)

33545 Repair of postinfarction ventricular septal defect, with or without myocardial resection

CORONARY ENDARTERECTOMY

+ **33572** Coronary endarterectomy, open, any method, of left anterior descending, circumflex, or right coronary artery performed in conjunction with coronary artery bypass graft procedure, each vessel (List separately in addition to primary procedure)

(Use 33572 in conjunction with 33510-33516, 33533-33536)

SINGLE VENTRICLE AND OTHER COMPLEX CARDIAC ANOMALIES

33600 Closure of atrioventricular valve (mitral or tricuspid) by suture or patch

33602 Closure of semilunar valve (aortic or pulmonary) by suture or patch

33606 Anastomosis of pulmonary artery to aorta (Damus-Kaye-Stansel procedure)

33608 Repair of complex cardiac anomaly other than pulmonary atresia with ventricular septal defect by construction or replacement of conduit from right or left ventricle to pulmonary artery

(For repair of pulmonary atresia with ventricular septal defect, see 33918, 33919, 33920)

33610 Repair of complex cardiac anomalies (eg, single ventricle with subaortic obstruction) by surgical enlargement of ventricular septal defect

(Do not report modifier '-63' in conjunction with 33610)

33611 Repair of double outlet right ventricle with intraventricular tunnel repair;

(Do not report modifier '-63' in conjunction with 33611)

33612   with repair of right ventricular outflow tract obstruction

33615   Repair of complex cardiac anomalies (eg, tricuspid atresia) by closure of atrial septal defect and anastomosis of atria or vena cava to pulmonary artery (simple Fontan procedure)

33617   Repair of complex cardiac anomalies (eg, single ventricle) by modified Fontan procedure

33619   Repair of single ventricle with aortic outflow obstruction and aortic arch hypoplasia (hypoplastic left heart syndrome) (eg, Norwood procedure)

(Do not report modifier '-63' in conjunction with 33619)

SEPTAL DEFECT

33641   Repair atrial septal defect, secundum, with cardiopulmonary bypass, with or without patch

33645   Direct or patch closure, sinus venosus, with or without anomalous pulmonary venous drainage

33647   Repair of atrial septal defect and ventricular septal defect, with direct or patch closure

(Do not report modifier '-63' in conjunction with 33647)

33660   Repair of incomplete or partial atrioventricular canal (ostium primum atrial septal defect), with or without atrioventricular valve repair

33665   Repair of intermediate or transitional atrioventricular canal, with or without atrioventricular valve repair

33670   Repair of complete atrioventricular canal, with or without prosthetic valve

(Do not report modifier '-63' in conjunction with 33670)

33681   Closure of ventricular septal defect, with or without patch;

33684   with pulmonary valvotomy or infundibular resection (acyanotic)

33688   with removal of pulmonary artery band, with or without gusset

33690   Banding of pulmonary artery

391

 Separate Procedure   Unlisted Procedure   CCI Comp. Code   Non-specific Procedure

(Do not report modifier '-63' in conjunction with 33690)

33692 Complete repair tetralogy of Fallot without pulmonary atresia;

33694   with transannular patch

(Do not report modifier '-63' in conjunction with 33694)

33697 Complete repair tetralogy of Fallot with pulmonary atresia including construction of conduit from right ventricle to pulmonary artery and closure of ventricular septal defect

SINUS OF VALSALVA

33702 Repair sinus of Valsalva fistula, with cardiopulmonary bypass;

33710   with repair of ventricular septal defect

33720 Repair sinus of Valsalva aneurysm, with cardiopulmonary bypass

33722 Closure of aortico-left ventricular tunnel

TOTAL ANOMALOUS PULMONARY VENOUS DRAINAGE

33730 Complete repair of anomalous venous return (supracardiac, intracardiac, or infracardiac types)

(Do not report modifier '-63' in conjunction with 33730)

(For partial anomalous return, see atrial septal defect)

33732 Repair of cor triatriatum or supravalvular mitral ring by resection of left atrial membrane

(Do not report modifier '-63' in conjunction with 33732)

SHUNTING PROCEDURES

33735 Atrial septectomy or septostomy; closed heart (Blalock-Hanlon type operation)

33736   open heart with cardiopulmonary bypass

(Do not report modifier '-63' in conjunction with 33735, 33736)

33737   open heart, with inflow occlusion

392

  ● New Code   ▲ Revised Code   + Add-On Code   ⊘ Modifier -51 Exempt

33750 Shunt; subclavian to pulmonary artery (Blalock-Taussig type operation)

33755 ascending aorta to pulmonary artery (Waterston type operation)

33762 descending aorta to pulmonary artery (Potts-Smith type operation)

(Do not report modifier '-63' in conjunction with 33750, 33755, 33762)

33764 central, with prosthetic graft

33766 superior vena cava to pulmonary artery for flow to one lung (classical Glenn procedure)

33767 superior vena cava to pulmonary artery for flow to both lungs (bidirectional Glenn procedure)

TRANSPOSITION OF THE GREAT VESSELS

33770 Repair of transposition of the great arteries with ventricular septal defect and subpulmonary stenosis; without surgical enlargement of ventricular septal defect

33771 with surgical enlargement of ventricular septal defect

33774 Repair of transposition of the great arteries, atrial baffle procedure (eg, Mustard or Senning type) with cardiopulmonary bypass;

33775 with removal of pulmonary band

33776 with closure of ventricular septal defect

33777 with repair of subpulmonic obstruction

33778 Repair of transposition of the great arteries, aortic pulmonary artery reconstruction (eg, Jatene type);

(Do not report modifier '-63' in conjunction with 33778)

33779 with removal of pulmonary band

33780 with closure of ventricular septal defect

393

 Separate Procedure   Unlisted Procedure   CCI Comp. Code   Non-specific Procedure

| 33781 | with repair of subpulmonic obstruction |

TRUNCUS ARTERIOSUS

| 33786 | Total repair, truncus arteriosus (Rastelli type operation) |

(Do not report modifier '-63' in conjunction with 33786)

| 33788 | Reimplantation of an anomalous pulmonary artery |

(For pulmonary artery band, use 33690)

AORTIC ANOMALIES

| 33800 | Aortic suspension (aortopexy) for tracheal decompression (eg, for tracheomalacia) (separate procedure) |

| 33802 | Division of aberrant vessel (vascular ring); |

| 33803 | with reanastomosis |

| 33813 | Obliteration of aortopulmonary septal defect; without cardiopulmonary bypass |

| 33814 | with cardiopulmonary bypass |

| 33820 | Repair of patent ductus arteriosus; by ligation |

| 33822 | by division, under 18 years |

| 33824 | by division, 18 years and older |

| 33840 | Excision of coarctation of aorta, with or without associated patent ductus arteriosus; with direct anastomosis |

| 33845 | with graft |

| 33851 | repair using either left subclavian artery or prosthetic material as gusset for enlargement |

| 33852 | Repair of hypoplastic or interrupted aortic arch using autogenous or prosthetic material; without cardiopulmonary bypass |

| 33853 | with cardiopulmonary bypass |

● New Code ▲ Revised Code ＋ Add-On Code ◯ Modifier -51 Exempt

THORACIC AORTIC ANEURYSM

33860 Ascending aorta graft, with cardiopulmonary bypass, with or without valve suspension;

33861 with coronary reconstruction

33863 with aortic root replacement using composite prosthesis and coronary reconstruction

33870 Transverse arch graft, with cardiopulmonary bypass

33875 Descending thoracic aorta graft, with or without bypass

33877 Repair of thoracoabdominal aortic aneurysm with graft, with or without cardiopulmonary bypass

PULMONARY ARTERY

33910 Pulmonary artery embolectomy; with cardiopulmonary bypass

33915 without cardiopulmonary bypass

33916 Pulmonary endarterectomy, with or without embolectomy, with cardiopulmonary bypass

33917 Repair of pulmonary artery stenosis by reconstruction with patch or graft

33918 Repair of pulmonary atresia with ventricular septal defect, by unifocalization of pulmonary arteries; without cardiopulmonary bypass

33919 with cardiopulmonary bypass

(Do not report modifier '-63' in conjunction with 33918, 33919)

33920 Repair of pulmonary atresia with ventricular septal defect, by construction or replacement of conduit from right or left ventricle to pulmonary artery

(For repair of other complex cardiac anomalies by construction or replacement of right or left ventricle to pulmonary artery conduit, use 33608)

33922 Transection of pulmonary artery with cardiopulmonary bypass

(Do not report modifier '-63' in conjunction with 33922)

395

| Separate Procedure | Unlisted Procedure | CCI Comp. Code | Non-specific Procedure |

+ **33924**   Ligation and takedown of a systemic-to-pulmonary artery shunt, performed in conjunction with a congenital heart procedure (List separately in addition to code for primary procedure)

(Use 33924 in conjunction with 33470-33475, 33600-33619, 33684-33688, 33692-33697, 33735-33767, 33770-33781, 33786, 33918-33922)

HEART/LUNG TRANSPLANTATION

(For implantation of a total replacement heart system (artificial heart) with recipient cardiectomy or heart replacement system components, see Category III codes 0051T-0053T)

33930   Donor cardiectomy-pneumonectomy, with preparation and maintenance of allograft

33935   Heart-lung transplant with recipient cardiectomy-pneumonectomy

33940   Donor cardiectomy, with preparation and maintenance of allograft

33945   Heart transplant, with or without recipient cardiectomy

CARDIAC ASSIST

(For percutaneous implantation of extracorporeal ventricular assist device or for removal of percutaneously implanted extracorporeal ventricular assist device, see Category III codes 0048T-0050T)

33960   Prolonged extracorporeal circulation for cardiopulmonary insufficiency; initial 24 hours

+ **33961**   each additional 24 hours (List separately in addition to code for primary procedure)

(Do not report modifier '-63' in conjunction with 33960, 33961)

(Use 33961 in conjunction with code 33960)

(For insertion of cannula for prolonged extracorporeal circulation, use 36822)

33967   Insertion of intra-aortic balloon assist device, percutaneous

33968   Removal of intra-aortic balloon assist device, percutaneous

● New Code   ▲ Revised Code   + Add-On Code   ⊘ Modifier -51 Exempt

33970 Insertion of intra-aortic balloon assist device through the femoral artery, open approach

33971 Removal of intra-aortic balloon assist device including repair of femoral artery, with or without graft

33973 Insertion of intra-aortic balloon assist device through the ascending aorta

33974 Removal of intra-aortic balloon assist device from the ascending aorta, including repair of the ascending aorta, with or without graft

33975 Insertion of ventricular assist device; extracorporeal, single ventricle

33976 extracorporeal, biventricular

33977 Removal of ventricular assist device; extracorporeal, single ventricle

33978 extracorporeal, biventricular

33979 Insertion of ventricular assist device, implantable intracorporeal, single ventricle

33980 Removal of ventricular assist device, implantable intracorporeal, single ventricle

OTHER PROCEDURES, CARDIAC SURGERY

33999 Unlisted procedure, cardiac surgery

ARTERIES AND VEINS

EMBOLECTOMY/THROMBECTOMY

Arterial, With or Without Catheter

34001 Embolectomy or thrombectomy, with or without catheter; carotid, subclavian or innominate artery, by neck incision

34051 innominate, subclavian artery, by thoracic incision

34101 axillary, brachial, innominate, subclavian artery, by arm incision

397

 Separate Procedure   Unlisted Procedure   CCI Comp. Code   Non-specific Procedure

34111   radial or ulnar artery, by arm incision

34151   renal, celiac, mesentery, aortoiliac artery, by abdominal incision

34201   femoropopliteal, aortoiliac artery, by leg incision

34203   popliteal-tibio-peroneal artery, by leg incision

Venous, Direct or With Catheter

34401   Thrombectomy, direct or with catheter; vena cava, iliac vein, by abdominal incision

34421   vena cava, iliac, femoropopliteal vein, by leg incision

34451   vena cava, iliac, femoropopliteal vein, by abdominal and leg incision

34471   subclavian vein, by neck incision

34490   axillary and subclavian vein, by arm incision

VENOUS RECONSTRUCTION

34501   Valvuloplasty, femoral vein

34502   Reconstruction of vena cava, any method

34510   Venous valve transposition, any vein donor

34520   Cross-over vein graft to venous system

34530   Saphenopopliteal vein anastomosis

ENDOVASCULAR REPAIR OF ABDOMINAL AORTIC ANEURYSM

34800   Endovascular repair of infrarenal abdominal aortic aneurysm or dissection; using aorto-aortic tube prosthesis

34802   using modular bifurcated prosthesis (one docking limb)

(For endovascular repair of infrarenal abdominal aortic aneurysm or dissection using a modular bifurcated prosthesis (two docking limbs), use Category III code 0001T)

● New Code   ▲ Revised Code   + Add-On Code   ⊘ Modifier -51 Exempt

34804   using unibody bifurcated prosthesis

(For endovascular repair of infrarenal abdominal aortic aneurysm or dissection using an aorto-uniiliac or aorto-unifemoral prosthesis, use Category III code 0002T)

● **34805**   using aorto-uniiliac or aorto-unifemoral prosthesis

+ **34808**   Endovascular placement of iliac artery occlusion device (List separately in addition to code for primary procedure)

(Use 34808 in conjunction with codes 34800, 34813, 34825, 34826)

(For radiological supervision and interpretation, use 75952 in conjunction with 34800, 34802, 34804, 34808)

(For open arterial exposure, report codes 34812, 34820, 34833, 34834 asappropriate, in addition to codes 34800, 34802, 34804, 34805, 34808)

34812   Open femoral artery exposure for delivery of endovascular prosthesis, by groin incision, unilateral

(For bilateral procedure, use modifier -50)

+ **34813**   Placement of femoral-femoral prosthetic graft during endovascular aortic aneurysm report (List separately in addition to code for primary procedure)

(Use 34813 in conjunction with code 34812)

(For femoral artery grafting, see 35521, 35533, 35546, 35551-35558, 35621, 35646, 35651-35661, 35666, 35700)

34820   Open iliac artery exposure for delivery of endovascular prosthesis or iliac occlusion during endovascular therapy, by abdominal or retroperitoneal incision, unilateral

(For bilateral procedure, use modifier -50)

34825   Placement of proximal or distal extension prosthesis for endovascular repair of infrarenal abdominal aortic or iliac aneurysm, false aneurysm, or dissection; initial vessel

+ **34826**   each additional vessel (List separately in addition to code for primary procedure)

(Use 34826 in conjunction with code 34825)

399

 Separate Procedure   Unlisted Procedure   CCI Comp. Code   Non-specific Procedure

(Use 34825, 34826 in addition to codes 34800-34808, 34900 as appropriate)

(For staged procedure, use modifier -58)

(For radiological supervision and interpretation, use 75953)

34830 Open repair of infrarenal aortic aneurysm or dissection, plus repair of associated arterial trauma, following unsuccessful endovascular repair; tube prosthesis

34831 aorto-bi-iliac prosthesis

34832 aorto-bifemoral prosthesis

34833 Open iliac artery exposure with creation of conduit for delivery of infrarenal aortic or iliac endovascular prosthesis, by abdominal or retroperitoneal incision, unilateral

(For bilateral procedure, use modifier '-50')

(Do not report 34833 in addition to 34820)

34834 Open brachial artery exposure to assist in the deployment of infrarenal aortic or iliac endovascular prosthesis by arm incision, unilateral

(For bilateral procedure, use modifier '-50')

ENDOVASCULAR REPAIR OF ILIAC ANEURYSM

34900 Endovascular graft replacement for repair of iliac artery (eg, aneurysm, pseudoaneurysm, arteriovenous malformation, trauma)

(For radiological supervision and interpretation, use 75954)

(For placement of extension prosthesis during endovascular iliac artery repair, use 34825)

(For bilateral procedure, use modifier '-50')

DIRECT REPAIR OF ANEURYSM OR EXCISION (PARTIAL OR TOTAL) AND GRAFT INSERTION FOR ANEURYSM, PSEUDOANEURYSM, RUPTURED ANEURYSM, AND ASSOCIATED OCCLUSIVE DISEASE

(For direct repairs associated with occlusive disease only, see 35201-35286)

(For intracranial aneurysm, see 61700 et seq)

● New Code   ▲ Revised Code   + Add-On Code   ⊘ Modifier -51 Exempt

(For endovascular repair of abdominal aortic aneurysm, see 34800-34826)

(For endovascular repair of iliac artery aneurysm, see 34900)

(For thoracic aortic aneurysm, see 33860-33875)

(For endovascular repair of thoracic aortic aneurysm, see Category III codes 0033T-0034T)

35001 Direct repair of aneurysm, pseudoaneurysm, or excision (partial or total) and graft insertion, with or without patch graft; for aneurysm and associated occlusive disease, carotid, subclavian artery, by neck incision

35002 for ruptured aneurysm, carotid, subclavian artery, by neck incision

35005 for aneurysm, pseudoaneurysm, and associated occlusive disease, vertebral artery

35011 for aneurysm and associated occlusive disease, axillary-brachial artery, by arm incision

35013 for ruptured aneurysm, axillary-brachial artery, by arm incision

35021 for aneurysm, pseudoaneurysm, and associated occlusive disease, innominate, subclavian artery, by thoracic incision

35022 for ruptured aneurysm, innominate, subclavian artery, by thoracic incision

35045 for aneurysm, pseudoaneurysm, and associated occlusive disease, radial or ulnar artery

35081 for aneurysm, pseudoaneurysm, and associated occlusive disease, abdominal aorta

35082 for ruptured aneurysm, abdominal aorta

35091 for aneurysm, pseudoaneurysm, and associated occlusive disease, abdominal aorta involving visceral vessels (mesenteric, celiac, renal)

35092 for ruptured aneurysm, abdominal aorta involving visceral vessels (mesenteric, celiac, renal)

401

 Separate Procedure   Unlisted Procedure   CCI Comp. Code   Non-specific Procedure

35102   for aneurysm, pseudoaneurysm, and associated occlusive disease, abdominal aorta involving iliac vessels (common, hypogastric, external)

35103   for ruptured aneurysm, abdominal aorta involving iliac vessels (common, hypogastric, external)

35111   for aneurysm, pseudoaneurysm, and associated occlusive disease, splenic artery

35112   for ruptured aneurysm, splenic artery

35121   for aneurysm, pseudoaneurysm, and associated occlusive disease, hepatic, celiac, renal, or mesenteric artery

35122   for ruptured aneurysm, hepatic, celiac, renal, or mesenteric artery

35131   for aneurysm, pseudoaneurysm, and associated occlusive disease, iliac artery (common, hypogastric, external)

35132   for ruptured aneurysm, iliac artery (common, hypogastric, external)

35141   for aneurysm, pseudoaneurysm, and associated occlusive disease, common femoral artery (profunda femoris, superficial femoral)

35142   for ruptured aneurysm, common femoral artery (profunda femoris, superficial femoral)

35151   for aneurysm, pseudoaneurysm, and associated occlusive disease, popliteal artery

35152   for ruptured aneurysm, popliteal artery

35161   for aneurysm, pseudoaneurysm, and associated occlusive disease, other arteries

35162   for ruptured aneurysm, other arteries

REPAIR ARTERIOVENOUS FISTULA

35180   Repair, congenital arteriovenous fistula; head and neck

35182   thorax and abdomen

● New Code   ▲ Revised Code   + Add-On Code   ⊘ Modifier -51 Exempt

| **35184** | extremities |

35188 Repair, acquired or traumatic arteriovenous fistula; head and neck

35189 thorax and abdomen

35190 extremities

REPAIR BLOOD VESSEL OTHER THAN FOR FISTULA, WITH OR WITHOUT PATCH ANGIOPLASTY

(For AV fistula repair, see 35180-35190)

35201 Repair blood vessel, direct; neck

35206 upper extremity

35207 hand, finger

35211 intrathoracic, with bypass

35216 intrathoracic, without bypass

35221 intra-abdominal

35226 lower extremity

35231 Repair blood vessel with vein graft; neck

35236 upper extremity

35241 intrathoracic, with bypass

35246 intrathoracic, without bypass

35251 intra-abdominal

35256 lower extremity

35261 Repair blood vessel with graft other than vein; neck

35266 upper extremity

35271 intrathoracic, with bypass

403

 Separate Procedure   Unlisted Procedure   CCI Comp. Code   Non-specific Procedure

| 35276 | intrathoracic, without bypass |

| 35281 | intra-abdominal |

| 35286 | lower extremity |

THROMBOENDARTERECTOMY

(For coronary artery, see 33510-33536 and 33572)

| 35301 | Thromboendarterectomy, with or without patch graft; carotid, vertebral, subclavian, by neck incision |

| 35311 | subclavian, innominate, by thoracic incision |

| 35321 | axillary-brachial |

| 35331 | abdominal aorta |

| 35341 | mesenteric, celiac, or renal |

| 35351 | iliac |

| 35355 | iliofemoral |

| 35361 | combined aortoiliac |

| 35363 | combined aortoiliofemoral |

| 35371 | common femoral |

| 35372 | deep (profunda) femoral |

| 35381 | femoral and/or popliteal, and/or tibioperoneal |

+ | 35390 | Reoperation, carotid, thromboendarterectomy, more than one month after original operation (List separately in addition to code for primary procedure)

(Use 35390 in conjunction with code 35301)

ANGIOSCOPY

+ | 35400 | Angioscopy (non-coronary vessels or grafts) during therapeutic intervention (List separately in addition to code for primary procedure)

404

● New Code   ▲ Revised Code   + Add-On Code   ⊘ Modifier -51 Exempt

TRANSLUMINAL ANGIOPLASTY

(For radiological supervision and interpretation, see 75962-75968 and 75978)

Open

35450   Transluminal balloon angioplasty, open; renal or other visceral artery

35452   aortic

35454   iliac

35456   femoral-popliteal

35458   brachiocephalic trunk or branches, each vessel

35459   tibioperoneal trunk and branches

35460   venous

Percutaneous

35470   Transluminal balloon angioplasty, percutaneous; tibioperoneal trunk or branches, each vessel

35471   renal or visceral artery

35472   aortic

35473   iliac

35474   femoral-popliteal

35475   brachiocephalic trunk or branches, each vessel

35476   venous

(For radiological supervision and interpretation, use 75978)

TRANSLUMINAL ATHERECTOMY

(For radiological supervision and interpretation, see 75992-75996)

405

 Separate Procedure   Unlisted Procedure   CCI Comp. Code   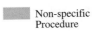 Non-specific Procedure

Open

35480	Transluminal peripheral atherectomy, open; renal or other visceral artery
35481	aortic
35482	iliac
35483	femoral-popliteal
35484	brachiocephalic trunk or branches, each vessel
35485	tibioperoneal trunk and branches

Percutaneous

35490	Transluminal peripheral atherectomy, percutaneous; renal or other visceral artery
35491	aortic
35492	iliac
35493	femoral-popliteal
35494	brachiocephalic trunk or branches, each vessel
35495	tibioperoneal trunk and branches

BYPASS GRAFT

Vein

+ **35500** Harvest of upper extremity vein, one segment, for lower extremity or coronary artery bypass procedure (List separately in addition to code for primary procedure)

(Use 35500 in conjunction with codes 33510-33536, 35556, 35566, 35571, 35583-35587)

(For harvest of more than one vein segment, see 35682, 35683)

(For endoscopic procedure, use 33508)

35501	Bypass graft, with vein; carotid
35506	carotid-subclavian

● New Code   ▲ Revised Code   + Add-On Code   ⊘ Modifier -51 Exempt

35507	subclavian-carotid
35508	carotid-vertebral
35509	carotid-carotid
● **35510**	carotid-brachial
35511	subclavian-subclavian
● **35512**	subclavian-brachial
35515	subclavian-vertebral
35516	subclavian-axillary
35518	axillary-axillary
35521	axillary-femoral

(For bypass graft performed with synthetic graft, use 35621)

● **35522**	axillary-brachial
● **35525**	brachial-brachial
35526	aortosubclavian or carotid

(For bypass graft performed with synthetic graft, use 35626)

35531	aortoceliac or aortomesenteric
35533	axillary-femoral-femoral

(For bypass graft performed with synthetic graft, use 35654)

35536	splenorenal
35541	aortoiliac or bi-iliac

(For bypass graft performed with synthetic graft, use 35641)

35546	aortofemoral or bifemoral

(For bypass graft performed with synthetic graft, use 35646)

35548	aortoiliofemoral, unilateral

407

	Separate Procedure		Unlisted Procedure		CCI Comp. Code		Non-specific Procedure

(For bypass graft performed with synthetic graft, use 37799)

35549   aortoiliofemoral, bilateral

(For bypass graft performed with synthetic graft, use 37799)

35551   aortofemoral-popliteal

35556   femoral-popliteal

35558   femoral-femoral

35560   aortorenal

35563   ilioiliac

35565   iliofemoral

35566   femoral-anterior tibial, posterior tibial, peroneal artery or other distal vessels

35571   popliteal-tibial, -peroneal artery or other distal vessels

+ 35572   Harvest of femoropopliteal vein, one segment, for vascular reconstruction procedure (eg, aortic, vena caval, coronary, peripheral artery) (List separately in addition to code for primary procedure)

(Use 35572 in conjunction with codes 33510-33516, 33517-33523, 34502, 34520, 35001-35002, 35011-35022, 35102-35103, 35121-35152, 35231-35256, 35501-35587, 35879-35881, 35901-35907)

(For bilateral procedure, use modifier '-50')

In-Situ Vein

35582   In-situ vein bypass; aortofemoral-popliteal (only femoral-popliteal portion in-situ)

35583   femoral-popliteal

35585   femoral-anterior tibial, posterior tibial, or peroneal artery

35587   popliteal-tibial, peroneal

● New Code   ▲ Revised Code   + Add-On Code   ⊘ Modifier -51 Exempt

Other Than Vein

⊘ **35600**   Harvest of upper extremity artery, one segment, for coronary artery bypass procedure

35601   Bypass graft, with other than vein; carotid

35606   carotid-subclavian

(For open subclavian to carotid artery transposition performed in conjunction with endovascular thoracic aneurysm repair, use Category III code 0037T)

35612   subclavian-subclavian

35616   subclavian-axillary

35621   axillary-femoral

35623   axillary-popliteal or -tibial

35626   aortosubclavian or carotid

35631   aortoceliac, aortomesenteric, aortorenal

35636   splenorenal (splenic to renal arterial anastomosis)

35641   aortoiliac or bi-iliac

(For open placement of aorto-bi-iliac prosthesis following unsuccessful endovascular repair, use 34831)

35642   carotid-vertebral

35645   subclavian-vertebral

35646   aortobifemoral

(For open placement of aortobifemoral prosthesis following unsuccessful endovascular repair, use 34832)

35647   aortofemoral

35650   axillary-axillary

35651   aortofemoral-popliteal

 Separate Procedure    Unlisted Procedure    CCI Comp. Code   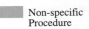 Non-specific Procedure

409

| 35654 | axillary-femoral-femoral |

35654 axillary-femoral-femoral

35656 femoral-popliteal

35661 femoral-femoral

35663 ilioiliac

35665 iliofemoral

35666 femoral-anterior tibial, posterior tibial, or peroneal artery

35671 popliteal-tibial or -peroneal artery

COMPOSITE GRAFTS

+ **35681** Bypass graft; composite, prosthetic and vein (List separately in addition to code for primary procedure)

(Do not report 35681 in addition to 35682, 35683)

+ **35682** autogenous composite, two segments of veins from two locations (List separately in addition to code for primary procedure)

(Do not report 35682 in addition to 35681, 35683)

+ **35683** autogenous composite, three or more segments of vein from two or more locations (List separately in addition to code for primary procedure)

(Do not report 35683 in addition to 35681, 35682)

ADJUVANT TECHNIQUES

(For composite graft(s), see 35681-35683)

+ **35685** Placement of vein patch or cuff at distal anastomosis of bypass graft, synthetic conduit (List separately in addition to code for primary procedure)

(Use 35685 in conjunction with codes 35656, 35666 or 35671)

+ **35686** Creation of distal arteriovenous fistula during lower extremity bypass surgery (non-hemodialysis) (List separately in addition to code for primary procedure)

(Use 35686 in conjunction with codes 35556, 35566, 35571, 35583-35587, 35623, 35656, 35666, 35671)

● New Code   ▲ Revised Code   + Add-On Code   ⊘ Modifier -51 Exempt

ARTERIAL TRANSPOSITION

35691 Transposition and/or reimplantation; vertebral to carotid artery

35693 vertebral to subclavian artery

35694 subclavian to carotid artery

(For open subclavian to carotid artery transposition performed in conjunction with endovascular thoracic aneurysm repair, use Category III code 0037T)

35695 carotid to subclavian artery

●+35697 Reimplantation, visceral artery to infrarenal aortic prosthesis, each artery (List separately in addition to code for primary procedure)

(Do not report 35697 in conjunction with 33877)

EXPLORATION/REVISION

+ 35700 Reoperation, femoral-popliteal or femoral (popliteal)-anterior tibial, posterior tibial, peroneal artery or other distal vessels, more than one month after original operation (List separately in addition to code for primary procedure)

(Use 35700 in conjunction with codes 35556, 35566, 35571, 35583, 35585, 35587, 35656, 35666, 35671)

35701 Exploration (not followed by surgical repair), with or without lysis of artery; carotid artery

35721 femoral artery

35741 popliteal artery

35761 other vessels

35800 Exploration for postoperative hemorrhage, thrombosis or infection; neck

35820 chest

35840 abdomen

35860 extremity

 Separate Procedure
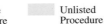 Unlisted Procedure
 CCI Comp. Code
 Non-specific Procedure

411

35870 Repair of graft-enteric fistula

35875 Thrombectomy of arterial or venous graft (other than hemodialysis graft or fistula);

35876 with revision of arterial or venous graft

(For thrombectomy of hemodialysis graft or fistula, see 36831, 36833)

35879 Revision, lower extremity arterial bypass, without thrombectomy, open; with vein patch angioplasty

35881 with segmental vein interposition

35901 Excision of infected graft; neck

35903 extremity

35905 thorax

35907 abdomen

VASCULAR INJECTION PROCEDURES

When using CPT codes from this section, note that the listed procedures include local anesthesia, introduction of needles or catheter, injection of contrast medium with or without automatic power injection, and pre- and post-injection care specifically related to the injection procedure.

Note that catheters, drugs and contrast media are not included in CPT codes listed in this section. These should be coded using CPT code 99070 or the appropriate HCPCS Level II code for Medicare patients.

CPT codes listed in this section do not cover radiological vascular injections, injection procedures for cardiac catheterization or chemotherapy. Refer to the RADIOLOGY or MEDICINE sections of CPT for the appropriate CPT codes for these procedures.

(For radiological supervision and interpretation, see RADIOLOGY)

(For injection procedures in conjunction with cardiac catheterization, see 93541-93545)

(For chemotherapy of malignant disease, see 96400-96549)

● New Code   ▲ Revised Code   + Add-On Code   ⊘ Modifier -51 Exempt

INTRAVENOUS

36000   Introduction of needle or intracatheter, vein

36002   Injection procedures (eg, thrombin) for percutaneous treatment of extremity pseudoaneurysm

(For imaging guidance, see 76003, 76360, 76393, or 76942)

(For ultrasound guided compression repair of pseudoaneurysms, use 76936)

(Do not report 36002 for vascular sealant of an arteriotomy site)

36005   Injection procedure for extremity venography (including introduction of needle or intracatheter)

(For radiological supervision and interpretation, see 75820, 75822)

36010   Introduction of catheter, superior or inferior vena cava

36011   Selective catheter placement, venous system; first order branch (eg, renal vein, jugular vein)

36012   second order, or more selective, branch (eg, left adrenal vein, petrosal sinus)

36013   Introduction of catheter, right heart or main pulmonary artery

36014   Selective catheter placement, left or right pulmonary artery

36015   Selective catheter placement, segmental or subsegmental pulmonary artery

(For insertion of flow directed catheter (eg, Swan-Ganz), use 93503)

(For venous catheterization for selective organ blood sampling, use 36500)

INTRA-ARTERIAL/INTRA-AORTIC

(For radiological supervision and interpretation, see RADIOLOGY)

36100   Introduction of needle or intracatheter, carotid or vertebral artery

413

 Separate Procedure    Unlisted Procedure   CCI Comp. Code   Non-specific Procedure

| 36120 | Introduction of needle or intracatheter; retrograde brachial artery |

36120 Introduction of needle or intracatheter; retrograde brachial artery

36140 extremity artery

36145 arteriovenous shunt created for dialysis (cannula, fistula, or graft)

(For insertion of arteriovenous cannula, see 36810-36821)

36160 Introduction of needle or intracatheter, aortic, translumbar

36200 Introduction of catheter, aorta

36215 Selective catheter placement, arterial system; each first order thoracic or brachiocephalic branch, within a vascular family

(For catheter placement for coronary angiography, use 93508)

36216 initial second order thoracic or brachiocephalic branch, within a vascular family

36217 initial third order or more selective thoracic or brachiocephalic branch, within a vascular family

+ 36218 additional second order, third order, and beyond, thoracic or brachiocephalic branch, within a vascular family (List in addition to code for initial second or third order vessel as appropriate)

(Use 36218 in conjunction with codes 36216, 36217)

(For angiography, see 75600-75790)

(For angioplasty, see 35470-35475)

(For transcatheter therapies, see 37200-37208, 61624, 61626)

36245 Selective catheter placement, arterial system; each first order abdominal, pelvic, or lower extremity artery branch, within a vascular family

36246 initial second order abdominal, pelvic, or lower extremity artery branch, within a vascular family

36247 initial third order or more selective abdominal, pelvic, or lower extremity artery branch, within a vascular family

● New Code   ▲ Revised Code   + Add-On Code   ⊘ Modifier -51 Exempt

+ 36248 additional second order, third order, and beyond, abdominal, pelvic, or lower extremity artery branch, within a vascular family (List in addition to code for initial second or third order vessel as appropriate)

(Use 36248 in conjunction with codes 36246, 36247)

36260 Insertion of implantable intra-arterial infusion pump (eg, for chemotherapy of liver)

36261 Revision of implanted intra-arterial infusion pump

36262 Removal of implanted intra-arterial infusion pump

36299 Unlisted procedure, vascular injection

VENOUS

▲ **36400** Venipuncture, under age 3 years, necessitating physician's skill, not to be used for routine venipuncture; femoral or jugular vein

36405 scalp vein

36406 other vein

▲ **36410** Venipuncture, age 3 years or older, necessitating physician's skill (separate procedure), for diagnostic or therapeutic purposes (not to be used for routine venipuncture)

36415 Collection of venous blood by venipuncture

(Do not report modifier '-63' in conjunction with 36415)

36416 Collection of capillary blood specimen (eg, finger, heel, ear stick)

36420 Venipuncture, cutdown; under age 1 year

(Do not report modifier '-63' in conjunction with 36420)

36425 age 1 or over

36430 Transfusion, blood or blood components

36440 Push transfusion, blood, 2 years or under

415

 Separate Procedure   Unlisted Procedure   CCI Comp. Code   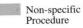 Non-specific Procedure

36450 Exchange transfusion, blood; newborn

(Do not report modifier '-63' in conjunction with 36450)

36455 other than newborn

36460 Transfusion, intrauterine, fetal

(Do not report modifier '-63' in conjunction with 36460)

(For radiological supervision and interpretation, use 76941)

36468 Single or multiple injections of sclerosing solutions, spider veins (telangiectasia); limb or trunk

36469 face

36470 Injection of sclerosing solution; single vein

36471 multiple veins, same leg

36481 Percutaneous portal vein catheterization by any method

(For radiological supervision and interpretation, see 75885, 75887)

(36488 deleted 2004 edition. To report, see 36555-36556, 36568-36569, 36580, 36584)

(36489 deleted 2004 edition. To report, see 36555-36556, 36568-36569, 36580, 36584)

(36490 deleted 2004 edition. To report, see 36555-36556, 36568-36569, 36580, 36584)

(36491 deleted 2004 edition. To report, see 36555-36556, 36568-36569, 36580, 36584)

(36493 deleted 2004 edition. To report, use 36597)

36500 Venous catheterization for selective organ blood sampling

(For catheterization in superior or inferior vena cava, use 36010)

(For radiological supervision and interpretation, use 75893)

● New Code ▲ Revised Code + Add-On Code ⊘ Modifier -51 Exempt

36510   Catheterization of umbilical vein for diagnosis or therapy, newborn

(Do not report modifier '-63' in conjunction with 36510)

36511   Therapeutic apheresis; for white blood cells

36512   for red blood cells

36513   for platelets

36514   for plasma pheresis

36515   with extracorporeal immunoadsorption and plasma reinfusion

36516   with extracorporeal selective adsorption or selective filtration and plasma reinfusion

(for physician evaluation, use modifier -26)

(36520   deleted 2003 edition. To report see 36511-36512)

(36521   deleted 2003 edition. To report, use 36516)

36522   Photopheresis, extracorporeal

(36530   deleted 2004 edition. To report, use 36563)

(36531   deleted 2004 edition. To report, see 36575-36576, 36578, 36581-36582, 36584-36585)

(36532   deleted 2004 edition. To report, use 36590)

(36533   deleted 2004 edition. To report, see 36557-36561, 36565-36566, 36570-36571)

(36534   deleted 2004 edition. To report, see 36575-36578, 36581-36583, 36585)

(36535   deleted 2004 edition. To report, use 36589)

(36536   deleted 2004 edition. To report, use 36595)

(36537   deleted 2004 edition. To report, use 36596)

 Separate Procedure    Unlisted Procedure   CCI Comp. Code   Non-specific Procedure

36540   Collection of blood specimen from a completely implantable venous access device

(Do not report 36540 in conjunction with 36415, 36416)

(For collection of venous blood specimen by venipuncture, use 36415)

(For collection of capillary blood specimen, use 36416)

36550   Declotting by thrombolytic agent of implanted vascular access device or catheter

CENTRAL VENOUS ACCESS PROCEDURES

To qualify as a central venous access catheter or device, the tip of the catheter/device must terminate in the subclavian, brachiocephalic (innominate) or iliac veins, the superior or inferior vena cava, or the right atrium. The venous access device may be either centrally inserted (jugular, subclavian, femoral vein or inferior vena cava catheter entry site) or peripherally inserted (eg, basilic or cephalic vein). The device may be accessed for use either via exposed catheter (external to the skin), via a subcutaneous port or via a subcutaneous pump.

The procedures involving these types of devices fall into five categories:

1) Insertion (placement of catheter through a newly established venous access)

2) Repair (fixing device without replacement of either catheter or port/pump, other than pharmacologic or mechanical correction of intracatheter or pericatheter occlusion (see 36595 or 36596))

3) Partial replacement of only the catheter component associated with a port/pump device, but not entire device

4) Complete replacement of entire device via same vanous access site (complete exchange)

5) Removal of entire device.

There is no coding distinction between venous access achieved percutaneously versus by cutdown or based on catheter size.

For the repair, partial (catheter only) replacement, complete replacement, or removal of both catheters (placed from separate venous access sites) of a multi-catheter device, with or without subcutaneous ports/pumps, use the appropriate code describing the service with a frequency of two.

If an existing central venous access device is removed and a new one placed via a separate venous access site, appropriate codes for both procedures (removal of old, if code exists, and insertion of new device) should be reported.

418

● New Code	▲ Revised Code	**+** Add-On Code	⊘ Modifier -51 Exempt

When imaging is used for these procedures, either for gaining access to the venous entry site or for manipulating the catheter into final central position, use 76937, 75998.

(For refilling and maintenance of an implantable pump or reservoir for intravenous or intra-arterial drug delivery, use 96530)

Insertion of Central Venous Access Device

● **36555**   Insertion of non-tunneled centrally inserted central venous catheter; under 5 years of age

(For peripherally inserted non-tunneled central venous catheter, under 5 years of age, use 36568)

● **36556**   age 5 years or older

(For peripherally inserted non-tunneled central venous catheter, age 5 years or older, use 36569)

● **36557**   Insertion of tunneled centrally inserted central venous catheter, without subcutaneous port or pump; under 5 years of age

● **36558**   age 5 years or older

(For peripherally inserted central venous catheter with port, age 5 years or older, use 36571)

● **36560**   Insertion of tunneled centrally inserted central venous access device, with subcutaneous port; under 5 years of age

(For peripherally inserted central venous access device with subcutaneous port, under 5 years of age, use 36570)

● **36561**   age 5 years or older

(For peripherally inserted central venous catheter with subcutaneous port, 5 years or older, use 36571)

● **36563**   Insertion of tunneled centrally inserted central venous access device with subcutaneous pump

● **36565**   Insertion of tunneled centrally inserted central venous access device, requiring two catheters via two separate venous access sites; without subcutaneous port or pump (eg, Tesio type catheter)

● **36566**   with subcutaneous port(s)

419

 Separate Procedure   Unlisted Procedure    CCI Comp. Code   Non-specific Procedure

● **36568**   Insertion of peripherally inserted central venous catheter (PICC), without subcutaneous port or pump; under 5 years of age

(For placement of centrally inserted non-tunneled central venous catheter, without subcutaneous port or pump, under 5 years of age, use 36555)

● **36569**   age 5 years or older

(For placement of centrally inserted non-tunneled central venous catheter, without subcutaneous port or pump, age 5 years or older, use 36556)

● **36570**   Insertion of peripherally inserted cetnral venous access device, with subcutaneous port; under 5 years of age

(For insertion of tunneled centrally inserted central venous access device with subcutaneous port, under 5 years of age, use 36560)

● **36571**   age 5 years or older

(For insertion of tunneled centrally inserted central venous access device with subcutaneous port, age 5 years or older, use 36561)

Repair of Central Venous Access Device

(For mechanical removal of pericatheter obstructive material, use 36595)

(For mechancial removal of intracatheter obstructive material, use 36596)

● **36575**   Repair of tunneled or non-tunneled central venous access catheter, without subcutaneous port or pump, central or peripheral insertion site

● **36576**   Repair of central venous access device, with subcutaneous port or pump, central or peripheral insertion site

Partial Replacement of Central Venous Access Device (Catheter Only)

● **36578**   Replacement, catheter only, of central venous access device, with subcutaneous port or pump, central or peripheral insertion site

(For complete replacement of entire device through same venous access, use 36582 or 36583)

---

420   ● New Code   ▲ Revised Code   **+** Add-On Code   ⃠ Modifier -51 Exempt

Complete Replacement of Central Venous Access Device Through Same Venous Access Site

- **36580**   Replacement, complete, of a non-tunneled centrally inserted central venous catheter, without subcutaneous port or pump, through same venous access

- **36581**   Replacement, complete, of a tunneled centrally inserted central venous catheter, without subcutaneous port of pump, through same venous access

- **36582**   Replacement, complete, of a tunneled centrally inserted central venous access device, with subcutaneous port, through same venous access

- **36583**   Replacement, complete, of a tunneled centrally inserted central venous access device, with subcutaneous pump, through same venous access

- **36584**   Replacement, complete, of a peripherally inserted central venous catheter (PICC), without subcutaneous port or pump, through same venous access

- **36585**   Replacement, complete, of a peripherally inserted central venous access device, with subcutaneous port, through same venous access

Removal of Central Venous Access Device

- **36589**   Removal of tunneled central venous catheter, without subcutaneous port or pump

- **36590**   Removal of tunneled central venous access device, with subcutaneous port or pump, central or peripheral insertion

    (Do not report 36589 or 36590 for removal of non-tunneled central venous catheters)

Mechanical Removal of Obstructive Material

- **36595**   Mechanical removal of pericatheter obstructive material (eg, fibrin sheath) from central venous device via separate venous access

    (Do not report 36550 in addition to 36595)

    (For venous catheterization, see 36010-36012)

    (For radiological supervision and interpretation, use 75901)

421

 Separate Procedure   Unlisted Procedure   CCI Comp. Code   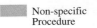 Non-specific Procedure

- **36596** Mechanical removal of intraluminal (intracatheter) obstructive material from central venous device through device lumen

  (Do not report 36550 in addition to 36596)

  (For venous catheterization, see 36010-36012)

  (For radiological supervision and interpretation, use 75902)

Other Central Venous Access Procedures

- **36597** Repositioning of previously placed central venous catheter under fluoroscopic guidance

  (For fluoroscopic guidance, use 76000)

ARTERIAL

36600 Arterial puncture, withdrawal of blood for diagnosis

⊘ **36620** Arterial catheterization or cannulation for sampling, monitoring or transfusion (separate procedure); percutaneous

36625 cutdown

36640 Arterial catheterization for prolonged infusion therapy (chemotherapy), cutdown

(See also 96420-96425)

(For arterial catheterization for occlusion therapy, see 75894)

⊘ **36660** Catheterization, umbilical artery, newborn, for diagnosis or therapy

(Do not report modifier '-63' in conjunction with 36660)

INTRAOSSEOUS

36680 Placement of needle for intraosseous infusion

HEMODIALYSIS ACCESS, INTERVASCULAR CANNULIZATION FOR EXTRACORPOREAL CIRCULATION, OR SHUNT INSERTION

36800 Insertion of cannula for hemodialysis, other purpose (separate procedure); vein to vein

36810 arteriovenous, external (Scribner type)

36815 arteriovenous, external revision, or closure

422

● New Code   ▲ Revised Code   + Add-On Code   ⊘ Modifier -51 Exempt

36819 Arteriovenous anastomosis, open; by upper arm basilic vein transposition

36820 by forearm vein transposition

36821 direct, any site (eg, Cimino type) (separate procedure)

36822 Insertion of cannula(s) for prolonged extracorporeal circulation for cardiopulmonary insufficiency (ECMO) (separate procedure)

(For maintenance of prolonged extracorporeal circulation, use 33960, 33961)

36823 Insertion of arterial and venous cannula(s) for isolated extracorporeal circulation including regional chemotherapy perfusion to an extremity, with or without hyperthermia, with removal of cannula(s) and repair of arteriotomy and venotomy sites

(36823 includes chemotherapy perfusion supported by a membrane oxygenator/perfusion pump. Do not report 96408-96425 in conjunction with 36823)

36825 Creation of arteriovenous fistula by other than direct arteriovenous anastomosis (separate procedure); autogenous graft

(For direct arteriovenous anastomosis, use 36821)

36830 nonautogenous graft (eg, biological collagen, thermoplastic graft)

(For direct arteriovenous anastomosis, use 36821)

36831 Thrombectomy, open, arteriovenous fistula without revision, autogenous or nonautogenous dialysis graft (separate procedure)

36832 Revision, open, arteriovenous fistula; without thrombectomy, autogenous or nonautogenous dialysis graft (separate procedure)

36833 with thrombectomy, autogenous or nonautogenous dialysis graft (separate procedure)

36834 Plastic repair of arteriovenous aneurysm (separate procedure)

36835 Insertion of Thomas shunt (separate procedure)

423

 Separate Procedure

Unlisted Procedure

 CCI Comp. Code

 Non-specific Procedure

● **36838**   Distal revascularization and interval ligation (DRIL), upper extremity hemodialysis access (steal syndrome)

(Do not report 36838 in conjunction with 35512, 35522, 36832, 37607, 37618)

36860   External cannula declotting (separate procedure); without balloon catheter

36861   with balloon catheter

(If imaging guidance is performed, use 76000)

36870   Thrombectomy, percutaneous, arteriovenous fistula, autogenous or nonautogenous graft (includes mechanical thrombus extraction and intro-graft thrombolysis)

(Do not report 36550 in conjunction with code 36870)

(For catheterization, use 36145)

(For radiological supervision and interpretation, use 75790)

PORTAL DECOMPRESSION PROCEDURES

37140   Venous anastomosis, open; portocaval

(For peritoneal-venous shunt, use 49425)

37145   renoportal

37160   caval-mesenteric

37180   splenorenal, proximal

37181   splenorenal, distal (selective decompression of esophagogastric varices, any technique)

(For percutaneous procedure, use 37182)

37182   Insertion of transvenous intrahepatic portosystemic shunt(s) (TIPS) (includes venous access, hepatic and portal vein catheterization, portography with hemodynamic evaluation, intrahepatic tract formation/dilatation, stent placement and all associated imaging guidance and documentation)

(Do not report 75885 or 75887 in conjunction with code 37182)

(For open procedure, use 37140)

424   ● New Code   ▲ Revised Code   + Add-On Code   ⊘ Modifier -51 Exempt

37183 Revision of transvenous intrahepatic portosystemic shunt(s) (TIPS) (includes venous access, hepatic and portal vein catheterization, portography with hemodynamic evaluation, intrahepatic tract recanulization/dilatation, stent placement and all associated imaging guidance and documentation)

(Do not report 75885 or 75887 in conjunction with code 37183)

TRANSCATHETER PROCEDURES

37195 Thrombolysis, cerebral, by intravenous infusion

37200 Transcatheter biopsy

(For radiological supervision and interpretation, use 75970)

37201 Transcatheter therapy, infusion for thrombolysis other than coronary

(For radiological supervision and interpretation, use 75896)

37202 Transcatheter therapy, infusion other than for thrombolysis, any type (eg, spasmolytic, vasoconstrictive)

(For thrombolysis of coronary vessels, see 92975, 92977)

(For radiological supervision and interpretation, use 75896)

37203 Transcatheter retrieval, percutaneous, of intravascular foreign body (eg, fractured venous or arterial catheter)

(For radiological supervision and interpretation, use 75961)

37204 Transcatheter occlusion or embolization (eg, for tumor destruction, to achieve hemostasis, to occlude a vascular malformation), percutaneous, any method, non-central nervous system, non-head or neck

(See also 61624, 61626)

(For radiological supervision and interpretation, use 75894)

37205 Transcatheter placement of an intravascular stent(s), (non-coronary vessel), percutaneous; initial vessel

(For radiological supervision and interpretation, use 75960)

+ 37206 each additional vessel (List separately in addition to code for primary procedure)

425

 Separate Procedure   Unlisted Procedure   CCI Comp. Code   Non-specific Procedure

(Use 37206 in conjunction with 37205)

(For transcatheter placement of extracranial cerebrovascular artery stent(s), see Category III codes 0005T, 0006T)

(For radiological supervision and interpretation, use 75960)

37207 Transcatheter placement of an intravascular stent(s), (non-coronary vessel), open; initial vessel

+ 37208   each additional vessel (List separately in addition to code for primary procedure)

(Use 37208 in conjunction with 37207)

(For radiological supervision and interpretation, use 75960)

(For catheterizations, see 36215-36248)

(For transcatheter placement of intracoronary stent(s), see 92980, 92981)

37209 Exchange of a previously placed arterial catheter during thrombolytic therapy

(For radiological supervision and interpretation, use 75900)

INTRAVASCULAR ULTRASOUND SERVICES

+ 37250 Intravascular ultrasound (non-coronary vessel) during diagnostic evaluation and/or therapeutic intervention; initial vessel (List separately in addition to code for primary procedure)

+ 37251   each additional vessel (List separately in addition to code for primary procedure)

(Use 37251 in conjunction with 37250)

(For catheterizations, see 36215-36248)

(For transcatheter therapies, see 37200-37208, 61624, 61626)

(For radiological supervision and interpretation, see 75945, 75946)

ENDOSCOPY

(Surgical vascular endoscopy always includes diagnostic endoscopy)

37500 Vascular endoscopy, surgical, with ligation or perforator veins, subfascial (SEPS)

426

● New Code   ▲ Revised Code   + Add-On Code   ⊘ Modifier -51 Exempt

(For open procedure, use 37760)

37501 Unlisted vascular endoscopy procedure

LIGATION AND OTHER PROCEDURES

37565 Ligation, internal jugular vein

37600 Ligation; external carotid artery

37605   internal or common carotid artery

37606   internal or common carotid artery, with gradual occlusion, as with Selverstone or Crutchfield clamp

(For transcatheter permanent arterial occlusion or embolization, see 61624-61626)

(For endovascular temporary arterial balloon occlusion, use 61623)

(For ligation treatment of intracranial aneurysm, use 61703)

37607 Ligation or banding of angioaccess arteriovenous fistula

37609 Ligation or biopsy, temporal artery

37615 Ligation, major artery (eg, post-traumatic, rupture); neck

37616   chest

37617   abdomen

37618   extremity

37620 Interruption, partial or complete, of inferior vena cava by suture, ligation, plication, clip, extravascular, intravascular (umbrella device)

(For radiological supervision and interpretation, use 75940)

37650 Ligation of femoral vein

37660 Ligation of common iliac vein

37700 Ligation and division of long saphenous vein at saphenofemoral junction, or distal interruptions

427

 Separate Procedure   Unlisted Procedure   CCI Comp. Code   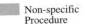 Non-specific Procedure

37720   Ligation and division and complete stripping of long or short saphenous veins

37730   Ligation and division and complete stripping of long and short saphenous veins

37735   Ligation and division and complete stripping of long or short saphenous veins with radical excision of ulcer and skin graft and/or interruption of communicating veins of lower leg, with excision of deep fascia

37760   Ligation of perforator veins, subfascial, radical (Linton type), with or without skin graft, open

        (For endoscopic procedure, use 37500)

● **37765**   Stab phlebectomy of varicose veins, one extremity; 10-20 stab incisions

        (For less than 10 incisions, use 37799)

        (For more than 20 incisions, use 37766)

● **37766**   more than 20 incisions

37780   Ligation and division of short saphenous vein at saphenopopliteal junction (separate procedure)

▲ **37785**   Ligation, division, and/or excision of varicose vein cluster(s), one leg

37788   Penile revascularization, artery, with or without vein graft

37790   Penile venous occlusive procedure

37799   Unlisted procedure, vascular surgery

This page intentionally left blank.

HEMIC AND LYMPHATIC SYSTEMS

CPT codes from this section of CPT are used to report invasive and surgical procedures performed on the spleen and lymph nodes. Bone marrow transplants are reported using CPT codes 38230-38241 from this section.

SPLEEN

EXCISION

38100   Splenectomy; total (separate procedure)

38101   partial (separate procedure)

+ **38102**   total, en bloc for extensive disease, in conjunction with other procedure (List in addition to code for primary procedure)

REPAIR

38115   Repair of ruptured spleen (splenorrhaphy) with or without partial splenectomy

LAPAROSCOPY

38120   Laparoscopy, surgical, splenectomy

38129   Unlisted laparoscopy procedure, spleen

INTRODUCTION

38200   Injection procedure for splenoportography

(For radiological supervision and interpretation, use 75810)

GENERAL

BONE MARROW OR STEM CELL SERVICES/PROCEDURES

CPT codes 38207-38215 may be reported once a day, regardless of the number of cells manipulated.

38204   Management of recipient hematopoietic progenitor cell donor search and cell acquisition

---

430

● New Code   ▲ Revised Code   + Add-On Code   ⊘ Modifier -51 Exempt

38205 Blood-derived hematopoietic progenitor cell harvesting for transplantation, per collection; allogenic

38206 autologous

38207 Transplant preparation of hematopoietic progenitor cells; cryopreservation and storage

(For diagnostic cryopreservation and storage, see 88240)

▲ **38208** thawing of previously frozen harvest, without washing

(For diagnostic thawing and expansion of frozen cells, see 88241)

▲ **38209** thawing of previuosly frozen harvest, with washing

38210 specific cell depletion within harvest, T-cell depletion

38211 tumor cell depletion

38212 red blood cell removal

38213 platelet depletion

38214 plasma (volume) depletion

38215 cell concentration in plasma, mononuclear, or buffy coat layer

(Do not report 88180, 88182 in conjunction with 38207-38215)

38220 Bone marrow; aspiration only

38221 biopsy, needle or trocar

(For bone marrow biopsy interpretation, use 88305)

38230 Bone marrow harvesting for transplantation

(38231 deleted 2003 edition. To report, use 38205-38206)

38240 Bone marrow or blood-derived peripheral stem cell transplantation; allogenic

38241 autologous

431

 Separate Procedure

 Unlisted Procedure

 CCI Comp. Code

 Non-specific Procedure

38242   allogeneic donor lymphocyte infusions

(For bone marrow aspiration, use 38220)

(For modification, treatment, and processing of bone marrow or blood-derived stem cell specimens for transplantation, see 38210-38213)

(For cryopreservation, freezing and storage of blood-derived stem cells for transplantation, use 88240)

(For thawing and expansion of blood-derived stem cells for transplantation, use 88241)

(For compatibility studies, see 86812-86822)

LYMPH NODES AND LYMPHATIC CHANNELS

INCISION

38300   Drainage of lymph node abscess or lymphadenitis; simple

38305   extensive

38308   Lymphangiotomy or other operations on lymphatic channels

38380   Suture and/or ligation of thoracic duct; cervical approach

38381   thoracic approach

38382   abdominal approach

EXCISION

(For injection for sentinel node identification, use 38792)

38500   Biopsy or excision of lymph node(s); open, superficial

(Do not report 38500 with 38700-38780)

38505   by needle, superficial (eg, cervical, inguinal, axillary)

(If imaging guidance is performed, see 76360, 76393, 76942)

(For fine needle aspiration, use 10021 or 10022)

(For evaluation of fine needle aspirate, see 88172, 88173)

38510   open, deep cervical node(s)

432

● New Code	▲ Revised Code	+ Add-On Code	⊘ Modifier -51 Exempt

38520   open, deep cervical node(s) with excision scalene fat pad

38525   open, deep axillary node(s)

38530   open, internal mammary node(s)

(Do not report 38530 with 38720-38746)

(For percutaneous needle biopsy, retroperitoneal lymph node or mass, use 49180. For fine needle aspiration, use 10022)

38542 Dissection, deep jugular node(s)

(For radical cervical neck dissection, use 38720)

38550 Excision of cystic hygroma, axillary or cervical; without deep neurovascular dissection

38555   with deep neurovascular dissection

LIMITED LYMPHADENECTOMY FOR STAGING

38562 Limited lymphadenectomy for staging (separate procedure); pelvic and para-aortic

(When combined with prostatectomy, use 55812 or 55842)

(When combined with insertion of radioactive substance into prostate, use 55862)

38564   retroperitoneal (aortic and/or splenic)

LAPAROSCOPY

38570 Laparoscopy, surgical; with retroperitoneal lymph node sampling (biopsy), single or multiple

38571   with bilateral total pelvic lymphadenectomy

38572   with bilateral total pelvic lymphadenectomy and peri-aortic lymph node sampling (biopsy), single or multiple

(For drainage of lymphocele to peritoneal cavity, use 49323)

38589 Unlisted laparoscopy procedure, lymphatic system

433

| | Separate Procedure | | Unlisted Procedure | | CCI Comp. Code | | Non-specific Procedure |

RADICAL LYMPHADENECTOMY (RADICAL RESECTION OF LYMPH NODES)

(For limited pelvic and retroperitoneal lymphadenectomies, see 38562, 38564)

38700 Suprahyoid lymphadenectomy

38720 Cervical lymphadenectomy (complete)

38724 Cervical lymphadenectomy (modified radical neck dissection)

38740 Axillary lymphadenectomy; superficial

38745 complete

+ **38746** Thoracic lymphadenectomy, regional, including mediastinal and peritracheal nodes (List separately in addition to code for primary procedure)

+ **38747** Abdominal lymphadenectomy, regional, including celiac, gastric, portal, peripancreatic, with or without para-aortic and vena caval nodes (List separately in addition to code for primary procedure)

38760 Inguinofemoral lymphadenectomy, superficial, including Cloquets node (separate procedure)

38765 Inguinofemoral lymphadenectomy, superficial, in continuity with pelvic lymphadenectomy, including external iliac, hypogastric, and obturator nodes (separate procedure)

38770 Pelvic lymphadenectomy, including external iliac, hypogastric, and obturator nodes (separate procedure)

38780 Retroperitoneal transabdominal lymphadenectomy, extensive, including pelvic, aortic, and renal nodes (separate procedure)

(For excision and repair of lymphedematous skin and subcutaneous tissue, see 15000, 15570-15650)

INTRODUCTION

38790 Injection procedure; lymphangiography

(For radiological supervision and interpretation, see 75801-75807)

● New Code   ▲ Revised Code   + Add-On Code   ⊘ Modifier -51 Exempt

⊘ **38792**   for identification of sentinel node

(For excision of sentinel node, see 38500-38542)

(For nuclear medicine lymphatics and lymph gland imaging, use 78195)

38794   Cannulation, thoracic duct

OTHER PROCEDURES

38999   Unlisted procedure, hemic or lymphatic system

MEDIASTINUM AND DIAPHRAGM

CPT codes from this section of CPT are used to report invasive and surgical procedures performed on the mediastinum and the diaphragm.

MEDIASTINUM

INCISION

39000 Mediastinotomy with exploration, drainage, removal of foreign body, or biopsy; cervical approach

39010 transthoracic approach, including either transthoracic or median sternotomy

EXCISION

39200 Excision of mediastinal cyst

39220 Excision of mediastinal tumor

(For substernal thyroidectomy, use 60270)

(For thymectomy, use 60520)

ENDOSCOPY

39400 Mediastinoscopy, with or without biopsy

OTHER PROCEDURES

39499 Unlisted procedure, mediastinum

DIAPHRAGM

REPAIR

39501 Repair, laceration of diaphragm, any approach

39502 Repair, paraesophageal hiatus hernia, transabdominal, with or without fundoplasty, vagotomy, and/or pyloroplasty, except neonatal

39503 Repair, neonatal diaphragmatic hernia, with or without chest tube insertion and with or without creation of ventral hernia

| ● | New Code | ▲ | Revised Code | + | Add-On Code | ⊘ | Modifier -51 Exempt |

(Do not report modifier '-63' in conjunction with 39503)

39520   Repair, diaphragmatic hernia (esophageal hiatal); transthoracic

39530   combined, thoracoabdominal

39531   combined, thoracoabdominal, with dilation of stricture (with or without gastroplasty)

39540   Repair, diaphragmatic hernia (other than neonatal), traumatic; acute

39541   chronic

39545   Imbrication of diaphragm for eventration, transthoracic or transabdominal, paralytic or nonparalytic

39560   Resection, diaphragm; with simple repair (eg, primary suture)

39561   with complex repair (eg, prosthetic material, local muscle flap)

OTHER PROCEDURES

39599   Unlisted procedure, diaphragm

 Separate
Procedure

 Unlisted
Procedure   CCI Comp.
Code

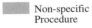 Non-specific
Procedure

437

DIGESTIVE SYSTEM

CPT codes from this section of the CPT coding system are used to report invasive and surgical procedures performed on the lips; mouth; tongue; dentoalveolar structures; palate; salivary gland; pharynx, adenoids and tonsils; esophagus; stomach; intestines; rectum; anus; liver; biliary tract; pancreas; and the abdomen, peritoneum, and omentum.

MISCELLANEOUS CODING RULES

Gastrointestinal endoscopy codes should be assigned based on the extent of visualization performed. HCFA's official guidelines for excision or destruction of a lesion are:

1. *use only the biopsy code if a single lesion is biopsied but not excised;*

2. *code only for the excision if a lesion is biopsied and the remaining portion is excised;*

3. *use the biopsy code once even if multiple biopsies are performed and none are excised; and*

4. *use both a biopsy and excision code if each lesion is taken from different sites.*

If the phrase "with or without biopsy" appears in the excision code's narrative, do not use a separate biopsy code. Diagnostic endoscopies are included in surgical endoscopies.

For upper gastrointestinal endoscopies, choose the appropriate code from documentation indicating whether the procedure was a simple exam, a diagnostic procedure or surgical procedure. Remember that code selection is based on the procedure(s) performed and the anatomical sites through which the scope passes. For example, if the scope is passed to the esophagus only, the code would be chosen from endoscopy codes beginning with 43200. If the scope is passed through the esophagus to the stomach, duodenum and/or the jejunum, the code selection would begin at 43235.

HERNIA REPAIR

Review the patient's age, the kind of hernia, the clinical presentation of the hernia, and method of repair documented in the medical record before assigning a hernia repair code.

APPENDECTOMY

To code appendectomies appropriately, review the documentation for an indicated purpose for the removal. If there is none, then it is probably incidental to a more serious surgery and should not be coded.

LIPS

(For procedures on skin of lips, see 10040 et seq)

EXCISION

40490 Biopsy of lip

40500 Vermilionectomy (lip shave), with mucosal advancement

40510 Excision of lip; transverse wedge excision with primary closure

40520 V-excision with primary direct linear closure

(For excision of mucous lesions, see 40810-40816)

40525 full thickness, reconstruction with local flap (eg, Estlander or fan)

40527 full thickness, reconstruction with cross lip flap (Abbe-Estlander)

40530 Resection of lip, more than one-fourth, without reconstruction

(For reconstruction, see 13131 et seq)

REPAIR (CHEILOPLASTY)

40650 Repair lip, full thickness; vermilion only

40652 up to half vertical height

40654 over one-half vertical height, or complex

40700 Plastic repair of cleft lip/nasal deformity; primary, partial or complete, unilateral

40701 primary bilateral, one stage procedure

40702 primary bilateral, one of two stages

439

 Separate Procedure   Unlisted Procedure   CCI Comp. Code Non-specific Procedure

40720   secondary, by recreation of defect and reclosure

(To report rhinoplasty only for nasal deformity secondary to congenital cleft lip, see 30460, 30462)

40761   with cross lip pedicle flap (Abbe-Estlander type), including sectioning and inserting of pedicle

(For repair cleft palate, see 42200 et seq)

(For other reconstructive procedures, see 14060, 14061, 15120-15261, 15574, 15576, 15630)

OTHER PROCEDURES

40799 Unlisted procedure, lips

VESTIBULE OF MOUTH

INCISION

40800 Drainage of abscess, cyst, hematoma, vestibule of mouth; simple

40801   complicated

40804 Removal of embedded foreign body, vestibule of mouth; simple

40805   complicated

40806 Incision of labial frenum (frenotomy)

EXCISION, DESTRUCTION

40808 Biopsy, vestibule of mouth

40810 Excision of lesion of mucosa and submucosa, vestibule of mouth; without repair

40812   with simple repair

40814   with complex repair

40816   complex, with excision of underlying muscle

40818 Excision of mucosa of vestibule of mouth as donor graft

---

440   ● New Code   ▲ Revised Code   + Add-On Code   ⊘ Modifier -51 Exempt

40819 Excision of frenum, labial or buccal (frenumectomy, frenulectomy, frenectomy)

40820 Destruction of lesion or scar of vestibule of mouth by physical methods (eg, laser, thermal, cryo, chemical)

REPAIR

40830 Closure of laceration, vestibule of mouth; 2.5 cm or less

40831   over 2.5 cm or complex

40840 Vestibuloplasty; anterior

40842   posterior, unilateral

40843   posterior, bilateral

40844   entire arch

40845   complex (including ridge extension, muscle repositioning)

(For skin grafts, see 15000 et seq)

OTHER PROCEDURES

40899 Unlisted procedure, vestibule of mouth

TONGUE AND FLOOR OF MOUTH

INCISION

41000 Intraoral incision and drainage of abscess, cyst, or hematoma of tongue or floor of mouth; lingual

41005   sublingual, superficial

41006   sublingual, deep, supramylohyoid

41007   submental space

41008   submandibular space

41009   masticator space

41010 Incision of lingual frenum (frenotomy)

441

| | Separate Procedure | | Unlisted Procedure | | CCI Comp. Code | | Non-specific Procedure |

41015 Extraoral incision and drainage of abscess, cyst, or hematoma of floor of mouth; sublingual

41016 submental

41017 submandibular

41018 masticator space

(For frenoplasty, use 41520)

EXCISION

41100 Biopsy of tongue; anterior two-thirds

41105 posterior one-third

41108 Biopsy of floor of mouth

41110 Excision of lesion of tongue without closure

41112 Excision of lesion of tongue with closure; anterior two-thirds

41113 posterior one-third

41114 with local tongue flap

(List 41114 in addition to code 41112 or 41113)

41115 Excision of lingual frenum (frenectomy)

41116 Excision, lesion of floor of mouth

41120 Glossectomy; less than one-half tongue

41130 hemiglossectomy

41135 partial, with unilateral radical neck dissection

41140 complete or total, with or without tracheostomy, without radical neck dissection

41145 complete or total, with or without tracheostomy, with unilateral radical neck dissection

---

442   ● New Code   ▲ Revised Code   ＋ Add-On Code   ⃠ Modifier -51 Exempt

41150 composite procedure with resection floor of mouth and mandibular resection, without radical neck dissection

41153 composite procedure with resection floor of mouth, with suprahyoid neck dissection

41155 composite procedure with resection floor of mouth, mandibular resection, and radical neck dissection (Commando type)

REPAIR

41250 Repair of laceration 2.5 cm or less; floor of mouth and/or anterior two-thirds of tongue

41251 posterior one-third of tongue

41252 Repair of laceration of tongue, floor of mouth, over 2.6 cm or complex

OTHER PROCEDURES

41500 Fixation of tongue, mechanical, other than suture (eg, K-wire)

41510 Suture of tongue to lip for micrognathia (Douglas type procedure)

41520 Frenoplasty (surgical revision of frenum, eg, with Z-plasty)

(For frenotomy, see 40806, 41010)

41599 Unlisted procedure, tongue, floor of mouth

DENTOALVEOLAR STRUCTURES

INCISION

41800 Drainage of abscess, cyst, hematoma from dentoalveolar structures

41805 Removal of embedded foreign body from dentoalveolar structures; soft tissues

41806 bone

443

 Separate Procedure   Unlisted Procedure   CCI Comp. Code   Non-specific Procedure

EXCISION, DESTRUCTION

41820 Gingivectomy, excision gingiva, each quadrant

41821 Operculectomy, excision pericoronal tissues

41822 Excision of fibrous tuberosities, dentoalveolar structures

41823 Excision of osseous tuberosities, dentoalveolar structures

41825 Excision of lesion or tumor (except listed above), dentoalveolar structures; without repair

41826   with simple repair

41827   with complex repair

(For nonexcisional destruction, use 41850)

41828 Excision of hyperplastic alveolar mucosa, each quadrant (specify)

41830 Alveolectomy, including curettage of osteitis or sequestrectomy

41850 Destruction of lesion (except excision), dentoalveolar structures

OTHER PROCEDURES

41870 Periodontal mucosal grafting

41872 Gingivoplasty, each quadrant (specify)

41874 Alveoloplasty, each quadrant (specify)

(For closure of lacerations, see 40830, 40831)

(For segmental osteotomy, use 21206)

(For reduction of fractures, see 21421-21490)

41899 Unlisted procedure, dentoalveolar structures

● New Code   ▲ Revised Code   + Add-On Code   ⊘ Modifier -51 Exempt

PALATE AND UVULA

INCISION

42000 Drainage of abscess of palate, uvula

EXCISION, DESTRUCTION

42100 Biopsy of palate, uvula

42104 Excision, lesion of palate, uvula; without closure

42106 with simple primary closure

42107 with local flap closure

(For skin graft, see 14040-14300)

(For mucosal graft, use 40818)

42120 Resection of palate or extensive resection of lesion

(For reconstruction of palate with extraoral tissue, see 14040-14300, 15050, 15120, 15240, 15576)

42140 Uvulectomy, excision of uvula

42145 Palatopharyngoplasty (eg, uvulopalatopharyngoplasty, uvulopharyngoplasty)

42160 Destruction of lesion, palate or uvula (thermal, cryo or chemical)

REPAIR

42180 Repair, laceration of palate; up to 2 cm

42182 over 2 cm or complex

42200 Palatoplasty for cleft palate, soft and/or hard palate only

42205 Palatoplasty for cleft palate, with closure of alveolar ridge; soft tissue only

42210 with bone graft to alveolar ridge (includes obtaining graft)

42215 Palatoplasty for cleft palate; major revision

445

 Separate Procedure

 Unlisted Procedure

CCI Comp. Code

 Non-specific Procedure

42220	secondary lengthening procedure
42225	attachment pharyngeal flap
42226	Lengthening of palate, and pharyngeal flap
42227	Lengthening of palate, with island flap
42235	Repair of anterior palate, including vomer flap
42260	Repair of nasolabial fistula
	(For repair of cleft lip, see 40700 et seq)
42280	Maxillary impression for palatal prosthesis
42281	Insertion of pin-retained palatal prosthesis

OTHER PROCEDURES

42299	Unlisted procedure, palate, uvula

SALIVARY GLAND AND DUCTS

INCISION

42300	Drainage of abscess; parotid, simple
42305	parotid, complicated
42310	submaxillary or sublingual, intraoral
42320	submaxillary, external
42325	Fistulization of sublingual salivary cyst (ranula);
42326	with prosthesis
42330	Sialolithotomy; submandibular (submaxillary), sublingual or parotid, uncomplicated, intraoral
42335	submandibular (submaxillary), complicated, intraoral
42340	parotid, extraoral or complicated intraoral

●	New Code	▲	Revised Code	+	Add-On Code	⊘	Modifier -51 Exempt

EXCISION

42400 Biopsy of salivary gland; needle

(For fine needle aspiration, see 10021, 10022)

(For evaluation of fine needle aspirate, see 88172, 88173)

(If imaging guidance, is performed, see 76003, 76360, 76393, 76942)

42405   incisional

(If imaging guidance is performed, see 76003, 76360, 76393, 76942)

42408 Excision of sublingual salivary cyst (ranula)

42409 Marsupialization of sublingual salivary cyst (ranula)

(For fistulization of sublingual salivary cyst, use 42325)

42410 Excision of parotid tumor or parotid gland; lateral lobe, without nerve dissection

42415   lateral lobe, with dissection and preservation of facial nerve

42420   total, with dissection and preservation of facial nerve

42425   total, en bloc removal with sacrifice of facial nerve

42426   total, with unilateral radical neck dissection

(For suture or grafting of facial nerve, see 64864, 64865, 69740, 69745)

42440 Excision of submandibular (submaxillary) gland

42450 Excision of sublingual gland

REPAIR

42500 Plastic repair of salivary duct, sialodochoplasty; primary or simple

42505   secondary or complicated

42507 Parotid duct diversion, bilateral (Wilke type procedure);

447

 Separate Procedure   Unlisted Procedure   CCI Comp. Code   Non-specific Procedure

42508	with excision of one submandibular gland
42509	with excision of both submandibular glands
42510	with ligation of both submandibular (Wharton's) ducts

OTHER PROCEDURES

42550	Injection procedure for sialography

(For radiological supervision and interpretation, use 70390)

42600	Closure salivary fistula
42650	Dilation salivary duct
42660	Dilation and catheterization of salivary duct, with or without injection
42665	Ligation salivary duct, intraoral
42699	Unlisted procedure, salivary glands or ducts

PHARYNX, ADENOIDS, AND TONSILS

INCISION

42700	Incision and drainage abscess; peritonsillar
42720	retropharyngeal or parapharyngeal, intraoral approach
42725	retropharyngeal or parapharyngeal, external approach

EXCISION, DESTRUCTION

42800	Biopsy; oropharynx
42802	hypopharynx
42804	nasopharynx, visible lesion, simple
42806	nasopharynx, survey for unknown primary lesion

(For laryngoscopic biopsy, see 31510, 31535, 31536)

42808	Excision or destruction of lesion of pharynx, any method

448

● New Code   ▲ Revised Code   + Add-On Code   ⊘ Modifier -51 Exempt

42809	Removal of foreign body from pharynx
42810	Excision branchial cleft cyst or vestige, confined to skin and subcutaneous tissues
42815	Excision branchial cleft cyst, vestige, or fistula, extending beneath subcutaneous tissues and/or into pharynx
42820	Tonsillectomy and adenoidectomy; under age 12
42821	age 12 or over
42825	Tonsillectomy, primary or secondary; under age 12
42826	age 12 or over
42830	Adenoidectomy, primary; under age 12
42831	age 12 or over
42835	Adenoidectomy, secondary; under age 12
42836	age 12 or over
42842	Radical resection of tonsil, tonsillar pillars, and/or retromolar trigone; without closure
42844	closure with local flap (eg, tongue, buccal)
42845	closure with other flap

(For closure with other flap(s), use appropriate number for flap(s))

(When combined with radical neck dissection, use also 38720)

42860	Excision of tonsil tags
42870	Excision or destruction lingual tonsil, any method (separate procedure)
42890	Limited pharyngectomy
42892	Resection of lateral pharyngeal wall or pyriform sinus, direct closure by advancement of lateral and posterior pharyngeal walls

449

Separate Procedure   Unlisted Procedure   CCI Comp. Code   Non-specific Procedure

(When combined with radical neck dissection, use also 38720)

42894 Resection of pharyngeal wall requiring closure with myocutaneous flap

(When combined with radical neck dissection, use also 38720)

REPAIR

42900 Suture pharynx for wound or injury

42950 Pharyngoplasty (plastic or reconstructive operation on pharynx)

(For pharyngeal flap, use 42225)

42953 Pharyngoesophageal repair

(For closure with myocutaneous or other flap, use appropriate number in addition)

OTHER PROCEDURES

42955 Pharyngostomy (fistulization of pharynx, external for feeding)

42960 Control oropharyngeal hemorrhage, primary or secondary (eg, post-tonsillectomy); simple

42961 complicated, requiring hospitalization

42962 with secondary surgical intervention

42970 Control of nasopharyngeal hemorrhage, primary or secondary (eg, postadenoidectomy); simple, with posterior nasal packs, with or without anterior packs and/or cautery

42971 complicated, requiring hospitalization

42972 with secondary surgical intervention

42999 Unlisted procedure, pharynx, adenoids, or tonsils

ESOPHAGUS

INCISION

(For esophageal intubation with laparotomy, use 43510)

43020 Esophagotomy, cervical approach, with removal of foreign body

43030   Cricopharyngeal myotomy

43045   Esophagotomy, thoracic approach, with removal of foreign body

EXCISION

(For gastrointestinal reconstruction for previous esophagectomy, see 43360, 43361)

43100   Excision of lesion, esophagus, with primary repair; cervical approach

43101   thoracic or abdominal approach

43107   Total or near total esophagectomy, without thoracotomy; with pharyngogastrostomy or cervical esophagogastrostomy, with or without pyloroplasty (transhiatal)

43108   with colon interposition or small intestine reconstruction, including intestine mobilization, preparation and anastomosis(es)

43112   Total or near total esophagectomy, with thoracotomy; with pharyngogastrostomy or cervical esophagogastrostomy, with or without pyloroplasty

43113   with colon interposition or small intestine reconstruction, including intestine mobilization, preparation, and anastomosis(es)

43116   Partial esophagectomy, cervical, with free intestinal graft, including microvascular anastomosis, obtaining the graft and intestinal reconstruction

(Do not report code 69990 in addition to code 43116)

(Report 43116 with the modifier -52 appended if intestinal or free jejunal graft with microvascular anastomosis is performed by another physician)

(For free jejunal graft with microvascular anastomosis performed by another physician, use 43496)

43117   Partial esophagectomy, distal two-thirds, with thoracotomy and separate abdominal incision, with or without proximal gastrectomy; with thoracic esophagogastrostomy, with or without pyloroplasty (Ivor Lewis)

451

	Separate Procedure		Unlisted Procedure		CCI Comp. Code		Non-specific Procedure

43118   with colon interposition or small intestine reconstruction, including intestine mobilization, preparation, and anastomosis(es)

43121   Partial esophagectomy, distal two-thirds, with thoracotomy only, with or without proximal gastrectomy, with thoracic esophagogastrostomy, with or without pyloroplasty

43122   Partial esophagectomy, thoracoabdominal or abdominal approach, with or without proximal gastrectomy; with esophagogastrostomy, with or without pyloroplasty

43123   with colon interposition or small intestine reconstruction, including intestine mobilization, preparation, and anastomosis(es)

43124   Total or partial esophagectomy, without reconstruction (any approach), with cervical esophagostomy

43130   Diverticulectomy of hypopharynx or esophagus, with or without myotomy; cervical approach

43135   thoracic approach

ENDOSCOPY

(To report endoscopic delivery of thermal energy to the muscle of lower esophageal sphincter and/or gastric cardia, use Category III code 0057T)

(For upper gastrointestinal endoscopy with suturing of the esophagogastric junction, use Category III code 0008T)

43200   Esophagoscopy, rigid or flexible; diagnostic, with or without collection of specimen(s) by brushing or washing (separate procedure)

43201   with directed submucosal injection(s), any substance

(For injection sclerosis of esophageal varices, use 43204)

43202   with biopsy, single or multiple

43204   with injection sclerosis of esophageal varices

43205   with band ligation of esophageal varices

43215   with removal of foreign body

452

● New Code   ▲ Revised Code   + Add-On Code   ⊘ Modifier -51 Exempt

SURGERY

(For radiological supervision and interpretation, use 74235)

43216 with removal of tumor(s), polyp(s), or other lesion(s) by hot biopsy forceps or bipolar cautery

43217 with removal of tumor(s), polyp(s), or other lesion(s) by snare technique

43219 with insertion of plastic tube or stent

43220 with balloon dilation (less than 30 mm diameter)

(If imaging guidance is performed, use 74360)

(For endoscopic dilation with balloon 30 mm diameter or larger, use 43458)

(For dilation without visualization, see 43450-43453)

43226 with insertion of guide wire followed by dilation over guide wire

(For radiological supervision and interpretation, use 74360)

43227 with control of bleeding (eg, injection, bipolar cautery, unipolar cautery, laser, heater probe, stapler, plasma coagulator)

43228 with ablation of tumor(s), polyp(s), or other lesion(s), not amenable to removal by hot biopsy forceps, bipolar cautery or snare technique

(For esophagoscopic photodynamic therapy, report 43228 in addition to 96570, 96571 as appropriate)

43231 with endoscopic ultrasound examination

43232 with transendoscopic ultrasound-guided intramural or transmural fine needle aspiration/biopsy(s)

(Do not report 43232 in conjunction with 76942)

(For interpretation of specimen, see 88172-88173)

43234 Upper gastrointestinal endoscopy, simple primary examination (eg, with small diameter flexible endoscope) (separate procedure)

| Separate Procedure | Unlisted Procedure | CCI Comp. Code | Non-specific Procedure |

43235 Upper gastrointestinal endoscopy including esophagus, stomach, and either the duodenum and/or jejunum as appropriate; diagnostic, with or without collection of specimen(s) by brushing or washing (separate procedure)

43236 with directed submucosal injection(s), any substance

(For injection sclerosis of esophageal and/or gastric varices, use 43243)

● **43237** with endoscopic ultrasound examination limited to the esophagus

(Do not report 43237 in conjunction with 76975)

● **43238** with transendoscopic ultrasound-guided intramural or transmural fine needle aspiration/biopsy(s), esophagus (includes endoscopic ultrasound examination limited to the esophagus)

(Do not report 43238 in conjunction with 76942 or 76975)

43239 with biopsy, single or multiple

(For upper gastrointestinal endoscopy with suturing of the esophagogastric junction, see Category III code 0008T)

43240 with transmural drainage of pseudocyst

43241 with transendoscopic intraluminal tube or catheter placement

▲ **43242** with transendoscopic ultrasound-guided intramural or transmural fine needle aspiration/biopsy(s) (includes endoscopic ultrasound examination of the esophagus, stomach, and either the duodenum and/or jejunum as appropriate

(Do not report 43242 in conjunction with 76942 or 76975)

(For transendoscopic fine needle aspiration/biopsy limited to esophagus, use 43238)

(For interpretation of specimen, see 88172-88173)

43243 with injection sclerosis of esophageal and/or gastric varices

43244 with band ligation of esophageal and/or gastric varices

● New Code ▲ Revised Code + Add-On Code ⊘ Modifier -51 Exempt

43245   with dilation of gastric outlet for obstruction (eg, balloon, guide wire, bougie)

(Do not report 43245 in conjunction with 43256)

43246   with directed placement of percutaneous gastrostomy tube

(For radiological supervision and interpretation, use 74350)

43247   with removal of foreign body

(For radiological supervision and interpretation, use 74235)

43248   with insertion of guide wire followed by dilation of esophagus over guide wire

43249   with balloon dilation of esophagus (less than 30 mm diameter)

43250   with removal of tumor(s), polyp(s), or other lesion(s) by hot biopsy forceps or bipolar cautery

43251   with removal of tumor(s), polyp(s), or other lesion(s) by snare technique

43255   with control of bleeding, any method

43256   with transendoscopic stent placement (includes predilation)

43258   with ablation of tumor(s), polyp(s), or other lesion(s) not amenable to removal by hot biopsy forceps, bipolar cautery or snare technique

(For injection sclerosis of esophageal varices, use 43204 or 43243)

▲ **43259**   with endoscopic ultrasound examination, including the esophagus, stomach, and either the duodenum and/or jejunum as appropriate

(Do not report 43259 in conjunction with 76975)

43260   Endoscopic retrograde cholangiopancreatography (ERCP); diagnostic, with or without collection of specimen(s) by brushing or washing (separate procedure)

(For radiological supervision and interpretation, see 74328, 74329, 74330)

455

| | Separate Procedure | | Unlisted Procedure | | CCI Comp. Code | | Non-specific Procedure |

43261   with biopsy, single or multiple

(For radiological supervision and interpretation, see 74328, 74329, 74330)

43262   with sphincterotomy/papillotomy

43263   with pressure measurement of sphincter of Oddi (pancreatic duct or common bile duct)

(For radiological supervision and interpretation, see 74328, 74329, 74330)

43264   with endoscopic retrograde removal of calculus/calculi from biliary and/or pancreatic ducts

(When done with sphincterotomy, also use 43262)

(For radiological supervision and interpretation, see 74328, 74329, 74330)

43265   with endoscopic retrograde destruction, lithotripsy of calculus/calculi, any method

(When done with sphincterotomy, also use 43262)

(For radiological supervision and interpretation, see 74328, 74329, 74330)

43267   with endoscopic retrograde insertion of nasobiliary or nasopancreatic drainage tube

(When done with sphincterotomy, also use 43262)

(For radiological supervision and interpretation, see 74328, 74329, 74330)

43268   with endoscopic retrograde insertion of tube or stent into bile or pancreatic duct

(When done with sphincterotomy, also use 43262)

(For radiological supervision and interpretation, see 74328, 74329, 74330)

43269   with endoscopic retrograde removal of foreign body and/or change of tube or stent

(When done with sphincterotomy, also use 43262)

● New Code   ▲ Revised Code   + Add-On Code   ⊘ Modifier -51 Exempt

(For radiological supervision and interpretation, see 74328, 74329, 74330)

43271   with endoscopic retrograde balloon dilation of ampulla, biliary and/or pancreatic duct(s)

(When done with sphincterotomy, also use 43262)

(For radiological supervision and interpretation, see 74328, 74329, 74330)

43272   with ablation of tumor(s), polyp(s), or other lesion(s) not amenable to removal by hot biopsy forceps, bipolar cautery or snare technique

(For radiological supervision and interpretation, see 74328, 74329, 74330)

LAPAROSCOPY

43280   Laparoscopy, surgical, esophagogastric fundoplasty (eg, Nissen, Toupet procedures)

(For open approach, use 43324)

43289   Unlisted laparoscopy procedure, esophagus

REPAIR

43300   Esophagoplasty, (plastic repair or reconstruction), cervical approach; without repair of tracheoesophageal fistula

43305   with repair of tracheoesophageal fistula

43310   Esophagoplasty, (plastic repair or reconstruction), thoracic approach; without repair of tracheoesophageal fistula

43312   with repair of tracheoesophageal fistula

43313   Esophagoplasty for congenital defect, (plastic repair or reconstruction), thoracic approach; without repair of congenital tracheoesophageal fistula

43314   with repair of congenital tracheoesophageal fistula

(Do not report modifier '-63' in conjunction with 43313, 43314)

43320   Esophagogastrostomy (cardioplasty), with or without vagotomy and pyloroplasty, transabdominal or transthoracic approach

457

 Separate Procedure   Unlisted Procedure   CCI Comp. Code   Non-specific Procedure

43324 Esophagogastric fundoplasty (eg, Nissen, Belsey IV, Hill procedures)

(For laparoscopic procedure, use 43280)

43325 Esophagogastric fundoplasty; with fundic patch (Thal-Nissen procedure)

(For cricopharyngeal myotomy, use 43030)

43326 with gastroplasty (eg, Collis)

43330 Esophagomyotomy (Heller type); abdominal approach

43331 thoracic approach

(For thoracoscopic esophagomyotomy, use 32665)

43340 Esophagojejunostomy (without total gastrectomy); abdominal approach

43341 thoracic approach

43350 Esophagostomy, fistulization of esophagus, external; abdominal approach

43351 thoracic approach

43352 cervical approach

43360 Gastrointestinal reconstruction for previous esophagectomy, for obstructing esophageal lesion or fistula, or for previous esophageal exclusion; with stomach, with or without pyloroplasty

43361 with colon interposition or small intestine reconstruction, including intestine mobilization, preparation, and anastomosis(es)

43400 Ligation, direct, esophageal varices

43401 Transection of esophagus with repair, for esophageal varices

43405 Ligation or stapling at gastroesophageal junction for pre-existing esophageal perforation

43410 Suture of esophageal wound or injury; cervical approach

458

● New Code　▲ Revised Code　+ Add-On Code　⊘ Modifier -51 Exempt

43415   transthoracic or transabdominal approach

43420 Closure of esophagostomy or fistula; cervical approach

43425   transthoracic or transabdominal approach

(For repair of esophageal hiatal hernia, see 39520 et seq)

MANIPULATION

(For associated esophagogram, use 74220)

43450 Dilation of esophagus, by unguided sound or bougie, single or multiple passes

43453 Dilation of esophagus, over guide wire

(For dilation with direct visualization, use 43220)

43456 Dilation of esophagus, by balloon or dilator, retrograde

43458 Dilation of esophagus with balloon (30 mm diameter or larger) for achalasia

(For dilation with balloon less than 30 mm diameter, use 43220)

(For radiological supervision and interpretation, use 74360)

43460 Esophagogastric tamponade, with balloon (Sengstaaken type)

(For removal of esophageal foreign body by balloon catheter, see 43215, 43247, 74235)

OTHER PROCEDURES

43496 Free jejunum transfer with microvascular anastomosis

(Do not report code 69990 in addition to code 43496)

43499 Unlisted procedure, esophagus

STOMACH

INCISION

43500 Gastrotomy; with exploration or foreign body removal

43501   with suture repair of bleeding ulcer

459

 Separate Procedure

Unlisted Procedure

 CCI Comp. Code

Non-specific Procedure

43502 with suture repair of pre-existing esophagogastric laceration (eg, Mallory-Weiss)

43510 with esophageal dilation and insertion of permanent intraluminal tube (eg, Celestin or Mousseaux-Barbin)

43520 Pyloromyotomy, cutting of pyloric muscle (Fredet-Ramstedt type operation)

(Do not report modifier '-63' in conjunction with 43520)

EXCISION

43600 Biopsy of stomach; by capsule, tube, peroral (one or more specimens)

43605 by laparotomy

43610 Excision, local; ulcer or benign tumor of stomach

43611 malignant tumor of stomach

43620 Gastrectomy, total; with esophagoenterostomy

43621 with Roux-en-Y reconstruction

43622 with formation of intestinal pouch, any type

43631 Gastrectomy, partial, distal; with gastroduodenostomy

43632 with gastrojejunostomy

43633 with Roux-en-Y reconstruction

43634 with formation of intestinal pouch

+ **43635** Vagotomy when performed with partial distal gastrectomy (List separately in addition to code(s) for primary procedure)

(Use 43635 in conjunction with codes 43631, 43632, 43633, 43634)

43638 Gastrectomy, partial, proximal, thoracic or abdominal approach including esophagogastrostomy, with vagotomy;

43639 with pyloroplasty or pyloromyotomy

460

● New Code ▲ Revised Code + Add-On Code ⊘ Modifier -51 Exempt

(For regional thoracic lymphadenectomy, use 38746)

(For regional abdominal lymphadenectomy, use 38747)

43640 Vagotomy including pyloroplasty, with or without gastrostomy; truncal or selective

(For pyloroplasty, use 43800)

(For vagotomy, see 64752-64760)

43641 parietal cell (highly selective)

(For upper gastrointestinal endoscopy, see 43234-43259)

LAPAROSCOPY

43651 Laparoscopy, surgical; transection of vagus nerves, truncal

43652 transection of vagus nerves, selective or highly selective

43653 gastrostomy, without construction of gastric tube (eg, Stamm procedure) (separate procedure)

43659 Unlisted laparoscopy procedure, stomach

INTRODUCTION

43750 Percutaneous placement of gastrostomy tube

(For radiological supervision and interpretation, use 74350)

▲ **43752** Naso- or oro-gastric tube placement, requiring physician's skill and fluoroscopic guidance (includes fluoroscopy, image documentation and report)

(For enteric tube placement, see 44500, 74340)

(Do not report 43752 in conjunction with critical care codes 99291-99292, neonatal critical care codes 99295-99296, pediatric critical care codes 99293-99294 or low birth weight intensive care service codes 99298-99299)

43760 Change of gastrostomy tube

(For endoscopic placement of gastrostomy tube, use 43246)

(For radiological supervision and interpretation, use 75984)

461

 Separate Procedure   Unlisted Procedure   CCI Comp. Code    Non-specific Procedure

43761 Repositioning of the gastric feeding tube, any method, through the duodenum for enteric nutrition

(If imaging guidance is performed, use 75984)

OTHER PROCEDURES

43800 Pyloroplasty

(For pyloroplasty and vagotomy, use 43640)

43810 Gastroduodenostomy

43820 Gastrojejunostomy; without vagotomy

43825 with vagotomy, any type

43830 Gastrostomy, open; without construction of gastric tube (eg, Stamm procedure) (separate procedure)

43831 neonatal, for feeding

(For change of gastrostomy tube, use 43760)

(Do not report modifier '-63' in conjunction with 43831)

43832 with construction of gastric tube (eg, Janeway procedure)

43840 Gastrorrhaphy, suture of perforated duodenal or gastric ulcer, wound, or injury

43842 Gastric restrictive procedure, without gastric bypass, for morbid obesity; vertical-banded gastroplasty

43843 other than vertical-banded gastroplasty

43846 Gastric restrictive procedure, with gastric bypass for morbid obesity; with short limb (less than 100 cm) Roux-en-Y gastroenterostomy

43847 with small intestine reconstruction to limit absorption

43848 Revision of gastric restrictive procedure for morbid obesity (separate procedure)

43850 Revision of gastroduodenal anastomosis (gastroduodenostomy) with reconstruction; without vagotomy

● New Code ▲ Revised Code + Add-On Code ⃠ Modifier -51 Exempt

43855   with vagotomy

43860   Revision of gastrojejunal anastomosis (gastrojejunostomy) with reconstruction, with or without partial gastrectomy or intestine resection; without vagotomy

43865   with vagotomy

43870   Closure of gastrostomy, surgical

43880   Closure of gastrocolic fistula

43999   Unlisted procedure, stomach

INTESTINES (EXCEPT RECTUM)

INCISION

44005   Enterolysis (freeing of intestinal adhesion) (separate procedure)

(Do not report 44005 in addition to 45136)

(For laparoscopic approach, use 44200)

44010   Duodenotomy, for exploration, biopsy(s), or foreign body removal

+ **44015**   Tube or needle catheter jejunostomy for enteral alimentation, intraoperative, any method (List separately in addition to primary procedure)

44020   Enterotomy, small intestine, other than duodenum; for exploration, biopsy(s), or foreign body removal

44021   for decompression (eg, Baker tube)

44025   Colotomy, for exploration, biopsy(s), or foreign body removal

44050   Reduction of volvulus, intussusception, internal hernia, by laparotomy

44055   Correction of malrotation by lysis of duodenal bands and/or reduction of midgut volvulus (eg, Ladd procedure)

(Do not report modifier '-63' in conjunction with 44055)

463

 Separate Procedure   Unlisted Procedure   CCI Comp. Code   Non-specific Procedure

EXCISION

44100 Biopsy of intestine by capsule, tube, peroral (one or more specimens)

44110 Excision of one or more lesions of small or large intestine not requiring anastomosis, exteriorization, or fistulization; single enterotomy

44111 multiple enterotomies

44120 Enterectomy, resection of small intestine; single resection and anastomosis

(Do not report 44120 in addition to 45136)

+ 44121 each additional resection and anastomosis (List separately in addition to code for primary procedure)

(Use 44121 in conjunction with code 44120)

44125 with enterostomy

44126 Enterectomy, resection of small intestine for congenital atresia, single resection and anastomosis of proximal segment of intestine; without tapering

44127 with tapering

+ 44128 each additional resection and anastomosis (List separately in addition to code for primary procedure)

(Use 44128 in conjunction with codes 44126, 44127)

(Do not report modifier '-63' in conjunction with 44126, 44127, 44128)

44130 Enteroenterostomy, anastomosis of intestine, with or without cutaneous enterostomy (separate procedure)

44132 Donor enterectomy, open, with preparation and maintenance of allograft; from cadaver donor

44133 partial, from living donor

44135 Intestinal allotransplantation; from cadaver donor

44136 from living donor

● New Code   ▲ Revised Code   ✚ Add-On Code   ⊘ Modifier -51 Exempt

+ **44139**   Mobilization (take-down) of splenic flexure performed in conjunction with partial colectomy (List separately in addition to primary procedure)

(Use 44139 in conjunction with codes 44140-44147)

44140   Colectomy, partial; with anastomosis

(For laparoscopic procedure, use 44204)

44141   with skin level cecostomy or colostomy

44143   with end colostomy and closure of distal segment (Hartmann type procedure)

(For laparoscopic procedure, use 44206)

44144   with resection, with colostomy or ileostomy and creation of mucofistula

44145   with coloproctostomy (low pelvic anastomosis)

(For laparoscopic procedure, use 44207)

44146   with coloproctostomy (low pelvic anastomosis), with colostomy

(For laparoscopic procedure, use 44208)

44147   abdominal and transanal approach

44150   Colectomy, total, abdominal, without proctectomy; with ileostomy or ileoproctostomy

(For laparoscopic procedure, use 44210)

44151   with continent ileostomy

44152   with rectal mucosectomy, ileoanal anastomosis, with or without loop ileostomy

(For laparoscopic procedure, use 44211)

44153   with rectal mucosectomy, ileoanal anastomosis, creation of ileal reservoir (S or J), with or without loop ileostomy

(For laparoscopic procedure, use 44211)

44155   Colectomy, total, abdominal, with proctectomy; with ileostomy

465

| ▨ Separate Procedure | ▨ Unlisted Procedure | ▨ CCI Comp. Code | ▨ Non-specific Procedure |

(For laparoscopic procedure, use 44212)

44156   with continent ileostomy

44160   Colectomy, partial, with removal of terminal ileum and ileocolostomy

(For laparoscopic procedure, use 44205)

LAPAROSCOPY

44200   Laparoscopy, surgical; enterolysis (freeing of intestinal adhesion) (separate procedure)

(For laparoscopy with salpingolysis, ovariolysis, use 58660)

44201   jejunostomy (eg, for decompression or feeding)

44202   enterectomy, resection of small intestine, single resection and anastomosis

+ **44203**   each additional small intestine resection and anastomosis (List separately in addition to code for primary procedure)

(Use 44203 in conjunction with code 44202)

(For open procedure, see 44120, 44121)

44204   colectomy, partial, with anastomosis

(For open procedure, use 44140)

44205   colectomy, partial, with removal of terminal ileum with ileocolostomy

(For open procedure, use 44160)

44206   colectomy, partial, with end colostomy and closure of distal segment (Hartmann type procedure)

(For open procedure, use 44143)

44207   colectomy, partial, with anastomosis, with coloproctostomy (low pelvic anastomosis)

(For open procedure, use 44145)

44208   colectomy, partial, with anastomosis, with coloproctostomy (low pelvic anastomosis) with colostomy

● New Code   ▲ Revised Code   + Add-On Code   ⊘ Modifier -51 Exempt

(For open procedure, use 44146)

(44209   deleted 2003 edition. To report, use 44238)

44210   colectomy, total, abdominal, without proctectomy, with ileostomy or ileoproctostomy

(For open procedure, use 44150)

44211   colectomy, total, abdominal, with proctectomy, with ileoanal anastomosis, creation of ileal reservoir (S or J), with loop ileostomy, with or without rectal mucosectomy

(For open procedure, see 44152, 44153)

44212   colectomy, total, abdominal, with proctectomy, with ileostomy

(For open procedure, use 44155)

44238   Unlisted laparoscopy procedure, intestine (except rectum)

44239   Unlisted laparoscopy procedure, rectum

ENTEROSTOMY—EXTERNAL FISTULIZATION OF INTESTINES

44300   Enterostomy or cecostomy, tube (eg, for decompression or feeding) (separate procedure)

44310   Ileostomy or jejunostomy, non-tube (separate procedure)

(Do not report 44310 in addition to 45136)

44312   Revision of ileostomy; simple (release of superficial scar) (separate procedure)

44314   complicated (reconstruction in-depth) (separate procedure)

44316   Continent ileostomy (Kock procedure) (separate procedure)

(For fiberoptic evaluation, use 44385)

44320   Colostomy or skin level cecostomy; (separate procedure)

44322   with multiple biopsies (eg, for congenital megacolon) (separate procedure)

467

 Separate Procedure   Unlisted Procedure   CCI Comp. Code   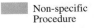 Non-specific Procedure

44340   Revision of colostomy; simple (release of superficial scar) (separate procedure)

44345   complicated (reconstruction in-depth) (separate procedure)

44346   with repair of paracolostomy hernia (separate procedure)

ENDOSCOPY, SMALL INTESTINE AND STOMAL

(For upper gastrointestinal endoscopy, see 43234-43258)

44360   Small intestinal endoscopy, enteroscopy beyond second portion of duodenum, not including ileum; diagnostic, with or without collection of specimen(s) by brushing or washing (separate procedure)

44361   with biopsy, single or multiple

44363   with removal of foreign body

44364   with removal of tumor(s), polyp(s), or other lesion(s) by snare technique

44365   with removal of tumor(s), polyp(s), or other lesion(s) by hot biopsy forceps or bipolar cautery

44366   with control of bleeding (eg, injection, bipolar cautery, unipolar cautery, laser, heater probe, stapler, plasma coagulator)

44369   with ablation of tumor(s), polyp(s), or other lesion(s) not amenable to removal by hot biopsy forceps, bipolar cautery or snare technique

44370   with transendoscopic stent placement (includes predilation)

44372   with placement of percutaneous jejunostomy tube

44373   with conversion of percutaneous gastrostomy tube to percutaneous jejunostomy tube

44376   Small intestinal endoscopy, enteroscopy beyond second portion of duodenum, including ileum; diagnostic, with or without collection of specimen(s) by brushing or washing (separate procedure)

44377   with biopsy, single or multiple

● New Code   ▲ Revised Code   + Add-On Code   ⊘ Modifier -51 Exempt

44378   with control of bleeding (eg, injection, bipolar cautery, unipolar cautery, laser, heater probe, stapler, plasma coagulator)

44379   with transendoscopic stent placement (includes predilation)

44380   Ileoscopy, through stoma; diagnostic, with or without collection of specimen(s) by brushing or washing (separate procedure)

44382   with biopsy, single or multiple

44383   with transendoscopic stent placement (includes predilation)

44385   Endoscopic evaluation of small intestinal (abdominal or pelvic) pouch; diagnostic, with or without collection of specimen(s) by brushing or washing (separate procedure)

44386   with biopsy, single or multiple

44388   Colonoscopy through stoma; diagnostic, with or without collection of specimen(s) by brushing or washing (separate procedure)

44389   with biopsy, single or multiple

44390   with removal of foreign body

44391   with control of bleeding (eg, injection, bipolar cautery, unipolar cautery, laser, heater probe, stapler, plasma coagulator)

44392   with removal of tumor(s), polyp(s), or other lesion(s) by hot biopsy forceps or bipolar cautery

44393   with ablation of tumor(s), polyp(s), or other lesion(s) not amenable to removal by hot biopsy forceps, bipolar cautery or snare technique

44394   with removal of tumor(s), polyp(s), or other lesion(s) by snare technique

(For colonoscopy per rectum, see 45330-45385)

44397   with transendoscopic stent placement (includes predilation)

469

 Separate Procedure   Unlisted Procedure    CCI Comp. Code   Non-specific Procedure

INTRODUCTION

⊘ **44500** Introduction of long gastrointestinal tube (eg, Miller-Abbott) (separate procedure)

(For radiological supervision and interpretation, use 74340)

(For naso- or oro-gastric tube placement, use 43752)

REPAIR

44602 Suture of small intestine (enterorrhaphy) for perforated ulcer, diverticulum, wound, injury or rupture; single perforation

44603 multiple perforations

44604 Suture of large intestine (colorrhaphy) for perforated ulcer, diverticulum, wound, injury, or rupture (single or multiple perforations); without colostomy

44605 with colostomy

44615 Intestinal stricturoplasty (enterotomy and enterorrhaphy) with or without dilation, for intestinal obstruction

44620 Closure of enterostomy, large or small intestine;

44625 with resection and anastomosis other than colorectal

44626 with resection and colorectal anastomosis (eg, closure of Hartmann type procedure)

44640 Closure of intestinal cutaneous fistula

44650 Closure of enteroenteric or enterocolic fistula

44660 Closure of enterovesical fistula; without intestinal or bladder resection

44661 with intestine and/or bladder resection

(For closure of renocolic fistula, see 50525, 50526)

(For closure of gastrocolic fistula, use 43880)

(For closure of rectovesical fistula, see 45800, 45805)

44680 Intestinal plication (separate procedure)

● New Code   ▲ Revised Code   + Add-On Code   ⊘ Modifier -51 Exempt

OTHER PROCEDURES

44700 Exclusion of small intestine from pelvis by mesh or other prosthesis, or native tissue (eg, bladder or omentum)

(For therapeutic radiation clinical treatment, see Radiation Oncology section)

+ 44701 Intraoperative colonic lavage (List separately in addition to code for primary procedure)

(Use 44701 in conjunction with codes 44140, 44145, 44150, or 44604 as appropriate)

(Do not report 44701 in conjunction with 44300, 44950-44960)

44799 Unlisted procedure, intestine

(For unlisted laparoscopic procedure, intestine except rectum, use 44238)

MECKEL'S DIVERTICULUM AND THE MESENTERY

EXCISION

44800 Excision of Meckel's diverticulum (diverticulectomy) or omphalomesenteric duct

44820 Excision of lesion of mesentery (separate procedure)

(With intestine resection, see 44120 or 44140 et seq)

SUTURE

44850 Suture of mesentery (separate procedure)

(For reduction and repair of internal hernia, use 44050)

OTHER PROCEDURES

44899 Unlisted procedure, Meckel's diverticulum and the mesentery

APPENDIX

INCISION

44900 Incision and drainage of appendiceal abscess; open

44901 percutaneous

471

 Separate Procedure   Unlisted Procedure   CCI Comp. Code   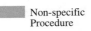 Non-specific Procedure

(For radiological supervision and interpretation, use 75989)

EXCISION

44950   Appendectomy;

(Incidental appendectomy during intra-abdominal surgery does not usually warrant a separate identification. If necessary to report, add modifier -52)

+ 44955   when done for indicated purpose at time of other major procedure (not as separate procedure) (List separately in addition to code for primary procedure)

44960   for ruptured appendix with abscess or generalized peritonitis

LAPAROSCOPY

44970   Laparoscopy, surgical, appendectomy

44979   Unlisted laparoscopy procedure, appendix

RECTUM

INCISION

45000   Transrectal drainage of pelvic abscess

45005   Incision and drainage of submucosal abscess, rectum

45020   Incision and drainage of deep supralevator, pelvirectal, or retrorectal abscess

(See also 46050, 46060)

EXCISION

45100   Biopsy of anorectal wall, anal approach (eg, congenital megacolon)

(For endoscopic biopsy, use 45305)

45108   Anorectal myomectomy

45110   Proctectomy; complete, combined abdominoperineal, with colostomy

45111   partial resection of rectum, transabdominal approach

472   ● New Code   ▲ Revised Code   + Add-On Code   ⊘ Modifier -51 Exempt

45112 Proctectomy, combined abdominoperineal, pull-through procedure (eg, colo-anal anastomosis)

(For colo-anal anastomosis with colonic reservoir or pouch, use 45119)

45113 Proctectomy, partial, with rectal mucosectomy, ileoanal anastomosis, creation of ileal reservoir (S or J), with or without loop ileostomy

45114 Proctectomy, partial, with anastomosis; abdominal and transsacral approach

45116 transsacral approach only (Kraske type)

45119 Proctectomy, combined abdominoperineal pull-through procedure (eg, colo-anal anastomosis), with creation of colonic reservoir (eg, J-pouch), with or without proximal diverting ostomy

45120 Proctectomy, complete (for congenital megacolon), abdominal and perineal approach; with pull-through procedure and anastomosis (eg, Swenson, Duhamel, or Soave type operation)

45121 with subtotal or total colectomy, with multiple biopsies

45123 Proctectomy, partial, without anastomosis, perineal approach

45126 Pelvic exenteration for colorectal malignancy, with proctectomy (with or without colostomy), with removal of bladder and ureteral transplantations, and/or hysterectomy, or cervicectomy, with or without removal of tube(s), with or without removal of ovary(s), or any combination thereof

45130 Excision of rectal procidentia, with anastomosis; perineal approach

45135 abdominal and perineal approach

45136 Excision of ileoanal reservoir with ileostomy

(Do not report 45136 in addition to 44005, 44120, 44310)

45150 Division of stricture of rectum

45160 Excision of rectal tumor by proctotomy, transsacral or transcoccygeal approach

473

 Separate Procedure   Unlisted Procedure   CCI Comp. Code   Non-specific Procedure

45170 Excision of rectal tumor, transanal approach

DESTRUCTION

45190 Destruction of rectal tumor (eg, electrodessiccation, electrosurgery, laser ablation, laser resection, cryosurgery) transanal approach

ENDOSCOPY

45300 Proctosigmoidoscopy, rigid; diagnostic, with or without collection of specimen(s) by brushing or washing (separate procedure)

45303 with dilation (eg, balloon, guide wire, bougie)

(For radiological supervision and interpretation, use 74360)

45305 with biopsy, single or multiple

45307 with removal of foreign body

45308 with removal of single tumor, polyp, or other lesion by hot biopsy forceps or bipolar cautery

45309 with removal of single tumor, polyp, or other lesion by snare technique

45315 with removal of multiple tumors, polyps, or other lesions by hot biopsy forceps, bipolar cautery or snare technique

45317 with control of bleeding (eg, injection, bipolar cutery, unipolar cautery, laser, heater probe, stapler, plasma coagulator)

45320 with ablation of tumor(s), polyp(s), or other lesion(s) not amenable to removal by hot biopsy forceps, bipolar cautery or snare technique (eg, laser)

45321 with decompression of volvulus

(45325 colonoscopy has been renumbered 45355 without change in terminology)

45327 with transendoscopic stent placement (includes predilation)

45330 Sigmoidoscopy, flexible; diagnostic, with or without collection of specimen(s) by brushing or washing (separate procedure)

474 ● New Code ▲ Revised Code ＋ Add-On Code ⊘ Modifier -51 Exempt

45331   with biopsy, single or multiple

45332   with removal of foreign body

45333   with removal of tumor(s), polyp(s), or other lesion(s) by hot biopsy forceps or bipolar cautery

45334   with control of bleeding (eg, injection, bipolar cutery, unipolar cautery, laser, heater probe, stapler, plasma coagulator)

45335   with directed submucosal injection(s), any substance

45337   with decompression of volvulus, any method

45338   with removal of tumor(s), polyp(s), or other lesion(s) by snare technique

45339   with ablation of tumor(s), polyp(s), or other lesion(s) not amenable to removal by hot biopsy forceps, bipolar cautery or snare technique

45340   with dilation by balloon, 1 or more strictures

(Do not report 45340 in conjunction with 45345)

45341   with endoscopic ultrasound examination

45342   with transendoscopic ultrasound guided intramural or transmural fine needle aspiration/biopsy(s)

(Do not report 76942 in conjunction with 45341, 45342)

(Do not report 76975 in conjunction with codes 45341, 45342)

(For interpretation of specimen, see 88172-88173)

(For transrectal ultrasound utilizing rigid probe device, use 76872)

45345   with transendoscopic stent placement (includes predilation)

45355   Colonoscopy, rigid or flexible, transabdominal via colotomy, single or multiple

475

 Separate Procedure    Unlisted Procedure    CCI Comp. Code   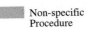 Non-specific Procedure

45378   Colonoscopy, flexible, proximal to splenic flexure; diagnostic, with or without collection of specimen(s) by brushing or washing, with or without colon decompression (separate procedure)

45379   with removal of foreign body

45380   with biopsy, single or multiple

45381   with directed submucosal injection(s), any substance

45382   with control of bleeding (eg, injection, bipolar cautery, unipolar cautery, laser, heater probe, stapler, plasma coagulator)

45383   with ablation of tumor(s), polyp(s), or other lesion(s) not amenable to removal by hot biopsy forceps, bipolar cautery or snare technique

45384   with removal of tumor(s), polyp(s), or other lesion(s) by hot biopsy forceps or bipolar cautery

45385   with removal of tumor(s), polyp(s), or other lesion(s) by snare technique

         (For small intestine and stomal endoscopy, see 44360-44393)

45386   with dilation by balloon, 1 or more strictures

         (Do not report 45386 in conjunction with 45387)

45387   with transendoscopic stent placement (includes predilation)

REPAIR

45500   Proctoplasty; for stenosis

45505   for prolapse of mucous membrane

45520   Perirectal injection of sclerosing solution for prolapse

45540   Proctopexy for prolapse; abdominal approach

45541   perineal approach

45550   Proctopexy combined with sigmoid resection, abdominal approach

● New Code   ▲ Revised Code   + Add-On Code   ⊘ Modifier -51 Exempt

45560 Repair of rectocele (separate procedure)

(For repair of rectocele with posterior colporrhaphy, use 57250)

45562 Exploration, repair, and presacral drainage for rectal injury;

45563 with colostomy

45800 Closure of rectovesical fistula;

45805 with colostomy

45820 Closure of rectourethral fistula;

45825 with colostomy

(For rectovaginal fistula closure, see 57300-57308)

MANIPULATION

45900 Reduction of procidentia (separate procedure) under anesthesia

45905 Dilation of anal sphincter (separate procedure) under anesthesia other than local

45910 Dilation of rectal stricture (separate procedure) under anesthesia other than local

45915 Removal of fecal impaction or foreign body (separate procedure) under anesthesia

OTHER PROCEDURES

45999 Unlisted procedure, rectum

(For unlisted laparoscopic procedure, rectum, use 44239)

ANUS

INCISION

46020 Placement of seton

(Do not report 46020 in addition to 46060, 46280, 46600)

46030 Removal of anal seton, other marker

477

 Separate Procedure
 Unlisted Procedure
 CCI Comp. Code
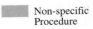 Non-specific Procedure

46040 Incision and drainage of ischiorectal and/or perirectal abscess (separate procedure)

46045 Incision and drainage of intramural, intramuscular, or submucosal abscess, transanal, under anesthesia

46050 Incision and drainage, perianal abscess, superficial

(See also 45020, 46060)

46060 Incision and drainage of ischiorectal or intramural abscess, with fistulectomy or fistulotomy, submuscular, with or without placement of seton

(Do not report 46060 in addition to 46020)

(See also 45020)

46070 Incision, anal septum (infant)

(For anoplasty, see 46700-46705)

(Do not report modifier '-63' in conjunction with 46070)

46080 Sphincterotomy, anal, division of sphincter (separate procedure)

46083 Incision of thrombosed hemorrhoid, external

EXCISION

46200 Fissurectomy, with or without sphincterotomy

46210 Cryptectomy; single

46211 multiple (separate procedure)

46220 Papillectomy or excision of single tag, anus (separate procedure)

46221 Hemorrhoidectomy, by simple ligature (eg, rubber band)

46230 Excision of external hemorrhoid tags and/or multiple papillae

46250 Hemorrhoidectomy, external, complete

46255 Hemorrhoidectomy, internal and external, simple;

46257 with fissurectomy

● New Code ▲ Revised Code + Add-On Code ⊘ Modifier -51 Exempt

46258   with fistulectomy, with or without fissurectomy

46260 Hemorrhoidectomy, internal and external, complex or extensive;

46261   with fissurectomy

46262   with fistulectomy, with or without fissurectomy

46270 Surgical treatment of anal fistula (fistulectomy/fistulotomy); subcutaneous

46275   submuscular

46280   complex or multiple, with or without placement of seton

(Do not report 46280 in addition to 46020)

(46281 has been renumbered to 46288 without change in terminology)

46285   second stage

46288 Closure of anal fistula with rectal advancement flap

46320 Enucleation or excision of external thrombotic hemorrhoid

INTRODUCTION

46500 Injection of sclerosing solution, hemorrhoids

ENDOSCOPY

46600 Anoscopy; diagnostic, with or without collection of specimen(s) by brushing or washing (separate procedure)

(Do not report 46600 in addition to 46020)

46604   with dilation (eg, balloon, guide wire, bougie)

46606   with biopsy, single or multiple

46608   with removal of foreign body

46610   with removal of single tumor, polyp, or other lesion by hot biopsy forceps or bipolar cautery

479

| | Separate Procedure | | Unlisted Procedure | CCI Comp. Code | Non-specific Procedure |

46611　　with removal of single tumor, polyp, or other lesion by snare technique

46612　　with removal of multiple tumors, polyps, or other lesions by hot biopsy forceps, bipolar cautery or snare technique

46614　　with control of bleeding (eg, injection, bipolar cautery, unipolar cautery, laser, heater probe, stapler, plasma coagulator)

46615　　with ablation of tumor(s), polyp(s), or other lesion(s) not amenable to removal by hot biopsy forceps, bipolar cautery or snare technique

REPAIR

46700　Anoplasty, plastic operation for stricture; adult

46705　　infant

(For simple incision of anal septum, use 46070)

(Do not report modifier '-63' in conjunction with 46705)

46706　Repair of anal fistula with fibrin glue

46715　Repair of low imperforate anus; with anoperineal fistula (cut-back procedure)

46716　　with transposition of anoperineal or anovestibular fistula

(Do not report modifier '-63' in conjunction with 46715, 46716)

46730　Repair of high imperforate anus without fistula; perineal or sacroperineal approach

46735　　combined transabdominal and sacroperineal approaches

(Do not report modifier '-63' in conjunction with 46730, 46735)

46740　Repair of high imperforate anus with rectourethral or rectovaginal fistula; perineal or sacroperineal approach

46742　　combined transabdominal and sacroperineal approaches

(Do not report modifier '-63' in conjunction with 46740, 46742)

● New Code ▲ Revised Code + Add-On Code ⊘ Modifier -51 Exempt

46744   Repair of cloacal anomaly by anorectovaginoplasty and urethroplasty, sacroperineal approach

(Do not report modifier '-63' in conjunction with 46744)

46746   Repair of cloacal anomaly by anorectovaginoplasty and urethroplasty, combined abdominal and sacroperineal approach;

46748   with vaginal lengthening by intestinal graft or pedicle flaps

46750   Sphincteroplasty, anal, for incontinence or prolapse; adult

46751   child

46753   Graft (Thiersch operation) for rectal incontinence and/or prolapse

46754   Removal of Thiersch wire or suture, anal canal

46760   Sphincteroplasty, anal, for incontinence, adult; muscle transplant

46761   levator muscle imbrication (Park posterior anal repair)

46762   implantation artificial sphincter

DESTRUCTION

46900   Destruction of lesion(s), anus (eg, condyloma, papilloma, molluscum contagiosum, herpetic vesicle), simple; chemical

46910   electrodesiccation

46916   cryosurgery

46917   laser surgery

46922   surgical excision

46924   Destruction of lesion(s), anus (eg, condyloma, papilloma, molluscum contagiosum, herpetic vesicle), extensive (eg, laser surgery, electrosurgery, cryosurgery, chemosurgery)

46934   Destruction of hemorrhoids, any method; internal

46935   external

481

 Separate Procedure   Unlisted Procedure   CCI Comp. Code   Non-specific Procedure

46936   internal and external

46937 Cryosurgery of rectal tumor; benign

46938   malignant

46940 Curettage or cautery of anal fissure, including dilation of anal sphincter (separate procedure); initial

46942   subsequent

SUTURE

46945 Ligation of internal hemorrhoids; single procedure

46946   multiple procedures

OTHER PROCEDURES

46999 Unlisted procedure, anus

LIVER

INCISION

47000 Biopsy of liver, needle; percutaneous

(If imaging guidance is performed, see 76003, 76360, 76393, 76942)

+ 47001   when done for indicated purpose at time of other major procedure (List separately in addition to code for primary procedure)

(If imaging guidance is performed, see 76003, 76942)

(For fine needle aspiration in conjunction with 47000, 47001, see 10021, 10022)

(For evaluation of fine needle aspirate in conjunction with 47000, 47001, see 88172, 88173)

47010 Hepatotomy; for open drainage of abscess or cyst, one or two stages

47011   for percutaneous drainage of abscess or cyst, one or two stages

(For radiological supervision and interpretation, use 75989)

47015 Laparotomy, with aspiration and/or injection of hepatic parasitic (eg, amoebic or echinococcal) cyst(s) or abscess(es)

EXCISION

47100 Biopsy of liver, wedge

47120 Hepatectomy, resection of liver; partial lobectomy

47122 trisegmentectomy

47125 total left lobectomy

47130 total right lobectomy

47133 Donor hepatectomy, with preparation and maintenance of allograft, from cadaver donor

(47134 deleted 2004 edition. To report, use 47140)

47135 Liver allotransplantation; orthotopic, partial or whole, from cadaver or living donor, any age

47136 heterotopic, partial or whole, from cadaver or living donor, any age

● **47140** Donor hepatectomy, with preparation and maintenance of allograft, from living donor; left lateral segment only (segments II and III)

● **47141** total left lobectomy (segments II, III, and IV)

● **47142** total right lobectomy (segments V, VI, VII, and VIII)

REPAIR

47300 Marsupialization of cyst or abscess of liver

47350 Management of liver hemorrhage; simple suture of liver wound or injury

47360 complex suture of liver wound or injury, with or without hepatic artery ligation

483

	Separate Procedure		Unlisted Procedure		CCI Comp. Code		Non-specific Procedure

47361   exploration of hepatic wound, extensive debridement, coagulation and/or suture, with or without packing of liver

47362   re-exploration of hepatic wound for removal of packing

LAPAROSCOPY

47370   Laparoscopy, surgical, ablation of one or more liver tumor(s); radiofrequency

(For imaging guidance, use 76490)

47371   cryosurgical

(For imaging guidance, use 76490)

47379   Unlisted laparoscopic procedure, liver

OTHER PROCEDURES

47380   Ablation, open, of one or more liver tumor(s); radiofrequency

(For imaging guidance, use 76490)

47381   cryosurgical

(For imaging guidance, use 76490)

47382   Ablation, one or more liver tumor(s), percutaneous, radiofrequency

(For imaging guidance and monitoring, see code 76362, 76394, or 76490)

47399   Unlisted procedure, liver

BILIARY TRACT

INCISION

47400   Hepaticotomy or hepaticostomy with exploration, drainage, or removal of calculus

47420   Choledochotomy or choledochostomy with exploration, drainage, or removal of calculus, with or without cholecystotomy; without transduodenal sphincterotomy or sphincteroplasty

47425   with transduodenal sphincterotomy or sphincteroplasty

484

●	New Code	▲ Revised Code	✛ Add-On Code	⊘ Modifier -51 Exempt

47460 Transduodenal sphincterotomy or sphincteroplasty, with or without transduodenal extraction of calculus (separate procedure)

47480 Cholecystotomy or cholecystostomy with exploration, drainage, or removal of calculus (separate procedure)

47490 Percutaneous cholecystostomy

(For radiological supervision and interpretation, use 75989)

INTRODUCTION

47500 Injection procedure for percutaneous transhepatic cholangiography

(For radiological supervision and interpretation, use 74320)

47505 Injection procedure for cholangiography through an existing catheter (eg, percutaneous transhepatic or T-tube)

(For radiological supervision and interpretation, use 74305)

47510 Introduction of percutaneous transhepatic catheter for biliary drainage

(For radiological supervision and interpretation, use 75980)

47511 Introduction of percutaneous transhepatic stent for internal and external biliary drainage

(For radiological supervision and interpretation, use 75982)

47525 Change of percutaneous biliary drainage catheter

(For radiological supervision and interpretation, use 75984)

47530 Revision and/or reinsertion of transhepatic tube

(For radiological supervision and interpretation, use 75984)

ENDOSCOPY

+ **47550** Biliary endoscopy, intraoperative (choledochoscopy) (List separately in addition to code for primary procedure)

47552 Biliary endoscopy, percutaneous via T-tube or other tract; diagnostic, with or without collection of specimen(s) by brushing and/or washing (separate procedure)

485

 Separate Procedure   Unlisted Procedure    CCI Comp. Code   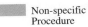 Non-specific Procedure

47553   with biopsy, single or multiple

47554   with removal of calculus/calculi

47555   with dilation of biliary duct stricture(s) without stent

(For ERCP, see 43260-43272, 74363)

(If imaging guidance is performed, see 74363, 75982)

47556   with dilation of biliary duct stricture(s) with stent

(If imaging guidance is performed, see 74363, 75982)

LAPAROSCOPY

47560 Laparoscopy, surgical; with guided transhepatic cholangiography, without biopsy

47561   with guided transhepatic cholangiography with biopsy

47562   cholecystectomy

47563   cholecystectomy with cholangiography

47564   cholecystectomy with exploration of common duct

47570   cholecystoenterostomy

47579 Unlisted laparoscopy procedure, biliary tract

EXCISION

47600 Cholecystectomy;

47605   with cholangiography

(For laparoscopic approach, see 47562-47564)

47610 Cholecystectomy with exploration of common duct;

47612   with choledochoenterostomy

47620   with transduodenal sphincterotomy or sphincteroplasty, with or without cholangiography

---

● New Code   ▲ Revised Code   ✚ Add-On Code   ⊘ Modifier -51 Exempt

47630 Biliary duct stone extraction, percutaneous via T-tube tract, basket, or snare (eg, Burhenne technique)

(For radiological supervision and interpretation, use 74327)

47700 Exploration for congenital atresia of bile ducts, without repair, with or without liver biopsy, with or without cholangiography

(Do not report modifier '-63' in conjunction with 47700)

47701 Portoenterostomy (eg, Kasai procedure)

(Do not report modifier '-63' in conjunction with 47701)

47711 Excision of bile duct tumor, with or without primary repair of bile duct; extrahepatic

47712 intrahepatic

(For anastomosis, see 47760-47800)

47715 Excision of choledochal cyst

47716 Anastomosis, choledochal cyst, without excision

REPAIR

47720 Cholecystoenterostomy; direct

(For laparoscopic approach, use 47570)

47721 with gastroenterostomy

47740 Roux-en-Y

47741 Roux-en-Y with gastroenterostomy

47760 Anastomosis, of extrahepatic biliary ducts and gastrointestinal tract

47765 Anastomosis, of intrahepatic ducts and gastrointestinal tract

47780 Anastomosis, Roux-en-Y, of extrahepatic biliary ducts and gastrointestinal tract

47785 Anastomosis, Roux-en-Y, of intrahepatic biliary ducts and gastrointestinal tract

487

 Separate Procedure

 Unlisted Procedure

 CCI Comp. Code

 Non-specific Procedure

47800 Reconstruction, plastic, of extrahepatic biliary ducts with end-to-end anastomosis

47801 Placement of choledochal stent

47802 U-tube hepaticoenterostomy

47900 Suture of extrahepatic biliary duct for pre-existing injury (separate procedure)

OTHER PROCEDURES

47999 Unlisted procedure, biliary tract

PANCREAS

(For peroral pancreatic endoscopic procedures, see 43260-43272)

INCISION

48000 Placement of drains, peripancreatic, for acute pancreatitis;

48001 with cholecystostomy, gastrostomy, and jejunostomy

48005 Resection or debridement of pancreas and peripancreatic tissue for acute necrotizing pancreatitis

48020 Removal of pancreatic calculus

EXCISION

48100 Biopsy of pancreas, open (eg, fine needle aspiration, needle core biopsy, wedge biopsy)

48102 Biopsy of pancreas, percutaneous needle

(For radiological supervision and interpretation, see 76003, 76360, 76393, 76942)

(For fine needle aspiration, use 10022)

(For evaluation of fine needle aspirate, see 88172, 88173)

48120 Excision of lesion of pancreas (eg, cyst, adenoma)

48140 Pancreatectomy, distal subtotal, with or without splenectomy; without pancreaticojejunostomy

● New Code   ▲ Revised Code   + Add-On Code   ⊘ Modifier -51 Exempt

48145   with pancreaticojejunostomy

48146 Pancreatectomy, distal, near-total with preservation of duodenum (Child-type procedure)

48148 Excision of ampulla of Vater

48150 Pancreatectomy, proximal subtotal with total duodenectomy, partial gastrectomy, choledochoenterostomy and gastrojejunostomy (Whipple-type procedure); with pancreatojejunostomy

48152   without pancreatojejunostomy

48153 Pancreatectomy, proximal subtotal with near-total duodenectomy, choledochoenterostomy, and duodenojejunostomy (pylorus-sparing, whipple-type procedure); with pancreatojejunostomy

48154   without pancreatojejunostomy

48155 Pancreatectomy, total

48160 Pancreatectomy, total or subtotal, with autologous transplantation of pancreas or pancreatic islet cells

48180 Pancreaticojejunostomy, side-to-side anastomosis (Puestow-type operation)

INTRODUCTION

+ 48400 Injection procedure for intraoperative pancreatography (List separately in addition to code for primary procedure)

(For radiological supervision and interpretation, see 74300-74305)

REPAIR

48500 Marsupialization of pancreatic cyst

48510 External drainage, pseudocyst of pancreas; open

48511   percutaneous

(For radiological supervision and interpretation, use 75989)

489

	Separate Procedure		Unlisted Procedure		CCI Comp. Code		Non-specific Procedure

48520   Internal anastomosis of pancreatic cyst to gastrointestinal tract; direct

48540   Roux-en-Y

48545   Pancreatorrhaphy for injury

48547   Duodenal exclusion with gastrojejunostomy for pancreatic injury

PANCREAS TRANSPLANTATION

48550   Donor pancreatectomy, with preparation and maintenance of allograft from cadaver donor, with or without duodenal segment for transplantation

48554   Transplantation of pancreatic allograft

48556   Removal of transplanted pancreatic allograft

OTHER PROCEDURES

48999   Unlisted procedure, pancreas

ABDOMEN, PERITONEUM, AND OMENTUM

INCISION

49000   Exploratory laparotomy, exploratory celiotomy with or without biopsy(s) (separate procedure)

(To report wound exploration due to penetrating trauma without laparatomy, use 20102)

49002   Reopening of recent laparotomy

(To report re-exploration of hepatic wound for removal of packing, use 47362)

49010   Exploration, retroperitoneal area with or without biopsy(s) (separate procedure)

(To report wound exploration due to penetrating trauma without laparotomy, use 20102)

49020   Drainage of peritoneal abscess or localized peritonitis, exclusive of appendiceal abscess; open

(For appendiceal abscess, use 44900)

● New Code   ▲ Revised Code   + Add-On Code   ⃠ Modifier -51 Exempt

49021 percutaneous

(For radiological supervision and interpretation, use 75989)

49040 Drainage of subdiaphragmatic or subphrenic abscess; open

49041 percutaneous

(For radiological supervision and interpretation, use 75989)

49060 Drainage of retroperitoneal abscess; open

49061 percutaneous

(For laparoscopic drainage, use 49323)

(For radiological supervision and interpretation, use 75989)

49062 Drainage of extraperitoneal lymphocele to peritoneal cavity, open

49080 Peritoneocentesis, abdominal paracentesis, or peritoneal lavage (diagnostic or therapeutic); initial

49081 subsequent

(If imaging guidance is performed, see 76360, 76942)

49085 Removal of peritoneal foreign body from peritoneal cavity

(For lysis of intestinal adhesions, use 44005)

EXCISION, DESTRUCTION

49180 Biopsy, abdominal or retroperitoneal mass, percutaneous needle

(If imaging guidance is performed, see 76003, 76360, 76393, 76942)

(For fine needle aspiration, use 10021 or 10022)

(For evaluation of fine needle aspirate, see 88172, 88173)

49200 Excision or destruction, open, intra-abdominal or retroperitoneal tumors or cysts or endometriomas;

49201 extensive

49215 Excision of presacral or sacrococcygeal tumor

 Separate Procedure   Unlisted Procedure   CCI Comp. Code   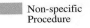 Non-specific Procedure

(Do not report modifier '-63' in conjunction with 49215)

49220 Staging laparotomy for Hodgkins disease or lymphoma (includes splenectomy, needle or open biopsies of both liver lobes, possibly also removal of abdominal nodes, abdominal node and/or bone marrow biopsies, ovarian repositioning)

49250 Umbilectomy, omphalectomy, excision of umbilicus (separate procedure)

49255 Omentectomy, epiploectomy, resection of omentum (separate procedure)

LAPAROSCOPY

49320 Laparoscopy, abdomen, peritoneum, and omentum; diagnostic, with or without collection of specimen(s) by brushing or washing (separate procedure)

49321 Laparoscopy, surgical; with biopsy (single or multiple)

49322 with aspiration of cavity or cyst (eg, ovarian cyst) (single or multiple)

49323 with drainage of lymphocele to peritoneal cavity

(For percutaneous or open drainage, see 49060, 49061)

49329 Unlisted laparoscopy procedure, abdomen, peritoneum and omentum

INTRODUCTION, REVISION, AND/OR REMOVAL

49400 Injection of air or contrast into peritoneal cavity (separate procedure)

(For radiological supervision and interpretation, use 74190)

49419 Insertion of intraperitoneal cannula or catheter, with subcutaneous reservoir, permanent (ie, totally implantable)

(For removal, use 49422)

49420 Insertion of intraperitoneal cannula or catheter for drainage or dialysis; temporary

49421 permanent

● New Code   ▲ Revised Code   + Add-On Code   ⊘ Modifier -51 Exempt

49422 Removal of permanent intraperitoneal cannula or catheter

(For removal of a temporary catheter/cannula, use appropriate E/M code)

49423 Exchange of previously placed abscess or cyst drainage catheter under radiological guidance (separate procedure)

(For radiological supervision and interpretation, use 75984)

49424 Contrast injection for assessment of abscess or cyst via previously placed drainage catheter or tube (separate procedure)

(For radiological supervision and interpretation, use 76080)

49425 Insertion of peritoneal-venous shunt

49426 Revision of peritoneal-venous shunt

(For shunt patency test, use 78291)

49427 Injection procedure (eg, contrast media) for evaluation of previously placed peritoneal-venous shunt

(For radiological supervision and interpretation, see 75809, 78291)

49428 Ligation of peritoneal-venous shunt

49429 Removal of peritoneal-venous shunt

REPAIR

Hernioplasty, Herniorrhaphy, Herniotomy

(For reduction and repair of intra-abdominal hernia, use 44050)

(For debridement of abdominal wall, see 11042, 11043)

49491 Repair, initial inguinal hernia, preterm infant (less than 37 weeks gestation at birth), performed from birth up to 50 weeks postconception age, with or without hydrocelectomy; reducible

49492 incarcerated or strangulated

(Do not report modifier '-63' in conjunction with 49491, 49492)

(Post-conception age equals gestational age at birth plus age of infant in weeks at the time of the hernia repair. Initial inguinal hernia repairs that are performed on preterm infants who are

493

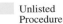 Separate Procedure
 Unlisted Procedure
CCI Comp. Code
 Non-specific Procedure

over 50 weeks postconceptual age and under age 6 months at the time of surgery, should be reported using codes 49495, 49496)

49495 Repair, initial inguinal hernia, full term infant under age 6 months, or preterm infant over 50 weeks postconception age and under age 6 months at the time of surgery, with or without hydrocelectomy; reducible

49496 incarcerated or strangulated

(Post-conception age equals gestational age at birth plus age in weeks at the time of the hernia repair. Initial inguinal hernia repairs that are performed on preterm infants who are under or up to 50 weeks postconceptual age but under 6 months of age since birth, should be reported using codes 49491, 49492. Inguinal hernia repairs on infants age 6 months to under 5 years should be reported using codes 49500-49501)

(Do not report modifier '-63' in conjunction with 49495, 49496)

49500 Repair initial inguinal hernia, age 6 months to under 5 years, with or without hydrocelectomy; reducible

49501 incarcerated or strangulated

49505 Repair initial inguinal hernia, age 5 years or over; reducible

49507 incarcerated or strangulated

49520 Repair recurrent inguinal hernia, any age; reducible

49521 incarcerated or strangulated

49525 Repair inguinal hernia, sliding, any age

49540 Repair lumbar hernia

49550 Repair initial femoral hernia, any age; reducible

49553 incarcerated or strangulated

49555 Repair recurrent femoral hernia; reducible

49557 incarcerated or strangulated

49560 Repair initial incisional or ventral hernia; reducible

● New Code ▲ Revised Code + Add-On Code ⊘ Modifier -51 Exempt

49561   incarcerated or strangulated

49565 Repair recurrent incisional or ventral hernia; reducible

49566   incarcerated or strangulated

+ **49568** Implantation of mesh or other prosthesis for incisional or ventral hernia repair (List separately in addition to code for the incisional or ventral hernia repair)

49570 Repair epigastric hernia (eg, preperitoneal fat); reducible (separate procedure)

49572   incarcerated or strangulated

49580 Repair umbilical hernia, under age 5 years; reducible

49582   incarcerated or strangulated

49585 Repair umbilical hernia, age 5 years or over; reducible

49587   incarcerated or strangulated

49590 Repair spigelian hernia

49600 Repair of small omphalocele, with primary closure

(Do not report modifier '-63' in conjunction with 49600)

49605 Repair of large omphalocele or gastroschisis; with or without prosthesis

49606   with removal of prosthesis, final reduction and closure, in operating room

(Do not report modifier '-63' in conjunction with 49605, 49606)

49610 Repair of omphalocele (Gross type operation); first stage

49611   second stage

(Do not report modifier '-63' in conjunction with 49610, 49611)

(For diaphragmatic or hiatal hernia repair, see 39502-39541)

 Separate Procedure   Unlisted Procedure   CCI Comp. Code   Non-specific Procedure

495

LAPAROSCOPY

49650 Laparoscopy, surgical; repair initial inguinal hernia

49651 repair recurrent inguinal hernia

49659 Unlisted laparoscopy procedure, hernioplasty, herniorrhaphy, herniotomy

SUTURE

49900 Suture, secondary, of abdominal wall for evisceration or dehiscence

(For suture of ruptured diaphragm, see 39540, 39541)

(For debridement of abdominal wall, see 11042, 11043)

OTHER PROCEDURES

49904 Omental flap, extra-abdominal (eg, for reconstruction of sternal and chest wall defects)

(Code 49904 includes harvest and transfer. If a second surgeon harvests the omental flap, then the two surgeons should code 49904 as co-surgeons, using modifier '-62')

+ 49905 Omental flap, intra-abdominal (List separately in addition to code for primary procedure)

(Do not report 49905 in conjunction with 47700)

49906 Free omental flap with microvascular anastomosis

(Do not report code 69990 in addition to code 49906)

49999 Unlisted procedure, abdomen, peritoneum and omentum

● New Code   ▲ Revised Code   + Add-On Code   ⊘ Modifier -51 Exempt

URINARY SYSTEM

CPT codes from this section of CPT are used to report invasive and surgical procedures performed on the kidney; ureter; bladder; prostate (resection); and urethra.

URODYNAMICS

CPT codes in this section may be used separately or in various combinations. When multiple procedures are performed in the same session, modifier -51 should be added to the second and all subsequent CPT codes. Procedures in this section are performed by, or under the direct supervision of, a physician.

In addition, all materials and supplies, used in the provision of these services, such as instruments, equipment, fluids, gases, probes, catheters, technician's fees, medications, gloves, trays, tubing and other sterile supplies are considered to be included in the base code. Use modifier -26 to code and report interpretation of results or operation of equipment only.

CYSTOSCOPY, URETHROSCOPY, and CYSTOURETHROSCOPY

The descriptions of CPT codes in this section are listed so that the main procedure can be identified without having to list all of the minor related procedures performed at the same time. For example:

52601   Transurethral electrosurgical resection of prostate, including control of postoperative bleeding, complete (vasectomy, meatotomy, cystourethroscopy, urethral calibration and/or dilation, and internal urethrotomy are included)

All of the secondary procedures are included in the single code 52601. If any of the secondary procedures requires significant additional time and effort, to the point of making the procedure "unusual", modifier -22 should be added with an appropriate increase in fee and a report explaining what made the procedure unusual.

KIDNEY

   (For provision of chemotherapeutic agents, use 96545 in addition to code for primary procedure)

INCISION

   (For retroperitoneal exploration, abscess, tumor, or cyst, see 49010, 49060, 49200, 49201)

497

| Separate Procedure | Unlisted Procedure | CCI Comp. Code | Non-specific Procedure |

50010   Renal exploration, not necessitating other specific procedures

(For laparoscopic ablation of renal mass lesion(s), use 50542)

50020   Drainage of perirenal or renal abscess; open

50021   percutaneous

(For radiological supervision and interpretation, use 75989)

50040   Nephrostomy, nephrotomy with drainage

50045   Nephrotomy, with exploration

(For renal endoscopy performed in conjunction with this procedure, see 50570-50580)

50060   Nephrolithotomy; removal of calculus

50065   secondary surgical operation for calculus

50070   complicated by congenital kidney abnormality

50075   removal of large staghorn calculus filling renal pelvis and calyces (including anatrophic pyelolithotomy)

50080   Percutaneous nephrostolithotomy or pyelostolithotomy, with or without dilation, endoscopy, lithotripsy, stenting, or basket extraction; up to 2 cm

50081   over 2cm

(For establishment of nephrostomy without nephrostolithotomy, see 50040, 50395, 52334)

(For fluoroscopic guidance, see 76000, 76001)

50100   Transection or repositioning of aberrant renal vessels (separate procedure)

50120   Pyelotomy; with exploration

(For renal endoscopy performed in conjunction with this procedure, see 50570-50580)

50125   with drainage, pyelostomy

● New Code   ▲ Revised Code   ✛ Add-On Code   ⊘ Modifier -51 Exempt

50130   with removal of calculus (pyelolithotomy, pelviolithotomy, including coagulum pyelolithotomy)

50135   complicated (eg, secondary operation, congenital kidney abnormality)

(For supply of anticarcinogenic agents, use 99070 in addition to code for primary procedure)

EXCISION

(For excision of retroperitoneal tumor or cyst, see 49200, 49201)

(For laparoscopic ablation of renal mass lesion(s), use 50542)

50200   Renal biopsy; percutaneous, by trocar or needle

(For radiological supervision and interpretation, see 76003, 76360, 76393, 76942)

(For fine needle aspiration, use 10022)

(For evaluation of fine needle aspirate, see 88172, 88173)

50205   by surgical exposure of kidney

50220   Nephrectomy, including partial ureterectomy, any open approach including rib resection;

50225   complicated because of previous surgery on same kidney

50230   radical, with regional lymphadenectomy and/or vena caval thrombectomy

(When vena caval resection with reconstruction is necessary, use 37799)

50234   Nephrectomy with total ureterectomy and bladder cuff; through same incision

50236   through separate incision

50240   Nephrectomy, partial

(For laparoscopic partial nephrectomy, use 50543)

50280   Excision or unroofing of cyst(s) of kidney

(For laparoscopic ablation of renal cysts, use 50541)

499

 Separate Procedure   Unlisted Procedure   CCI Comp. Code   Non-specific Procedure

50290   Excision of perinephric cyst

RENAL TRANSPLANTATION

(For dialysis, see 90935-90999)

(For laparoscopic donor nephrectomy, use 50547)

(For laparoscopic drainage of lymphocele to peritoneal cavity, use 49323)

50300   Donor nephrectomy, with preparation and maintenance of allograft, from cadaver donor, unilateral or bilateral

50320   Donor nephrectomy, open from living donor (excluding preparation and maintenance of allograft)

50340   Recipient nephrectomy (separate procedure)

50360   Renal allotransplantation, implantation of graft; excluding donor and recipient nephrectomy

50365   with recipient nephrectomy

50370   Removal of transplanted renal allograft

50380   Renal autotransplantation, reimplantation of kidney

(For extra-corporeal "bench" surgery, use autotransplantation as the primary procedure and add the secondary procedure (eg, partial nephrectomy, nephrolithotomy), and use the modifier -51)

INTRODUCTION

50390   Aspiration and/or injection of renal cyst or pelvis by needle, percutaneous

(For radiological supervision and interpretation, see 74425, 74470, 76003, 76360, 76393, 76942)

(For evaluation of fine needle aspirate, see 88172, 88173)

50392   Introduction of intracatheter or catheter into renal pelvis for drainage and/or injection, percutaneous

(For radiological supervision and interpretation, see 74475, 76360, 76942)

● New Code   ▲ Revised Code   + Add-On Code   ⊘ Modifier -51 Exempt

50393 Introduction of ureteral catheter or stent into ureter through renal pelvis for drainage and/or injection, percutaneous

(For radiological supervision and interpretation, see 74480, 76003, 76360, 76942)

50394 Injection procedure for pyelography (as nephrostogram, pyelostogram, antegrade pyeloureterograms) through nephrostomy or pyelostomy tube, or indwelling ureteral catheter

(For radiological supervision and interpretation, use 74425)

50395 Introduction of guide into renal pelvis and/or ureter with dilation to establish nephrostomy tract, percutaneous

(For radiological supervision and interpretation, see 74475, 74480, 74485)

(For nephrostolithotomy, see 50080, 50081)

(For retrograde percutaneous nephrostomy, use 52334)

(For endoscopic surgery, see 50551-50561)

50396 Manometric studies through nephrostomy or pyelostomy tube, or indwelling ureteral catheter

(For radiological supervision and interpretation, see 74425, 74475, 74480)

50398 Change of nephrostomy or pyelostomy tube

(For radiological supervision and interpretation, use 75984)

REPAIR

50400 Pyeloplasty (Foley Y-pyeloplasty), plastic operation on renal pelvis, with or without plastic operation on ureter, nephropexy, nephrostomy, pyelostomy, or ureteral splinting; simple

50405 complicated (congenital kidney abnormality, secondary pyeloplasty, solitary kidney, calycoplasty)

(For laparoscopic approach, use 50544)

50500 Nephrorrhaphy, suture of kidney wound or injury

50520 Closure of nephrocutaneous or pyelocutaneous fistula

501

| Separate Procedure | Unlisted Procedure | CCI Comp. Code | Non-specific Procedure |

50525 Closure of nephrovisceral fistula (eg, renocolic), including visceral repair; abdominal approach

50526 thoracic approach

50540 Symphysiotomy for horseshoe kidney with or without pyeloplasty and/or other plastic procedure, unilateral or bilateral (one operation)

LAPAROSCOPY

50541 Laparoscopy, surgical; ablation of renal cysts

50542 ablation of renal mass lesion(s)

(For open procedure, see 50220-50240)

50543 partial nephrectomy

(For open procedure, use 50240)

50544 pyeloplasty

50545 radical nephrectomy (includes removal of Gerota's fascia and surrounding fatty tissue, removal of regional lymph nodes, and adrenalectomy

(For open procedure, use 50230)

50546 nephrectomy including partial ureterectomy

50547 donor nephrectomy from living donor (excluding preparation and maintenance of allograft)

(For open procedure, use 50320)

50548 nephrectomy with total ureterectomy

(For open procedure, see 50234, 50236)

50549 Unlisted laparoscopy procedure, renal

(For laparoscopic drainage of lymphocele to peritoneal cavity, use 49323)

● New Code ▲ Revised Code + Add-On Code ⊘ Modifier -51 Exempt

ENDOSCOPY

(For supplies and materials, use 99070)

50551 Renal endoscopy through established nephrostomy or pyelostomy, with or without irrigation, instillation, or ureteropyelography, exclusive of radiologic service;

50553 with ureteral catheterization, with or without dilation of ureter

50555 with biopsy

50557 with fulguration and/or incision, with or without biopsy

50559 with insertion of radioactive substance with or without biopsy and/or fulguration

50561 with removal of foreign body or calculus

50562 with resection of tumor

(When procedures 50570-50580 provide a significant identifiable service, they may be added to 50045 and 50120)

50570 Renal endoscopy through nephrotomy or pyelotomy, with or without irrigation, instillation, or ureteropyelography, exclusive of radiologic service;

(For nephrotomy, use 50045)

(For pyelotomy, use 50120)

50572 with ureteral catheterization, with or without dilation of ureter

50574 with biopsy

50575 with endopyelotomy (includes cystoscopy, ureteroscopy, dilation of ureter and ureteral pelvic junction, incision of ureteral pelvic junction and insertion of endopyelotomy stent)

50576 with fulguration and/or incision, with or without biopsy

50578 with insertion of radioactive substance, with or without biopsy and/or fulguration

---

503

 Separate Procedure   Unlisted Procedure   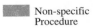 CCI Comp. Code   Non-specific Procedure

| 50580 | with removal of foreign body or calculus |

OTHER PROCEDURES

| 50590 | Lithotripsy, extracorporeal shock wave |

URETER

INCISION

| 50600 | Ureterotomy with exploration or drainage (separate procedure) |

(For ureteral endoscopy performed in conjunction with this procedure, see 50970-50980)

| 50605 | Ureterotomy for insertion of indwelling stent, all types |

| 50610 | Ureterolithotomy; upper one-third of ureter |

| 50620 | middle one-third of ureter |

| 50630 | lower one-third of ureter |

(For laparoscopic approach, use 50945)

(For transvesical ureterolithotomy, use 51060)

(For cystotomy with stone basket extraction of ureteral calculus, use 51065)

(For endoscopic extraction or manipulation of ureteral calculus, see 50080, 50081, 50561, 50961, 50980, 52320-52330, 52352, 52353)

EXCISION

(For ureterocele, see 51535, 52300)

| 50650 | Ureterectomy, with bladder cuff (separate procedure) |

| 50660 | Ureterectomy, total, ectopic ureter, combination abdominal, vaginal and/or perineal approach |

● New Code ▲ Revised Code + Add-On Code ⃠ Modifier -51 Exempt

INTRODUCTION

50684 Injection procedure for ureterography or ureteropyelography through ureterostomy or indwelling ureteral catheter

(For radiological supervision and interpretation, use 74425)

50686 Manometric studies through ureterostomy or indwelling ureteral catheter

50688 Change of ureterostomy tube

(If imaging guidance is performed, use 75984)

50690 Injection procedure for visualization of ileal conduit and/or ureteropyelography, exclusive of radiologic service

(For radiological supervision and interpretation, use 74425)

REPAIR

50700 Ureteroplasty, plastic operation on ureter (eg, stricture)

50715 Ureterolysis, with or without repositioning of ureter for retroperitoneal fibrosis

50722 Ureterolysis for ovarian vein syndrome

50725 Ureterolysis for retrocaval ureter, with reanastomosis of upper urinary tract or vena cava

50727 Revision of urinary-cutaneous anastomosis (any type urostomy);

50728 with repair of fascial defect and hernia

50740 Ureteropyelostomy, anastomosis of ureter and renal pelvis

50750 Ureterocalycostomy, anastomosis of ureter to renal calyx

50760 Ureteroureterostomy

50770 Transureteroureterostomy, anastomosis of ureter to contralateral ureter

(Codes 50780-50785 include minor procedures to prevent vesicoureteral reflux)

50780 Ureteroneocystostomy; anastomosis of single ureter to bladder

505

| 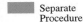 Separate Procedure | Unlisted Procedure | CCI Comp. Code | Non-specific Procedure |

(When combined with cystourethroplasty or vesical neck revision, use 51820)

50782 anastomosis of duplicated ureter to bladder

50783 with extensive ureteral tailoring

50785 with vesico-psoas hitch or bladder flap

50800 Ureteroenterostomy, direct anastomosis of ureter to intestine

50810 Ureterosigmoidostomy, with creation of sigmoid bladder and establishment of abdominal or perineal colostomy, including intestine anastomosis

50815 Ureterocolon conduit, including intestine anastomosis

50820 Ureteroileal conduit (ileal bladder), including intestine anastomosis (Bricker operation)

(For combination of 50800-50820 with cystectomy, see 51580-51595)

50825 Continent diversion, including intestine anastomosis using any segment of small and/or large intestine (Kock pouch or Camey enterocystoplasty)

50830 Urinary undiversion (eg, taking down of ureteroileal conduit, ureterosigmoidostomy or ureteroenterostomy with ureteroureterostomy or ureteroneocystostomy)

50840 Replacement of all or part of ureter by intestine segment, including intestine anastomosis

50845 Cutaneous appendico-vesicostomy

50860 Ureterostomy, transplantation of ureter to skin

50900 Ureterorrhaphy, suture of ureter (separate procedure)

50920 Closure of ureterocutaneous fistula

50930 Closure of ureterovisceral fistula (including visceral repair)

50940 Deligation of ureter

(For ureteroplasty, ureterolysis, see 50700-50860)

● New Code   ▲ Revised Code   + Add-On Code   ⊘ Modifier -51 Exempt

LAPAROSCOPY

50945 Laparoscopy, surgical; ureterolithotomy

50947 ureteroneocystostomy with cystoscopy and ureteral stent placement

50948 ureteroneocystostomy without cystoscopy and ureteral stent placement

(For open ureteroneocystostomy, see 50780-50785)

50949 Unlisted laparoscopy procedure, ureter

ENDOSCOPY

50951 Ureteral endoscopy through established ureterostomy, with or without irrigation, instillation, or ureteropyelography, exclusive of radiologic service;

50953 with ureteral catheterization, with or without dilation of ureter

50955 with biopsy

50957 with fulguration and/or incision, with or without biopsy

50959 with insertion of radioactive substance, with or without biopsy and/or fulguration (not including provision of material)

50961 with removal of foreign body or calculus

(When procedures 50970-50980 provide a significant identifiable service, they may be added to 50600)

50970 Ureteral endoscopy through ureterotomy, with or without irrigation, instillation, or ureteropyelography, exclusive of radiologic service;

(For ureterotomy, use 50600)

50972 with ureteral catheterization, with or without dilation of ureter

50974 with biopsy

50976 with fulguration and/or incision, with or without biopsy

 Separate Procedure   Unlisted Procedure  CCI Comp. Code 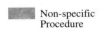 Non-specific Procedure

507

50978   with insertion of radioactive substance, with or without biopsy and/or fulguration (not including provision of material)

50980   with removal of foreign body or calculus

BLADDER

INCISION

51000   Aspiration of bladder by needle

51005   Aspiration of bladder; by trocar or intracatheter

51010   with insertion of suprapubic catheter

(If imaging guidance is performed, see 76003, 76360, 76942)

51020   Cystotomy or cystostomy; with fulguration and/or insertion of radioactive material

51030   with cryosurgical destruction of intravesical lesion

51040   Cystostomy, cystotomy with drainage

51045   Cystotomy, with insertion of ureteral catheter or stent (separate procedure)

51050   Cystolithotomy, cystotomy with removal of calculus, without vesical neck resection

51060   Transvesical ureterolithotomy

51065   Cystotomy, with calculus basket extraction and/or ultrasonic or electrohydraulic fragmentation of ureteral calculus

51080   Drainage of perivesical or prevesical space abscess

EXCISION

51500   Excision of urachal cyst or sinus, with or without umbilical hernia repair

51520   Cystotomy; for simple excision of vesical neck (separate procedure)

---

508   ● New Code   ▲ Revised Code   ✚ Add-On Code   ⊘ Modifier -51 Exempt

51525 for excision of bladder diverticulum, single or multiple (separate procedure)

51530 for excision of bladder tumor

(For transurethral resection, see 52234-52240, 52305)

51535 Cystotomy for excision, incision, or repair of ureterocele

(For transurethral excision, use 52300)

51550 Cystectomy, partial; simple

51555 complicated (eg, postradiation, previous surgery, difficult location)

51565 Cystectomy, partial, with reimplantation of ureter(s) into bladder (ureteroneocystostomy)

51570 Cystectomy, complete; (separate procedure)

51575 with bilateral pelvic lymphadenectomy, including external iliac, hypogastric, and obturator nodes

51580 Cystectomy, complete, with ureterosigmoidostomy or ureterocutaneous transplantations;

51585 with bilateral pelvic lymphadenectomy, including external iliac, hypogastric, and obturator nodes

51590 Cystectomy, complete, with ureteroileal conduit or sigmoid bladder, including intestine anastomosis;

51595 with bilateral pelvic lymphadenectomy, including external iliac, hypogastric, and obturator nodes

51596 Cystectomy, complete, with continent diversion, any open technique, using any segment of small and/or large intestine to construct neobladder

51597 Pelvic exenteration, complete, for vesical, prostatic or urethral malignancy, with removal of bladder and ureteral transplantations, with or without hysterectomy and/or abdominoperineal resection of rectum and colon and colostomy, or any combination thereof

(For pelvic exenteration for gynecologic malignancy, use 58240)

509

	Separate Procedure		Unlisted Procedure		CCI Comp. Code		Non-specific Procedure

INTRODUCTION

(For bladder catheterization, see 51701-51703)

51600 Injection procedure for cystography or voiding urethrocystography

(For radiological supervision and interpretation, see 74430, 74455)

51605 Injection procedure and placement of chain for contrast and/or chain urethrocystography

(For radiological supervision and interpretation, use 74430)

51610 Injection procedure for retrograde urethrocystography

(For radiological supervision and interpretation, use 74450)

51700 Bladder irrigation, simple, lavage and/or instillation

(Codes 51701-51702 are reported only when performed independently. Do not report 51701-51702 when catheter insertion is an inclusive component of another procedure.)

51701 Insertion of non-indwelling bladder catheter (eg, straight catheterization of residual urine)

51702 Insertion of temporary indwelling bladder catheter; simple (eg, Foley)

51703 complicated (eg, altered anatomy, fractured catheter/balloon)

51705 Change of cystostomy tube; simple

51710 complicated

(If imaging guidance is performed, use 75984)

51715 Endoscopic injection of implant material into the submucosal tissues of the urethra and/or bladder neck

51720 Bladder instillation of anticarcinogenic agent (including detention time)

URODYNAMICS

51725 Simple cystometrogram (CMG) (eg, spinal manometer)

● New Code	▲ Revised Code	+ Add-On Code	⊘ Modifier -51 Exempt

51726 Complex cystometrogram (eg, calibrated electronic equipment)

51736 Simple uroflowmetry (UFR) (eg, stop-watch flow rate, mechanical uroflowmeter)

51741 Complex uroflowmetry (eg, calibrated electronic equipment)

51772 Urethral pressure profile studies (UPP) (urethral closure pressure profile), any technique

51784 Electromyography studies (EMG) of anal or urethral sphincter, other than needle, any technique

51785 Needle electromyography studies (EMG) of anal or urethral sphincter, any technique

51792 Stimulus evoked response (eg, measurement of bulbocavernosus reflex latency time)

51795 Voiding pressure studies (VP); bladder voiding pressure, any technique

51797 intra-abdominal voiding pressure (AP) (rectal, gastric, intraperitoneal)

51798 Measurement of post-voiding residual urine and/or bladder capacity by ultrasound, non-imaging

REPAIR

51800 Cystoplasty or cystourethroplasty, plastic operation on bladder and/or vesical neck (anterior Y-plasty, vesical fundus resection), any procedure, with or without wedge resection of posterior vesical neck

51820 Cystourethroplasty with unilateral or bilateral ureteroneocystostomy

51840 Anterior vesicourethropexy, or urethropexy (eg, Marshall-Marchetti-Krantz, Burch); simple

51841 complicated (eg, secondary repair)

(For urethropexy (Pereyra type), use 57289)

51845 Abdomino-vaginal vesical neck suspension, with or without endoscopic control (eg, Stamey, Raz, modified Pereyra)

511

Separate Procedure / Unlisted Procedure / CCI Comp. Code / Non-specific Procedure

51860 Cystorrhaphy, suture of bladder wound, injury or rupture; simple

51865 complicated

51880 Closure of cystostomy (separate procedure)

51900 Closure of vesicovaginal fistula, abdominal approach

(For vaginal approach, see 57320-57330)

51920 Closure of vesicouterine fistula;

51925 with hysterectomy

(For closure of vesicoenteric fistula, see 44660, 44661)

(For closure of rectovesical fistula, see 45800-45805)

51940 Closure, exstrophy of bladder

(See also 54390)

51960 Enterocystoplasty, including intestinal anastomosis

51980 Cutaneous vesicostomy

LAPAROSCOPY

51990 Laparoscopy, surgical; urethral suspension for stress incontinence

51992 sling operation for stress incontinence (eg, fascia or synthetic)

(For open sling operation for stress incontinence, use 57288)

(For reversal or removal of sling operation for stress incontinence, use 57287)

ENDOSCOPY—CYSTOSCOPY, URETHROSCOPY, CYSTOURETHROSCOPY

52000 Cystourethroscopy (separate procedure)

52201 Cystourethroscopy with irrigation and evacuation of multiple obstructing clots

(Do not report 52001 in addition to 52000)

512

● New Code	▲ Revised Code	+ Add-On Code	⊘ Modifier -51 Exempt

52005 Cystourethroscopy, with ureteral catheterization, with or without irrigation, instillation, or ureteropyelography, exclusive of radiologic service;

52007 with brush biopsy of ureter and/or renal pelvis

52010 Cystourethroscopy, with ejaculatory duct catheterization, with or without irrigation, instillation, or duct radiography, exclusive of radiologic service

(For radiological supervision and interpretation, use 74440)

TRANSURETHRAL SURGERY

Urethra and Bladder

52204 Cystourethroscopy, with biopsy

52214 Cystourethroscopy, with fulguration (including cryosurgery or laser surgery) of trigone, bladder neck, prostatic fossa, urethra, or periurethral glands

52224 Cystourethroscopy, with fulguration (including cryosurgery or laser surgery) or treatment of MINOR (less than 0.5 cm) lesion(s) with or without biopsy

52234 Cystourethroscopy, with fulguration (including cryosurgery or laser surgery) and/or resection of; SMALL bladder tumor(s) (0.5 to 2.0 cm)

52235 MEDIUM bladder tumor(s) (2.0 to 5.0 cm)

52240 LARGE bladder tumor(s)

52250 Cystourethroscopy with insertion of radioactive substance, with or without biopsy or fulguration

52260 Cystourethroscopy, with dilation of bladder for interstitial cystitis; general or conduction (spinal) anesthesia

52265 local anesthesia

52270 Cystourethroscopy, with internal urethrotomy; female

52275 male

52276 Cystourethroscopy with direct vision internal urethrotomy

513

 Separate Procedure

 Unlisted Procedure

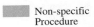 CCI Comp. Code

Non-specific Procedure

52277 Cystourethroscopy, with resection of external sphincter (sphincterotomy)

52281 Cystourethroscopy, with calibration and/or dilation of urethral stricture or stenosis, with or without meatotomy, with or without injection procedure for cystography, male or female

52282 Cystourethroscopy, with insertion of urethral stent

52283 Cystourethroscopy, with steroid injection into stricture

52285 Cystourethroscopy for treatment of the female urethral syndrome with any or all of the following: urethral meatotomy, urethral dilation, internal urethrotomy, lysis of urethrovaginal septal fibrosis, lateral incisions of the bladder neck, and fulguration of polyp(s) of urethra, bladder neck, and/or trigone

52290 Cystourethroscopy; with ureteral meatotomy, unilateral or bilateral

52300   with resection or fulguration of orthotopic ureterocele(s), unilateral or bilateral

52301   with resection or fulguration of ectopic ureterocele(s), unilateral or bilateral

52305   with incision or resection of orifice of bladder diverticulum, single or multiple

52310 Cystourethroscopy, with removal of foreign body, calculus, or ureteral stent from urethra or bladder (separate procedure); simple

52315   complicated

52317 Litholapaxy: crushing or fragmentation of calculus by any means in bladder and removal of fragments; simple or small (less than 2.5 cm)

52318   complicated or large (over 2.5 cm)

● New Code   ▲ Revised Code   + Add-On Code   ⊘ Modifier -51 Exempt

URETER AND PELVIS

52320 Cystourethroscopy (including ureteral catheterization); with removal of ureteral calculus

52325 with fragmentation of ureteral calculus (eg, ultrasonic or electro-hydraulic technique)

52327 with subureteric injection of implant material

52330 with manipulation, without removal of ureteral calculus

52332 Cystourethroscopy, with insertion of indwelling ureteral stent (eg, Gibbons or double-J type)

52334 Cystourethroscopy with insertion of ureteral guide wire through kidney to establish a percutaneous nephrostomy, retrograde

(For percutaneous nephrostolithotomy, see 50080, 50081; for establishment of nephrostomy tract only, use 50395)

52341 Cystourethroscopy; with treatment of ureteral stricture (eg, balloon dilation, laser, electrocautery, and incision)

52342 with treatment of ureteropelvic junction stricture (eg, balloon dilation, laser, electrocautery, and incision)

52343 with treatment of intra-renal stricture (eg, balloon dilation, laser, electrocautery, and incision)

52344 Cystourethroscopy with ureteroscopy; with treatment of ureteral stricture (eg, balloon dilation, laser, electrocautery, and incision)

52345 with treatment of ureteropelvic junction stricture (eg, balloon dilation, laser, electrocautery, and incision)

52346 with treatment of intra-renal stricture (eg, balloon dilation, laser, electrocautery, and incision)

52347 Cystourethroscopy with transurethral resection or incision of ejaculatory ducts

52351 Cystourethroscopy, with ureteroscopy and/or pyeloscopy; diagnostic

(For radiological supervision and interpretation, use 74485)

515

 Separate Procedure    Unlisted Procedure   CCI Comp. Code   Non-specific Procedure

(Do not report 52351 in conjunction with 52341-52346, 52352-52355)

52352 with removal or manipulation of calculus (ureteral catheterization is included)

52353 with lithotripsy (ureteral catheterization is included)

52354 with biopsy and/or fulguration of ureteral or renal pelvic lesion

52355 with resection of ureteral or renal pelvic tumor

VESICAL NECK AND PROSTATE

52400 Cystourethroscopy with incision, fulguration, or resection of congenital posterior urethral valves, or congenital obstructive hypertrophic mucosal folds

52450 Transurethral incision of prostate

52500 Transurethral resection of bladder neck (separate procedure)

52510 Transurethral balloon dilation of the prostatic urethra

52601 Transurethral electrosurgical resection of prostate, including control of postoperative bleeding, complete (vasectomy, meatotomy, cystourethroscopy, urethral calibration and/or dilation, and internal urethrotomy are included)

(For other approaches, see 55801-55845)

52606 Transurethral fulguration for postoperative bleeding occurring after the usual follow-up time

52612 Transurethral resection of prostate; first stage of two-stage resection (partial resection)

52614 second stage of two-stage resection (resection completed)

52620 Transurethral resection; of residual obstructive tissue after 90 days postoperative

52630 of regrowth of obstructive tissue longer than one year postoperative

52640 of postoperative bladder neck contracture

● New Code ▲ Revised Code + Add-On Code ⊘ Modifier -51 Exempt

52647 Non-contact laser coagulation of prostate, including control of postoperative bleeding, complete (vasectomy, meatotomy, cystourethroscopy, urethral calibration and/or dilation, and internal urethrotomy are included)

52648 Contact laser vaporization with or without transurethral resection of prostate, including control of postoperative bleeding, complete (vasectomy, meatotomy, cystourethroscopy, urethral calibration and/or dilation, and internal urethrotomy are included)

52700 Transurethral drainage of prostatic abscess

URETHRA

(For endoscopy, see cystoscopy, urethroscopy, cystourethroscopy, 52000-52700)

(For injection procedure for urethrocystography, see 51600-51610)

INCISION

53000 Urethrotomy or urethrostomy, external (separate procedure); pendulous urethra

53010 perineal urethra, external

53020 Meatotomy, cutting of meatus (separate procedure); except infant

53025 infant

(Do not report modifier '-63' in conjunction with 53025)

53040 Drainage of deep periurethral abscess

(For subcutaneous abscess, see 10060, 10061)

53060 Drainage of Skene's gland abscess or cyst

53080 Drainage of perineal urinary extravasation; uncomplicated (separate procedure)

53085 complicated

517

 Separate Procedure    Unlisted Procedure   CCI Comp. Code   Non-specific Procedure

EXCISION

53200 Biopsy of urethra

53210 Urethrectomy, total, including cystostomy; female

53215 male

53220 Excision or fulguration of carcinoma of urethra

53230 Excision of urethral diverticulum (separate procedure); female

53235 male

53240 Marsupialization of urethral diverticulum, male or female

53250 Excision of bulbourethral gland (Cowper's gland)

53260 Excision or fulguration; urethral polyp(s), distal urethra

(For endoscopic approach, see 52214, 52224)

53265 urethral caruncle

53270 Skene's glands

53275 urethral prolapse

REPAIR

(For hypospadias, see 54300-54352)

53400 Urethroplasty; first stage, for fistula, diverticulum, or stricture (eg, Johannsen type)

53405 second stage (formation of urethra), including urinary diversion

53410 Urethroplasty, one-stage reconstruction of male anterior urethra

53415 Urethroplasty, transpubic or perineal, one stage, for reconstruction or repair of prostatic or membranous urethra

53420 Urethroplasty, two-stage reconstruction or repair of prostatic or membranous urethra; first stage

53425 second stage

● New Code   ▲ Revised Code   + Add-On Code   ⊘ Modifier -51 Exempt

53430 Urethroplasty, reconstruction of female urethra

53431 Urethroplasty with tubularization of posterior urethra and/or lower bladder for incontinence (eg, Tenago, Leadbetter procedure)

53440 Sling operation for correction of male urinary incontinence (eg, fascia or synthetic)

53442 Removal or revision of sling for male urinary incontinence (eg, fascia or synthetic)

(53443 deleted 2002 edition. To report, use 53431)

53444 Insertion of tandem cuff (dual cuff)

53445 Insertion of inflatable urethral/bladder neck sphincter, including placement of pump, reservoir, and cuff

53446 Removal of inflatable urethral/bladder neck sphincter, including pump, reservoir, and cuff

53447 Removal and replacement of inflatable urethral/bladder neck sphincter including pump, reservoir, and cuff at the same operative session

53448 Removal and replacement of inflatable urethral/bladder neck sphincter including pump, reservoir, and cuff through an infected field at the same operative session including irrigation and debridement of infected tissue

(Do not report 11040-11043 in addition to 53448)

53449 Repair of inflatable urethral/bladder neck sphincter, including pump, reservoir, and cuff

53450 Urethromeatoplasty, with mucosal advancement

(For meatotomy, see 53020, 53025)

53460 Urethromeatoplasty, with partial excision of distal urethral segment (Richardson type procedure)

● **53500** Urethrolysis, transvaginal, secondary, open, including cystourethroscopy (eg, postsurgical obstruction, scarring)

(For urethrolysis by retropubic approach, use 53899)

519

| | Separate Procedure | | Unlisted Procedure |  | CCI Comp. Code | | Non-specific Procedure |

(Do not report 53500 in conjunction with 52000)

53502 Urethrorrhaphy, suture of urethral wound or injury; female

53505 penile

53510 perineal

53515 prostatomembranous

53520 Closure of urethrostomy or urethrocutaneous fistula, male (separate procedure)

(For closure of urethrovaginal fistula, use 57310)

(For closure of urethrorectal fistula, see 45820, 45825)

MANIPULATION

(For radiological supervision and interpretation, use 74485)

53600 Dilation of urethral stricture by passage of sound or urethral dilator, male; initial

53601 subsequent

53605 Dilation of urethral stricture or vesical neck by passage of sound or urethral dilator, male, general or conduction (spinal) anesthesia

53620 Dilation of urethral stricture by passage of filiform and follower, male; initial

53621 subsequent

53660 Dilation of female urethra including suppository and/or instillation; initial

53661 subsequent

53665 Dilation of female urethra, general or conduction (spinal) anesthesia

(53670 deleted 2003 edition. To report, see 51701, 51702)

(53675 deleted 2003 edition. To report, use 51703)

OTHER PROCEDURES

53850   Transurethral destruction of prostate tissue; by microwave thermotherapy

53852   by radiofrequency thermotherapy

53853   by water-induced thermotherapy

53899   Unlisted procedure, urinary system

Separate Procedure   Unlisted Procedure   CCI Comp. Code   Non-specific Procedure

This page intentionally left blank.

● New
Code

▲ Revised
Code

✚ Add-On
Code

⊘ Modifier -51
Exempt

MALE GENITAL SYSTEM

CPT codes from this section of CPT are used to report invasive and surgical procedures performed on the penis; testis; epididymis; scrotum; spermatic cord and prostate. There are several starred procedures in this section.

PENIS

INCISION

54000 Slitting of prepuce, dorsal or lateral (separate procedure); newborn

(Do not report modifier '-63' in conjunction with 54000)

54001 except newborn

54015 Incision and drainage of penis, deep

(For skin and subcutaneous abscess, see 10060-10160)

DESTRUCTION

54050 Destruction of lesion(s), penis (eg, condyloma, papilloma, molluscum contagiosum, herpetic vesicle), simple; chemical

54055 electrodesiccation

54056 cryosurgery

54057 laser surgery

54060 surgical excision

54065 Destruction of lesion(s), penis (eg, condyloma, papilloma, molluscum contagiosum, herpetic vesicle), extensive (eg, laser surgery, electosurgery, cryosurgery, chemosurgery)

(For destruction or excision of other lesions, see Integumentary System)

EXCISION

54100 Biopsy of penis; (separate procedure)

54105 deep structures

523

	Separate Procedure		Unlisted Procedure		CCI Comp. Code		Non-specific Procedure

54110   Excision of penile plaque (Peyronie disease);

54111   with graft to 5 cm in length

54112   with graft greater than 5 cm in length

54115   Removal foreign body from deep penile tissue (eg, plastic implant)

54120   Amputation of penis; partial

54125   complete

54130   Amputation of penis, radical; with bilateral inguinofemoral lymphadenectomy

54135   in continuity with bilateral pelvic lymphadenectomy, including external iliac, hypogastric and obturator nodes

(For lymphadenectomy (separate procedure) see 38760-38770)

54150   Circumcision, using clamp or other device; newborn

(Do not report modifier '-63' in conjunction with 54150)

54152   except newborn

54160   Circumcision, surgical excision other than clamp, device or dorsal slit; newborn

(Do not report modifier '-63' in conjunction with 54160)

54161   except newborn

54162   Lysis or excision of penile post-circumcision adhesions

54163   Repair incomplete circumcision

54164   Frenulotomy of penis

(Do not report with circumcision codes 54150-54161, 54162, 54163)

INTRODUCTION

54200   Injection procedure for Peyronie disease;

● New Code	▲ Revised Code	+ Add-On Code	⊘ Modifier -51 Exempt

54205   with surgical exposure of plaque

54220 Irrigation of corpora cavernosa for priapism

54230 Injection procedure for corpora cavernosography

(For radiological supervision and interpretation, use 74445)

54231 Dynamic cavernosometry, including intracavernosal injection of vasoactive drugs (eg, papaverine, phentolamine)

54235 Injection of corpora cavernosa with pharmacologic agent(s) (eg, papaverine, phentolamine)

54240 Penile plethysmography

54250 Nocturnal penile tumescence and/or rigidity test

REPAIR

(For other urethroplasties, see 53400-53430)

(For penile revascularization, use 37788)

54300 Plastic operation of penis for straightening of chordee (eg, hypospadias), with or without mobilization of urethra

54304 Plastic operation on penis for correction of chordee or for first stage hypospadias repair with or without transplantation of prepuce and/or skin flaps

54308 Urethroplasty for second stage hypospadias repair (including urinary diversion); less than 3 cm

54312   greater than 3 cm

54316 Urethroplasty for second stage hypospadias repair (including urinary diversion) with free skin graft obtained from site other than genitalia

54318 Urethroplasty for third stage hypospadias repair to release penis from scrotum (eg, third stage Cecil repair)

54322 One stage distal hypospadias repair (with or without chordee or circumcision); with simple meatal advancement (eg, Magpi, V-flap)

525

 Separate Procedure
 Unlisted Procedure
 CCI Comp. Code
 Non-specific Procedure

54324   with urethroplasty by local skin flaps (eg, flip-flap, prepucial flap)

54326   with urethroplasty by local skin flaps and mobilization of urethra

54328   with extensive dissection to correct chordee and urethroplasty with local skin flaps, skin graft patch, and/or island flap

54332 One stage proximal penile or penoscrotal hypospadias repair requiring extensive dissection to correct chordee and urethroplasty by use of skin graft tube and/or island flap

54336 One stage perineal hypospadias repair requiring extensive dissection to correct chordee and urethroplasty by use of skin graft tube and/or island flap

54340 Repair of hypospadias complications (ie, fistula, stricture, diverticula); by closure, incision, or excision, simple

54344   requiring mobilization of skin flaps and urethroplasty with flap or patch graft

54348   requiring extensive dissection and urethroplasty with flap, patch or tubed graft (includes urinary diversion)

54352 Repair of hypospadias cripple requiring extensive dissection and excision of previously constructed structures including re-release of chordee and reconstruction of urethra and penis by use of local skin as grafts and island flaps and skin brought in as flaps or grafts

54360 Plastic operation on penis to correct angulation

54380 Plastic operation on penis for epispadias distal to external sphincter;

54385   with incontinence

54390   with exstrophy of bladder

54400 Insertion of penile prosthesis; non-inflatable (semi-rigid)

54401   inflatable (self-contained)

(54402   deleted 2002 edition. To report, see 54415, 54416)

● New Code   ▲ Revised Code   + Add-On Code   ⊘ Modifier -51 Exempt

54405   Insertion of multi-component inflatable penile prosthesis, including placement of pump, cylinders, and reservoir

(For reduced services, report 54405 with modifier -52)

54406   Removal of all components of a multi-component inflatable penile prosthesis without replacement of prosthesis

(For reduced services, report 54406 with modifier -52)

(54407   deleted 2002 edition. To report, see 54406, 54408, 54410)

54408   Repair of component(s) of a multi-component, inflatable penile prosthesis

(54409   deleted 2002 edition. To report, use 54408)

54410   Removal and replacement of all component(s) of a multi-component inflatable penile prosthesis at the same operative session

54411   Removal and replacement of all components of a multi-component inflatable penile prosthesis through an infected field at the same operative session, including irrigation and debridement of infected tissue

(For reduced services, report 54411 with modifier -52)

(Do not report 11040-11043 in addition to 54411)

54415   Removal of non-inflatable (semi-rigid) or inflatable (self-contained) penile prosthesis, without replacement of prosthesis

54416   Removal and replacement of non-inflatable (semi-rigid) or inflatable (self-contained) penile prosthesis at the same operative session

54417   Removal and replacement of non-inflatable (semi-rigid) or inflatable (self-contained) penile prosthesis through an infected field at the same operative session, including irrigation and debridement of infected tissue

(Do not report 11040-11043 in addition to 54417)

54420   Corpora cavernosa-saphenous vein shunt (priapism operation), unilateral or bilateral

527

 Separate Procedure   Unlisted Procedure   CCI Comp. Code   Non-specific Procedure

54430 Corpora cavernosa-corpus spongiosum shunt (priapism operation), unilateral or bilateral

54435 Corpora cavernosa-glans penis fistulization (eg, biopsy needle, Winter procedure, rongeur, or punch) for priapism

54440 Plastic operation of penis for injury

MANIPULATION

54450 Foreskin manipulation including lysis of preputial adhesions and stretching

TESTIS

EXCISION

54500 Biopsy of testis, needle (separate procedure)

(For fine needle aspiration, see 10021, 10022)

(For evaluation of fine needle aspirate, see 88172, 88173)

54505 Biopsy of testis, incisional (separate procedure)

(When combined with vasogram, seminal vesiculogram, or epididymogram, use 55300)

(54510 deleted 2002 edition. To report, use 54512)

54512 Excision of extraparenchymal lesion of testis

54520 Orchiectomy, simple (including subcapsular), with or without testicular prosthesis, scrotal or inguinal approach

54522 Orchiectomy, partial

54530 Orchiectomy, radical, for tumor; inguinal approach

54535 with abdominal exploration

(For orchiectomy with repair of hernia, see 49505 or 49507 and 54520)

(For radical retroperitoneal lymphadenectomy, use 38780)

54550 Exploration for undescended testis (inguinal or scrotal area)

54560   Exploration for undescended testis with abdominal exploration

REPAIR

54600   Reduction of torsion of testis, surgical, with or without fixation of contralateral testis

54620   Fixation of contralateral testis (separate procedure)

54640   Orchiopexy, inguinal approach, with or without hernia repair

(For inguinal hernia repair performed in conjunction with inguinal orchiopexy, see 49495-49525)

54650   Orchiopexy, abdominal approach, for intra-abdominal testis (eg, Fowler-Stephens)

(For laparoscopic approach, use 54692)

54660   Insertion of testicular prosthesis (separate procedure)

54670   Suture or repair of testicular injury

54680   Transplantation of testis(es) to thigh (because of scrotal destruction)

LAPAROSCOPY

54690   Laparoscopy, surgical; orchiectomy

54692   orchiopexy for intra-abdominal testis

54699   Unlisted laparoscopy procedure, testis

EPIDIDYMIS

INCISION

54700   Incision and drainage of epididymis, testis and/or scrotal space (eg, abscess or hematoma)

EXCISION

54800   Biopsy of epididymis, needle

(For fine needle aspiration, see 10021, 10022)

(For evaluation of fine needle aspirate, see 88172, 88173)

529

	Separate Procedure		Unlisted Procedure		CCI Comp. Code		Non-specific Procedure

54820	Exploration of epididymis, with or without biopsy
54830	Excision of local lesion of epididymis
54840	Excision of spermatocele, with or without epididymectomy
54860	Epididymectomy; unilateral
54861	bilateral

REPAIR

54900	Epididymovasostomy, anastomosis of epididymis to vas deferens; unilateral
54901	bilateral

(For operating microscope, use 69990)

TUNICA VAGINALIS

INCISION

55000	Puncture aspiration of hydrocele, tunica vaginalis, with or without injection of medication

EXCISION

55040	Excision of hydrocele; unilateral
55041	bilateral

(With hernia repair, see 49495-49501)

REPAIR

55060	Repair of tunica vaginalis hydrocele (Bottle type)

SCROTUM

INCISION

55100	Drainage of scrotal wall abscess

(See also 54700)

55110	Scrotal exploration

530

● New Code   ▲ Revised Code   + Add-On Code   ⃠ Modifier -51 Exempt

55120 Removal of foreign body in scrotum

EXCISION

(For excision of local lesion of skin of scrotum, see Integumentary System)

55150 Resection of scrotum

REPAIR

55175 Scrotoplasty; simple

55180 complicated

VAS DEFERENS

INCISION

55200 Vasotomy, cannulization with or without incision of vas, unilateral or bilateral (separate procedure)

EXCISION

55250 Vasectomy, unilateral or bilateral (separate procedure), including postoperative semen examination(s)

INTRODUCTION

55300 Vasotomy for vasograms, seminal vesiculograms, or epididymograms, unilateral or bilateral

(For radiological supervision and interpretation, use 74440)

(When combined with biopsy of testis, see 54505 and use modifier -51)

REPAIR

55400 Vasovasostomy, vasovasorrhaphy

(For operating microscope, use 69990)

SUTURE

55450 Ligation (percutaneous) of vas deferens, unilateral or bilateral (separate procedure)

531

 Separate Procedure

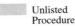 Unlisted Procedure

 CCI Comp. Code

 Non-specific Procedure

SPERMATIC CORD

EXCISION

55500 Excision of hydrocele of spermatic cord, unilateral (separate procedure)

55520 Excision of lesion of spermatic cord (separate procedure)

55530 Excision of varicocele or ligation of spermatic veins for varicocele; (separate procedure)

55535 abdominal approach

55540 with hernia repair

LAPAROSCOPY

55550 Laparoscopy, surgical, with ligation of spermatic veins for varicocele

55559 Unlisted laparoscopy procedure, spermatic cord

SEMINAL VESICLES

INCISION

55600 Vesiculotomy;

55605 complicated

EXCISION

55650 Vesiculectomy, any approach

55680 Excision of Mullerian duct cyst

(For injection procedure, see 52010, 55300)

PROSTATE

INCISION

55700 Biopsy, prostate; needle or punch, single or multiple, any approach

(If imaging guidance is performed, use 76942)

532

- ● New Code
- ▲ Revised Code
- ✚ Add-On Code
- ⊘ Modifier -51 Exempt

(For fine needle aspiration, see 10021, 10022)

(For evaluation of fine needle aspirate, see 88172, 88173)

55705   incisional, any approach

55720   Prostatotomy, external drainage of prostatic abscess, any approach; simple

55725   complicated

(For transurethral drainage, use 52700)

EXCISION

(For transurethral removal of prostate, see 52601-52640)

(For transurethral destruction of prostate, see 53850-53852)

(For limited pelvic lymphadenectomy for staging (separate procedure), use 38562)

(For independent node dissection, see 38770-38780)

55801   Prostatectomy, perineal, subtotal (including control of postoperative bleeding, vasectomy, meatotomy, urethral calibration and/or dilation, and internal urethrotomy)

55810   Prostatectomy, perineal radical;

55812   with lymph node biopsy(s) (limited pelvic lymphadenectomy)

55815   with bilateral pelvic lymphadenectomy, including external iliac, hypogastric and obturator nodes

(If 55815 is carried out on separate days, use 38770 with modifier -50 and 55810)

55821   Prostatectomy (including control of postoperative bleeding, vasectomy, meatotomy, urethral calibration and/or dilation, and internal urethrotomy); suprapubic, subtotal, one or two stages

55831   retropubic, subtotal

55840   Prostatectomy, retropubic radical, with or without nerve sparing;

55842   with lymph node biopsy(s) (limited pelvic lymphadenectomy)

533

 Separate Procedure   Unlisted Procedure   CCI Comp. Code   Non-specific Procedure

55845   with bilateral pelvic lymphadenectomy, including external iliac, hypogastric, and obturator nodes

(If 55845 is carried out on separate days, use 38770 with modifier -50 and 55840)

(For laparoscopic retropubic radical prostatectomy, use 55866)

55859   Transperineal placement of needles or catheters into prostate for interstitial radioelement application, with or without cystoscopy

(For interstitial radioelement application, see 77776-77778)

(For ultrasonic guidance for interstitial radioelement application, use 76965)

55860   Exposure of prostate, any approach, for insertion of radioactive substance;

(For application of interstitial radioelement, see 77776-77778)

55862   with lymph node biopsy(s) (limited pelvic lymphadenectomy)

55865   with bilateral pelvic lymphadenectomy, including external iliac, hypogastric and obturator nodes

LAPAROSCOPY

55866   Laparoscopy, surgical prostatectomy, retropubic radical, including nerve sparing

(For open procedure, use 55840)

OTHER PROCEDURES

(For artificial insemination, see 58321, 58322)

55870   Electroejaculation

55873   Cryosurgical ablation of the prostate (includes ultrasonic guidance for interstitial cryosurgical probe placement)

55899   Unlisted procedure, male genital system

● New Code   ▲ Revised Code   + Add-On Code   ⊘ Modifier -51 Exempt

INTERSEX SURGERY

55970   Intersex surgery; male to female

55980   female to male

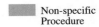

| Separate Procedure | Unlisted Procedure | CCI Comp. Code | Non-specific Procedure |

This page intentionally left blank.

● New
Code

▲ Revised
Code

+ Add-On
Code

⊘ Modifier -51
Exempt

FEMALE GENITAL SYSTEM

CPT codes from this section of the CPT coding system are used to report invasive and surgical procedures performed on the perineum; vulva and introitus; vagina; cervix uteri; corpus uteri; oviduct and ovarium. In vitro fertilization is also coded using CPT codes 58970-58976 from this section.

When coding the removal of multiple vulva or perineal lesions, multiple lesions are coded with multiple codes.

When coding for the insertion of vaginal pessaries, code for the pessary itself (A4560) if purchased by the physician's office.

Select the code describing the excision procedure performed on the specific anatomic site to report LEEP (Loop Electrosurgical Excision Procedure) performed on an anatomic site other than the cervix (57460 and 57522).

Do not code pelvic examination under anesthesia (57410) when D & C or cervical circumferential biopsies with D & Cs are performed. In fact, pelvic examinations under anesthesia (57410) should not be coded separately when any other procedures are performed.

> (For pelvic laparotomy, use 49000)
>
> (For excision or destruction of endometriomas, open method, see 49200, 49201)
>
> (For paracentesis, see 49080, 49081)
>
> (For secondary closure of abdominal wall evisceration or disruption, use 49900)
>
> (For fulguration or excision of lesions, laparoscopic approach, use 58662)
>
> (For chemotherapy, see 96400-96549)

VULVA, PERINEUM AND INTROITUS

INCISION

> (For incision and drainage of sebaceous cyst, furuncle, or abscess, see 10040, 10060, 10061)

56405 Incision and drainage of vulva or perineal abscess

56420 Incision and drainage of Bartholin's gland abscess

537

 Separate Procedure    Unlisted Procedure   CCI Comp. Code   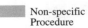 Non-specific Procedure

(For incision and drainage of Skene's gland abscess or cyst, use 53060)

56440 Marsupialization of Bartholin's gland cyst

56441 Lysis of labial adhesions

DESTRUCTION

56501 Destruction of lesion(s), vulva; simple (eg, laser surgery, electrosurgery, cryosurgery, chemosurgery)

56515 extensive (eg, laser surgery, electrosurgery, cryosurgery, chemosurgery)

(For destruction of Skene's gland cyst or abscess, use 53270)

(For cautery destruction of urethral caruncle, use 53265)

EXCISION

56605 Biopsy of vulva or perineum (separate procedure); one lesion

+ **56606** each separate additional lesion (List separately in addition to code for primary procedure)

(Use 56606 in conjunction with code 56605)

(For excision of local lesion, see 11420-11426, 11620-11626)

56620 Vulvectomy simple; partial

56625 complete

(For skin graft, see 15000 et seq)

56630 Vulvectomy, radical, partial;

(For skin graft, if used, see 15000, 15120, 15121, 15240, 15241)

56631 with unilateral inguinofemoral lymphadenectomy

56632 with bilateral inguinofemoral lymphadenectomy

56633 Vulvectomy, radical, complete;

56634 with unilateral inguinofemoral lymphadenectomy

538 ● New Code   ▲ Revised Code   + Add-On Code   ⊘ Modifier -51 Exempt

56637   with bilateral inguinofemoral lymphadenectomy

56640   Vulvectomy, radical, complete, with inguinofemoral, iliac, and pelvic lymphadenectomy

(For lymphadenectomy, see 38760-38780)

56700   Partial hymenectomy or revision of hymenal ring

56720   Hymenotomy, simple incision

56740   Excision of Bartholin's gland or cyst

(For excision of Skene's gland, use 53270)

(For excision of urethral caruncle, use 53265)

(For excision or fulguration of urethral carcinoma, use 53220)

(For excision or marsupialization of urethral diverticulum, see 53230, 53240)

REPAIR

(For repair of urethra for mucosal prolapse, use 53275)

56800   Plastic repair of introitus

56805   Clitoroplasty for intersex state

56810   Perineoplasty, repair of perineum, nonobstetrical (separate procedure)

(See also 56800)

(For repair of wounds to genitalia, see 12001-12007, 12041-12047, 13131-13133)

(For repair of recent injury of vagina and perineum, nonobstetrical, use 57210)

(For anal sphincteroplasty, see 46750, 46751)

(For episiorrhaphy, episioperineorrhaphy for recent injury of vulva and/or perineum, nonobstetrical, use 57210)

ENDOSCOPY

56820   Colposcopy of the vulva

56821   with biopsy(s)

539

 Separate Procedure   Unlisted Procedure    CCI Comp. Code   Non-specific Procedure

(For colposcopic examinations/procedures involving the vagina, see 57420, 57421; cervix, see 57452-57461)

VAGINA

INCISION

57000 Colpotomy; with exploration

57010   with drainage of pelvic abscess

57020 Colpocentesis (separate procedure)

57022 Incision and drainage of vaginal hematoma; obstetrical/postpartum

57023   non-obstetrical (eg, post-trauma, spontaneous bleeding)

DESTRUCTION

57061 Destruction of vaginal lesion(s); simple (eg, laser surgery, electrosurgery, cryosurgery, chemosurgery)

57065   extensive (eg, laser surgery, electrosurgery, cryosurgery, chemosurgery)

EXCISION

57100 Biopsy of vaginal mucosa; simple (separate procedure)

57105   extensive, requiring suture (including cysts)

57106 Vaginectomy, partial removal of vaginal wall;

57107   with removal of paravaginal tissue (radical vaginectomy)

57109   with removal of paravaginal tissue (radical vaginectomy) with bilateral total pelvic lymphadenectomy and para-aortic lymph node sampling (biopsy)

57110 Vaginectomy, complete removal of vaginal wall;

57111   with removal of paravaginal tissue (radical vaginectomy)

57112   with removal of paravaginal tissue (radical vaginectomy) with bilateral total pelvic lymphadenectomy and para-aortic lymph node sampling (biopsy)

● New Code   ▲ Revised Code   + Add-On Code   ⊘ Modifier -51 Exempt

57120 Colpocleisis (Le Fort type)

57130 Excision of vaginal septum

57135 Excision of vaginal cyst or tumor

INTRODUCTION

57150 Irrigation of vagina and/or application of medicament for treatment of bacterial, parasitic, or fungoid disease

57155 Insertion of uterine tandems and/or vaginal ovoids for clinical brachytherapy

(For insertion of radioelement sources or ribbons, see 77761-77763, 77781-77784)

57160 Fitting and insertion of pessary or other intravaginal support device

57170 Diaphragm or cervical cap fitting with instructions

57180 Introduction of any hemostatic agent or pack for spontaneous or traumatic nonobstetrical vaginal hemorrhage (separate procedure)

REPAIR

(For urethral suspension, Marshall-Marchetti-Krantz type, abdominal approach, see 51840, 51841)

(For laparoscopic suspension, use 51990)

57200 Colporrhaphy, suture of injury of vagina (nonobstetrical)

57210 Colpoperineorrhaphy, suture of injury of vagina and/or perineum (nonobstetrical)

57220 Plastic operation on urethral sphincter, vaginal approach (eg, Kelly urethral plication)

57230 Plastic repair of urethrocele

57240 Anterior colporrhaphy, repair of cystocele with or without repair of urethrocele

57250 Posterior colporrhaphy, repair of rectocele with or without perineorrhaphy

541

	Separate Procedure		Unlisted Procedure		CCI Comp. Code		Non-specific Procedure

(For repair of rectocele (separate procedure) without posterior colporrhaphy, use 45560)

57260 Combined anteroposterior colporrhaphy;

57265   with enterocele repair

57268 Repair of enterocele, vaginal approach (separate procedure)

57270 Repair of enterocele, abdominal approach (separate procedure)

57280 Colpopexy, abdominal approach

57282 Sacrospinous ligament fixation for prolapse of vagina

57284 Paravaginal defect repair (including repair of cystocele, stress urinary incontinence, and/or incomplete vaginal prolapse)

57287 Removal or revision of sling for stress incontinence (eg, fascia or synthetic)

57288 Sling operation for stress incontinence (eg, fascia or synthetic)

(For laparoscopic approach, use 51992)

57289 Pereyra procedure, including anterior colporrhaphy

57291 Construction of artificial vagina; without graft

57292   with graft

57300 Closure of rectovaginal fistula; vaginal or transanal approach

57305   abdominal approach

57307   abdominal approach, with concomitant colostomy

57308   transperineal approach, with perineal body reconstruction, with or without levator plication

57310 Closure of urethrovaginal fistula;

57311   with bulbocavernosus transplant

57320 Closure of vesicovaginal fistula; vaginal approach

542

● New Code   ▲ Revised Code   + Add-On Code   ⊘ Modifier -51 Exempt

(For concomitant cystostomy, see 51005-51040)

57330   transvesical and vaginal approach

(For abdominal approach, use 51900)

57335   Vaginoplasty for intersex state

MANIPULATION

57400   Dilation of vagina under anesthesia

57410   Pelvic examination under anesthesia

57415   Removal of impacted vaginal foreign body (separate procedure) under anesthesia

(For removal without anesthesia of an impacted vaginal foreign body, use the appropriate E/M code)

ENDOSCOPY

(For speculoscopy, see Category III codes 0030T, 0031T)

57420   Colposcopy of the entire vagina, with cervix if present;

57421   with biopsy(s)

(For colposcopic visualization of cervix and adjacent upper vagina, use 57452)

(When reporting colposcopies of multiple sites, use modifier '-51' as appropriate. For colposcopic examinations/procedures involving the vulva, see 56820, 56821; cervix, see 57452-57461)

● **57425**   Laparoscopy, surgical, colpopexy (suspension of vaginal apex)

CERVIX UTERI

(For cervicography, see Category III code 0003T)

ENDOSCOPY

(For colposcopic examinations/procedures involving the vulva, see 56820, 56821; vagina, see 57420, 57421)

57452   Colposcopy of the cervix including upper/adjacent vagina

(Do not report 57452 in addition to 57454-57461)

543

| Separate Procedure | Unlisted Procedure | CCI Comp. Code | Non-specific Procedure |

57454	with biopsy(s) of the cervix and endocervical curettage
57455	with biopsy(s) of the cervix
57456	with endocervical curettage
57460	with loop electrode biopsy(s) of the cervix
57461	with loop electrode conization of the cervix

(Do not report 57456 in addition to 57461)

EXCISION

(For radical surgical procedures, see 58200-58240)

57500 Biopsy, single or multiple, or local excision of lesion, with or without fulguration (separate procedure)

57505 Endocervical curettage (not done as part of a dilation and curettage)

57510 Cautery of cervix; electro or thermal

57511 cryocautery, initial or repeat

57513 laser ablation

57520 Conization of cervix, with or without fulguration, with or without dilation and curettage, with or without repair; cold knife or laser

(See also 58120)

57522 loop electrode excision

57530 Trachelectomy (cervicectomy), amputation of cervix (separate procedure)

57531 Radical trachelectomy, with bilateral total pelvic lymphadenectomy and para-aortic lymph node sampling biopsy, with or without removal of tube(s), with or without removal of ovary(s)

(For radical abdominal hysterectomy, use 58210)

57540 Excision of cervical stump, abdominal approach;

57545   with pelvic floor repair

57550 Excision of cervical stump, vaginal approach;

57555   with anterior and/or posterior repair

57556   with repair of enterocele

(For insertion of intrauterine device, use 58300)

REPAIR

57700 Cerclage of uterine cervix, nonobstetrical

57720 Trachelorrhaphy, plastic repair of uterine cervix, vaginal approach

MANIPULATION

57800 Dilation of cervical canal, instrumental (separate procedure)

57820 Dilation and curettage of cervical stump

CORPUS UTERI

EXCISION

58100 Endometrial sampling (biopsy) with or without endocervical sampling (biopsy), without cervical dilation, any method (separate procedure)

(For endocervical curettage only, use 57505)

58120 Dilation and curettage, diagnostic and/or therapeutic (nonobstetrical)

(For postpartum hemorrhage, use 59160)

58140 Myomectomy, excision of fibroid tumor(s) of uterus, 1 to 4 intramural myoma(s) with total weight of 250 grams or less and/or removal of surface myomas; abdominal approach

58145   vaginal approach

58146 Myomectomy, excision of fibroid tumor(s) of uterus, 5 or more intramural myomas and/or intramural myomas with total weight greater than 250 grams, abdominal approach

545

 Separate Procedure   Unlisted Procedure   CCI Comp. Code   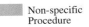 Non-specific Procedure

(Do not report 58146 in addition to 58140-58145, 58150-58240)

58150 Total abdominal hysterectomy (corpus and cervix), with or without removal of tube(s), with or without removal of ovary(s);

58152   with colpo-urethrocystopexy (eg, Marshall-Marchetti-Krantz, Burch)

(For urethrocystopexy without hysterectomy, see 51840, 51841)

58180 Supracervical abdominal hysterectomy (subtotal hysterectomy), with or without removal of tube(s), with or without removal of ovary(s)

58200 Total abdominal hysterectomy, including partial vaginectomy, with para-aortic and pelvic lymph node sampling, with or without removal of tube(s), with or without removal of ovary(s)

58210 Radical abdominal hysterectomy, with bilateral total pelvic lymphadenectomy and para-aortic lymph node sampling (biopsy), with or without removal of tube(s), with or without removal of ovary(s)

(For radical hysterectomy with ovarian transposition, use also 58825)

58240 Pelvic exenteration for gynecologic malignancy, with total abdominal hysterectomy or cervicectomy, with or without removal of tube(s), with or without removal of ovary(s), with removal of bladder and ureteral transplantations, and/or abdominoperineal resection of rectum and colon and colostomy, or any combination thereof

(For pelvic exenteration for lower urinary tract or male genital malignancy, use 51597)

58260 Vaginal hysterectomy, for uterus 250 grams or less;

58262   with removal of tube(s), and/or ovary(s)

58263   with removal of tube(s), and/or ovary(s), with repair of enterocele

58267   with colpo-urethrocystopexy (Marshall-Marchetti-Krantz type, Pereyra type) with or without endoscopic control

58270   with repair of enterocele

546

● New Code   ▲ Revised Code   + Add-On Code   ⊘ Modifier -51 Exempt

(For repair of enterocele with removal of tubes and/or ovaries, use 58263)

58275 Vaginal hysterectomy, with total or partial vaginectomy;

58280   with repair of enterocele

58285 Vaginal hysterectomy, radical (Schauta type operation)

58290 Vaginal hysterectomy, for uterus greater than 250 grams;

58291   with removal of tube(s) and/or ovary(s)

58292   with removal of tube(s) and/or ovary(s), with repair of enterocele

58293   with colpo-urethrocystopexy (Marshall-Marchetti-Krantz type, Pereyra type) with or without endoscopic control

58294   with repair of enterocele

INTRODUCTION

(For insertion/removal of implantable contraceptive capsules, see 11975, 11976, 11977)

58300 Insertion of intrauterine device (IUD)

58301 Removal of intrauterine device (IUD)

58321 Artificial insemination; intra-cervical

58322   intra-uterine

58323 Sperm washing for artificial insemination

▲ **58340** Catheterization and introduction of saline or contrast material for saline infusion sonohysterography (SIS) or hysterosalpingography

(For radiological supervision and interpretation of saline infusion sonohysterography, use 76831)

(For radiological supervision and interpretation of hysterosalpingography, use 74740)

(For endometrial cryoablation with ultrasonic guidance, use Category III code 0009T)

547

| Separate Procedure | Unlisted Procedure |  CCI Comp. Code | Non-specific Procedure |

58345   Transcervical introduction of fallopian tube catheter for diagnosis and/or re-establishing patency (any method), with or without hysterosalpingography

(For radiological supervision and interpretation, use 74742)

58346   Insertion of Heyman capsules for clinical brachytherapy

(For insertion of radioelement sources or ribbons, see 77761-77763, 77781-77784)

58350   Chromotubation of oviduct, including materials

(For materials supplied by physician, use 99070)

58353   Endometrial ablation, thermal, without hysteroscopic guidance

(For hysteroscopic procedure, use 58563)

REPAIR

58400   Uterine suspension, with or without shortening of round ligaments, with or without shortening of sacrouterine ligaments; (separate procedure)

58410   with presacral sympathectomy

58520   Hysterorrhaphy, repair of ruptured uterus (nonobstetrical)

58540   Hysteroplasty, repair of uterine anomaly (Strassman type)

(For closure of vesicouterine fistula, use 51920)

LAPAROSCOPY-HYSTEROSCOPY

The descriptions of CPT codes in this section are listed so that the main procedure can be identified without having to list all of the minor related procedures performed at the same time. For example:

58558   Hysterscopy, surgical; with sampling (biopsy) of endometrium and/or polypectomy, with or without D & C

The secondary procedure(s) is/are included in the single code 58558. If any of the secondary procedures require significant additional time and effort, to the point of making the procedure "unusual," modifier -22 should be added with an appropriate increase in fee and a report explaining why the procedure was unusual.

● New Code   ▲ Revised Code   + Add-On Code   ⊘ Modifier -51 Exempt

58545 Laparoscopy, surgical, myomectomy, excision; 1 to 4 intramural myomas with total weight of 250 grams or less and/or removal of surface myomas

58546 5 or more intramural myomas and/or intramural myomas with total weight greater than 250 grams

58550 Laparoscopy, surgical with vaginal hysterectomy, for uterus 250 grams or less;

(58551 deleted 2003 edition. To report see 58545, 58546)

58552 with removal of tube(s) and/or ovary(s)

58553 Laparoscopy, surgical, with vaginal hysterectomy, for uterus greater than 250 grams;

58554 with removal of tube(s) and/or ovary(s)

58555 Hysteroscopy, diagnostic (separate procedure)

58558 Hysteroscopy, surgical; with sampling (biopsy) of endometrium and/or polypectomy, with or without D & C

58559 with lysis of intrauterine adhesions (any method)

58560 with division or resection of intrauterine septum (any method)

58561 with removal of leiomyomata

58562 with removal of impacted foreign body

58563 with endometrial ablation (eg, endometrial resection, electrosurgical ablation, thermoablation)

58578 Unlisted laparoscopy procedure, uterus

58579 Unlisted hysteroscopy procedure, uterus

OVIDUCT/OVARY

INCISION

58600 Ligation or transection of fallopian tube(s), abdominal or vaginal approach, unilateral or bilateral

549

 Separate Procedure

 Unlisted Procedure

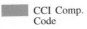 CCI Comp. Code

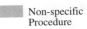 Non-specific Procedure

58605 Ligation or transection of fallopian tube(s), abdominal or vaginal approach, postpartum, unilateral or bilateral, during same hospitalization (separate procedure)

(For laparoscopic procedures, use 58670, 58671)

+ 58611 Ligation or transection of fallopian tube(s) when done at the time of cesarean delivery or intra-abdominal surgery (not a separate procedure) (List separately in addition to code for primary procedure)

58615 Occlusion of fallopian tube(s) by device (eg, band, clip, Falope ring) vaginal or suprapubic approach

(For laparoscopic approach, use 58671)

LAPAROSCOPY

(For laparoscopic biopsy of the ovary or fallopian tube, use 49321)

58660 Laparoscopy, surgical; with lysis of adhesions (salpingolysis, ovariolysis) (separate procedure)

58661 with removal of adnexal structures (partial or total oophorectomy and/or salpingectomy)

58662 with fulguration or excision of lesions of the ovary, pelvic viscera, or peritoneal surface by any method

58670 with fulguration of oviducts (with or without transection)

58671 with occlusion of oviducts by device (eg, band, clip, or Falope ring)

58672 with fimbrioplasty

58673 with salpingostomy (salpingoneostomy)

(Codes 58672 and 58673 are used to report unilateral procedures. For bilateral procedure, use modifier -50)

58679 Unlisted laparoscopy procedure, oviduct, ovary

EXCISION

58700 Salpingectomy, complete or partial, unilateral or bilateral (separate procedure)

● New Code ▲ Revised Code + Add-On Code ⊘ Modifier -51 Exempt

58720 Salpingo-oophorectomy, complete or partial, unilateral or bilateral (separate procedure)

REPAIR

58740 Lysis of adhesions (salpingolysis, ovariolysis)

(For laparoscopic approach, use 58660)

(For excision or destruction of endometriomas, open method, see 49200, 49201)

(For fulguration or excision of lesions, laparscopic approach, use 58662)

58750 Tubotubal anastomosis

58752 Tubouterine implantation

58760 Fimbrioplasty

(For laparoscopic approach, use 58672)

58770 Salpingostomy (salpingoneostomy)

(For laparscopic approach, use 58673)

OVARY

INCISION

58800 Drainage of ovarian cyst(s), unilateral or bilateral, (separate procedure); vaginal approach

58805 abdominal approach

58820 Drainage of ovarian abscess; vaginal approach, open

58822 abdominal approach

58823 Drainage of pelvic abscess, transvaginal or transrectal approach, percutaneous (eg, ovarian, pericolic)

(For radiological supervision and interpretation, use 75989)

58825 Transposition, ovary(s)

551

 Separate Procedure    Unlisted Procedure   CCI Comp. Code   Non-specific Procedure

EXCISION

58900 Biopsy of ovary, unilateral or bilateral (separate procedure)

(For laparoscopic biopsy of the ovary or fallopian tube, use 49321)

58920 Wedge resection or bisection of ovary, unilateral or bilateral

58925 Ovarian cystectomy, unilateral or bilateral

58940 Oophorectomy, partial or total, unilateral or bilateral;

58943 for ovarian, tubal or primary peritoneal malignancy, with para-aortic and pelvic lymph node biopsies, peritoneal washings, peritoneal biopsies, diaphragmatic assessments, with or without salpingectomy(s), with or without omentectomy

58950 Resection of ovarian, tubal or primary peritoneal malignancy with bilateral salpingo-oophorectomy and omentectomy;

58951 with total abdominal hysterectomy, pelvic and limited para-aortic lymphadenectomy

58952 with radical dissection for debulking (ie, radical excision or destruction, intra-abdominal or retroperitoneal tumors)

58953 Bilateral salpingo-oophorectomy with omentectomy, total abdominal hysterectomy and radical dissection for debulking;

58954 with pelvic lymphadenectomy and limited para-aortic lymphadenectomy

58960 Laparotomy, for staging or restaging of ovarian, tubal or primary peritoneal malignancy (second look), with or without omentectomy, peritoneal washing, biopsy of abdominal and pelvic peritoneum, diaphragmatic assessment with pelvic and limited para-aortic lymphadenectomy

IN VITRO FERTILIZATION

58970 Follicle puncture for oocyte retrieval, any method

(For radiological supervision and interpretation, use 76948)

58974 Embryo transfer, intrauterine

● New Code   ▲ Revised Code   + Add-On Code   ⊘ Modifier -51 Exempt

58976 Gamete, zygote, or embryo intrafallopian transfer, any method

OTHER PROCEDURES

58999 Unlisted procedure, female genital system (nonobstetrical)

	Separate Procedure		Unlisted Procedure		CCI Comp. Code		Non-specific Procedure

This page intentionally left blank.

● New
Code

▲ Revised
Code

+ Add-On
Code

⊘ Modifier -51
Exempt

MATERNITY CARE AND DELIVERY

CPT codes from this section are used to report routine maternity care and invasive and surgical procedures performed as part of prenatal, delivery and post-partum care. The services normally provided in uncomplicated maternity cases include antepartum care, delivery, and postpartum care.

ANTEPARTUM CARE

The definition of antepartum care for coding purposes includes the initial and subsequent history, physical examinations, recording of weight, blood pressures, fetal heart tones, routine chemical urinalysis, and routine visits. Routine antepartum visits are defined as:

- *Monthly visits up to 28 weeks gestation*

- *Biweekly visits up to 36 weeks gestation, and*

- *Weekly visits until delivery*

Any other visits or services provided within this time period should be coded separately. Using 6 to 8 weeks gestation as the typical starting point, the above definition translates into between 9 and 11 routine visits per patient.

DELIVERY

Delivery services are defined as including hospital admission, the admission history and physical examination, management of uncomplicated labor, and vaginal or cesarean delivery.

- *The definition of delivery services includes the hospital admission, and admission history and physical.*

- *Resuscitation of newborn infants when necessary, defined in previous editions, is not included in the delivery services. If the delivering physician has to resuscitate the newborn infant, he/she may code this service as a separate procedure.*

- *Medical problems "complicating labor and delivery management" may require additional resources and should be reported using evaluation and management service codes.*

555

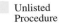 Separate Procedure   Unlisted Procedure   CCI Comp. Code   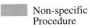 Non-specific Procedure

POSTPARTUM CARE

Postpartum care is defined as hospital and office visits following vaginal or cesarean delivery. No number of visits is defined by CPT; however, the typical fee for total obstetrical care includes a single office follow-up visit six weeks postpartum.

COMPLICATIONS OF PREGNANCY

The services defined previously are for normal, uncomplicated maternity care. For medical complications of pregnancy, for example, cardiac problems, neurological problems, diabetes, hypertension, toxemia, hyperemesis, pre-term labor and premature rupture of membranes, use evaluation and management service codes.

For surgical complications of pregnancy, such as appendectomy, hernia, ovarian cyst, Bartholin cysts, etc., use CPT codes from the SURGERY section of CPT. Note that in either case, complications are not considered to be part of routine maternity care and should be coded and reported in addition to maternity CPT codes.

PARTIAL MATERNITY SERVICES

Occasionally a physician may provide all or part of the antepartum and/or postpartum care but does not perform the actual delivery due to termination of the pregnancy by abortion, or referral to another physician for delivery. In this circumstance, the physician has the option of using the inclusive CPT codes 59420 or 59430 from the Maternity Care and Delivery section reporting each visit using evaluation and management service codes 99201-99215.

MISCELLANEOUS CODING RULES

Obstetric care can be coded as a global package or can be broken down when necessary into antepartum, delivery and postpartum care.

Complicated pregnancies and deliveries need to be coded appropriately to indicate the increased work on the physician's part during the patient's care. There are several options for recording these circumstances.

(For circumcision of newborn, see 54150, 54160)

ANTEPARTUM SERVICES

(For insertion of transcervical or transvaginal fetal oximetry sensor, use Category III code 0021T)

59000 Amniocentesis, diagnostic

(For radiological supervision and interpretation, use 76946)

| ● | New Code | ▲ | Revised Code | + | Add-On Code | ⊘ | Modifier -51 Exempt |

59001   therapeutic amniotic fluid reduction (includes ultrasound guidance)

59012 Cordocentesis (intrauterine), any method

(For radiological supervision and interpretation, use 76941)

59015 Chorionic villus sampling, any method

(For radiological supervision and interpretation, use 76945)

59020 Fetal contraction stress test

59025 Fetal non-stress test

59030 Fetal scalp blood sampling

59050 Fetal monitoring during labor by consulting physician (ie, non-attending physician) with written report; supervision and interpretation

59051   interpretation only

● **59070** Transabdominal amnioinfusion, including ultrasound guidance

● **59072** Fetal umbilical cord occlusion, including ultrasound guidance

● **59074** Fetal fluid drainage (eg, vesicocentesis, thoracocentesis, paracentesis), including ultrasound guidance

● **59076** Fetal shunt placement, including ultrasound guidance

(For unlisted fetal invasive procedure, use 59897)

EXCISION

59100 Hysterotomy, abdominal (eg, for hydatidiform mole, abortion)

(When tubal ligation is performed at the same time as hysterotomy, use 58611 in addition to 59100)

59120 Surgical treatment of ectopic pregnancy; tubal or ovarian, requiring salpingectomy and/or oophorectomy, abdominal or vaginal approach

59121   tubal or ovarian, without salpingectomy and/or oophorectomy

557

| ▮ Separate Procedure | ▮ Unlisted Procedure |  CCI Comp. Code | Non-specific Procedure |

59130 abdominal pregnancy

59135 interstitial, uterine pregnancy requiring total hysterectomy

59136 interstitial, uterine pregnancy with partial resection of uterus

59140 cervical, with evacuation

59150 Laparoscopic treatment of ectopic pregnancy; without salpingectomy and/or oophorectomy

59151 with salpingectomy and/or oophorectomy

59160 Curettage, postpartum

INTRODUCTION

(For intrauterine fetal transfusion, use 36460)

(For introduction of hypertonic solution and/or prostaglandins to initiate labor, see 59850-59857)

59200 Insertion of cervical dilator (eg, laminaria, prostaglandin) (separate procedure)

REPAIR

(For tracheoplasty, use 57700)

59300 Episiotomy or vaginal repair, by other than attending physician

59320 Cerclage of cervix, during pregnancy; vaginal

59325 abdominal

59350 Hysterorrhaphy of ruptured uterus

VAGINAL DELIVERY, ANTEPARTUM AND POSTPARTUM CARE

(For insertion of transcervical or transvaginal fetal oximetry sensor, use Category III code 0021T)

59400 Routine obstetric care including antepartum care, vaginal delivery (with or without episiotomy, and/or forceps) and postpartum care

59409 Vaginal delivery only (with or without episiotomy and/or forceps);

59410   including postpartum care

59412 External cephalic version, with or without tocolysis

(Use 59412 in addition to code(s) for delivery)

59414 Delivery of placenta (separate procedure)

(For 1-3 antepartum care visits, see appropriate E/M code(s))

59425 Antepartum care only; 4-6 visits

59426   7 or more visits

59430 Postpartum care only (separate procedure)

CESAREAN DELIVERY

(For standby attendance for infant, use 99360)

(For insertion of transcervical or transvaginal fetal oximetry sensor, use Category III code 0021T)

59510 Routine obstetric care including antepartum care, cesarean delivery, and postpartum care

59514 Cesarean delivery only;

59515   including postpartum care

+ **59525** Subtotal or total hysterectomy after cesarean delivery (List separately in addition to code for primary procedure)

(Use 59525 in conjunction with codes 59510, 59514, 59515, 59618, 59620, 59622)

DELIVERY AFTER PREVIOUS CESAREAN DELIVERY

(For insertion of transcervical or transvaginal fetal oximetry sensor, use Category III code 0021T)

59610 Routine obstetric care including antepartum care, vaginal delivery (with or without episiotomy, and/or forceps) and postpartum care, after previous cesarean delivery

559

 Separate Procedure    Unlisted Procedure   CCI Comp. Code   Non-specific Procedure

| 59612 | Vaginal delivery only, after previous cesarean delivery (with or without episiotomy and/or forceps); |

59614   including postpartum care

59618 Routine obstetric care including antepartum care, cesarean delivery, and postpartum care, following attempted vaginal delivery after previous cesarean delivery

59620 Cesarean delivery only, following attempted vaginal delivery after previous cesarean delivery;

59622   including postpartum care

ABORTION

(For medical treatment of spontaneous complete abortion, any trimester, use E/M codes 99201-99233)

59812 Treatment of incomplete abortion, any trimester, completed surgically

59820 Treatment of missed abortion, completed surgically; first trimester

59821   second trimester

59830 Treatment of septic abortion, completed surgically

59840 Induced abortion, by dilation and curettage

59841 Induced abortion, by dilation and evacuation

59850 Induced abortion, by one or more intra-amniotic injections (amniocentesis-injections), including hospital admission and visits, delivery of fetus and secundines;

59851   with dilation and curettage and/or evacuation

59852   with hysterotomy (failed intra-amniotic injection)

(For insertion of cervical dilator, use 59200)

59855 Induced abortion, by one or more vaginal suppositories (eg, prostaglandin) with or without cervical dilation (eg, laminaria), including hospital admission and visits, delivery of fetus and secundines;

560   ● New Code   ▲ Revised Code   **+** Add-On Code   ⊘ Modifier -51 Exempt

59856   with dilation and curettage and/or evacuation

59857   with hysterotomy (failed medical evacuation)

OTHER PROCEDURES

59866   Multifetal pregnancy reduction(s) (MPR)

59870   Uterine evacuation and curettage for hydatidiform mole

59871   Removal of cerclage suture under anesthesia (other than local)

● **59897**   Unlisted fetal invasive procedure, including ultrasound guidance

59898   Unlisted laparoscopy procedure, maternity care and delivery

59899   Unlisted procedure, maternity care and delivery

| | Separate Procedure | | Unlisted Procedure | | CCI Comp. Code | | Non-specific Procedure |

This page intentionally left blank.

● New
Code

▲ Revised
Code

✛ Add-On
Code

⊘ Modifier -51
Exempt

ENDOCRINE SYSTEM

CPT codes from this section of CPT are used to report invasive and surgical procedures performed on the thyroid gland, parathyroid, thymus, adrenal glands and carotid body.

(For pituitary and pineal surgery, see Nervous System)

THYROID GLAND

INCISION

60000 Incision and drainage of thyroglossal duct cyst, infected

EXCISION

60001 Aspiration and/or injection, thyroid cyst

(For fine needle aspiration, see 10021, 10022)

(If imaging guidance is performed, see 76360, 76942)

60100 Biopsy thyroid, percutaneous core needle

(If imaging guidance is performed, see 76003, 76360, 76393, 76942)

(For fine needle aspiration, use 10021 or 10022)

(For evaluation of fine needle aspirate, see 88172, 88173)

60200 Excision of cyst or adenoma of thyroid, or transection of isthmus

60210 Partial thyroid lobectomy, unilateral; with or without isthmusectomy

60212 with contralateral subtotal lobectomy, including isthmusectomy

60220 Total thyroid lobectomy, unilateral; with or without isthmusectomy

60225 with contralateral subtotal lobectomy, including isthmusectomy

60240 Thyroidectomy, total or complete

563

 Separate Procedure   Unlisted Procedure    CCI Comp. Code   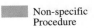 Non-specific Procedure

| 60252 | Thyroidectomy, total or subtotal for malignancy; with limited neck dissection |

| 60254 | with radical neck dissection |

| 60260 | Thyroidectomy, removal of all remaining thyroid tissue following previous removal of a portion of thyroid |

| 60270 | Thyroidectomy, including substernal thyroid; sternal split or transthoracic approach |

| 60271 | cervical approach |

| 60280 | Excision of thyroglossal duct cyst or sinus; |

| 60281 | recurrent |

(For thyroid ultrasonography, use 76536)

PARATHYROID, THYMUS, ADRENAL GLANDS, PANCREAS, AND CAROTID BODY

EXCISION

(For pituitary and pineal surgery, see Nervous System)

| 60500 | Parathyroidectomy or exploration of parathyroid(s); |

| 60502 | re-exploration |

| 60505 | with mediastinal exploration, sternal split or transthoracic approach |

+ **60512** Parathyroid autotransplantation (List separately in addition to code for primary procedure)

(Use 60512 in conjunction with codes 60500, 60502, 60505, 60212, 60225, 60240, 60252, 60254, 60260, 60270, 60271)

| 60520 | Thymectomy, partial or total; transcervical approach (separate procedure) |

| 60521 | sternal split or transthoracic approach, without radical mediastinal dissection (separate procedure) |

| 60522 | sternal split or transthoracic approach, with radical mediastinal dissection (separate procedure) |

● New Code   ▲ Revised Code   + Add-On Code   ⊘ Modifier -51 Exempt

60540 Adrenalectomy, partial or complete, or exploration of adrenal gland with or without biopsy, transabdominal, lumbar or dorsal (separate procedure);

60545 with excision of adjacent retroperitoneal tumor

(For excision of remote or disseminated pheochromocytoma, see 49200, 49201)

(For laparoscopic approach, use 56321)

60600 Excision of carotid body tumor; without excision of carotid artery

60605 with excision of carotid artery

LAPAROSCOPY

60650 Laparoscopy, surgical, with adrenalectomy, partial or complete, or exploration of adrenal gland with or without biopsy, transabdominal, lumbar or dorsal

60659 Unlisted laparoscopy procedure, endocrine system

OTHER PROCEDURES

60699 Unlisted procedure, endocrine system

 Separate Procedure   Unlisted Procedure   CCI Comp. Code   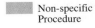 Non-specific Procedure

This page intentionally left blank.

● New
Code

▲ Revised
Code

✚ Add-On
Code

⊘ Modifier -51
Exempt

NERVOUS SYSTEM

CPT codes from this section of the CPT coding system are used to report invasive and surgical procedures on the skull; meninges and brain; spine and spinal cord; and the extracranial nerves, peripheral nerves and autonomic nervous system.

There are numerous codes for spinal injections found in this section. Review documentation for whether the injection is a single one, differential one or continuous. Also determine the number of levels involved when a regional block is administered.

CNS
61000

SKULL, MENINGES, AND BRAIN

(For injection procedure for cerebral angiography, see 36100-36218)

(For injection procedure for ventriculography, see 61026, 61120, 61130)

(For injection procedure for pneumoencephalography, use 61055)

INJECTION, DRAINAGE OR ASPIRATION

61000 Subdural tap through fontanelle, or suture, infant, unilateral or bilateral; initial

61001 subsequent taps

61020 Ventricular puncture through previous burr hole, fontanelle, suture, or implanted ventricular catheter/reservoir; without injection

61026 with injection of medication or other substance for diagnosis or treatment

61050 Cisternal or lateral cervical (C1-C2) puncture; without injection (separate procedure)

61055 with injection of medication or other substance for diagnosis or treatment (eg, C1-C2)

(For radiological supervision and interpretation, see Radiology)

61070 Puncture of shunt tubing or reservoir for aspiration or injection procedure

567

 Separate Procedure

 Unlisted Procedure

 CCI Comp. Code

 Non-specific Procedure

(For radiological supervision and interpretation, use 75809)

TWIST DRILL, BURR HOLE(S), OR TREPHINE

61105 Twist drill hole for subdural or ventricular puncture;

⊘ **61107** for implanting ventricular catheter or pressure recording device

(For intracranial neuroendoscopic ventricular catheter placement, use 62160)

61108 for evacuation and/or drainage of subdural hematoma

61120 Burr hole(s) for ventricular puncture (including injection of gas, contrast media, dye, or radioactive material)

61140 Burr hole(s) or trephine; with biopsy of brain or intracranial lesion

61150 with drainage of brain abscess or cyst

61151 with subsequent tapping (aspiration) of intracranial abscess or cyst

61154 Burr hole(s) with evacuation and/or drainage of hematoma, extradural or subdural

61156 Burr hole(s); with aspiration of hematoma or cyst, intracerebral

⊘ **61210** for implanting ventricular catheter, reservoir, EEG electrode(s) or pressure recording device (separate procedure)

(For intracranial neuroendoscopic ventricular catheter placement, use 62160)

61215 Insertion of subcutaneous reservoir, pump or continuous infusion system for connection to ventricular catheter

(For refilling and maintenance of an implantable infusion pump for spinal or brain drug therapy, use 95990)

(For chemotherapy, use 96450)

61250 Burr hole(s) or trephine, supratentorial, exploratory, not followed by other surgery

● New Code   ▲ Revised Code   + Add-On Code   ⊘ Modifier -51 Exempt

61253 Burr hole(s) or trephine, infratentorial, unilateral or bilateral

(If burr hole(s) or trephine are followed by craniotomy at same operative session, use 61304-61321; do not use 61250 or 61253)

CRANIECTOMY OR CRANIOTOMY

61304 Craniectomy or craniotomy, exploratory; supratentorial

61305 infratentorial (posterior fossa)

61312 Craniectomy or craniotomy for evacuation of hematoma, supratentorial; extradural or subdural

61313 intracerebral

61314 Craniectomy or craniotomy for evacuation of hematoma, infratentorial; extradural or subdural

61315 intracerebellar

+ **61316** Incision and subcutaneous placement of cranial bone graft (List separately in addition to code for primary procedure)

(Use 61316 in conjunction with codes 61304, 61312, 61313, 61322, 61323, 61340, 31570, 31571, 61680-61705)

61320 Craniectomy or craniotomy, drainage of intracranial abscess; supratentorial

61321 infratentorial

61322 Craniectomy or craniotomy, decompressive, with or without duraplasty, for treatment of intracranial hypertension, without evacuation of associated intraparenchymal hematoma; without lobectomy

(Do not report 61313 in addition to 61322)

(For subtemporal decompression, use 61340)

61323 with lobectomy

(Do not report 61313 in addition to 61323)

(For subtemporal decompression, use 61340)

61330 Decompression of orbit only, transcranial approach

569

 Separate Procedure   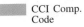 Unlisted Procedure   CCI Comp. Code   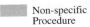 Non-specific Procedure

61332 Exploration of orbit (transcranial approach); with biopsy

61333   with removal of lesion

61334   with removal of foreign body

61340 Subtemporal cranial decompression (pseudotumor cerebri, slit ventricle syndrome)

(For decompressive craniotomy or craniectomy for intracranial hypertension, without hematoma evacuation, see 61322, 61323)

61343 Craniectomy, suboccipital with cervical laminectomy for decompression of medulla and spinal cord, with or without dural graft (eg, Arnold-Chiari malformation)

61345 Other cranial decompression, posterior fossa

(For orbital decompression by lateral wall approach, Kroenlein type, use 67445)

61440 Craniotomy for section of tentorium cerebelli (separate procedure)

61450 Craniectomy, subtemporal, for section, compression, or decompression of sensory root of gasserian ganglion

61458 Craniectomy, suboccipital; for exploration or decompression of cranial nerves

61460   for section of one or more cranial nerves

61470   for medullary tractotomy

61480   for mesencephalic tractotomy or pedunculotomy

61490 Craniotomy for lobotomy, including cingulotomy

61500 Craniectomy; with excision of tumor or other bone lesion of skull

61501   for osteomyelitis

61510 Craniectomy, trephination, bone flap craniotomy; for excision of brain tumor, supratentorial, except meningioma

61512   for excision of meningioma, supratentorial

570

| ● | New Code | ▲ | Revised Code | + | Add-On Code | ⊘ | Modifier -51 Exempt |

61514   for excision of brain abscess, supratentorial

61516   for excision or fenestration of cyst, supratentorial

(For excision of pituitary tumor or craniopharyngioma, see 61545, 61546, 61548)

+ **61517**   Implantation of brain intracavitary chemotherapy agent (List separately in addition to code for primary procedure)

(Use 61517 only in conjunction with codes 61510 or 61518)

(Do not report 61517 for brachytherapy insertion. For intracavitary insertion of radioelement sources or ribbons, see 77781-77784)

61518   Craniectomy for excision of brain tumor, infratentorial or posterior fossa; except meningioma, cerebellopontine angle tumor, or midline tumor at base of skull

61519   meningioma

61520   cerebellopontine angle tumor

61521   midline tumor at base of skull

61522   Craniectomy, infratentorial or posterior fossa; for excision of brain abscess

61524   for excision or fenestration of cyst

61526   Craniectomy, bone flap craniotomy, transtemporal (mastoid) for excision of cerebellopontine angle tumor;

61530   combined with middle/posterior fossa craniotomy/craniectomy

61531   Subdural implantation of strip electrodes through one or more burr or trephine hole(s) for long term seizure monitoring

(For stereotactic implantation of electrodes, use 61760)

61533   Craniotomy with elevation of bone flap; for subdural implantation of an electrode array, for long term seizure monitoring

(For continuous EEG monitoring, see 95950-95954)

571

 Separate Procedure   Unlisted Procedure   CCI Comp. Code   Non-specific Procedure

61534   for excision of epileptogenic focus without electrocorticography during surgery

61535   for removal of epidural or subdural electrode array, without excision of cerebral tissue (separate procedure)

61536   for excision of cerebral epileptogenic focus, with electrocorticography during surgery (includes removal of electrode array)

● **61537**   for lobectomy, temporal lobe, without electrocorticography during surgery

▲ **61538**   for lobectomy, temporal lobe, with electrocorticography during surgery

▲ **61539**   for lobectomy, other than temporal lobe, partial or total, with electrocorticography during surgery

● **61540**   for lobectomy, other than temporal lobe, partial or total, without electrocorticography during surgery

61541   for transection of corpus callosum

61542   for total hemispherectomy

▲ **61543**   for partial or subtotal (functional) hemispherectomy

61544   for excision or coagulation of choroid plexus

61545   for excision of craniopharyngioma

(For craniotomy for selective amygdalohippocampectomy, use 61566)

(For craniotomy for multiple subpial transections during surgery, use 61567)

61546 Craniotomy for hypophysectomy or excision of pituitary tumor, intracranial approach

61548 Hypophysectomy or excision of pituitary tumor, transnasal or transseptal approach, nonstereotactic

(Do not report code 69990 in addition to code 61548)

61550 Craniectomy for craniosynostosis; single cranial suture

● New Code   ▲ Revised Code   + Add-On Code   ⊘ Modifier -51 Exempt

61552   multiple cranial sutures

(For cranial reconstruction for orbital hypertelorism, see 21260-21263)

61556 Craniotomy for craniosynostosis; frontal or parietal bone flap

61557   bifrontal bone flap

61558 Extensive craniectomy for multiple cranial suture craniosynostosis (eg, cloverleaf skull); not requiring bone grafts

61559   recontouring with multiple osteotomies and bone autografts (eg, barrel-stave procedure) (includes obtaining grafts)

61563 Excision, intra and extracranial, benign tumor of cranial bone (eg, fibrous dysplasia); without optic nerve decompression

61564   with optic nerve decompression

(For reconstruction, see 21181-21183)

● **61566** Craniotomy with elevation of bone flap; for selective amygdalohippocampectomy

● **61567**   for multiple subpial transections, with electrocorticography during surgery

61570 Craniectomy or craniotomy; with excision of foreign body from brain

61571   with treatment of penetrating wound of brain

(For sequestrectomy for osteomyelitis, use 61501)

61575 Transoral approach to skull base, brain stem or upper spinal cord for biopsy, decompression or excision of lesion;

61576   requiring splitting of tongue and/or mandible (including tracheostomy)

(For arthrodesis, use 22548)

573

 Separate Procedure   Unlisted Procedure   CCI Comp. Code   Non-specific Procedure

APPROACH PROCEDURES

Anterior Cranial Fossa

61580   Craniofacial approach to anterior cranial fossa; extradural, including lateral rhinotomy, ethmoidectomy, sphenoidectomy, without maxillectomy or orbital exenteration

61581   extradural, including lateral rhinotomy, orbital exenteration, ethmoidectomy, sphenoidectomy and/or maxillectomy

61582   extradural, including unilateral or bifrontal craniotomy, elevation of frontal lobe(s), osteotomy of base of anterior cranial fossa

61583   intradural, including unilateral or bifrontal craniotomy, elevation or resection of frontal lobe, osteotomy of base of anterior cranial fossa

61584   Orbitocranial approach to anterior cranial fossa, extradural, including supraorbital ridge osteotomy and elevation of frontal and/or temporal lobe(s); without orbital exenteration

61585   with orbital exenteration

61586   Bicoronal, transzygomatic and/or LeFort I osteotomy approach to anterior cranial fossa with or without internal fixation, without bone graft

Middle Cranial Fossa

61590   Infratemporal pre-auricular approach to middle cranial fossa (parapharyngeal space, infratemporal and midline skull base, nasopharynx), with or without disarticulation of the mandible, including parotidectomy, craniotomy, decompression and/or mobilization of the facial nerve and/or petrous carotid artery

61591   Infratemporal post-auricular approach to middle cranial fossa (internal auditory meatus, petrous apex, tentorium, cavernous sinus, parasellar area, infratemporal fossa) including mastoidectomy, resection of sigmoid sinus, with or without decompression and/or mobilization of contents of auditory canal or petrous carotid artery

61592   Orbitocranial zygomatic approach to middle cranial fossa (cavernous sinus and carotid artery, clivus, basilar artery or petrous apex) including osteotomy of zygoma, craniotomy, extra- or intradural elevation of temporal lobe

● New Code   ▲ Revised Code   + Add-On Code   ⊘ Modifier -51 Exempt

Posterior Cranial Fossa

61595   Transtemporal approach to posterior cranial fossa, jugular foramen or midline skull base, including mastoidectomy, decompression of sigmoid sinus and/or facial nerve, with or without mobilization

61596   Transcochlear approach to posterior cranial fossa, jugular foramen or midline skull base, including labyrinthectomy, decompression, with or without mobilization of facial nerve and/or petrous carotid artery

61597   Transcondylar (far lateral) approach to posterior cranial fossa, jugular foramen or midline skull base, including occipital condylectomy, mastoidectomy, resection of C1-C3 vertebral body(s), decompression of vertebral artery, with or without mobilization

61598   Transpetrosal approach to posterior cranial fossa, clivus or foramen magnum, including ligation of superior petrosal sinus and/or sigmoid sinus

DEFINITIVE PROCEDURES

Base of Anterior Cranial Fossa

61600   Resection or excision of neoplastic, vascular or infectious lesion of base of anterior cranial fossa; extradural

61601   intradural, including dural repair, with or without graft

Base of Middle Cranial Fossa

61605   Resection or excision of neoplastic, vascular or infectious lesion of infratemporal fossa, parapharyngeal space, petrous apex; extradural

61606   intradural, including dural repair, with or without graft

61607   Resection or excision of neoplastic, vascular or infectious lesion of parasellar area, cavernous sinus, clivus or midline skull base; extradural

61608   intradural, including dural repair, with or without graft

(Codes 61609-61612 are reported in addition to code(s) for primary procedure(s) 61605-61608. Report only one transection or ligation of carotid artery code per operative session.)

575

 Separate Procedure    Unlisted Procedure   CCI Comp. Code   Non-specific Procedure

+ 61609   Transection or ligation, carotid artery in cavernous sinus; without repair (List separately in addition to code for primary procedure)

+ 61610   with repair by anastomosis or graft (List separately in addition to code for primary procedure)

+ 61611   Transection or ligation, carotid artery in petrous canal; without repair (List separately in addition to code for primary procedure)

+ 61612   with repair by anastomosis or graft (List separately in addition to code for primary procedure)

61613   Obliteration of carotid aneurysm, arteriovenous malformation, or carotid-cavernous fistula by dissection within cavernous sinus

Base of Posterior Cranial Fossa

61615   Resection or excision of neoplastic, vascular or infectious lesion of base of posterior cranial fossa, jugular foramen, foramen magnum, or C1-C3 vertebral bodies; extradural

61616   intradural, including dural repair, with or without graft

REPAIR AND/OR RECONSTRUCTION OF SURGICAL DEFECTS OF SKULL BASE

61618   Secondary repair of dura for cerebrospinal fluid leak, anterior, middle or posterior cranial fossa following surgery of the skull base; by free tissue graft (eg, pericranium, fascia, tensor fascia lata, adipose tissue, homologous or synthetic grafts)

61619   by local or regionalized vascularized pedicle flap or myocutaneous flap (including galea, temporalis, frontalis or occipitalis muscle)

ENDOVASCULAR THERAPY

61623   Endovascular temporary balloon arterial occlusion, head or neck (extracranial/intracranial) including selective catheterization of vessel to be occluded, positioning and inflation of occlusion balloon, concomitant neurological monitoring, and radiologic supervision and interpretation of all angiography required for balloon occlusion and to exclude vascular injury post occlusion

● New Code   ▲ Revised Code   + Add-On Code   ⊘ Modifier -51 Exempt

(If selective catheterization and angiography of arteries other than artery to be occluded is performed, use appropriate catheterization and radiologic supervision and interpretation codes)

(If complete diagnostic angiography of the artery to be occluded is performed immediately prior to temporary occlusion, use appropriate radiologic supervision and interpretation codes only)

61624 Transcatheter permanent occlusion or embolization (eg, for tumor destruction, to achieve hemostasis, to occlude a vascular malformation), percutaneous, any method; central nervous system (intracranial, spinal cord)

(See also 37204)

(For radiological supervision and interpretation, use 75894)

61626 non-central nervous system, head or neck (extracranial, brachiocephalic branch)

(See also 37204)

(For radiological supervision and interpretation, use 75894)

SURGERY FOR ANEURYSM, ARTERIOVENOUS MALFORMATION OR VASCULAR DISEASE

61680 Surgery of intracranial arteriovenous malformation; supratentorial, simple

61682 supratentorial, complex

61684 infratentorial, simple

61686 infratentorial, complex

61690 dural, simple

61692 dural, complex

61697 Surgery of complex intracranial aneurysm, intracranial approach; carotid circulation

61698 vertebrobasilar circulation

577

 Separate Procedure

 Unlisted Procedure

 CCI Comp. Code

 Non-specific Procedure

(61697, 61698 involve aneurysms that are larger than 15 mm or with calcification of the aneurysm neck, or with incorporation of normal vessels into the aneurysm neck, or a procedure requiring temporary vessel occlusion, trapping or cardiopulmonary bypass to successfully treat the aneurysm)

61700 Surgery of simple intracranial aneurysm, intracranial approach; carotid circulation

61702 vertebrobasilar circulation

61703 Surgery of intracranial aneurysm, cervical approach by application of occluding clamp to cervical carotid artery (Selverstone-Crutchfield type)

(For cervical approach for direct ligation of carotid artery, see 37600-37606)

61705 Surgery of aneurysm, vascular malformation or carotid-cavernous fistula; by intracranial and cervical occlusion of carotid artery

61708 by intracranial electrothrombosis

(For ligation or gradual occlusion of internal/common carotid artery, see 37605, 37606)

61710 by intra-arterial embolization, injection procedure, or balloon catheter

61711 Anastomosis, arterial, extracranial-intracranial (eg, middle cerebral/cortical) arteries

(For carotid or vertebral thromboendarterectomy, use 35301)

STEREOTAXIS

61720 Creation of lesion by stereotactic method, including burr hole(s) and localizing and recording techniques, single or multiple stages; globus pallidus or thalamus

61735 subcortical structure(s) other than globus pallidus or thalamus

61750 Stereotactic biopsy, aspiration, or excision, including burr hole(s), for intracranial lesion;

61751 with computed tomography and/or magnetic resonance guidance

● New Code ▲ Revised Code + Add-On Code ⊘ Modifier -51 Exempt

(For radiological supervision and interpretation of computerized tomography, see 70450, 70460, or 70470 as appropriate)

(For radiological supervision and interpretation of magnetic resonance imaging, see 70551, 70552, or 70553 as appropriate)

61760 Stereotactic implantation of depth electrodes into the cerebrum for long term seizure monitoring

61770 Stereotactic localization, including burr hole(s), with insertion of catheter(s) or probe(s) for placement of radiation source

61790 Creation of lesion by stereotactic method, percutaneous, by neurolytic agent (eg, alcohol, thermal, electrical, radiofrequency); gasserian ganglion

61791 trigeminal medullary tract

61793 Stereotactic radiosurgery (particle beam, gamma ray or linear accelerator), one or more sessions

(For intensity modulated beam delivery plan and treatment, see 77301, 77418)

+ 61795 Stereotactic computer assisted volumetric (navigational) procedure, intracranial, extracranial, or spinal (List separately in addition to code for primary procedure)

NEUROSTIMULATORS (INTRACRANIAL)

61850 Twist drill or burr hole(s) for implantation of neurostimulator electrodes, cortical

61860 Craniectomy or craniotomy for implantation of neurostimulator electrodes, cerebral, cortical

(61862 deleted 2004 edition. To report, see 61867, 61868)

● **61863** Twist drill, burr hole, craniotomy, or craniectomy with stereotactic implantation of neurostimulator electrode array in subcortical site (eg, thalamus, globus pallidus, subthalamic nucleus, periventricular, periaqueductal gray), without use of intraoperative microelectrode recording; first array

●**+61864** each additional array (List separately in addition to primary procedure)

(Use 61864 in conjuncition with 61863)

 Separate Procedure   Unlisted Procedure   CCI Comp. Code   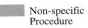 Non-specific Procedure

(61865 has been deleted. To report, use 61867, 61868)

● **61867** Twist drill, burr hole, craniotomy, or craniectomy with stereotactic implantation of neurostimulator electrode array in subcortical site (eg, thalamus, globus pallidus, subthalamic nucleus, periventricular, periaqueductal gray), with use of intraoperative microelectrode recording; first array

●+**61868** each additional array (List separately in addition to primary procedure)

(Use 61868 in conjunciton with 61867)

61870 Craniectomy for implantation of neurostimulator electrodes, cerebellar; cortical

61875 subcortical

61880 Revision or removal of intracranial neurostimulator electrodes

61885 Incision and subcutaneous placement of cranial neurostimulator pulse generator or receiver, direct or inductive coupling; with connection to a single electrode array

61886 with connection to two or more electrode arrays

(For open placement of cranial nerve (eg, vagal, trigeminal) neurostimulator electrode(s), use 64573)

(For percutaneous placement of cranial nerve (eg, vagal, trigeminal) neurostimulator electrode(s), use 64553)

(For revision or removal of cranial nerve (eg, vagal, trigeminal) neurostimulator electrode(s), use 64585)

61888 Revision or removal of cranial neurostimulator pulse generator or receiver

REPAIR

62000 Elevation of depressed skull fracture; simple, extradural

62005 compound or comminuted, extradural

62010 with repair of dura and/or debridement of brain

62100 Craniotomy for repair of dural/cerebrospinal fluid leak, including surgery for rhinorrhea/otorrhea

● New Code   ▲ Revised Code   + Add-On Code   ⊘ Modifier -51 Exempt

(For repair of spinal dural/CSF leak, see 63707, 63709)

62115 Reduction of craniomegalic skull (eg, treated hydrocephalus); not requiring bone grafts or cranioplasty

62116 with simple cranioplasty

62117 requiring craniotomy and reconstruction with or without bone graft (includes obtaining grafts)

62120 Repair of encephalocele, skull vault, including cranioplasty

62121 Craniotomy for repair of encephalocele, skull base

62140 Cranioplasty for skull defect; up to 5 cm diameter

62141 larger than 5 cm diameter

62142 Removal of bone flap or prosthetic plate of skull

62143 Replacement of bone flap or prosthetic plate of skull

62145 Cranioplasty for skull defect with reparative brain surgery

62146 Cranioplasty with autograft (includes obtaining bone grafts); up to 5 cm diameter

62147 larger than 5 cm diameter

+ **62148** Incision and retrieval of subcutaneous cranial bone graft for cranioplasty (List separately in addition to code for primary procedure)

(Use 62148 in conjunction with codes 62140-62147)

NEUROENDOSCOPY

(Surgical endoscopy always includes diagnostic endoscopy)

+ **62160** Neuroendoscopy, intracranial, for placement or replacement of ventricular catheter and attachment to shunt system or external drainage (List separately in addition to code for primary procedure)

(Use 62160 only in conjuction with codes 61107, 61210, 62220, 62223, 62225, or 62230)

581

| | Separate Procedure | | Unlisted Procedure | CCI Comp. Code | 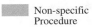 Non-specific Procedure |

62161   Neuroendoscopy, intracranial; with dissection of adhesions, fenestration of septum pellucidum or intraventricular cysts (including placement, replacement, or removal of ventricular catheter)

62162   with fenestration or excision of colloid cyst, including placement of external ventricular catheter for drainage

62163   with retrieval of foreign body

62164   with excision of brain tumor, including placement of external ventricular catheter for drainage

62165   with excision of pituitary tumor, transnasal or transsphenoidal approach

CEREBROSPINAL FLUID (CSF) SHUNT

62180   Ventriculocisternostomy (Torkildsen type operation)

62190   Creation of shunt; subarachnoid/subdural-atrial, -jugular, -auricular

62192   subarachnoid/subdural-peritoneal, -pleural, other terminus

62194   Replacement or irrigation, subarachnoid/subdural catheter

62200   Ventriculocisternostomy, third ventricle;

62201   stereotactic, neuroendoscopic method

       (For intracranial neuroendoscopic procedures, see 62161-62165)

62220   Creation of shunt; ventriculo-atrial, -jugular, -auricular

       (For intracranial neuroendoscopic ventricular catheter placement, use 62160)

62223   ventriculo-peritoneal, -pleural, other terminus

       (For intracranial neuroendoscopic ventricular catheter placement, use 62160)

62225   Replacement or irrigation, ventricular catheter

       (For intracranial neuroendoscopic ventricular catheter placement, use 62160)

● New Code   ▲ Revised Code   + Add-On Code   ⊘ Modifier -51 Exempt

62230 Replacement or revision of cerebrospinal fluid shunt, obstructed valve, or distal catheter in shunt system

(For intracranial neuroendoscopic ventricular catheter placement, use 62160)

62252 Reprogramming of programmable cerebrospinal shunt

62256 Removal of complete cerebrospinal fluid shunt system; without replacement

62258 with replacement by similar or other shunt at same operation

(For percutaneous irrigation or aspiration of shunt reservoir, use 61070)

(For reprogramming of programmable CSF shunt, use 62252)

SPINE AND SPINAL CORD

(For application of caliper or tongs, use 20660)

(For treatment of fracture or dislocation of spine, see 22305-22327)

INJECTION, DRAINAGE, OR ASPIRATION

(Report 01996 for daily hospital management of continuous epidural or subarachnoid drug administration performed in conjunction with 62318-62319)

(For endoscopic lysis of epidural adhesions, use Category III code 0027T)

62263 Percutaneous lysis of epidural adhesions using solution injection (eg, hypertonic saline, enzyme) or mechanical means (eg, catheter) including radiologic localization (includes contrast when administered), multiple adhesiolysis sessions; 2 or more days

(62263 includes codes 76005 and 72275)

62264 1 day

(Do not report 62264 with 62263)

(62264 includes codes 76005 and 72275)

62268 Percutaneous aspiration, spinal cord cyst or syrinx

583

 Separate Procedure   Unlisted Procedure   CCI Comp. Code   Non-specific Procedure

(For radiological supervision and interpretation, see 76003, 76360, 76942)

62269 Biopsy of spinal cord, percutaneous needle

(For radiological supervision and interpretation, see 76003, 76360, 76942)

(For fine needle aspiration, see 10021, 10022)

(For evaluation of fine needle aspirate, see 88172, 88173)

62270 Spinal puncture, lumbar, diagnostic

62272 Spinal puncture, therapeutic, for drainage of cerebrospinal fluid (by needle or catheter)

62273 Injection, epidural, of blood or clot patch

62280 Injection/infusion of neurolytic substance (eg, alcohol, phenol, iced saline solutions), with or without other therapeutic substance; subarachnoid

62281 epidural, cervical or thoracic

62282 epidural, lumbar, sacral (caudal)

⊘ **62284** Injection procedure for myelography and/or computed tomography, spinal (other than C1-C2 and posterior fossa)

(For injection procedure at C1-C2, use 61055)

(For radiological supervision and interpretation, see Radiology)

62287 Aspiration or decompression procedure, percutaneous, of nucleus pulposus of intervertebral disk, any method, single or multiple levels, lumbar (eg, manual or automated percutaneous diskectomy, percutaneous laser diskectomy)

(For fluoroscopic guidance, use 76003)

62290 Injection procedure for diskography, each level; lumbar

62291 cervical or thoracic

(For radiological supervision or interpretation, see 72285, 72295)

● New Code ▲ Revised Code + Add-On Code ⊘ Modifier -51 Exempt

62292 Injection procedure for chemonucleolysis, including diskography, intervertebral disk, single or multiple levels, lumbar

62294 Injection procedure, arterial, for occlusion of arteriovenous malformation, spinal

62310 Injection, single (not via indwelling catheter), not including neurolytic substances, with or without contrast (for either localization or epidurography), of diagnostic or therapeutic substance(s) (including anesthetic, antispasmodic, opioid, steroid, other solution), epidural or subarachnoid; cervical or thoracic

62311   lumbar, sacral (caudal)

62318 Injection, including catheter placement, continuous infusion with intermittent bolus not including neurolytic substances, with or without contrast (for either localization or epidurography), of diagnostic or therapeutic substance(s) (including anesthetic, antispasmodic, opioid, steroid, other solution), epidural or subarachnoid; cervical or thoracic

62319   lumbar, sacral (caudal)

(For transforaminal epidural injection, see 64479-64484)

(Report 01996 for daily hospital management of continuous epidural or subarachnoid drug administration performed in conjunction with codes 62318-62319)

CATHETER IMPLANTATION

(For percutaneous placement of intrathecal or epidural catheter, see codes 62270-62273, 62280-62284, 62310-62319)

62350 Implantation, revision or repositioning of tunneled intrathecal or epidural catheter, for long-term medication administration via an external pump or implantable reservoir/infusion pump; without laminectomy

62351   with laminectomy

(For refilling and maintenance of an implantable infusion pump for spinal or brain drug therapy, use 95990)

62355 Removal of previously implanted intrathecal or epidural catheter

585

| Separate Procedure | Unlisted Procedure | CCI Comp. Code | Non-specific Procedure |

RESERVOIR/PUMP IMPLANTATION

62360 Implantation or replacement of device for intrathecal or epidural drug infusion; subcutaneous reservoir

62361 non-programmable pump

62362 programmable pump, including preparation of pump, with or without programming

62365 Removal of subcutaneous reservoir or pump, previously implanted for intrathecal or epidural infusion

62367 Electronic analysis of programmable, implanted pump for intrathecal or epidural drug infusion (includes evaluation of reservoir status, alarm status, drug prescription status); without reprogramming

62368 with reprogramming

(For refilling and maintenance of an implantable infusion pump for spinal or brain drug therapy, use 95990)

POSTERIOR EXTRADURAL LAMINOTOMY OR LAMINECTOMY FOR EXPLORATION/DECOMPRESSION OF NEURAL ELEMENTS OR EXCISION OF HERNIATED INTERVERTEBRAL DISKS

(When 63001-63048 are followed by arthrodesis, see 22590-22614)

63001 Laminectomy with exploration and/or decompression of spinal cord and/or cauda equina, without facetectomy, foraminotomy or diskectomy, (eg, spinal stenosis), one or two vertebral segments; cervical

63003 thoracic

63005 lumbar, except for spondylolisthesis

63011 sacral

63012 Laminectomy with removal of abnormal facets and/or pars inter-articularis with decompression of cauda equina and nerve roots for spondylolisthesis, lumbar (Gill type procedure)

● New Code   ▲ Revised Code   + Add-On Code   ⊘ Modifier -51 Exempt

63015 Laminectomy with exploration and/or decompression of spinal cord and/or cauda equina, without facetectomy, foraminotomy or diskectomy, (eg, spinal stenosis), more than 2 vertebral segments; cervical

63016 thoracic

63017 lumbar

63020 Laminotomy (hemilaminectomy), with decompression of nerve root(s), including partial facetectomy, foraminotomy and/or excision of herniated intervertebral disk; one interspace, cervical

63030 one interspace, lumbar (including open or endoscopically assisted approach)

+ 63035 each additional interspace, cervical or lumbar (List separately in addition to code for primary procedure)

(Use 63035 in conjunction with codes 63020-63030)

(63020, 63030, 63035 are unilateral procedures. For bilateral procedures, use modifier '-50')

63040 Laminotomy (hemilaminectomy), with decompression of nerve root(s), including partial facetectomy, foraminotomy and/or excision of herniated intervertebral disk, reexploration, single interspace; cervical

63042 lumbar

(Codes 63040-63044 are unilateral procedures. For bilateral procedures, use modifier -50)

+ 63043 each additional cervical interspace (List separately in addition to code for primary procedure)

(Use 63043 in conjunction with code 63040)

+ 63044 each additional lumbar interspace (List separately in addition to code for primary procedure)

(Use 63044 in conjunction with code 63042)

63045 Laminectomy, facetectomy and foraminotomy (unilateral or bilateral with decompression of spinal cord, cauda equina and/or nerve root(s), (eg, spinal or lateral recess stenosis)), single vertebral segment; cervical

587

 Separate Procedure Unlisted Procedure CCI Comp. Code 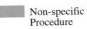 Non-specific Procedure

| 63046 | thoracic |
| 63047 | lumbar |

+ **63048**   each additional segment, cervical, thoracic, or lumbar (List separately in addition to code for primary procedure)

(Use 63048 in conjunction with codes 63045-63047)

TRANSPEDICULAR OR COSTOVERTEBRAL APPROACH FOR POSTEROLATERAL EXTRADURAL EXPLORATION/ DECOMPRESSION

63055   Transpedicular approach with decompression of spinal cord, equina and/or nerve root(s) (eg, herniated intervertebral disk), single segment; thoracic

63056   lumbar (including transfacet, or lateral extraforaminal approach) (eg, far lateral herniated intervertebral disk)

+ **63057**   each additional segment, thoracic or lumbar (List separately in addition to code for primary procedure)

(Use 63057 in conjunction with codes 63055, 63056)

63064   Costovertebral approach with decompression of spinal cord or nerve root(s), (eg, herniated intervertebral disk), thoracic; single segment

+ **63066**   each additional segment (List separately in addition to code for primary procedure)

(Use 63066 in conjunction with code 63064)

(For excision of thoracic intraspinal lesions by laminectomy, see 63266, 63271, 63276, 63281, 63286)

ANTERIOR OR ANTEROLATERAL APPROACH FOR EXTRADURAL EXPLORATION/DECOMPRESSION

63075   Diskectomy, anterior, with decompression of spinal cord and/or nerve root(s), including osteophytectomy; cervical, single interspace

+ **63076**   cervical, each additional interspace (List separately in addition to code for primary procedure)

(Use 63076 in conjunction with code 63075)

588

| ● | New Code | ▲ | Revised Code | + | Add-On Code | ⊘ | Modifier -51 Exempt |

63077   thoracic, single interspace

+ 63078   thoracic, each additional interspace (List separately in addition to code for primary procedure)

(Use 63078 in conjunction with code 63077)

(Do not report code 69990 in addition to codes 63075-63078)

63081   Vertebral corpectomy (vertebral body resection), partial or complete, anterior approach with decompression of spinal cord and/or nerve root(s); cervical, single segment

+ 63082   cervical, each additional segment (List separately in addition to code for primary procedure)

(Use 63082 in conjunction with code 63081)

(For transoral approach, see 61575, 61576)

63085   Vertebral corpectomy (vertebral body resection), partial or complete, transthoracic approach with decompression of spinal cord and/or nerve root(s); thoracic, single segment

+ 63086   thoracic, each additional segment (List separately in addition to code for primary procedure)

(Use 63086 in conjunction with code 63085)

63087   Vertebral corpectomy (vertebral body resection), partial or complete, combined thoracolumbar approach with decompression of spinal cord, cauda equina or nerve root(s), lower thoracic or lumbar; single segment

+ 63088   each additional segment (List separately in addition to code for primary procedure)

(Use 63088 in conjunction with code 63087)

63090   Vertebral corpectomy (vertebral body resection), partial or complete, transperitoneal or retroperitoneal approach with decompression of spinal cord, cauda equina or nerve root(s), lower thoracic, lumbar, or sacral; single segment

+ 63091   each additional segment (List separately in addition to code for primary procedure)

(Use 63091 in conjunction with code 63090)

589

 Separate Procedure   Unlisted Procedure   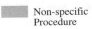 CCI Comp. Code   Non-specific Procedure

(Procedures 63081-63091 include diskectomy above and/or below vertebral segment)

(If followed by arthrodesis, see 22548-22812)

(For reconstruction of spine, use appropriate vertebral corpectomy codes 63081-63091, bone graft codes 20930-20938, arthrodesis codes 22548-22812, and spinal instrumentation codes 22840-22855)

LATERAL EXTRACAVITARY APPROACH FOR EXTRADURAL EXPLORATION/DECOMPRESSION

● **63101**   Vertebral corpectomy (vertebral body resection), partial or complete, lateral extracavitary approach with decompression of spinal cord and/or nerve root(s) (eg, for tumor or retropulsed bone fragments); thoracic, single segment

● **63102**   lumbar, single segment

●+**63103**   thoracic or lumbar, each additional segment (List separately in addition to code for primary procedure)

(Use 63103 in conjunction with 63101 and 63102)

INCISION

63170   Laminectomy with myelotomy (eg, Bischof or DREZ type), cervical, thoracic, or thoracolumbar

63172   Laminectomy with drainage of intramedullary cyst/syrinx; to subarachnoid space

▲ **63173**   to peritoneal or pleural space

63180   Laminectomy and section of dentate ligaments, with or without dural graft, cervical; one or two segments

63182   more than two segments

63185   Laminectomy with rhizotomy; one or two segments

63190   more than two segments

63191   Laminectomy with section of spinal accessory nerve

(For resection of sternocleidomastoid muscle, use 21720)

---

590   ● New Code   ▲ Revised Code   + Add-On Code   ⊘ Modifier -51 Exempt

63194 Laminectomy with cordotomy, with section of one spinothalamic tract, one stage; cervical

63195 thoracic

63196 Laminectomy with cordotomy, with section of both spinothalamic tracts, one stage; cervical

63197 thoracic

63198 Laminectomy with cordotomy with section of both spinothalamic tracts, two stages within 14 days; cervical

63199 thoracic

63200 Laminectomy, with release of tethered spinal cord, lumbar

EXCISION BY LAMINECTOMY OF LESION OTHER THAN HERNIATED DISK

63250 Laminectomy for excision or occlusion of arteriovenous malformation of spinal cord; cervical

63251 thoracic

63252 thoracolumbar

63265 Laminectomy for excision or evacuation of intraspinal lesion other than neoplasm, extradural; cervical

63266 thoracic

63267 lumbar

63268 sacral

63270 Laminectomy for excision of intraspinal lesion other than neoplasm, intradural; cervical

63271 thoracic

63272 lumbar

63273 sacral

591

 Separate Procedure    Unlisted Procedure   CCI Comp. Code   Non-specific Procedure

63275 Laminectomy for biopsy/excision of intraspinal neoplasm; extradural, cervical

63276 extradural, thoracic

63277 extradural, lumbar

63278 extradural, sacral

63280 intradural, extramedullary, cervical

63281 intradural, extramedullary, thoracic

63282 intradural, extramedullary, lumbar

63283 intradural, sacral

63285 intradural, intramedullary, cervical

63286 intradural, intramedullary, thoracic

63287 intradural, intramedullary, thoracolumbar

63290 combined extradural-intradural lesion, any level

(For drainage of intramedullary cyst/syrinx, use 63172, 63173)

EXCISION, ANTERIOR OR ANTEROLATERAL APPROACH, INTRASPINAL LESION

(For arthrodesis, see 22548-22585)

(For reconstruction of spine, see 20930-20938)

63300 Vertebral corpectomy (vertebral body resection), partial or complete, for excision of intraspinal lesion, single segment; extradural, cervical

63301 extradural, thoracic by transthoracic approach

63302 extradural, thoracic by thoracolumbar approach

63303 extradural, lumbar or sacral by transperitoneal or retroperitoneal approach

63304 intradural, cervical

592

● New Code	▲ Revised Code	+ Add-On Code	⊘ Modifier -51 Exempt

63305   intradural, thoracic by transthoracic approach

63306   intradural, thoracic by thoracolumbar approach

63307   intradural, lumbar or sacral by transperitoneal or retroperitoneal approach

+ 63308   each additional segment (List separately in addition to codes for single segment)

(Use 63308 in conjunction with codes 63300-63307)

STEREOTAXIS

63600   Creation of lesion of spinal cord by stereotactic method, percutaneous, any modality (including stimulation and/or recording)

63610   Stereotactic stimulation of spinal cord, percutaneous, separate procedure not followed by other surgery

63615   Stereotactic biopsy, aspiration, or excision of lesion, spinal cord

NEUROSTIMULATORS (SPINAL)

63650   Percutaneous implantation of neurostimulator electrode array, epidural

63655   Laminectomy for implantation of neurostimulator electrodes, plate/paddle, epidural

63660   Revision or removal of spinal neurostimulator electrode percutaneous array(s) or plate/paddle(s)

63685   Incision and subcutaneous placement of spinal neurostimulator pulse generator or receiver, direct or inductive coupling

63688   Revision or removal of implanted spinal neurostimulator pulse generator or receiver

REPAIR

63700   Repair of meningocele; less than 5 cm diameter

63702   larger than 5 cm diameter

(Do not use modifier '-63' in conjunction with 63700, 63702)

593

 Separate Procedure   Unlisted Procedure   CCI Comp. Code   Non-specific Procedure

63704 Repair of myelomeningocele; less than 5 cm diameter

63706   larger than 5 cm diameter

(Do not use modifier '-63' in conjunction with 63704, 63706)

(For complex skin closure, see Integumentary System)

63707 Repair of dural/cerebrospinal fluid leak, not requiring laminectomy

63709 Repair of dural/cerebrospinal fluid leak or pseudomeningocele, with laminectomy

63710 Dural graft, spinal

(For laminectomy and section of dentate ligaments, with or without dural graft, cervical, see 63180, 63182)

SHUNT, SPINAL CSF

63740 Creation of shunt, lumbar, subarachnoid-peritoneal, -pleural, or other; including laminectomy

63741   percutaneous, not requiring laminectomy

63744 Replacement, irrigation or revision of lumbosubarachnoid shunt

63746 Removal of entire lumbosubarachnoid shunt system without replacement

EXTRACRANIAL NERVES, PERIPHERAL NERVES, AND AUTONOMIC NERVOUS SYSTEM

(For intracranial surgery on cranial nerves, see 61450, 61460, 61790)

INTRODUCTION/INJECTION OF ANESTHETIC AGENT (NERVE BLOCK), DIAGNOSTIC OR THERAPEUTIC

Somatic Nerves

64400 Injection, anesthetic agent; trigeminal nerve, any division or branch

64402   facial nerve

64405   greater occipital nerve

● New Code   ▲ Revised Code   + Add-On Code   ⊘ Modifier -51 Exempt

64408   vagus nerve

64410   phrenic nerve

64412   spinal accessory nerve

64413   cervical plexus

64415   brachial plexus, single

64416   brachial plexus, continuous infusion by catheter (including catheter placement) including daily management for anesthetic agent administration

(Do not report 01996 in addition to 64416)

64417   axillary nerve

64418   suprascapular nerve

64420   intercostal nerve, single

64421   intercostal nerves, multiple, regional block

64425   ilioinguinal, iliohypogastric nerves

64430   pudendal nerve

64435   paracervical (uterine) nerve

64445   sciatic nerve, single

64446   sciatic nerve, continuous infusion by catheter, (including catheter placement) including daily management for anesthetic agent administration

(Do not report 01996 in addition to 64446)

64447   femoral nerve, single

(Do not report 01996 in addition to 64447)

64448   femoral nerve, continuous infusion by catheter (including catheter placement) including daily management for anesthetic agent administration

(Do not report 01996 in addition to 64448)

595

	Separate Procedure		Unlisted Procedure		CCI Comp. Code		Non-specific Procedure

● **64449**   lumbar plexus, posterior approach, continuous infusion by catheter (including catheter placement) including daily managemnt for anesthetic agent administration

(Do not report 01996 in conjunction with 64449)

64450   other peripheral nerve or branch

(For phenol destruction, see 64622-64627)

(For subarachnoid or subdural injection, see 62280, 62310-62319)

(For epidural or caudal injection, see 62273, 62281-62282, 62310-62319)

(Codes 64470-64484 are unilateral procedures. For bilateral procedures, use modifier -50)

(For fluoroscopic guidance and localization for needle placement and injection in conjunction with codes 64470-64484, use code 76005)

64470 Injection, anesthetic agent and/or steroid, paravertebral facet joint or facet joint nerve; cervical or thoracic, single level

+ **64472**   cervical or thoracic, each additional level (List separately in addition to code for primary procedure)

(Use code 64472 in conjunction with code 64470)

64475   lumbar or sacral, single level

+ **64476**   lumbar or sacral, each additional level (List separately in addition to code for primary procedure)

(Use code 64476 in conjunction with code 64475)

64479 Injection, anesthetic agent and/or steroid, transforaminal epidural; cervical or thoracic, single level

+ **64480**   cervical or thoracic, each additional level (List separately in addition to code for primary procedure)

(Use code 64480 in conjunction with code 64479)

64483   lumbar or sacral, single level

+ **64484**   lumbar or sacral, each additional level (List separately in addition to code for primary procedure)

● New Code   ▲ Revised Code   + Add-On Code   ⊘ Modifier -51 Exempt

(Use code 64484 in conjunction with code 64483)

Sympathetic Nerves

64505 Injection, anesthetic agent; sphenopalatine ganglion

64508 carotid sinus (separate procedure)

64510 stellate ganglion (cervical sympathetic)

● **64517** superior hypogastric plexus

64520 lumbar or thoracic (paravertebral sympathetic)

64530 celiac plexus, with or without radiologic monitoring

NEUROSTIMULATORS (PERIPHERAL NERVE)

64550 Application of surface (transcutaneous) neurostimulator

64553 Percutaneous implantation of neurostimulator electrodes; cranial nerve

(For open placement of cranial nerve (eg, vagal, trigeminal) neurostimulator pulse generator or receiver, see 61885, 61886, as appropriate)

64555 peripheral nerve (excludes sacral nerve)

64560 autonomic nerve

64561 sacral nerve (transforaminal placement)

64565 neuromuscular

64573 Incision for implantation of neurostimulator electrodes; cranial nerve

(For open placement of cranial nerve (eg, vagal, trigeminal) neurostimulator pulse generator or receiver, see 61885, 61886, as appropriate)

(For revision or removal of cranial nerve (eg, vagal, trigeminal) neurostimulator pulse generator or receiver, use 61888)

64575 peripheral nerve (excludes sacral nerve)

597

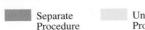 Separate Procedure  Unlisted Procedure   CCI Comp. Code Non-specific Procedure

64577	autonomic nerve
64580	neuromuscular
64581	sacral nerve (transforaminal placement)

64585 Revision or removal of peripheral neurostimulator electrodes

64590 Incision and subcutaneous placement of peripheral neurostimulator pulse generator or receiver, direct or inductive coupling

64595 Revision or removal of peripheral neurostimulator pulse generator or receiver

DESTRUCTION BY NEUROLYTIC AGENT (eg, CHEMICAL, THERMAL, ELECTRICAL, OR RADIOFREQUENCY)

(Codes 64600-64681 include the injection of other therapeutic agents (eg, corticosteroids).

Somatic Nerves

64600 Destruction by neurolytic agent, trigeminal nerve; supraorbital, infraorbital, mental, or inferior alveolar branch

64605 second and third division branches at foramen ovale

64610 second and third division branches at foramen ovale under radiologic monitoring

64612 Chemodenervation of muscle(s); muscle(s) innervated by facial nerve (eg, for blepharospasm, hemifacial spasm)

64613 cervical spinal muscle(s) (eg, for spasmodic torticollis)

64614 extremity(s) and/or trunk muscle(s) (eg, for dystonia, cerebral palsy, multiple sclerosis)

(For chemodenervation for strabismus involving the extraocular muscles, use 67345)

64620 Destruction by neurolytic agent, intercostal nerve

(Codes 64622-64627 are unilateral procedures. For bilateral procedures, use modifier -50)

598

● New Code ▲ Revised Code ✛ Add-On Code ⊘ Modifier -51 Exempt

(For fluoroscopic guidance and localization for needle placement and neurolysis in conjunction with codes 64622-64627, use 76005)

64622 Destruction by neurolytic agent, paravertebral facet joint nerve; lumbar or sacral, single level

+ 64623 lumbar or sacral, each additional level (List separately in addition to code for primary procedure)

(Use 64623 in conjunction with code 64622)

64626 cervical or thoracic, single level

+ 64627 cervical or thoracic, each additional level (List separately in addition to code for primary procedure)

(Use 64627 in conjunction with code 64626)

64630 Destruction by neurolytic agent; pudendal nerve

64640 other peripheral nerve or branch

Sympathetic Nerves

▲ **64680** Destruction by neurolytic agent, with or without radiologic monitoring; celiac plexus

● **64681** superior hypogastric plexus

NEUROPLASTY (EXPLORATION, NEUROLYSIS OR NERVE DECOMPRESSION)

(For internal neurolysis requiring use of operating microscope, use 64727)

(For facial nerve decompression, use 69720)

64702 Neuroplasty; digital, one or both, same digit

64704 nerve of hand or foot

64708 Neuroplasty, major peripheral nerve, arm or leg; other than specified

64712 sciatic nerve

64713 brachial plexus

599

 Separate Procedure   Unlisted Procedure   CCI Comp. Code   Non-specific Procedure

64714   lumbar plexus

64716   Neuroplasty and/or transposition; cranial nerve (specify)

64718   ulnar nerve at elbow

64719   ulnar nerve at wrist

64721   median nerve at carpal tunnel

     (For arthroscopic procedure, use 29848)

64722   Decompression; unspecified nerve(s) (specify)

64726   plantar digital nerve

+ 64727   Internal neurolysis, requiring use of operating microscope (List separately in addition to code for neuroplasty) (Neuroplasty includes external neurolysis)

     (Do not report code 69990 in addition to code 64727)

TRANSECTION OR AVULSION

     (For stereotactic lesion of gasserian ganglion, use 61790)

64732   Transection or avulsion of; supraorbital nerve

64734   infraorbital nerve

64736   mental nerve

64738   inferior alveolar nerve by osteotomy

64740   lingual nerve

64742   facial nerve, differential or complete

64744   greater occipital nerve

64746   phrenic nerve

     (For section of recurrent laryngeal nerve, use 31595)

64752   vagus nerve (vagotomy), transthoracic

600

●   New Code   ▲   Revised Code   +   Add-On Code   ⊘   Modifier -51 Exempt

64755   vagus nerves limited to proximal stomach (selective proximal vagotomy, proximal gastric vagotomy, parietal cell vagotomy, supra- or highly selective vagotomy)

(For laparoscopic approach, use 43652)

64760   vagus nerve (vagotomy), abdominal

(For laparoscopic approach, use 43651)

64761   pudendal nerve

64763   Transection or avulsion of obturator nerve, extrapelvic, with or without adductor tenotomy

64766   Transection or avulsion of obturator nerve, intrapelvic, with or without adductor tenotomy

64771   Transection or avulsion of other cranial nerve, extradural

64772   Transection or avulsion of other spinal nerve, extradural

(For excision of tender scar, skin and subcutaneous tissue, with or without tiny neuroma, see 11400-11446, 13100-13153)

EXCISION

Somatic Nerves

(For Morton neurectomy, use 28080)

64774   Excision of neuroma; cutaneous nerve, surgically identifiable

64776   digital nerve, one or both, same digit

+ 64778   digital nerve, each additional digit (List separately in addition to code for primary procedure)

(Use 64778 in conjunction with code 64776)

64782   hand or foot, except digital nerve

+ 64783   hand or foot, each additional nerve, except same digit (List separately in addition to code for primary procedure)

(Use 64783 in conjunction with code 64782)

64784   major peripheral nerve, except sciatic

601

 Separate Procedure   Unlisted Procedure   CCI Comp. Code    Non-specific Procedure

64786   sciatic nerve

+ 64787   Implantation of nerve end into bone or muscle (List separately in addition to neuroma excision)

(Use 64787 in conjunction with codes 64774-64786)

64788   Excision of neurofibroma or neurolemmoma; cutaneous nerve

64790   major peripheral nerve

64792   extensive (including malignant type)

64795   Biopsy of nerve

Sympathetic Nerves

64802   Sympathectomy, cervical

64804   Sympathectomy, cervicothoracic

64809   Sympathectomy, thoracolumbar

64818   Sympathectomy, lumbar

64820   Sympathectomy; digital arteries, each digit

(Do not report 69990 in addition to code 64820)

64821   radial artery

(Do not report 69990 in addition to code 64821)

64822   ulnar artery

(Do not report 69990 in addition to code 64822)

64823   superficial palmar arch

(Do not report 69990 in addition to code 64823)

NEURORRHAPHY

64831   Suture of digital nerve, hand or foot; one nerve

+ 64832   each additional digital nerve (List separately in addition to code for primary procedure)

602   ● New Code   ▲ Revised Code   **+** Add-On Code   ⊘ Modifier -51 Exempt

(Use 64832 in conjunction with code 64831)

64834 Suture of one nerve, hand or foot; common sensory nerve

64835   median motor thenar

64836   ulnar motor

+ 64837 Suture of each additional nerve, hand or foot (List separately in addition to code for primary procedure)

(Use 64837 in conjunction with codes 64834-64836)

64840 Suture of posterior tibial nerve

64856 Suture of major peripheral nerve, arm or leg, except sciatic; including transposition

64857   without transposition

64858 Suture of sciatic nerve

+ 64859 Suture of each additional major peripheral nerve (List separately in addition to code for primary procedure)

(Use 64859 in conjunction with codes 64856, 64857)

64861 Suture of; brachial plexus

64862   lumbar plexus

64864 Suture of facial nerve; extracranial

64865   infratemporal, with or without grafting

64866 Anastomosis; facial-spinal accessory

64868   facial-hypoglossal

64870   facial-phrenic

+ 64872 Suture of nerve; requiring secondary or delayed suture (List separately in addition to code for primary neurorrhaphy)

(Use 64872 in conjunction with codes 64831-64865)

603

 Separate
Procedure

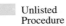 Unlisted
Procedure

 CCI Comp.
Code

 Non-specific
Procedure

+ 64874   requiring extensive mobilization, or transposition of nerve (List separately in addition to code for nerve suture)

(Use 64874 in conjunction with codes 64831-64865)

+ 64876   requiring shortening of bone of extremity (List separately in addition to code for nerve suture)

(Use 64876 in conjunction with codes 64831-64865)

NEURORRHAPHY WITH NERVE GRAFT

64885 Nerve graft (includes obtaining graft), head or neck; up to 4 cm in length

64886   more than 4 cm length

64890 Nerve graft (includes obtaining graft), single strand, hand or foot; up to 4 cm length

64891   more than 4 cm length

64892 Nerve graft (includes obtaining graft), single strand, arm or leg; up to 4 cm length

64893   more than 4 cm length

64895 Nerve graft (includes obtaining graft), multiple strands (cable), hand or foot; up to 4 cm length

64896   more than 4 cm length

64897 Nerve graft (includes obtaining graft), multiple strands (cable), arm or leg; up to 4 cm length

64898   more than 4 cm length

+ 64901 Nerve graft, each additional nerve; single strand (List separately in addition to code for primary procedure)

(Use 64901 in conjunction with codes 64885-64893)

+ 64902   multiple strands (cable) (List separately in addition to code for primary procedure)

(Use 64902 in conjunction with codes 64885, 64886, 64895-64898)

● New Code   ▲ Revised Code   + Add-On Code   ⊘ Modifier -51 Exempt

64905 Nerve pedicle transfer; first stage

64907 second stage

OTHER PROCEDURES

64999 Unlisted procedure, nervous system

| Separate Procedure | Unlisted Procedure | CCI Comp. Code | Non-specific Procedure |

This page intentionally left blank.

● New
Code

▲ Revised
Code

✛ Add-On
Code

⊘ Modifier -51
Exempt

EYE AND OCULAR ADNEXA

CPT codes from this section of the CPT coding system are used to report surgical procedures on the eye and ocular adnexa. Diagnostic services and medical treatment of the eye are defined in the Medicine Section of the CPT manual.

If surgical procedures are performed only on the eyelid, code from the Integumentary System subsection of the CPT coding system. Cataract codes are selected on the type of procedure performed. Whenever injections are performed during cataract surgery, do not report them separately.

(For diagnostic and treatment ophthalmological services, see Medicine, Ophthalmology, and 92002 et seq)

(Do not report code 69990 in addition to codes 65091-68850)

EYEBALL

REMOVAL OF EYE

65091 Evisceration of ocular contents; without implant

65093 with implant

65101 Enucleation of eye; without implant

65103 with implant, muscles not attached to implant

65105 with implant, muscles attached to implant

(For conjunctivoplasty after enucleation, see 68320 et seq)

65110 Exenteration of orbit (does not include skin graft), removal of orbital contents; only

65112 with therapeutic removal of bone

65114 with muscle or myocutaneous flap

(For skin graft to orbit (split skin), see 15120, 15121; free, full thickness, see 15260, 15261)

(For eyelid repair involving more than skin, see 67930 et seq)

607

	Separate Procedure		Unlisted Procedure		CCI Comp. Code		Non-specific Procedure

SECONDARY IMPLANT(S) PROCEDURES

65125 Modification of ocular implant with placement or replacement of pegs (eg, drilling receptacle for prosthesis appendage) (separate procedure)

65130 Insertion of ocular implant secondary; after evisceration, in scleral shell

65135 after enucleation, muscles not attached to implant

65140 after enucleation, muscles attached to implant

65150 Reinsertion of ocular implant; with or without conjunctival graft

65155 with use of foreign material for reinforcement and/or attachment of muscles to implant

65175 Removal of ocular implant

(For orbital implant (implant outside muscle cone) insertion, use 67550; removal, use 67560)

REMOVAL OF FOREIGN BODY

(For removal of implanted material: ocular implant, use 65175; anterior segment implant, use 65920; posterior segment implant, use 67120; orbital implant, use 67560)

(For diagnostic x-ray for foreign body, use 70030)

(For diagnostic echography for foreign body, use 76529)

(For removal of foreign body from orbit: frontal approach, use 67413; lateral approach, use 67430; transcranial approach, use 61334)

(For removal of foreign body from eyelid, embedded, use 67938)

(For removal of foreign body from lacrimal system, use 68530)

65205 Removal of foreign body, external eye; conjunctival superficial

65210 conjunctival embedded (includes concretions), subconjunctival, or scleral nonperforating

65220 corneal, without slit lamp

● New Code	▲ Revised Code	+ Add-On Code	⊘ Modifier -51 Exempt

65222 corneal, with slit lamp

(For repair of corneal laceration with foreign body, use 65275)

65235 Removal of foreign body, intraocular; from anterior chamber of eye or lens

(For removal of implanted material from anterior segment, use 65920)

65260 from posterior segment, magnetic extraction, anterior or posterior route

65265 from posterior segment, nonmagnetic extraction

(For removal of implanted material from posterior segment, use 67120)

REPAIR OF LACERATION

(For fracture of orbit, see 21385 et seq)

(For repair of wound of eyelid, skin, linear, simple, see 12011-12018; intermediate, layered closure, see 12051-12057; linear, complex, see 13150-13160; other, see 67930, 67935)

(For repair of wound of lacrimal system, use 68700)

(For repair of operative wound, use 66250)

65270 Repair of laceration; conjunctiva, with or without nonperforating laceration sclera, direct closure

65272 conjunctiva, by mobilization and rearrangement, without hospitalization

65273 conjunctiva, by mobilization and rearrangement, with hospitalization

65275 cornea, nonperforating, with or without removal foreign body

65280 cornea and/or sclera, perforating, not involving uveal tissue

65285 cornea and/or sclera, perforating, with reposition or resection of uveal tissue

65286 application of tissue glue, wounds of cornea and/or sclera

609

 Separate Procedure   Unlisted Procedure   CCI Comp. Code   Non-specific Procedure

(Repair of laceration includes use of conjunctival flap and restoration of anterior chamber, by air or saline injection when indicated)

(For repair of iris or ciliary body, use 66680)

65290   Repair of wound, extraocular muscle, tendon and/or Tenon's capsule

ANTERIOR SEGMENT

CORNEA

Excision

65400   Excision of lesion, cornea (keratectomy, lamellar, partial), except pterygium

65410   Biopsy of cornea

65420   Excision or transposition of pterygium; without graft

65426   with graft

Removal or Destruction

65430   Scraping of cornea, diagnostic, for smear and/or culture

65435   Removal of corneal epithelium; with or without chemocauterization (abrasion, curettage)

65436   with application of chelating agent (eg, EDTA)

65450   Destruction of lesion of cornea by cryotherapy, photocoagulation or thermocauterization

65600   Multiple punctures of anterior cornea (eg, for corneal erosion, tattoo)

Keratoplasty

(Keratoplasty excludes refractive keratoplasty procedures, 65760, 65765, and 65767)

65710   Keratoplasty (corneal transplant); lamellar

65730   penetrating (except in aphakia)

| ● | New Code | ▲ | Revised Code | + | Add-On Code | ⊘ | Modifier -51 Exempt |

65750 penetrating (in aphakia)

65755 penetrating (in pseudophakia)

Other Procedures

65760 Keratomileusis

65765 Keratophakia

65767 Epikeratoplasty

65770 Keratoprosthesis

65771 Radial keratotomy

65772 Corneal relaxing incision for correction of surgically induced astigmatism

65775 Corneal wedge resection for correction of surgically induced astigmatism

(For fitting of contact lens for treatment of disease, use 92070)

(For unlisted procedures on cornea, use 66999)

● **65780** Ocular surface reconstruction; amniotic membrane transplantation

● **65781** limbal stem cell allograft (eg, cadaveric or living donor)

● **65782** limbal conjunctival autograft (includes obtaining graft)

(For harvesting conjunctival allograft, living donor, use 68371)

ANTERIOR CHAMBER

Incision

65800 Paracentesis of anterior chamber of eye (separate procedure); with diagnostic aspiration of aqueous

65805 with therapeutic release of aqueous

65810 with removal of vitreous and/or discission of anterior hyaloid membrane, with or without air injection

---

611

| | Separate Procedure | | Unlisted Procedure | | CCI Comp. Code | | Non-specific Procedure |

65815   with removal of blood, with or without irrigation and/or air injection

(For injection, see 66020-66030)

(For removal of blood clot, use 65930)

65820   Goniotomy

(Do not report modifier '-63' in conjunction with 65820)

65850   Trabeculotomy ab externo

65855   Trabeculoplasty by laser surgery, one or more sessions (defined treatment series)

(If re-treatment is necessary after several months because of disease progression, a new treatment or treatment series should be reported with a modifier, if necessary, to indicate lesser or greater complexity)

(For trabeculectomy, use 66170)

65860   Severing adhesions of anterior segment, laser technique (separate procedure)

Other Procedures

65865   Severing adhesions of anterior segment of eye, incisional technique (with or without injection of air or liquid) (separate procedure); goniosynechiae

(For trabeculoplasty by laser surgery, use 65855)

65870   anterior synechiae, except goniosynechiae

65875   posterior synechiae

65880   corneovitreal adhesions

(For laser surgery, use 66821)

65900   Removal of epithelial downgrowth, anterior chamber of eye

65920   Removal of implanted material, anterior segment of eye

65930   Removal of blood clot, anterior segment of eye

● New Code   ▲ Revised Code   + Add-On Code   ⊘ Modifier -51 Exempt

66020   Injection, anterior chamber of eye (separate procedure); air or liquid

66030   medication

(For unlisted procedures on anterior segment, use 66999)

ANTERIOR SCLERA

Excision

(For removal of intraocular foreign body, use 65235)

(For operations on posterior sclera, use 67250, 67255)

66130   Excision of lesion, sclera

66150   Fistulization of sclera for glaucoma; trephination with iridectomy

66155   thermocauterization with iridectomy

66160   sclerectomy with punch or scissors, with iridectomy

66165   iridencleisis or iridotasis

66170   trabeculectomy ab externo in absence of previous surgery

(For trabeculotomy ab externo, use 65850)

(For repair of operative wound, use 66250)

66172   trabeculectomy ab externo with scarring from previous ocular surgery or trauma (includes injection of antifibrotic agents)

66180   Aqueous shunt to extraocular reservoir (eg, Molteno, Schocket, Denver-Krupin)

66185   Revision of aqueous shunt to extraocular reservoir

(For removal of implanted shunt, use 67120)

Repair or Revision

(For scleral procedures in retinal surgery, see 67101 et seq)

66220   Repair of scleral staphyloma; without graft

613

 Separate Procedure    Unlisted Procedure   CCI Comp. Code   Non-specific Procedure

66225	with graft

(For scleral reinforcement, see 67250, 67255)

66250	Revision or repair of operative wound of anterior segment, any type, early or late, major or minor procedure

(For unlisted procedures on anterior sclera, use 66999)

IRIS, CILIARY BODY

Incision

66500	Iridotomy by stab incision (separate procedure); except transfixion

66505	with transfixion as for iris bombe

(For iridotomy by photocoagulation, use 66761)

Excision

66600	Iridectomy, with corneoscleral or corneal section; for removal of lesion

66605	with cyclectomy

66625	peripheral for glaucoma (separate procedure)

66630	sector for glaucoma (separate procedure)

66635	optical (separate procedure)

(For coreoplasty by photocoagulation, use 66762)

Repair

66680	Repair of iris, ciliary body (as for iridodialysis)

(For reposition or resection of uveal tissue with perforating wound of cornea or sclera, use 65285)

66682	Suture of iris, ciliary body (separate procedure) with retrieval of suture through small incision (eg, McCannel suture)

Destruction

66700	Ciliary body destruction; diathermy

614

● New Code　　▲ Revised Code　　✛ Add-On Code　　⊘ Modifier -51 Exempt

66710   cyclophotocoagulation

66720   cryotherapy

66740   cyclodialysis

66761   Iridotomy/iridectomy by laser surgery (eg, for glaucoma) (one or more sessions)

66762   Iridoplasty by photocoagulation (one or more sessions) (eg, for improvement of vision, for widening of anterior chamber angle)

66770   Destruction of cyst or lesion iris or ciliary body (nonexcisional procedure)

(For excision lesion iris, ciliary body, see 66600, 66605; for removal of epithelial downgrowth, use 65900)

(For unlisted procedures on iris, ciliary body, use 66999)

LENS

Incision

66820   Discission of secondary membranous cataract (opacified posterior lens capsule and/or anterior hyaloid); stab incision technique (Ziegler or Wheeler knife)

66821   laser surgery (eg, YAG laser) (one or more stages)

66825   Repositioning of intraocular lens prosthesis, requiring an incision (separate procedure)

Removal Cataract

66830   Removal of secondary membranous cataract (opacified posterior lens capsule and/or anterior hyaloid) with corneo-scleral section, with or without iridectomy (iridocapsulotomy, iridocapsulectomy)

66840   Removal of lens material; aspiration technique, one or more stages

66850   phacofragmentation technique (mechanical or ultrasonic) (eg, phacoemulsification), with aspiration

66852   pars plana approach, with or without vitrectomy

615

 Separate Procedure   Unlisted Procedure   CCI Comp. Code   Non-specific Procedure

66920   intracapsular

66930   intracapsular, for dislocated lens

66940   extracapsular (other than 66840, 66850, 66852)

(For removal of intralenticular foreign body without lens extraction, use 65235)

(For repair of operative wound, use 66250)

66982   Extracapsular cataract removal with insertion of intraocular lens prosthesis (one stage procedure), manual or mechanical technique (eg, irrigation and aspiration or phacoemulsification), complex, requiring devices or techniques not generally used in routine cataract surgery (eg, iris expansion device, suture support for intraocular lens, or primary posterior capsulorrhexis) or performed on patients in the amblyogenic developmental stage

66983   Intracapsular cataract extraction with insertion of intraocular lens prosthesis (one stage procedure)

66984   Extracapsular cataract removal with insertion of intraocular lens prosthesis (one stage procedure), manual or mechanical technique (eg, irrigation and aspiration or phacoemulsification)

(For complex extracapsular cataract removal, use 66982)

66985   Insertion of intraocular lens prosthesis (secondary implant), not associated with concurrent cataract removal

(To code implant at time of concurrent cataract surgery, see 66982, 66983, 66984)

(For intraocular lens prosthesis supplied by physician, use 99070)

(For ultrasonic determination of intraocular lens power, use 76519)

(For removal of implanted material from anterior segment, use 65920)

(For secondary fixation (separate procedure), use 66682)

66986   Exchange of intraocular lens

+ **66990**   Use of ophthalmic endoscope (List separately in addition to code for primary procedure)

---

616   ● New Code   ▲ Revised Code   + Add-On Code   ⊘ Modifier -51 Exempt

(66990 may be used only with codes 65820, 65875, 65920, 66985, 66986, 67038, 67039, 67040)

OTHER PROCEDURES

66999 Unlisted procedure, anterior segment of eye

POSTERIOR SEGMENT

VITREOUS

67005 Removal of vitreous, anterior approach (open sky technique or limbal incision); partial removal

67010 subtotal removal with mechanical vitrectomy

(For removal of vitreous by paracentesis of anterior chamber, use 65810)

(For removal of corneovitreal adhesions, use 65880)

67015 Aspiration or release of vitreous, subretinal or choroidal fluid, pars plana approach (posterior sclerotomy)

67025 Injection of vitreous substitute, pars plana or limbal approach, (fluid-gas exchange), with or without aspiration (separate procedure)

67027 Implantation of intravitreal drug delivery system (eg, ganciclovir implant), includes concomitant removal of vitreous

(For removal, use 67121)

67028 Intravitreal injection of a pharmacologic agent (separate procedure)

67030 Discission of vitreous strands (without removal), pars plana approach

67031 Severing of vitreous strands, vitreous face adhesions, sheets, membranes or opacities, laser surgery (one or more stages)

67036 Vitrectomy, mechanical, pars plana approach;

67038 with epiretinal membrane stripping

67039 with focal endolaser photocoagulation

617

	Separate Procedure		Unlisted Procedure		CCI Comp. Code		Non-specific Procedure

67040   with endolaser panretinal photocoagulation

(For use of ophthalmic endoscope with 67038, 67039, 67040, use 66990)

(For associated lensectomy, use 66850)

(For use of vitrectomy in retinal detachment surgery, use 67108)

(For associated removal of foreign body, see 65260, 65265)

(For unlisted procedures on vitreous, use 67299)

RETINA OR CHOROID

Repair

(If diathermy, cryotherapy and/or photocoagulation are combined, report under principal modality used)

67101   Repair of retinal detachment, one or more sessions; cryotherapy or diathermy, with or without drainage of subretinal fluid

67105   photocoagulation, with or without drainage of subretinal fluid

67107   Repair of retinal detachment; scleral buckling (such as lamellar scleral dissection, imbrication or encircling procedure), with or without implant, with or without cryotherapy, photocoagulation, and drainage of subretinal fluid

67108   with vitrectomy, any method, with or without air or gas tamponade, focal endolaser photocoagulation, cryotherapy, drainage of subretinal fluid, scleral buckling, and/or removal of lens by same technique

67110   by injection of air or other gas (eg, pneumatic retinopexy)

67112   by scleral buckling or vitrectomy, on patient having previous ipsilateral retinal detachment repair(s) using scleral buckling or vitrectomy techniques

(For aspiration of drainage of subretinal or subchoroidal fluid, use 67015)

67115   Release of encircling material (posterior segment)

67120   Removal of implanted material, posterior segment; extraocular

67121   intraocular

618   ● New Code   ▲ Revised Code   + Add-On Code   ⊘ Modifier -51 Exempt

(For removal from anterior segment, use 65920)

(For removal of foreign body, see 65260, 65265)

Prophylaxis

67141 Prophylaxis of retinal detachment (eg, retinal break, lattice degeneration) without drainage, one or more sessions; cryotherapy, diathermy

67145 photocoagulation (laser or xenon arc)

Destruction

67208 Destruction of localized lesion of retina (eg, macular edema, tumors), one or more sessions; cryotherapy, diathermy

67210 photocoagulation

67218 radiation by implantation of source (includes removal of source)

67220 Destruction of localized lesion of choroid (eg, choroidal neovascularization); photocoagulation (eg, laser), one or more sessions

(For destruction of macular drusen, photocoagulation, use Category III code 0017T)

(For destruction of localized lesion of choroid by transpupillary thermotherapy, use Category III code 0016T)

67221 photodynamic therapy (includes intravenous infusion)

+ 67225 photodynamic therapy, second eye, at single session (List separately in addition to code for primary eye treatment)

(Use 67225 in conjunction with code 67221)

67227 Destruction of extensive or progressive retinopathy (eg, diabetic retinopathy), one or more sessions; cryotherapy, diathermy

67228 photocoagulation (laser or xenon arc)

(For unlisted procedures on retina, use 67299)

619

 Separate Procedure

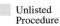 Unlisted Procedure

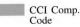 CCI Comp. Code

 Non-specific Procedure

SCLERA

Repair

(For excision lesion sclera, use 66130)

67250 Scleral reinforcement (separate procedure); without graft

67255 with graft

(For repair scleral staphyloma, see 66220, 66225)

OTHER PROCEDURES

67299 Unlisted procedure, posterior segment

OCULAR ADNEXA

EXTRAOCULAR MUSCLES

67311 Strabismus surgery, recession or resection procedure; one horizontal muscle

67312 two horizontal muscles

67314 one vertical muscle (excluding superior oblique)

67316 two or more vertical muscles (excluding superior oblique)

(For adjustable sutures, use 67335 in addition to codes 67311-67334 for primary procedure reflecting number of muscles operated on)

67318 Strabismus surgery, any procedure, superior oblique muscle

+ **67320** Transposition procedure (eg, for paretic extraocular muscle), any extraocular muscle (specify) (List separately in addition to code for primary procedure)

(Use 67320 in conjunction with codes 67311-67318)

+ **67331** Strabismus surgery on patient with previous eye surgery or injury that did not involve the extraocular muscles (List separately in addition to code for primary procedure)

(Use 67331 in conjunction with codes 67311-67318)

● New Code   ▲ Revised Code   + Add-On Code   ⊘ Modifier -51 Exempt

+ 67332 Strabismus surgery on patient with scarring of extraocular muscles (eg, prior ocular injury, strabismus or retinal detachment surgery) or restrictive myopathy (eg, dysthyroid ophthalmopathy) (List separately in addition to code for primary procedure)

(Use 67332 in conjunction with codes 67311-67318)

+ 67334 Strabismus surgery by posterior fixation suture technique, with or without muscle recession (List separately in addition to code for primary procedure)

(Use 67334 in conjunction with codes 67311-67318)

+ 67335 Placement of adjustable suture(s) during strabismus surgery, including postoperative adjustment(s) of suture(s) (List separately in addition to code for specific strabismus surgery)

(Use 67335 in conjunction with codes 67311-67334)

+ 67340 Strabismus surgery involving exploration and/or repair of detached extraocular muscle(s) (List separately in addition to code for primary procedure)

(Use 67340 in conjunction with codes 67311-67334)

67343 Release of extensive scar tissue without detaching extraocular muscle (separate procedure)

(Use 67343 in conjunction with codes 67311-67340, when such procedures are performed other than on the affected muscle)

67345 Chemodenervation of extraocular muscle

(For chemodenervation for blepharospasm and other neurological disorders, see 64612 and 64613)

Other Procedures

67350 Biopsy of extraocular muscle

(For repair of wound, extraocular muscle, tendon or Tenon's capsule, use 65290)

67399 Unlisted procedure, ocular muscle

621

Separate Procedure	Unlisted Procedure	CCI Comp. Code	Non-specific Procedure

ORBIT

Exploration, Excision, Decompression

67400 Orbitotomy without bone flap (frontal or transconjunctival approach); for exploration, with or without biopsy

67405 with drainage only

67412 with removal of lesion

67413 with removal of foreign body

67414 with removal of bone for decompression

67415 Fine needle aspiration of orbital contents

(For exenteration, enucleation, and repair, see 65101 et seq; for optic nerve decompression, use 67570)

67420 Orbitotomy with bone flap or window, lateral approach (eg, Kroenlein); with removal of lesion

67430 with removal of foreign body

67440 with drainage

67445 with removal of bone for decompression

(For optic nerve sheath decompression, use 67570)

67450 for exploration, with or without biopsy

(For orbitotomy, transcranial approach, see 61330-61334)

(For orbital implant, see 67550, 67560)

(For removal of eyeball or for repair after removal, see 65091-65175)

Other Procedures

67500 Retrobulbar injection; medication (separate procedure, does not include supply of medication)

67505 alcohol

67515 Injection of medication or other substance into Tenon's capsule

622

| ● | New Code | ▲ | Revised Code | ✚ | Add-On Code | ⊘ | Modifier -51 Exempt |

(For subconjunctival injection, use 68200)

67550 Orbital implant (implant outside muscle cone); insertion

67560   removal or revision

(For ocular implant (implant inside muscle cone), see 65093-65105, 65130-65175)

(For treatment of fractures of malar area, orbit, see 21355 et seq)

67570 Optic nerve decompression (eg, incision or fenestration of optic nerve sheath)

67599 Unlisted procedure, orbit

EYELIDS

Incision

67700 Blepharotomy, drainage of abscess, eyelid

67710 Severing of tarsorrhaphy

67715 Canthotomy (separate procedure)

(For canthoplasty, use 67950)

(For division of symblepharon, use 68340)

Excision

(For removal of lesion, involving mainly skin of eyelid, see 11310-11313; 11440-11446, 11640-11646; 17000-17004)

(For repair of wounds, blepharoplasty, grafts, reconstructive surgery, see 67930-67975)

67800 Excision of chalazion; single

67801   multiple, same lid

67805   multiple, different lids

67808   under general anesthesia and/or requiring hospitalization, single or multiple

67810 Biopsy of eyelid

623

| Separate Procedure | Unlisted Procedure |  CCI Comp. Code | Non-specific Procedure |

67820 Correction of trichiasis; epilation, by forceps only

67825 epilation by other than forceps (eg, by electrosurgery, cryotherapy, laser surgery)

67830 incision of lid margin

67835 incision of lid margin, with free mucous membrane graft

67840 Excision of lesion of eyelid (except chalazion) without closure or with simple direct closure

(For excision and repair of eyelid by reconstructive surgery, see 67961, 67966)

67850 Destruction of lesion of lid margin (up to 1 cm)

(For Mohs micrographic surgery, see 17304-17310)

(For initiation or follow-up care of topical chemotherapy (eg, 5-FU or similar agents), see appropriate office visits)

Tarsorrhaphy

67875 Temporary closure of eyelids by suture (eg, Frost suture)

67880 Construction of intermarginal adhesions, median tarsorrhaphy, or canthorrhaphy;

67882 with transposition of tarsal plate

(For severing of tarsorrhaphy, use 67710)

(For canthoplasty, reconstruction canthus, use 67950)

(For canthotomy, use 67715)

Repair (Brow Ptosis, Blepharoptosis, Lid Retraction, Ectropion, Entropion)

67900 Repair of brow ptosis (supraciliary, mid-forehead or coronal approach)

(For forehead rhytidectomy, use 15824)

67901 Repair of blepharoptosis; frontalis muscle technique with suture or other material

● New Code　　▲ Revised Code　　+ Add-On Code　　⊘ Modifier -51 Exempt

67902   frontalis muscle technique with fascial sling (includes obtaining fascia)

67903   (tarso) levator resection or advancement, internal approach

67904   (tarso) levator resection or advancement, external approach

67906   superior rectus technique with fascial sling (includes obtaining fascia)

67908   conjunctivo-tarso-Muller's muscle-levator resection (eg, Fasanella-Servat type)

67909   Reduction of overcorrection of ptosis

67911   Correction of lid retraction

(For obtaining autogenous graft materials, see 20920, 20922, or 20926)

(For correction of trichiasis by mucous membrane graft, use 67835)

● **67912**   Correction of lagophthalmos, with implantation of upper eyelid load (eg, gold weight)

67914   Repair of ectropion; suture

67915   thermocauterization

▲ **67916**   excision tarsal wedge

▲ **67917**   extensive (eg, tarsal strip operations)

(For correction of everted punctum, use 68705)

67921   Repair of entropion; suture

67922   thermocauterization

▲ **67923**   excision tarsal wedge

▲ **67924**   extensive (eg, tarsal strip or capsulopalpebral fascia repairs operation)

(For repair of cicatricial ectropion or entropion requiring scar excision or skin graft, see also 67961 et seq)

625

	Separate Procedure		Unlisted Procedure		CCI Comp. Code		Non-specific Procedure

Reconstruction

67930 Suture of recent wound, eyelid, involving lid margin, tarsus, and/or palpebral conjunctiva direct closure; partial thickness

67935 full thickness

67938 Removal of embedded foreign body, eyelid

(For repair of skin of eyelid, see 12011-12018; 12051-12057; 13150-13153)

(For tarsorrhaphy, canthorrhaphy, see 67880, 67882)

(For repair of blepharoptosis and lid retraction, see 67901-67911)

(For blepharoplasty for entropion, ectropion, see 67916, 67917, 67923, 67924)

(For correction of blepharochalasis (blepharorhytidectomy), see 15820-15823)

(For repair of skin of eyelid, adjacent tissue transfer, see 14060, 14061; preparation for graft, use 15000; free graft, see 15120, 15121, 15260, 15261)

(For excision of lesion of eyelid, use 67800 et seq)

(For repair of lacrimal canaliculi, use 68700)

67950 Canthoplasty (reconstruction of canthus)

67961 Excision and repair of eyelid, involving lid margin, tarsus, conjunctiva, canthus, or full thickness, may include preparation for skin graft or pedicle flap with adjacent tissue transfer or rearrangement; up to one-fourth of lid margin

67966 over one-fourth of lid margin

(For canthoplasty, use 67950)

(For free skin grafts, see 15120, 15121, 15260, 15261)

(For tubed pedicle flap preparation, use 15576; for delay, use 15630; for attachment, use 15650)

67971 Reconstruction of eyelid, full thickness by transfer of tarsoconjunctival flap from opposing eyelid; up to two-thirds of eyelid, one stage or first stage

● New Code   ▲ Revised Code   + Add-On Code   ⊘ Modifier -51 Exempt

67973   total eyelid, lower, one stage or first stage

67974   total eyelid, upper, one stage or first stage

67975   second stage

Other Procedures

67999   Unlisted procedure, eyelids

CONJUNCTIVA

(For removal of foreign body, see 65205 et seq)

INCISION AND DRAINAGE

68020   Incision of conjunctiva, drainage of cyst

68040   Expression of conjunctival follicles (eg, for trachoma)

EXCISION AND/OR DESTRUCTION

68100   Biopsy of conjunctiva

68110   Excision of lesion, conjunctiva; up to 1 cm

68115   over 1 cm

68130   with adjacent sclera

68135   Destruction of lesion, conjunctiva

INJECTION

(For injection into Tenon's capsule or retrobulbar injection, see 67500-67515)

68200   Subconjunctival injection

CONJUNCTIVOPLASTY

(For wound repair, see 65270-65273)

68320   Conjunctivoplasty; with conjunctival graft or extensive rearrangement

68325   with buccal mucous membrane graft (includes obtaining graft)

627

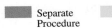 Separate Procedure   Unlisted Procedure   CCI Comp. Code   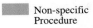 Non-specific Procedure

| 68326 | Conjunctivoplasty, reconstruction cul-de-sac; with conjunctival graft or extensive rearrangement |

68326 Conjunctivoplasty, reconstruction cul-de-sac; with conjunctival graft or extensive rearrangement

68328 with buccal mucous membrane graft (includes obtaining graft)

68330 Repair of symblepharon; conjunctivoplasty, without graft

68335 with free graft conjunctiva or buccal mucous membrane (includes obtaining graft)

68340 division of symblepharon, with or without insertion of conformer or contact lens

OTHER PROCEDURES

68360 Conjunctival flap; bridge or partial (separate procedure)

68362 total (such as Gunderson thin flap or purse string flap)

(For conjunctival flap for perforating injury, see 65280, 65285)

(For repair of operative wound, use 66250)

(For removal of conjunctival foreign body, see 65205, 65210)

● **68371** Harvesting conjunctival allograft, living donor

68399 Unlisted procedure, conjunctiva

LACRIMAL SYSTEM

Incision

68400 Incision, drainage of lacrimal gland

68420 Incision, drainage of lacrimal sac (dacryocystotomy or dacryocystostomy)

68440 Snip incision of lacrimal punctum

Excision

68500 Excision of lacrimal gland (dacryoadenectomy), except for tumor; total

68505 partial

● New Code　　▲ Revised Code　　+ Add-On Code　　⊘ Modifier -51 Exempt

68510 Biopsy of lacrimal gland

68520 Excision of lacrimal sac (dacryocystectomy)

68525 Biopsy of lacrimal sac

68530 Removal of foreign body or dacryolith, lacrimal passages

68540 Excision of lacrimal gland tumor; frontal approach

68550 involving osteotomy

Repair

68700 Plastic repair of canaliculi

68705 Correction of everted punctum, cautery

68720 Dacryocystorhinostomy (fistulization of lacrimal sac to nasal cavity)

68745 Conjunctivorhinostomy (fistulization of conjunctiva to nasal cavity); without tube

68750 with insertion of tube or stent

68760 Closure of the lacrimal punctum; by thermocauterization, ligation, or laser surgery

68761 by plug, each

68770 Closure of lacrimal fistula (separate procedure)

Probing and/or Related Procedures

68801 Dilation of lacrimal punctum, with or without irrigation

(To report a bilateral procedure, use 68801 with modifier -50)

68810 Probing of nasolacrimal duct, with or without irrigation;

68811 requiring general anesthesia

68815 with insertion of tube or stent

(See also 92018)

629

 Separate Procedure    Unlisted Procedure   CCI Comp. Code   Non-specific Procedure

(To report a bilateral procedure, use 68810, 68811, or 68815 with modifier -50)

68840   Probing of lacrimal canaliculi, with or without irrigation

68850   Injection of contrast medium for dacryocystography

(For radiological supervision and interpretation, see 70170, 78660)

Other Procedures

68899   Unlisted procedure, lacrimal system

● New Code   ▲ Revised Code   ✚ Add-On Code   ⊘ Modifier -51 Exempt

AUDITORY SYSTEM

CPT codes from this subsection of the CPT coding system are used to report invasive and surgical procedures performed on the external ear; middle ear; inner ear and temporal bone. Includes procedures performed on the inner, outer and middle ear and to the temporal bone.

Diagnostic services, such as otoscopy under general anesthesia, audiometry and vestibular tests, are defined in the Medicine Section of the CPT manual.

Wound repairs to the external ear are located in the Integumentary Subsection of the CPT coding system.

> (For diagnostic services (eg, audiometry, vestibular tests), see 92502 et seq)

EXTERNAL EAR

INCISION

69000 Drainage external ear, abscess or hematoma; simple

69005   complicated

69020 Drainage external auditory canal, abscess

69090 Ear piercing

EXCISION

69100 Biopsy external ear

69105 Biopsy external auditory canal

69110 Excision external ear; partial, simple repair

69120   complete amputation

(For reconstruction of ear, see 15120 et seq)

69140 Excision exostosis(es), external auditory canal

69145 Excision soft tissue lesion, external auditory canal

69150 Radical excision external auditory canal lesion; without neck dissection

631

 Separate Procedure   Unlisted Procedure    CCI Comp. Code   Non-specific Procedure

69155   with neck dissection

(For resection of temporal bone, use 69535)

(For skin grafting, see 15000-15261)

REMOVAL OF FOREIGN BODY

69200   Removal foreign body from external auditory canal; without general anesthesia

69205   with general anesthesia

69210   Removal impacted cerumen (separate procedure), one or both ears

69220   Debridement, mastoidectomy cavity, simple (eg, routine cleaning)

69222   Debridement, mastoidectomy cavity, complex (eg, with anesthesia or more than routine cleaning)

REPAIR

(For suture of wound or injury of external ear, see 12011-14300)

69300   Otoplasty, protruding ear, with or without size reduction

69310   Reconstruction of external auditory canal (meatoplasty) (eg, for stenosis due to injury, infection) (separate procedure)

69320   Reconstruction external auditory canal for congenital atresia, single stage

(For combination with middle ear reconstruction, see 69631, 69641)

(For other reconstructive procedures with grafts (eg, skin, cartilage, bone), see 13150-15760, 21230-21235)

OTHER PROCEDURES

(For otoscopy under general anesthesia, use 92502)

69399   Unlisted procedure, external ear

●	New Code	▲ Revised Code	+ Add-On Code	⃠ Modifier -51 Exempt

MIDDLE EAR

INTRODUCTION

69400 Eustachian tube inflation, transnasal; with catheterization

69401   without catheterization

69405 Eustachian tube catheterization, transtympanic

69410 Focal application of phase control substance, middle ear (baffle technique)

INCISION

69420 Myringotomy including aspiration and/or eustachian tube inflation

69421 Myringotomy including aspiration and/or eustachian tube inflation requiring general anesthesia

69424 Ventilating tube removal requiring general anesthesia

(69424 is a unilateral procedure. To report a bilateral procedure, use 69424 with modifier '-50')

(Do not report code 69424 in conjunction with codes 69205, 69210, 69420, 69421, 69433-69676, 69710-69745, 69801-69930)

69433 Tympanostomy (requiring insertion of ventilating tube), local or topical anesthesia

69436 Tympanostomy (requiring insertion of ventilating tube), general anesthesia

69440 Middle ear exploration through postauricular or ear canal incision

(For atticotomy, see 69601 et seq)

69450 Tympanolysis, transcanal

EXCISION

69501 Transmastoid antrotomy (simple mastoidectomy)

69502 Mastoidectomy; complete

633

 Separate Procedure   Unlisted Procedure   CCI Comp. Code   Non-specific Procedure

| 69505 | modified radical |

| 69511 | radical |

(For skin graft, see 15000 et seq)

(For mastoidectomy cavity debridement, see 69220, 69222)

| 69530 | Petrous apicectomy including radical mastoidectomy |

| 69535 | Resection temporal bone, external approach |

(For middle fossa approach, see 69950-69970)

| 69540 | Excision aural polyp |

| 69550 | Excision aural glomus tumor; transcanal |

| 69552 | transmastoid |

| 69554 | extended (extratemporal) |

REPAIR

| 69601 | Revision mastoidectomy; resulting in complete mastoidectomy |

| 69602 | resulting in modified radical mastoidectomy |

| 69603 | resulting in radical mastoidectomy |

| 69604 | resulting in tympanoplasty |

(For planned secondary tympanoplasty after mastoidectomy, see 69631, 69632)

| 69605 | with apicectomy |

(For skin graft, see 15120, 15121, 15260, 15261)

| 69610 | Tympanic membrane repair, with or without site preparation or perforation for closure, with or without patch |

| 69620 | Myringoplasty (surgery confined to drumhead and donor area) |

| 69631 | Tympanoplasty without mastoidectomy (including canalplasty, atticotomy and/or middle ear surgery), initial or revision; without ossicular chain reconstruction |

● New Code   ▲ Revised Code   + Add-On Code   ⊘ Modifier -51 Exempt

69632   with ossicular chain reconstruction (eg, postfenestration)

69633   with ossicular chain reconstruction and synthetic prosthesis (eg, partial ossicular replacement prosthesis (PORP), total ossicular replacement prosthesis (TORP))

69635   Tympanoplasty with antrotomy or mastoidotomy (including canalplasty, atticotomy, middle ear surgery, and/or tympanic membrane repair); without ossicular chain reconstruction

69636   with ossicular chain reconstruction

69637   with ossicular chain reconstruction and synthetic prosthesis (eg, partial ossicular replacement prosthesis (PORP), total ossicular replacement prosthesis (TORP))

69641   Tympanoplasty with mastoidectomy (including canalplasty, middle ear surgery, tympanic membrane repair); without ossicular chain reconstruction

69642   with ossicular chain reconstruction

69643   with intact or reconstructed wall, without ossicular chain reconstruction

69644   with intact or reconstructed canal wall, with ossicular chain reconstruction

69645   radical or complete, without ossicular chain reconstruction

69646   radical or complete, with ossicular chain reconstruction

69650   Stapes mobilization

69660   Stapedectomy or stapedotomy with reestablishment of ossicular continuity, with or without use of foreign material;

69661   with footplate drill out

69662   Revision of stapedectomy or stapedotomy

69666   Repair oval window fistula

69667   Repair round window fistula

69670   Mastoid obliteration (separate procedure)

635

| | Separate Procedure | | Unlisted Procedure | | CCI Comp. Code | | Non-specific Procedure |

69676 Tympanic neurectomy

OTHER PROCEDURES

69700 Closure postauricular fistula, mastoid (separate procedure)

69710 Implantation or replacement of electromagnetic bone conduction hearing device in temporal bone

(Replacement procedure includes removal of old device)

69711 Removal or repair of electromagnetic bone conduction hearing device in temporal bone

69714 Implantation, osseointegrated implant, temporal bone, with percutaneous attachment to external speech processor/cochlear stimulator; without mastoidectomy

69715 with mastoidectomy

69717 Replacement (including removal of existing device), osseointegrated implant, temporal bone, with percutaneous attachment to external speech processor/cochlear stimulator; without mastoidectomy

69718 with mastoidectomy

69720 Decompression facial nerve, intratemporal; lateral to geniculate ganglion

69725 including medial to geniculate ganglion

69740 Suture facial nerve, intratemporal, with or without graft or decompression; lateral to geniculate ganglion

69745 including medial to geniculate ganglion

(For extracranial suture of facial nerve, use 64864)

69799 Unlisted procedure, middle ear

| ● | New Code | ▲ | Revised Code | + | Add-On Code | ⊘ | Modifier -51 Exempt |

INNER EAR

INCISION AND/OR DESTRUCTION

69801 Labyrinthotomy, with or without cryosurgery including other nonexcisional destructive procedures or perfusion of vestibuloactive drugs (single or multiple perfusions); transcanal

(69801 includes all required infusions performed on initial and subsequent days of treatment)

69802 with mastoidectomy

69805 Endolymphatic sac operation; without shunt

69806 with shunt

69820 Fenestration semicircular canal

69840 Revision fenestration operation

EXCISION

69905 Labyrinthectomy; transcanal

69910 with mastoidectomy

69915 Vestibular nerve section, translabyrinthine approach

(For transcranial approach, use 69950)

INTRODUCTION

69930 Cochlear device implantation, with or without mastoidectomy

OTHER PROCEDURES

69949 Unlisted procedure, inner ear

TEMPORAL BONE, MIDDLE FOSSA APPROACH

(For external approach, use 69535)

69950 Vestibular nerve section, transcranial approach

69955 Total facial nerve decompression and/or repair (may include graft)

637

 Separate Procedure

Unlisted Procedure

 CCI Comp. Code

 Non-specific Procedure

69960 Decompression internal auditory canal

69970 Removal of tumor, temporal bone

OTHER PROCEDURES

69979 Unlisted procedure, temporal bone, middle fossa approach

● New Code   ▲ Revised Code   ✛ Add-On Code   ⊘ Modifier -51 Exempt

OPERATING MICROSCOPE

+ **69990**   Microsurgical techniques, requiring use of operating microscope
(List separately in addition to code for primary procedure)

 Separate
Procedure
 Unlisted
Procedure
 CCI Comp.
Code
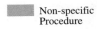 Non-specific
Procedure

This page intentionally left blank.

● New
Code

▲ Revised
Code

✛ Add-On
Code

⊘ Modifier -51
Exempt

RADIOLOGY

RADIOLOGY SECTION OVERVIEW

The fourth section of the CPT coding system is the radiology section, which includes diagnostic and therapeutic radiology, nuclear medicine and diagnostic ultrasound services. Within each subsection, the CPT codes are arranged by anatomical site.

Diagnostic radiology uses all modalities of radiant energy in medical diagnosis and therapeutic procedures requiring radiologic guidance. This includes imaging techniques and methodologies using radiation emitted by x-ray tubes, radionuclides, ultrasonographic devices, and radiofrequency electromagnetic radiation.

RADIOLOGY SUBSECTIONS

The RADIOLOGY section of the CPT coding system is divided into 4 subsections; namely:

Diagnostic Radiology (Diagnostic Imaging)	70010-76499
Diagnostic Ultrasound	76506-76999
Radiation Oncology	77261-77799
Nuclear Medicine	78000-79999

COMPLETE PROCEDURES

Interventional radiologic procedures or diagnostic studies involving injection of contrast media include all usual preinjection and postinjection services, for example, necessary local anesthesia, placement of needle or catheter, injection of contrast media, supervision of the study, and interpretation of results. When one of these procedures is performed in full by a single physician, it is designated as a "complete procedure."

SUPERVISION AND INTERPRETATION ONLY

When a procedure is performed by a radiologist-clinician team, it is designated as "supervision and interpretation only" and the separate injection procedure is listed in the appropriate section of the SURGERY section of the CPT coding system. These CPT codes are used only when a procedure is performed by more than one physician, for example, a radiologist-clinician team.

641

 Separate Procedure
 Unlisted Procedure
 CCI Comp. Code
 Non-specific Procedure

RADIOLOGY SERVICE MODIFIERS

Listed surgical services and procedures may be modified under certain circumstances. When applicable, the modifying circumstance is identified by adding the appropriate two digit modifier to the base procedure code(s). Modifiers commonly used to report RADIOLOGY services include:

-22 Unusual services

-26 Professional component

-32 Mandated services

-51 Multiple procedures

-52 Reduced services

-62 Two surgeons

-66 Surgical team

-76 Repeat procedure by same physician

-77 Repeat procedure by another physician

-78 Return to the operating room for a related procedure during the postoperative period

-79 Unrelated procedure or service by the same physician during the postoperative period

-80 Assistant surgeon

-90 Reference (outside) laboratory

-99 Multiple modifiers

-LT Left side of body

-RT Right side of body

BILATERAL PROCEDURE CODES

The RADIOLOGY section includes some CPT codes which include the term "bilateral" in the definition. When reporting these services, do not add the modifier -50, because the procedure is already defined as "bilateral."

● New Code ▲ Revised Code + Add-On Code ⊘ Modifier -51 Exempt

RADIOLOGY SERVICES MEDICARE CONSIDERATIONS

Most of the CPT codes in this section are subject to Medicare Purchased Diagnostic Services guidelines. Coding and reporting should be as instructed by your local Medicare carrier.

| Separate Procedure | Unlisted Procedure | CCI Comp. Code | Non-specific Procedure |

This page intentionally left blank.

● New
Code

▲ Revised
Code

✚ Add-On
Code

⊘ Modifier -51
Exempt

RADIOLOGY CODES

DIAGNOSTIC RADIOLOGY (DIAGNOSTIC IMAGING)

HEAD AND NECK

(70002, 70003 have been deleted. To report, use 76499)

70010 Myelography, posterior fossa, radiological supervision and interpretation

70015 Cisternography, positive contrast, radiological supervision and interpretation

70030 Radiologic examination, eye, for detection of foreign body

70100 Radiologic examination, mandible; partial, less than four views

70110 complete, minimum of four views

70120 Radiologic examination, mastoids; less than three views per side

70130 complete, minimum of three views per side

70134 Radiologic examination, internal auditory meati, complete

70140 Radiologic examination, facial bones; less than three views

70150 complete, minimum of three views

70160 Radiologic examination, nasal bones, complete, minimum of three views

70170 Dacryocystography, nasolacrimal duct, radiological supervision and interpretation

70190 Radiologic examination; optic foramina

70200 orbits, complete, minimum of four views

70210 Radiologic examination, sinuses, paranasal, less than three views

| 70220 | Radiologic examination, sinuses, paranasal, complete, minimum of three views |

70240 Radiologic examination, sella turcica

▲ **70250** Radiologic examination, skull; less than four views

▲ 70260 complete, minimum of four views

70300 Radiologic examination, teeth; single view

70310 partial examination, less than full mouth

70320 complete, full mouth

70328 Radiologic examination, temporomandibular joint, open and closed mouth; unilateral

70330 bilateral

70332 Temporomandibular joint arthrography, radiological supervision and interpretation

(Do not report 76003 in addition to 70332)

70336 Magnetic resonance (eg, proton) imaging, temporomandibular joint(s)

70350 Cephalogram, orthodontic

70355 Orthopantogram

70360 Radiologic examination; neck, soft tissue

70370 pharynx or larynx, including fluoroscopy and/or magnification technique

70371 Complex dynamic pharyngeal and speech evaluation by cine or video recording

70373 Laryngography, contrast, radiological supervision and interpretation

70380 Radiologic examination, salivary gland for calculus

70390 Sialography, radiological supervision and interpretation

● New Code ▲ Revised Code + Add-On Code ⊘ Modifier -51 Exempt

70450   Computed tomography, head or brain; without contrast material

70460   with contrast material(s)

70470   without contrast material, followed by contrast material(s) and further sections

    (For coronal, sagittal, and/or oblique sections, use 76375)

70480   Computed tomography, orbit, sella, or posterior fossa or outer, middle, or inner ear; without contrast material

70481   with contrast material(s)

70482   without contrast material, followed by contrast material(s) and further sections

    (For coronal, sagittal, and/or oblique sections, use 76375)

70486   Computed tomography, maxillofacial area; without contrast material

70487   with contrast material(s)

70488   without contrast material, followed by contrast material(s) and further sections

    (For coronal, sagittal, and/or oblique sections, use 76375)

70490   Computed tomography, soft tissue neck; without contrast material

70491   with contrast material(s)

70492   without contrast material followed by contrast material(s) and further sections

    (For coronal, sagittal, and/or oblique sections, use 76375)

    (For cervical spine, see 72125, 72126)

70496   Computed tomographic angiography, head, without contrast material(s), followed by contrast material(s) and further sections, including image post-processing

70498   Computed tomographic angiography, neck, without contrast material(s), followed by contrast material(s) and further sections, including image post-processing

647

	Separate Procedure		Unlisted Procedure		CCI Comp. Code		Non-specific Procedure

70540   Magnetic resonance (eg, proton) imaging, orbit, face, and neck; without contrast material(s)

70542   with contrast material(s)

70543   without contrast material(s), followed by contrast material(s) and further sequences

70544   Magnetic resonance angiography, head; without contrast materials

70545   with contrast materials

70546   without contrast material(s), followed by contrast material(s) and further sequences

70547   Magnetic resonance angiography, neck; without contrast materials

70548   with contrast materials

70549   without contrast material(s), followed by contrast material(s) and further sequences

70551   Magnetic resonance (eg, proton) imaging, brain (including brain stem); without contrast material

70552   with contrast material(s)

70553   without contrast material, followed by contrast material(s) and further sequences

        (For magnetic spectroscopy, use 76390)

● **70557**   Magnetic resonance (eg, proton) imaging, brain (including brain stem and skull base), during open intracranial procedure (eg, to assess for residual tumor or residual vascular malformation); without contrast material

● **70558**   with contrast material(s)

● **70559**   without contrast material(s), followed by contrast material(s) and further sequences

---

648   ● New Code   ▲ Revised Code   + Add-On Code   ⊘ Modifier -51 Exempt

(For stereotactic biopsy of intracranial lesion with magnetic resonance guidance, use 61751. 70557, 70558 or 70559 may be reported only if a separate report is generated. Report only one of the above codes once per operative session. Do not use these codes in conjunction with 61751, 76393, 76394)

CHEST

(71000 has been deleted)

71010   Radiologic examination, chest; single view, frontal

71015   stereo, frontal

71020   Radiologic examination, chest, two views, frontal and lateral;

71021   with apical lordotic procedure

71022   with oblique projections

71023   with fluoroscopy

71030   Radiologic examination, chest, complete, minimum of four views;

71034   with fluoroscopy

(For separate chest fluoroscopy, use 76000)

71035   Radiologic examination, chest, special views (eg, lateral decubitus, Bucky studies)

71040   Bronchography, unilateral, radiological supervision and interpretation

71060   Bronchography, bilateral, radiological supervision and interpretation

71090   Insertion pacemaker, fluoroscopy and radiography, radiological supervision and interpretation

(For procedure, see appropriate organ or site)

71100   Radiologic examination, ribs, unilateral; two views

71101   including posteroanterior chest, minimum of three views

649

 Separate Procedure   Unlisted Procedure    CCI Comp. Code   Non-specific Procedure

71110   Radiologic examination, ribs, bilateral; three views

71111   including posteroanterior chest, minimum of four views

71120   Radiologic examination; sternum, minimum of two views

71130   sternoclavicular joint or joints, minimum of three views

71250   Computed tomography, thorax; without contrast material

71260   with contrast material(s)

71270   without contrast material, followed by contrast material(s) and further sections

(For coronal, sagittal, and/or oblique sections, use 76375)

71275   Computed tomographic angiography, chest, without contrast material(s), followed by contrast material(s) and further sections, including image post-processing

71550   Magnetic resonance (eg, proton) imaging, chest (eg, for evaluation of hilar and mediastinal lymphadenopathy); without contrast material(s)

71551   with contrast material(s)

71552   without contrast material(s), followed by contrast material(s) and further sequences

(For breast MRI, see 76093 and 76094)

71555   Magnetic resonance angiography, chest (excluding myocardium), with or without contrast material(s)

SPINE AND PELVIS

72010   Radiologic examination, spine, entire, survey study, anteroposterior and lateral

72020   Radiologic examination, spine, single view, specify level

72040   Radiologic examination, spine, cervical; two or three views

72050   minimum of four views

650   ● New Code   ▲ Revised Code   ✚ Add-On Code   ⊘ Modifier -51 Exempt

72052   complete, including oblique and flexion and/or extension studies

72069   Radiologic examination, spine, thoracolumbar, standing (scoliosis)

72070   Radiologic examination, spine; thoracic, two views

72072   thoracic, three views

72074   thoracic, minimum of four views

72080   thoracolumbar, two views

72090   scoliosis study, including supine and erect studies

72100   Radiologic examination, spine, lumbosacral; two or three views

72110   minimum of four views

72114   complete, including bending views

72120   Radiologic examination, spine, lumbosacral, bending views only, minimum of four views

(Contrast material in CT of spine is either by intrathecal or intravenous injection. For intrathecal injection, use also 61055 or 62284. IV injection of contrast material is part of the CT procedure)

72125   Computed tomography, cervical spine; without contrast material

72126   with contrast material

72127   without contrast material, followed by contrast material(s) and further sections

(For intrathecal injection procedure, see 61055, 62284)

72128   Computed tomography, thoracic spine; without contrast material

72129   with contrast material

(For intrathecal injection procedure, see 61055, 62284)

72130   without contrast material, followed by contrast material(s) and further sections

651

Separate Procedure	Unlisted Procedure	CCI Comp. Code	Non-specific Procedure

(For intrathecal injection procedure, see 61055, 62284)

72131 Computed tomography, lumbar spine; without contrast material

72132 with contrast material

72133 without contrast material, followed by contrast material(s) and further sections

(For intrathecal injection procedure, see 61055, 62284)

(For coronal, sagittal, and/or oblique sections, use 76375)

72141 Magnetic resonance (eg, proton) imaging, spinal canal and contents, cervical; without contrast material

72142 with contrast material(s)

(For cervical spinal canal imaging without contrast material followed by contrast material, use 72156)

72146 Magnetic resonance (eg, proton) imaging, spinal canal and contents, thoracic; without contrast material

72147 with contrast material(s)

(For thoracic spinal canal imaging without contrast material followed by contrast material, use 72157)

72148 Magnetic resonance (eg, proton) imaging, spinal canal and contents, lumbar; without contrast material

72149 with contrast material(s)

(For lumbar spinal canal imaging without contrast material followed by contrast material, use 72158)

72156 Magnetic resonance (eg, proton) imaging, spinal canal and contents, without contrast material, followed by contrast material(s) and further sequences; cervical

72157 thoracic

72158 lumbar

72159 Magnetic resonance angiography, spinal canal and contents, with or without contrast material(s)

● New Code   ▲ Revised Code   + Add-On Code   ⊘ Modifier -51 Exempt

72170   Radiologic examination, pelvis; one or two views

72190   complete, minimum of three views

(For pelvimetry, use 74710)

72191   Computed tomographic angiography, pelvis; without contrast material(s), followed by contrast material(s) and further sections, including image post-processing

(For CTA aorto-iliofemoral runoff, use 75635)

72192   Computed tomography, pelvis; without contrast material

72193   with contrast material(s)

72194   without contrast material, followed by contrast material(s) and further sections

(For coronal, sagittal, and/or oblique sections, use 76375)

72195   Magnetic resonance (eg, proton) imaging, pelvis; without contrast material(s)

72196   with contrast material(s)

72197   without contrast material(s), followed by contrast material(s) and further sequences

72198   Magnetic resonance angiography, pelvis, with or without contrast material(s)

72200   Radiologic examination, sacroiliac joints; less than three views

72202   three or more views

72220   Radiologic examination, sacrum and coccyx, minimum of two views

72240   Myelography, cervical, radiological supervision and interpretation

72255   Myelography, thoracic, radiological supervision and interpretation

72265   Myelography, lumbosacral, radiological supervision and interpretation

653

	Separate Procedure		Unlisted Procedure		CCI Comp. Code		Non-specific Procedure

▲ **72270** Myelography, two or more regions (eg, lumbar/thoracic, cervical/thoracic, lumbar/cervical, lumbar/thoracic/cervical), radiological supervision and interpretation

72275 Epidurography, radiological supervision and interpretation

(72275 includes 76005)

(For injection procedure, see 62280-62282, 62310-62319, 64479-64484, 0027T)

(Use 72275 only when an epidurogram is performed, images documented, and a formal radiologic report is issued)

72285 Diskography, cervical or thoracic, radiological supervision and interpretation

72295 Diskography, lumbar, radiological supervision and interpretation

UPPER EXTREMITIES

(For stress views, any joint, use 76006)

73000 Radiologic examination; clavicle, complete

73010 scapula, complete

73020 Radiologic examination, shoulder; one view

73030 complete, minimum of two views

73040 Radiologic examination, shoulder, arthrography, radiological supervision and interpretation

(Do not report 76003 in addition to 73040)

73050 Radiologic examination; acromioclavicular joints, bilateral, with or without weighted distraction

73060 humerus, minimum of two views

73070 Radiologic examination, elbow; two views

73080 complete, minimum of three views

73085 Radiologic examination, elbow, arthrography, radiological supervision and interpretation

(Do not report 76003 in addition to 73085)

73090   Radiologic examination; forearm, two views

73092   upper extremity, infant, minimum of two views

73100   Radiologic examination, wrist; two views

73110   complete, minimum of three views

73115   Radiologic examination, wrist, arthrography, radiological supervision and interpretation

(Do not report 76003 in addition to 73115)

73120   Radiologic examination, hand; two views

73130   minimum of three views

73140   Radiologic examination, finger(s), minimum of two views

73200   Computed tomography, upper extremity; without contrast material

73201   with contrast material(s)

73202   without contrast material, followed by contrast material(s) and further sections

(For coronal, sagittal, and/or oblique sections, use 76375)

73206   Computed tomographic angiography, upper extremity, without contrast material(s), followed by contrast material(s) and further sections, including image post-processing

73218   Magnetic resonance (eg, proton) imaging, upper extremity, other than joint; without contrast material(s)

73219   with contrast material(s)

73220   without contrast material(s), followed by contrast material(s) and further sequences

73221   Magnetic resonance (eg, proton) imaging, any joint of upper extremity; without contrast material(s)

73222   with contrast material(s)

655

| | Separate Procedure | | Unlisted Procedure | | CCI Comp. Code | | Non-specific Procedure |

73223   without contrast material(s), followed by contrast material(s) and further sequences

73225   Magnetic resonance angiography, upper extremity, with or without contrast material(s)

LOWER EXTREMITIES

(For stress views, any joint, use 76006)

73500   Radiologic examination, hip, unilateral; one view

73510   complete, minimum of two views

73520   Radiologic examination, hips, bilateral, minimum of two views of each hip, including anteroposterior view of pelvis

73525   Radiologic examination, hip, arthrography, radiological supervision and interpretation

(Do not report 76003 in addition to 73525)

73530   Radiologic examination, hip, during operative procedure

73540   Radiologic examination, pelvis and hips, infant or child, minimum of two views

73542   Radiological examination, sacroiliac joint arthrography, radiological supervision and interpretation

(Do not report 76003 in addition to 73542)

(For procedure, use 27096. If formal arthrography is not performed, recorded, and a formal radiologic report is not issued, use 76005 for fluoroscopic guidance for sacroiliac joint injections)

73550   Radiologic examination, femur, two views

73560   Radiologic examination, knee; one or two views

73562   three views

73564   complete, four or more views

73565   both knees, standing, anteroposterior

● New Code   ▲ Revised Code   + Add-On Code   ⊘ Modifier -51 Exempt

73580   Radiologic examination, knee, arthrography, radiological supervision and interpretation

(Do not report 76003 in addition to 73580)

73590   Radiologic examination; tibia and fibula, two views

73592   lower extremity, infant, minimum of two views

73600   Radiologic examination, ankle; two views

73610   complete, minimum of three views

73615   Radiologic examination, ankle, arthrography, radiological supervision and interpretation

(Do not report 76003 in addition to 73615)

73620   Radiologic examination, foot; two views

73630   complete, minimum of three views

73650   Radiologic examination; calcaneus, minimum of two views

73660   toe(s), minimum of two views

73700   Computed tomography, lower extremity; without contrast material

73701   with contrast material(s)

73702   without contrast material, followed by contrast material(s) and further sections

(For coronal, sagittal, and/or oblique sections, use 76375)

73706   Computed tomographic angiography, lower extremity, without contrast material(s), followed by contrast material(s) and further sections, including image post-processing

(For CTA aorto-iliofemoral runoff, use 75635)

73718   Magnetic resonance (eg, proton) imaging, lower extremity, other than joint; without contrast material(s)

73719   with contrast material(s)

657

 Separate Procedure

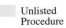 Unlisted Procedure

 CCI Comp. Code

 Non-specific Procedure

73720   without contrast material(s), followed by contrast material(s) and further sequences

73721   Magnetic resonance (eg, proton) imaging, any joint of lower extremity; without contrast material

73722   with contrast material

73723   without contrast material followed by contrast material(s) and further sequences

73725   Magnetic resonance angiography, lower extremity, with or without contrast material(s)

ABDOMEN

74000   Radiologic examination, abdomen; single anteroposterior view

74010   anteroposterior and additional oblique and cone views

74020   complete, including decubitus and/or erect views

74022   complete acute abdomen series, including supine, erect, and/or decubitus views, single view chest

74150   Computed tomography, abdomen; without contrast material

74160   with contrast material(s)

74170   without contrast material, followed by contrast material(s) and further sections

(For coronal, sagittal, and/or oblique sections, use 76375)

74175   Computed tomographic angiography, abdomen, without contrast material(s), followed by contrast material(s) and further sections, including image post-processing

(For CTA aorto-iliofemoral runoff, use 75635)

74181   Magnetic resonance (eg, proton) imaging, abdomen; without contrast material(s)

74182   with contrast material(s)

74183   without contrast material, followed by contrast material(s) and further sequences

● New Code   ▲ Revised Code   + Add-On Code   ⊘ Modifier -51 Exempt

74185   Magnetic resonance angiography, abdomen, with or without contrast material(s)

74190   Peritoneogram (eg, after injection of air or contrast), radiological supervision and interpretation

(For procedure, use 49400)

(For computerized axial tomography, see 72192 or 74150)

GASTROINTESTINAL TRACT

(For percutaneous placement of gastrostomy tube, use 43750)

74210   Radiologic examination; pharynx and/or cervical esophagus

74220   esophagus

74230   Swallowing function, with cineradiography/videoradiography

74235   Removal of foreign body(s), esophageal, with use of balloon catheter, radiological supervision and interpretation

(For procedure, see 43215, 43247)

74240   Radiologic examination, gastrointestinal tract, upper; with or without delayed films, without KUB

74241   with or without delayed films, with KUB

74245   with small intestine, includes multiple serial films

74246   Radiological examination, gastrointestinal tract, upper, air contrast, with specific high density barium, effervescent agent, with or without glucagon; with or without delayed films, without KUB

74247   with or without delayed films, with KUB

74249   with small intestine follow-through

74250   Radiologic examination, small intestine, includes multiple serial films;

74251   via enteroclysis tube

74260   Duodenography, hypotonic

659

	Separate Procedure		Unlisted Procedure		CCI Comp. Code		Non-specific Procedure

74270   Radiologic examination, colon; barium enema, with or without KUB

74280   air contrast with specific high density barium, with or without glucagon

74283   Therapeutic enema, contrast or air, for reduction of intussusception or other intraluminal obstruction (eg, meconium ileus)

74290   Cholecystography, oral contrast;

74291   additional or repeat examination or multiple day examination

74300   Cholangiography and/or pancreatography; intraoperative, radiological supervision and interpretation

+ 74301   additional set intraoperative, radiological supervision and interpretation (List separately in addition to code for primary procedure)

(Use 74301 in conjunction with code 74300)

74305   through existing catheter, radiological supervision and interpretation

(For procedure, see 47505, 48400, 47560-47561, 47563)

(For biliary duct stone extraction, percutaneous, see 47630, 74327)

74320   Cholangiography, percutaneous, transhepatic, radiological supervision and interpretation

74327   Postoperative biliary duct calculus removal, percutaneous via T-tube tract, basket, or snare (eg, Burhenne technique), radiological supervision and interpretation

(For procedure, use 47630)

74328   Endoscopic catheterization of the biliary ductal system, radiological supervision and interpretation

(For procedure, see 43260-43272 as appropriate)

74329   Endoscopic catheterization of the pancreatic ductal system, radiological supervision and interpretation

660   ● New Code   ▲ Revised Code   + Add-On Code   ⊘ Modifier -51 Exempt

(For procedure, see 43260-43272 as appropriate)

74330 Combined endoscopic catheterization of the biliary and pancreatic ductal systems, radiological supervision and interpretation

(For procedure, see 43260-43272 as appropriate)

74340 Introduction of long gastrointestinal tube (eg, Miller-Abbott), including multiple fluoroscopies and films, radiological supervision and interpretation

(For tube placement, use 44500)

74350 Percutaneous placement of gastrostomy tube, radiological supervision and interpretation

74355 Percutaneous placement of enteroclysis tube, radiological supervision and interpretation

74360 Intraluminal dilation of strictures and/or obstructions (eg, esophagus), radiological supervision and interpretation

74363 Percutaneous transhepatic dilation of biliary duct stricture with or without placement of stent, radiological supervision and interpretation

(For procedure, see 47510, 47511, 47555, 47556)

URINARY TRACT

74400 Urography (pyelography), intravenous, with or without KUB, with or without tomography

74410 Urography, infusion, drip technique and/or bolus technique;

74415 with nephrotomography

74420 Urography, retrograde, with or without KUB

74425 Urography, antegrade, (pyelostogram, nephrostogram, loopogram), radiological supervision and interpretation

74430 Cystography, minimum of three views, radiological supervision and interpretation

74440 Vasography, vesiculography, or epididymography, radiological supervision and interpretation

661

| | Separate Procedure | | Unlisted Procedure | | CCI Comp. Code | | Non-specific Procedure |

74445   Corpora cavernosography, radiological supervision and interpretation

74450   Urethrocystography, retrograde, radiological supervision and interpretation

74455   Urethrocystography, voiding, radiological supervision and interpretation

74470   Radiologic examination, renal cyst study, translumbar, contrast visualization, radiological supervision and interpretation

74475   Introduction of intracatheter or catheter into renal pelvis for drainage and/or injection, percutaneous, radiological supervision and interpretation

74480   Introduction of ureteral catheter or stent into ureter through renal pelvis for drainage and/or injection, percutaneous, radiological supervision and interpretation

(For transurethral surgery (ureter and pelvis), see 52320-52355)

74485   Dilation of nephrostomy, ureters, or urethra, radiological supervision and interpretation

(For dilation of ureter without radiologic guidance, use 52341, 52344)

(For change of nephrostomy or pyelostomy tube, use 50398)

GYNECOLOGICAL AND OBSTETRICAL

(For abdomen and pelvis, see 72170-72190, 74000-74170)

74710   Pelvimetry, with or without placental localization

74740   Hysterosalpingography, radiological supervision and interpretation

(For introduction of saline or contrast for hysterosalpingography, see 58340)

74742   Transcervical catheterization of fallopian tube, radiological supervision and interpretation

(For procedure, use 58345)

74775   Perineogram (eg, vaginogram, for sex determination or extent of anomalies)

| ● | New Code | ▲ | Revised Code | + | Add-On Code | ⊘ | Modifier -51 Exempt |

HEART

(For separate injection procedures for vascular radiology, see Surgery section, 36000-36299)

(For cardiac catheterization procedures, see 93501-93556)

75552 Cardiac magnetic resonance imaging for morphology; without contrast material

75553 with contrast material

75554 Cardiac magnetic resonance imaging for function, with or without morphology; complete study

75555 limited study

75556 Cardiac magnetic resonance imaging for velocity flow mapping

AORTA AND ARTERIES

(For intravenous procedure, see 36000-36013, 36400-36425 and 36100-36248 for intra-arterial procedure)

(For radiological supervision and interpretation, see 75600-75978)

75600 Aortography, thoracic, without serialography, radiological supervision and interpretation

(For injection procedure, use 93544)

75605 Aortography, thoracic, by serialography, radiological supervision and interpretation

(For injection procedure, use 93544)

(75620, 75621, 75622, 75623 have been deleted. To report, use 76499)

75625 Aortography, abdominal, by serialography, radiological supervision and interpretation

(For injection procedure, use 93544)

75630 Aortography, abdominal plus bilateral iliofemoral lower extremity, catheter, by serialography, radiological supervision and interpretation

 Separate Procedure
 Unlisted Procedure
 CCI Comp. Code
 Non-specific Procedure

663

75635   Computed tomographic angiography, abdominal aorta and bilateral iliofemoral lower extremity runoff, radiological supervision and interpretation, without contrast material(s), followed by contrast material(s) and further sections, including image post-processing

75650   Angiography, cervicocerebral, catheter, including vessel origin, radiological supervision and interpretation

75658   Angiography, brachial, retrograde, radiological supervision and interpretation

75660   Angiography, external carotid, unilateral, selective, radiological supervision and interpretation

75662   Angiography, external carotid, bilateral, selective, radiological supervision and interpretation

75665   Angiography, carotid, cerebral, unilateral, radiological supervision and interpretation

75671   Angiography, carotid, cerebral, bilateral, radiological supervision and interpretation

75676   Angiography, carotid, cervical, unilateral, radiological supervision and interpretation

75680   Angiography, carotid, cervical, bilateral, radiological supervision and interpretation

75685   Angiography, vertebral, cervical, and/or intracranial, radiological supervision and interpretation

75705   Angiography, spinal, selective, radiological supervision and interpretation

75710   Angiography, extremity, unilateral, radiological supervision and interpretation

75716   Angiography, extremity, bilateral, radiological supervision and interpretation

75722   Angiography, renal, unilateral, selective (including flush aortogram), radiological supervision and interpretation

75724   Angiography, renal, bilateral, selective (including flush aortogram), radiological supervision and interpretation

---

664
-   New Code
- ▲   Revised Code
- +   Add-On Code
- ⊘   Modifier -51 Exempt

75726 Angiography, visceral, selective or supraselective, (with or without flush aortogram), radiological supervision and interpretation

(For selective angiography, each additional visceral vessel studied after basic examination, use 75774)

75731 Angiography, adrenal, unilateral, selective, radiological supervision and interpretation

75733 Angiography, adrenal, bilateral, selective, radiological supervision and interpretation

75736 Angiography, pelvic, selective or supraselective, radiological supervision and interpretation

75741 Angiography, pulmonary, unilateral, selective, radiological supervision and interpretation

(For injection procedure, use 93541)

75743 Angiography, pulmonary, bilateral, selective, radiological supervision and interpretation

(For injection procedure, use 93541)

75746 Angiography, pulmonary, by nonselective catheter or venous injection, radiological supervision and interpretation

(For injection procedure, use 93541)

(For introduction of catheter, injection procedure, see 93501-93533, 93539, 93540, 93545, 93556)

75756 Angiography, internal mammary, radiological supervision and interpretation

(For introduction of catheter, injection procedure, see 93501-93533, 93545, 93556)

+ **75774** Angiography, selective, each additional vessel studied after basic examination, radiological supervision and interpretation (List separately in addition to code for primary procedure)

(Use 75774 in addition to code for specific initial vessel studied)

(For angiography, see codes 75600-75790)

(For catheterizations, see codes 36215-36248)

665

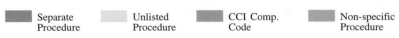

Separate Procedure

Unlisted Procedure

CCI Comp. Code

Non-specific Procedure

(For introduction of catheter, injection procedure, see 93501-93533, 93545, 93555, 93556)

75790 Angiography, arteriovenous shunt (eg, dialysis patient), radiological supervision and interpretation

(For introduction of catheter, use 36140, 36145, 36215-36217, 36245-36247)

VEINS AND LYMPHATICS

(For injection procedure for venous system, see 36000-36015, 36400-36510)

(For injection procedure for lymphatic system, use 38790)

75801 Lymphangiography, extremity only, unilateral, radiological supervision and interpretation

75803 Lymphangiography, extremity only, bilateral, radiological supervision and interpretation

75805 Lymphangiography, pelvic/abdominal, unilateral, radiological supervision and interpretation

75807 Lymphangiography, pelvic/abdominal, bilateral, radiological supervision and interpretation

75809 Shuntogram for investigation of previously placed indwelling nonvascular shunt (eg, LeVeen shunt, ventriculoperitoneal shunt, indwelling infusion pump), radiological supervision and interpretation

(For procedure, see 49427 or 61070)

75810 Splenoportography, radiological supervision and interpretation

75820 Venography, extremity, unilateral, radiological supervision and interpretation

75822 Venography, extremity, bilateral, radiological supervision and interpretation

75825 Venography, caval, inferior, with serialography, radiological supervision and interpretation

75827 Venography, caval, superior, with serialography, radiological supervision and interpretation

666 ● New Code   ▲ Revised Code   + Add-On Code   ⊘ Modifier -51 Exempt

75831 Venography, renal, unilateral, selective, radiological supervision and interpretation

75833 Venography, renal, bilateral, selective, radiological supervision and interpretation

75840 Venography, adrenal, unilateral, selective, radiological supervision and interpretation

75842 Venography, adrenal, bilateral, selective, radiological supervision and interpretation

▲ **75860** Venography, venous sinus (eg, petrosal and inferior sagittal) or jugular, catheter, radiological supervision and interpretation

75870 Venography, superior sagittal sinus, radiological supervision and interpretation

75872 Venography, epidural, radiological supervision and interpretation

75880 Venography, orbital, radiological supervision and interpretation

75885 Percutaneous transhepatic portography with hemodynamic evaluation, radiological supervision and interpretation

75887 Percutaneous transhepatic portography without hemodynamic evaluation, radiological supervision and interpretation

75889 Hepatic venography, wedged or free, with hemodynamic evaluation, radiological supervision and interpretation

75891 Hepatic venography, wedged or free, without hemodynamic evaluation, radiological supervision and interpretation

75893 Venous sampling through catheter, with or without angiography (eg, for parathyroid hormone, renin), radiological supervision and interpretation

(For procedure, use 36500)

TRANSCATHETER PROCEDURES

75894 Transcatheter therapy, embolization, any method, radiological supervision and interpretation

75896 Transcatheter therapy, infusion, any method (eg, thrombolysis other than coronary), radiological supervision and interpretation

667

Separate Procedure   Unlisted Procedure   CCI Comp. Code   Non-specific Procedure

(For infusion for coronary disease, see 92975, 92977)

75898 Angiography through existing catheter for follow-up study for transcatheter therapy, embolization or infusion

75900 Exchange of a previously placed arterial catheter during thrombolytic therapy with contrast monitoring, radiological supervision and interpretation

(For procedure, use 37209)

75901 Mechanical removal of pericatheter obstructive material (eg., fibrin sheath) from central venous device via separate venous access, radiologic supervision and interpretation

(For procedure, use 36595)

(For venous catheterization, see 36010-36012)

75902 Mechanical removal of intraluminal (intracatheter) obstructive material from central venous device through device lumen, radiologic supervision and interpretation

(For procedure, use 36596)

(For venous catheterization, see 36010-36012)

75940 Percutaneous placement of IVC filter, radiological supervision and interpretation

75945 Intravascular ultrasound (non-coronary vessel), radiological supervision and interpretation; initial vessel

+ **75946** each additional non-coronary vessel (List separately in addition to code for primary procedure)

(Use 75946 in conjunction with code 75945)

(For catheterizations, see codes 36215-36248)

(For transcatheter therapies, see codes 37200-37208, 61624, 61626)

(For procedure, see 37250, 37251)

75952 Endovascular repair of infrarenal abdominal aortic aneurysm or dissection, radiological supervision and interpretation

(For implantation of endovascular grafts, see 34800-34808)

● New Code   ▲ Revised Code   + Add-On Code   ⊘ Modifier -51 Exempt

75953   Placement of proximal or distal extension prosthesis for endovascular repair of infrarenal aortic or iliac artery aneurysm, pseudoaneurysm, or dissection, radiological supervision and interpretation

(For implantation of endovascular extension prostheses, see 34825, 34826)

75954   Endovascular repair of iliac artery aneurysm, psuedoaneurysm, arteriovenous malformation, or trauma, radiological supervision and interpretation

(For implantation of endovascular graft, see 34900)

75960   Transcatheter introduction of intravascular stent(s), (non-coronary vessel), percutaneous and/or open, radiological supervision and interpretation, each vessel

(For procedure, see 37205-37208)

(For radiologic supervision and interpretation for transcatheter placement of extracranial cerebrovascular artery stent(s), use Category III code 0007T)

75961   Transcatheter retrieval, percutaneous, of intravascular foreign body (eg, fractured venous or arterial catheter), radiological supervision and interpretation

(For procedure, use 37203)

75962   Transluminal balloon angioplasty, peripheral artery, radiological supervision and interpretation

+ 75964   Transluminal balloon angioplasty, each additional peripheral artery, radiological supervision and interpretation (List separately in addition to code for primary procedure)

(Use 75964 in conjunction with code 75962)

75966   Transluminal balloon angioplasty, renal or other visceral artery, radiological supervision and interpretation

+ 75968   Transluminal balloon angioplasty, each additional visceral artery, radiological supervision and interpretation (List separately in addition to code for primary procedure)

(Use 75968 in conjunction with code 75966)

(For percutaneous transluminal coronary angioplasty, see 92982-92984)

669

	Separate Procedure		Unlisted Procedure		CCI Comp. Code		Non-specific Procedure

75970 Transcatheter biopsy, radiological supervision and interpretation

(For injection procedure only for transcatheter therapy or biopsy, see 36100-36299)

(For transcatheter renal and ureteral biopsy, use 52007)

(For percutaneous needle biopsy of pancreas, use 48102; of retroperitoneal lymph node or mass, use 49180)

75978 Transluminal balloon angioplasty, venous (eg, subclavian stenosis), radiological supervision and interpretation

75980 Percutaneous transhepatic biliary drainage with contrast monitoring, radiological supervision and interpretation

75982 Percutaneous placement of drainage catheter for combined internal and external biliary drainage or of a drainage stent for internal biliary drainage in patients with an inoperable mechanical biliary obstruction, radiological supervision and interpretation

75984 Change of percutaneous tube or drainage catheter with contrast monitoring (eg, gastrointestinal system, genitourinary system, abscess), radiological supervision and interpretation

(For change of nephrostomy or pyelostomy tube only, use 50398)

(For introduction procedure only for percutaneous biliary drainage, see 47510, 47511)

(For percutaneous choloecystostomy, use 47490)

(For change of percutaneous biliary drainage catheter only, use 47525)

(For percutaneous nephrostolithotomy or pyelostolithotomy, see 50080, 50081)

75989 Radiological guidance (ie, fluoroscopy, ultrasound, or computed tomography), for percutaneous drainage (eg., abscess, specimen collection), with placement of catheter, radiological supervision and interpretation

TRANSLUMINAL ATHERECTOMY

75992 Transluminal atherectomy, peripheral artery, radiological supervision and interpretation

(For procedure, see 35481-35485, 35491-35495)

670   ● New Code   ▲ Revised Code   + Add-On Code   ⊘ Modifier -51 Exempt

+ 75993 Transluminal atherectomy, each additional peripheral artery, radiological supervision and interpretation (List separately in addition to code for primary procedure)

(Use 75993 in conjunction with code 75992)

(For procedure, see 35481-35485, 35491-35495)

75994 Transluminal atherectomy, renal, radiological supervision and interpretation

(For procedure, see 35480, 35490)

75995 Transluminal atherectomy, visceral, radiological supervision and interpretation

(For procedure, see 35480, 35490)

+ 75996 Transluminal atherectomy, each additional visceral artery, radiological supervision and interpretation (List separately in addition to code for primary procedure)

(Use 75996 in conjunction with code 75995)

(For procedure, see 35480, 35490)

OTHER PROCEDURES

(For computed tomography cerebral perfusion analysis, see Category III code 0042T)

(For arthrography of shoulder, use 73040; elbow, use 73085; wrist, use 73115; hip, use 73525; knee, use 73580; ankle, use 73615)

●+75998 Fluoroscopic guidance for central venous access device placement, replacement (catheter only or complete), or removal (includes fluoroscopic guidance for vascular access and catheter manipulation, any necessary contrast injections through access site or catheter with related venography radiologic supervision and interpretation, and radiographic documentation of final catheter position) (List separately in addition to code for primary procedure)

(Do not use 76003 in conjunction with 75998)

(If formal extremity venography is performed from separate venous access and separately interpreted, use 36005 and 75820, 75822, 75825 or 75827)

 Separate Procedure

 Unlisted Procedure

CCI Comp. Code

 Non-specific Procedure

76000 Fluoroscopy (separate procedure), up to one hour physician time, other than 71023 or 71034 (eg, cardiac fluoroscopy)

76001 Fluoroscopy, physician time more than one hour, assisting a non-radiologic physician (eg, nephrostolithotomy, ERCP, bronchoscopy, transbronchial biopsy)

76003 Fluoroscopic guidance for needle placement (eg, biopsy, aspiration, injection, localization device)

(See appropriate surgical code for procedure and anatomic location)

(Fluoroscopy 76003 is considered inclusive of all radiographic arthrography with the exception of supervision and interpretation for CT and MR arthrography)

(Do not report 76003 in addition to 70332, 73040, 73085, 73115, 73525, 73580, 73615)

(Fluoroscopy 76003 is considered inclusive of organ/anatomic specific radiological supervision and interpretation procedures 74320, 74350, 74355, 74445, 74470, 74475, 75809, 75810, 75885, 75887, 75980, 75982, 75989)

76005 Fluoroscopic guidance and localization of needle or catheter tip for spine or paraspinous diagnostic or therapeutic injection procedures (epidural, transforaminal epidural, subarachnoid, paravertebral facet joint, paravertebral facet joint nerve or sacroiliac joint), including neurolytic agent destruction

(Injection of contrast during fluoroscopic guidance and localization is an inclusive component of codes 62263, 62264, 62270-62273, 62280-62282, 62310-32319, 0027T)

(Fluoroscopic guidance for subarachnoid puncture for diagnostic radiographic myelography is included in supervision and interpretation codes 72240, 72255, 72265, 72270)

(For epidural or subarachnoid needle or catheter placement and injection, see codes 62270-62273, 62280-62282, 62310-62319)

(For sacroiliac joint arthrography, see 27096, 73542. If formal arthrography is not performed, recorded, and a formal radiographic report is not issued, use 76005 for fluoroscopic guidance for sacroiliac joint injections)

(For paravertebral facet joint injection, see 64470-64476. For transforaminal epidural needle placement and injection, see 64479-64484)

● New Code   ▲ Revised Code   + Add-On Code   ⊘ Modifier -51 Exempt

(For destruction by neurolytic agent, see 64600-64680)

(For percutaneous or endoscopic lysis of epidural adhesions, codes 62263, 62264, 0027T include fluoroscopic guidance and localization)

76006 Manual application of stress performed by physician for joint radiography, including contralateral joint if indicated

(For radiographic interpretation of stressed images, see appropriate anatomic site and number of views)

76010 Radiologic examination from nose to rectum for foreign body, single view, child

76012 Radiological supervision and interpretation, percutaneous vertebroplasty, per vertebral body; under fluoroscopic guidance

76013 under CT guidance

(For procedure, see 22520-22522)

76020 Bone age studies

76040 Bone length studies (orthoroentgenogram, scanogram)

76061 Radiologic examination, osseous survey; limited (eg, for metastases)

76062 complete (axial and appendicular skeleton)

76065 Radiologic examination, osseous survey, infant

76066 Joint survey, single view, two or more joints (specify)

76070 Computed tomography, bone mineral density study, one or more sites; axial skeleton (eg., hips, pelvis, spine)

76071 appendicular skeleton (peripheral) (eg., radius, wrist, heel)

76075 Dual energy x-ray absorptiometry (DEXA), bone density study, one or more sites; axial skeleton (eg, hips, pelvis, spine)

76076 appendicular skeleton (peripheral) (eg, radius, wrist, heel)

(To report dual energy x-ray absorptiometry (DEXA) body composition study, one or more sites, use Category III code 0028T)

673

 Separate Procedure   Unlisted Procedure   CCI Comp. Code   Non-specific Procedure

76078   Radiographic absorptiometry (eg, photodensitometry, radiogrammetry), one or more sites

76080   Radiologic examination, abscess, fistula or sinus tract study, radiological supervision and interpretation

●+**76082**   Computer aided detection (computer algorithm analysis of digital image data for lesion detection) with further physician review for interpretation, with or without digitization of film radiographic images; diagnostic mammography (List separately in addition to code for primary procedure)

(Use 76082 in conjunction with 76090 or 76091)

●+**76083**   screening mammography (List separately in addition to code for primary procedure)

(Use 76083 in conjunction with 76092)

(**76085**   deleted. To report, see 76082, 76083)

76086   Mammary ductogram or galactogram, single duct, radiological supervision and interpretation

76088   Mammary ductogram or galactogram, multiple ducts, radiological supervision and interpretation

76090   Mammography; unilateral

76091   bilateral

(Use 76082 in conjunction with 76090 or 76091 for computer aided detection applied to a diagnostic mammogram)

76092   Screening mammography, bilateral (two view film study of each breast)

(Use 76083 in conjunction with 76092 for computer aided detection applied to a screening mammogram)

(To report electrical impedance scan of the breast, bilateral, use Category III code 0060T)

76093   Magnetic resonance imaging, breast, without and/or with contrast material(s); unilateral

76094   bilateral

● New Code   ▲ Revised Code   + Add-On Code   ⊘ Modifier -51 Exempt

76095   Stereotactic localization for breast biopsy or needle placement (eg, for wire localization or for injection), each lesion, radiological supervision and interpretation

(For procedure, see 10022, 19000, 19001, 19102, 19103, 19290, 19291)

(For injection for sentinel node localization without lymphoscintigraphy, use 38792)

76096   Mammographic guidance for needle placement, breast, (eg, for wire localization or for injection), each lesion, radiological supervision and interpretation

(For procedure, see 10022, 19000, 19102, 19103, 19290, 19291)

(For injection for sentinel node localization without lymphoscintigraphy, use 38792)

76098   Radiological examination, surgical specimen

76100   Radiologic examination, single plane body section (eg, tomography), other than with urography

76101   Radiologic examination, complex motion (ie, hypercycloidal) body section (eg, mastoid polytomography), other than with urography; unilateral

76102   bilateral

(For nephrotomography, use 74415)

76120   Cineradiography/videoradiography, except where specifically included

+ **76125**   Cineradiography/videoradiography to complement routine examination (List separately in addition to code for primary procedure)

76140   Consultation on x-ray examination made elsewhere, written report

76150   Xeroradiography

(76150 is to be used for non-mammographic studies only)

76350   Subtraction in conjunction with contrast studies

76355   Computed tomography guidance for stereotactic localization

675

 Separate Procedure   Unlisted Procedure   CCI Comp. Code   Non-specific Procedure

76360   Computed tomography guidance for needle placement (eg., biopsy, aspiration, injection, localization device), radiological supervision and interpretation

▲ **76362**   Computed tomography guidance for, and monitoring of, visceral tissue ablation

(For percutaneous radiofrequency ablation, use 47382)

76370   Computed tomography guidance for placement of radiation therapy fields

76375   Coronal, sagittal, multiplanar, oblique, 3-dimensional and/or holographic reconstruction of computed tomography, magnetic resonance imaging, or other tomographic modality

(Use 76375 in addition to code for imaging procedure)

76380   Computed tomography, limited or localized follow-up study

76390   Magnetic resonance spectroscopy

(For magnetic resonance imaging, use appropriate MRI body site code)

76393   Magnetic resonance guidance for needle placement (eg, for biopsy, needle aspiration, injection, or placement of localization device) radiological supervision and interpretation

(For procedure see appropriate organ or site)

▲ **76394**   Magnetic resonance guidance for, and monitoring of, visceral tissue ablation

(For percutaneous radiofrequency ablation, use 47382)

76400   Magnetic resonance (eg, proton) imaging, bone marrow blood supply

(**76490**   deleted 2004 edition. To report, use 76940)

76496   Unlisted fluoroscopic procedure (eg., diagnostic, interventional)

76497   Unlisted computed tomography procedure (eg., diagnostic, interventional)

76498   Unlisted magnetic resonance procedure (eg., diagnostic, interventional)

---

676   ● New Code   ▲ Revised Code   + Add-On Code   ⊘ Modifier -51 Exempt

76499   Unlisted diagnostic radiographic procedure

DIAGNOSTIC ULTRASOUND

Diagnostic ultrasound is a non-invasive medical imaging technology that uses high frequency sound waves to form an image of body tissues. Information obtained from these images can be utilized along with other patient data in order to arrive at a medical diagnosis. Ultrasound, when compared to other imaging modalities like MRI (Magnetic Resonance Imaging) and CT (Computed Tomography), is a relatively low cost non-invasive procedure that does not utilize either magnetic fields or ionizing radiation (x-rays).

The following definitions are important when choosing CPT codes for diagnostic ultrasound services and procedures.

A-MODE   Implies a one-dimensional ultrasonic measurement procedure.

M-MODE   Implies a one-dimensional ultrasonic measurement procedure with movement of the trace to record amplitude and velocity of moving echo-producing structures.

B-SCAN   Implies a two-dimensional ultrasonic scanning procedure with a two-dimensional display.

REAL-TIME   Implies a two-dimensional ultrasonic scanning procedure with display of both two-dimensional structure and motion with time.

(To report diagnostic vascular ultrasound studies, see 93875-93990)

HEAD AND NECK

76506   Echoencephalography, B-scan and/or real time with image documentation (gray scale) (for determination of ventricular size, delineation of cerebral contents and detection of fluid masses or other intracranial abnormalities), including A-mode encephalography as secondary component where indicated

76511   Ophthalmic ultrasound, echography, diagnostic; A-scan only, with amplitude quantification

76512   contact B-scan (with or without simultaneous A-scan)

76513   anterior segment ultrasound, immersion (water bath) B-scan or high resolution biomicroscopy

677

 Separate Procedure   Unlisted Procedure   CCI Comp. Code   Non-specific Procedure

- **76514**   corneal pachymetry, unilateral or bilateral (determination of corneal thickness)

76516   Ophthalmic biometry by ultrasound echography, A-scan;

76519   with intraocular lens power calculation

(For partial coherence interferometry, use 92136)

76529   Ophthalmic ultrasonic foreign body localization

76536   Ultrasound, soft tissues of head and neck (eg, thyroid, parathyroid, parotid), B-scan and/or real time with image documentation

CHEST

76604   Ultrasound, chest, B-scan (includes mediastinum) and/or real time with image documentation

76645   Ultrasound, breast(s) (unilateral or bilateral), B-scan and/or real time with image documentation

ABDOMEN AND PERITONEUM

76700   Ultrasound, abdominal, B-scan and/or real time with image documentation; complete

76705   limited (eg, single organ, quadrant, follow-up)

76770   Ultrasound, retroperitoneal (eg, renal, aorta, nodes), B-scan and/or real time with image documentation; complete

76775   limited

76778   Ultrasound, transplanted kidney, B-scan and/or real time with image documentation, with or without duplex Doppler study

SPINAL CANAL

76800   Ultrasound, spinal canal and contents

PELVIS

OBSTETRICAL

76801 Ultrasound, pregnant uterus, real time with image documentation, fetal and maternal evaluation, first trimester (<14 weeks 0 days), transabdominal approach; single or first gestation

+ 76802 each additional gestation (List separately in addition to code for primary procedure)

(Use 76802 in conjunction with code 76801)

76805 Ultrasound, pregnant uterus, real time with image documentation, fetal and maternal evaluation, after first trimester (> or = 14 weeks 0 days), transabdominal approach; single or first gestation

+ 76810 each additional gestation (List separately in addition to code for primary procedure)

(Use 76810 in conjunction with code 76805)

76811 Ultrasound, pregnant uterus, real time with image documentation, fetal and maternal evaluation plus detailed fetal anatomic examination, transabdominal approach; single or first gestation

+ 76812 each additional gestation (List separately in addition to code for primary procedure)

(Use 76812 in conjunction with code 76811)

76815 Ultrasound, pregnant uterus, real time with image documentation, limited (eg., fetal heart beat, placental location, fetal position, and/or qualitative amniotic fluid volume), one or more fetuses

(Use 76815 only once per exam and not per element)

76816 Ultrasound, pregnant uterus, real time with image documentation, follow-up (eg., re-evaluation of fetal size by measuring standard growth parameters and amniotic fluid volume, re-evaluation of organ system(s) suspected or confirmed to be abnormal on a previous scan), transabdominal approach, per fetus

(Report 76816 with modifier -59 for each additional fetus examined in a multiple pregnancy)

679

 Separate Procedure   Unlisted Procedure    CCI Comp. Code   Non-specific Procedure

76817 Ultrasound, pregnant uterus, real time with image documentation, transvaginal

(For non-obstetrical transvaginal ultrasound, use 76830)

(If transvaginal examination is done in addition to transabdominal obstetrical ultrasound exam, use 76817 in addition to appropriate transabdominal exam code)

76818 Fetal biophysical profile; with non-stress testing

76819   without non-stress testing

(Fetal biophysical profile assessments for the second and any additional fetuses, should be reported separately by code 76818 or 76819 with the modifier -59 appended)

(For amniotic fluid index without non-stress test, use 76815)

76825 Echocardiography, fetal, cardiovascular system, real time with image documentation (2D), with or without M-mode recording;

76826   follow-up or repeat study

76827 Doppler echocardiography, fetal, cardiovascular system, pulsed wave and/or continuous wave with spectral display; complete

76828   follow-up or repeat study

(To report the use of color mapping, use 93325)

NON-OBSTETRICAL

76830 Ultrasound, transvaginal

(For obstetrical transvaginal ultrasound, use 76817)

(If transvaginal examination is done in addition to transabdominal non-obstetrical ultrasound exam, use 76830 in addition to appropriate transabdominal exam code)

▲ **76831** Saline infusion sonohysterography (SIS), including color flow Doppler, when performed

(For introduction of saline for saline infusion sonohysterography, use 58340)

76856 Ultrasound, pelvic (nonobstetric), B-scan and/or real time with image documentation; complete

● New Code   ▲ Revised Code   + Add-On Code   ⊘ Modifier -51 Exempt

76857   limited or follow-up (eg, for follicles)

GENITALIA

76870   Ultrasound, scrotum and contents

▲ **76872**   Ultrasound, transrectal;

76873   prostate volume study for brachytherapy treatment planning (separate procedure)

EXTREMITIES

76880   Ultrasound, extremity, non-vascular, B-scan and/or real time with image documentation

76885   Ultrasound of infant hips, real time with imaging documentation; dynamic (requiring physician manipulation)

76886   limited, static (not requiring physician manipulation)

ULTRASONIC GUIDANCE PROCEDURES

76930   Ultrasonic guidance for pericardiocentesis, imaging supervision and interpretation

76932   Ultrasonic guidance for endomyocardial biopsy, imaging supervision and interpretation

76936   Ultrasound guided compression repair of arterial pseudoaneurysm or arteriovenous fistulae (includes diagnostic ultrasound evaluation, compression of lesion and imaging)

●+**76937**   Ultrasound guidance for vascular access requiring ultrasound evaluation of potential access sites, documentation of selected vessel patency, concurrent realtime ultrasound visualization of vascular needle entry, with permanent recording and reporting (List separately in addition to code for primary procedure)

(Do not use 76937 in conjunction with 76942)

(If extremity venous non-invasive vascular diagnostic study is performed separate from venous access guidance, use 93965, 93970, or 93971)

● **76940**   Ultrasound guidance for, and monitoring of, visceral tissue ablation

 Separate Procedure   Unlisted Procedure   CCI Comp. Code   Non-specific Procedure

(Do not report 76940 in conjunction with 76986)

(For ablation, see 47370-47382)

76941 Ultrasonic guidance for intrauterine fetal transfusion or cordocentesis, imaging supervision and interpretation

(For procedure, see 36460, 59012)

76942 Ultrasonic guidance for needle placement (eg, biopsy, aspiration, injection, localization device) imaging supervision and interpretation

(Do not report 76942 in conjunction with 43232, 43237, 43242, 45341, 45342, or 76975)

(For microwave thermotherapy of the breast, use Category III code 0061T)

76945 Ultrasonic guidance for chorionic villus sampling, imaging supervision and interpretation

(For procedure, use 59015)

76946 Ultrasonic guidance for amniocentesis, imaging supervision and interpretation

76948 Ultrasonic guidance for aspiration of ova, imaging supervision and interpretation

76950 Ultrasonic guidance for placement of radiation therapy fields

76965 Ultrasonic guidance for interstitial radioelement application

OTHER PROCEDURES

76970 Ultrasound study follow-up (specify)

76975 Gastrointestinal endoscopic ultrasound, imaging supervision and interpretation

(Do not report 76975 in conjunction with 43231, 43232, 43237, 43238, 43242, 43259, 45341, 45342, or 76942)

76977 Ultrasound bone density measurement and interpretation, peripheral site(s), any method

76986 Ultrasonic guidance, intraoperative

● New Code   ▲ Revised Code   + Add-On Code   ⊘ Modifier -51 Exempt

(Do not report 76986 in addition to 47370-47382)

(For ultrasound guidance for open and laparoscopic radiofrequency tissue ablation, use 76490)

76999 Unlisted ultrasound procedure (eg., diagnostic, interventional)

RADIATION ONCOLOGY

Radiation therapy is the use of high level radiation to destroy cancer cells. Both tumor cells and healthy cells may be affected by this radiation. The radiation injures the cancer cells so they can no longer continue to divide or multiply. With each treatment, more of the cells die and the tumor shrinks. The dead cells are broken down, carried away by the blood and excreted by the body. Most of the healthy cells are able to recover from this injury. However, the damage to the healthy cells is the reason for the side effects of radiation therapy.

The dose of radiation is determined by the size, extent, type and grade of tumor along with its response to radiation therapy. Complex calculations are done to determine the dose and timing of radiation in treatment planning. Often, the treatment is given over several different angles in order to deliver the maximum amount of radiation to the tumor and the minimum amount to normal tissues.

Services defined in this section of the CPT book coding system teletherapy and brachytherapy. To report Radiation Oncology services, the following must be performed and documented:

- *The initial consultation*

- *Clinical treatment planning with/without simulation*

- *Medical radiation physics, dosimetry, treatment devices and special services*

- *Clinical treatment management procedures*

- *Normal follow-up care during treatment and for three months following completion of treatment*

CONSULTATION OR CLINICAL MANAGEMENT

All consultations, pre-treatment patient evaluations, and/or medical care services are coded using evaluation and management service codes

CLINICAL TREATMENT PLANNING

Clinical treatment planning includes test interpretation, localization of tumor(s), treatment determination, and choice of treatment modality and treatment devices. Clinical treatment planning may be simple, intermediate or complex.

683

 Separate Procedure   Unlisted Procedure   CCI Comp. Code   Non-specific Procedure

(77260, 77265, 77270, 77275 have been deleted. To report, see 77261-77263)

77261 Therapeutic radiology treatment planning; simple

77262 intermediate

77263 complex

77280 Therapeutic radiology simulation-aided field setting; simple

77285 intermediate

77290 complex

77295 three-dimensional

77299 Unlisted procedure, therapeutic radiology clinical treatment planning

MEDICAL RADIATION PHYSICS, DOSIMETRY, TREATMENT DEVICES, AND SPECIAL SERVICES

77300 Basic radiation dosimetry calculation, central axis depth dose calculation, TDF, NSD, gap calculation, off axis factor, tissue inhomogeneity factors, calculation of non-ionizing radiation surface and depth dose, as required during course of treatment, only when prescribed by the treating physician

77301 Intensity modulated radiotherapy plan, including dose-volume histograms for target and critical structure partial tolerance specifications

(Dose plan is optimized using inverse or forward planning technique for modulated beam delivery (eg, binary, dynamic MLC) to create highly conformal dose distribution. Computer plan distribution must be verified for positional accuracy based on dosimetric verification of the intensity map with verification of treatment set up and interpretation of verification methodology)

77305 Teletherapy, isodose plan (whether hand or computer calculated); simple (one or two parallel opposed unmodified ports directed to a single area of interest)

77310 intermediate (three or more treatment ports directed to a single area of interest)

● New Code ▲ Revised Code + Add-On Code ⊘ Modifier -51 Exempt

77315 complex (mantle or inverted Y, tangential ports, the use of wedges, compensators, complex blocking, rotational beam, or special beam considerations)

(Only one teletherapy isodose plan may be reported for a given course of therapy to a specific treatment area)

77321 Special teletherapy port plan, particles, hemibody, total body

77326 Brachytherapy isodose plan; simple (calculation made from single plane, one to four sources/ribbon application, remote afterloading brachytherapy, 1 to 8 sources)

(For definition of source/ribbon, see Clinical Brachytherapy)

77327 intermediate (multiplane dosage calculations, application involving 5 to 10 sources/ribbons, remote afterloading brachytherapy, 9 to 12 sources)

77328 complex (multiplane isodose plan, volume implant calculations, over 10 sources/ribbons used, special spatial reconstruction, remote afterloading brachytherapy, over 12 sources)

77331 Special dosimetry (eg, TLD, microdosimetry) (specify), only when prescribed by the treating physician

77332 Treatment devices, design and construction; simple (simple block, simple bolus)

77333 intermediate (multiple blocks, stents, bite blocks, special bolus)

77334 complex (irregular blocks, special shields, compensators, wedges, molds or casts)

77336 Continuing medical physics consultation, including assessment of treatment parameters, quality assurance of dose delivery, and review of patient treatment documentation in support of the radiation oncologist, reported per week of therapy

77370 Special medical radiation physics consultation

77399 Unlisted procedure, medical radiation physics, dosimetry and treatment devices, and special services

685

| Separate Procedure | Unlisted Procedure | CCI Comp. Code | Non-specific Procedure |

RADIATION TREATMENT DELIVERY

(Radiation treatment delivery (77401-77416) recognizes the technical component and the various energy levels.)

(77400 has been deleted.)

77401 Radiation treatment delivery, superficial and/or ortho voltage

77402 Radiation treatment delivery, single treatment area, single port or parallel opposed ports, simple blocks or no blocks; up to 5 MeV

77403 6-10 MeV

77404 11-19 MeV

77406 20 MeV or greater

77407 Radiation treatment delivery, two separate treatment areas, three or more ports on a single treatment area, use of multiple blocks; up to 5 MeV

77408 6-10 MeV

77409 11-19 MeV

77411 20 MeV or greater

77412 Radiation treatment delivery, three or more separate treatment areas, custom blocking, tangential ports, wedges, rotational beam, compensators, special particle beam (eg, electron or neutrons); up to 5 MeV

77413 6-10 MeV

77414 11-19 MeV

77416 20 MeV or greater

77417 Therapeutic radiology port film(s)

77418 Intensity modulated treatment delivery, single or multiple fields/arcs, via narrow spatially and temporally modulated beams (eg, binary, dynamic MLC), per treatment session

(For intensity modulated treatment planning, use 77301)

686 ● New Code ▲ Revised Code + Add-On Code ⊘ Modifier -51 Exempt

RADIATION TREATMENT MANAGEMENT

CPT codes in this section presume treatment on a daily basis (4 or 5 fractions per week) with the use of megavoltage photon or high energy particle sources. Daily and weekly clinical treatment management are mutually exclusive for the same dates. CPT defines three distinct levels of clinical treatment management: simple, intermediate and complex. Review this section of CPT for detailed definitions of these levels of service.

77427 Radiation treatment management, five treatments

77431 Radiation therapy management with complete course of therapy consisting of one or two fractions only

(77431 is not to be used to fill in the last week of a long course of therapy)

77432 Stereotactic radiation treatment management of cerebral lesion(s) (complete course of treatment consisting of one session)

77470 Special treatment procedure (eg, total body irradiation, hemibody irradiation, per oral, endocavitary or vaginal cone irradiation)

(77470 assumes that the procedure is performed one or more times during the course of therapy, in addition to daily or weekly patient management)

77499 Unlisted procedure, therapeutic radiology treatment management

PROTON BEAM TREATMENT DELIVERY

77520 Proton treatment delivery; simple, without compensation

77522 simple, with compensation

77523 intermediate

77525 complex

HYPERTHERMIA

77600 Hyperthermia, externally generated; superficial (ie, heating to a depth of 4 cm or less)

77605 deep (ie, heating to depths greater than 4 cm)

 Separate Procedure   Unlisted Procedure   CCI Comp. Code   Non-specific Procedure

687

77610 Hyperthermia generated by interstitial probe(s); 5 or fewer interstitial applicators

77615 more than 5 interstitial applicators

CLINICAL INTRACAVITARY HYPERTHERMIA

77620 Hyperthermia generated by intracavitary probe(s)

CLINICAL BRACHYTHERAPY

(77700-77749 have been deleted. To report, see 77761-77799)

77750 Infusion or instillation of radioelement solution

(For administration of radiolabeled monoclonal antibodies see 79403)

77761 Intracavitary radiation source application; simple

77762 intermediate

77763 complex

77776 Interstitial radiation source application; simple

77777 intermediate

77778 complex

77781 Remote afterloading high intensity brachytherapy; 1-4 source positions or catheters

77782 5-8 source positions or catheters

77783 9-12 source positions or catheters

77784 over 12 source positions or catheters

77789 Surface application of radiation source

77790 Supervision, handling, loading of radiation source

77799 Unlisted procedure, clinical brachytherapy

● New Code   ▲ Revised Code   + Add-On Code   ⊘ Modifier -51 Exempt

NUCLEAR MEDICINE

Nuclear medicine is used in the diagnosis, management, treatment, and prevention of serious disease. Nuclear medicine imaging procedures often identify abnormalities very early in the progression of a disease. This early detection allows a disease to be treated early in its course when there may be a more successful prognosis.

Nuclear medicine uses very small amounts of radioactive materials or radiopharmaceuticals to diagnose and treat disease. Radiopharmaceuticals are substances that are attracted to specific organs, bones, or tissues. The radiopharmaceuticals used in nuclear medicine emit gamma rays that can be detected externally by special types of cameras: gamma or PET cameras. These cameras work in conjunction with computers used to form images that provide data and information about the area of body being imaged. The amount of radiation from a nuclear medicine procedure is comparable to that received during a diagnostic x-ray.

Nuclear medicine procedures may be performed independently or in the course of overall medical care. If the physician providing nuclear medicine services is also responsible for the diagnostic work-up and/or follow-up care of the patient, evaluation and management service codes should be coded in addition to the nuclear medicine procedures.

Radioimmunoassay tests are located in the clinical pathology section, code series 82000-84999. These CPT codes can be used by any specialist performing such tests in a laboratory licensed and/or certified for radioimmunoassays. The reporting of these tests is not confined to clinical pathology laboratories alone.

Note that the services listed in this section do not include the provision of radium or other elements. When those materials are supplied by the physician they should be listed as separate procedures using code 78990 for diagnostic radionuclide(s) and 79900 for therapeutic radionuclide.

DIAGNOSTIC NUCLEAR MEDICINE

ENDOCRINE SYSTEM

78000   Thyroid uptake; single determination

78001   multiple determinations

78003   stimulation, suppression or discharge (not including initial uptake studies)

78006   Thyroid imaging, with uptake; single determination

689

 Separate Procedure

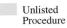 Unlisted Procedure

 CCI Comp. Code

 Non-specific Procedure

78007	multiple determinations
78010	Thyroid imaging; only
78011	with vascular flow
78015	Thyroid carcinoma metastases imaging; limited area (eg, neck and chest only)
78016	with additional studies (eg, urinary recovery)
78018	whole body

+ **78020**   Thyroid carcinoma metastases uptake (List separately in addition to code for primary procedure)

(Use 78020 in conjunction with code 78018 only)

78070	Parathyroid imaging
78075	Adrenal imaging, cortex and/or medulla
78099	Unlisted endocrine procedure, diagnostic nuclear medicine

(For chemical analysis, see Chemistry section)

HEMATOPOIETIC, RETICULOENDOTHELIAL AND LYMPHATIC SYSTEM

78102	Bone marrow imaging; limited area
78103	multiple areas
78104	whole body
78110	Plasma volume, radiopharmaceutical volume-dilution technique (separate procedure); single sampling
78111	multiple samplings
78120	Red cell volume determination (separate procedure); single sampling
78121	multiple samplings

● New Code   ▲ Revised Code   + Add-On Code   ⃠ Modifier -51 Exempt

78122 Whole blood volume determination, including separate measurement of plasma volume and red cell volume (radiopharmaceutical volume-dilution technique)

78130 Red cell survival study;

78135 differential organ/tissue kinetics, (eg, splenic and/or hepatic sequestration)

78140 Labeled red cell sequestration, differential organ/tissue, (eg, splenic and/or hepatic)

78160 Plasma radioiron disappearance (turnover) rate

78162 Radioiron oral absorption

78170 Radioiron red cell utilization

78172 Chelatable iron for estimation of total body iron

78185 Spleen imaging only, with or without vascular flow

(If combined with liver study, use procedures 78215 and 78216)

78190 Kinetics, study of platelet survival, with or without differential organ/tissue localization

78191 Platelet survival study

78195 Lymphatics and lymph nodes imaging

(For sentinel node identification without scintigraphy imaging, use 38792)

(For sentinel node excision, see 38500-38542)

78199 Unlisted hematopoietic, reticuloendothelial and lymphatic procedure, diagnostic nuclear medicine

(For chemical analysis, see Chemistry section)

GASTROINTESTINAL SYSTEM

78201 Liver imaging; static only

78202 with vascular flow

(For spleen imaging only, use 78185)

| | Separate Procedure | | Unlisted Procedure | | CCI Comp. Code | | Non-specific Procedure |

78205 Liver imaging (SPECT);

78206   with vascular flow

78215 Liver and spleen imaging; static only

78216   with vascular flow

78220 Liver function study with hepatobiliary agents, with serial images

78223 Hepatobiliary ductal system imaging, including gallbladder, with or without pharmacologic intervention, with or without quantitative measurement of gallbladder function

78230 Salivary gland imaging;

78231   with serial images

78232 Salivary gland function study

78258 Esophageal motility

78261 Gastric mucosa imaging

78262 Gastroesophageal reflux study

78264 Gastric emptying study

78267 Urea breath test, C-14; acquisition for analysis

78268   analysis

78270 Vitamin B-12 absorption study (eg, Schilling test); without intrinsic factor

78271   with intrinsic factor

78272 Vitamin B-12 absorption studies combined, with and without intrinsic factor

78278 Acute gastrointestinal blood loss imaging

78282 Gastrointestinal protein loss

| ● | New Code | ▲ | Revised Code | + | Add-On Code | ⊘ | Modifier -51 Exempt |

78290 Intestine imaging (eg, ectopic gastric mucosa, Meckels localization, volvulus)

78291 Peritoneal-venous shunt patency test (eg, for LeVeen, Denver shunt)

(For injection procedure, use 49427)

78299 Unlisted gastrointestinal procedure, diagnostic nuclear medicine

(For chemical analysis, see Chemistry section)

MUSCULOSKELETAL SYSTEM

78300 Bone and/or joint imaging; limited area

78305 multiple areas

78306 whole body

78315 three phase study

78320 tomographic (SPECT)

78350 Bone density (bone mineral content) study, one or more sites; single photon absorptiometry

78351 dual photon absorptiometry, one or more sites

(For radiographic bone density (photodensitometry), use 76078)

78399 Unlisted musculoskeletal procedure, diagnostic nuclear medicine

CARDIOVASCULAR SYSTEM

(78401-78412 have been deleted. To report, see 78472-78483)

78414 Determination of central c-v hemodynamics (non-imaging) (eg, ejection fraction with probe technique) with or without pharmacologic intervention or exercise, single or multiple determinations

78428 Cardiac shunt detection

78445 Non-cardiac vascular flow imaging (ie, angiography, venography)

78455 Venous thrombosis study (eg, radioactive fibrinogen)

693

	Separate Procedure		Unlisted Procedure		CCI Comp. Code		Non-specific Procedure

78456   Acute venous thrombosis imaging, peptide

78457   Venous thrombosis imaging, venogram; unilateral

78458   bilateral

78459   Myocardial imaging, positron emission tomography (PET), metabolic evaluation

(For myocardial perfusion study, see 78491-78492)

78460   Myocardial perfusion imaging; (planar) single study, at rest or stress (exercise and/or pharmacologic), with or without quantification

78461   multiple studies, (planar) at rest and/or stress (exercise and/or pharmacologic), and redistribution and/or rest injection, with or without quantification

78464   tomographic (SPECT), single study at rest or stress (exercise and/or pharmacologic), with or without quantification

78465   tomographic (SPECT), multiple studies, at rest and/or stress (exercise and/or pharmacologic) and redistribution and/or rest injection, with or without quantification

78466   Myocardial imaging, infarct avid, planar; qualitative or quantitative

78468   with ejection fraction by first pass technique

78469   tomographic SPECT with or without quantification

78472   Cardiac blood pool imaging, gated equilibrium; planar, single study at rest or stress (exercise and/or pharmacologic), wall motion study plus ejection fraction, with or without additional quantitative processing

(For assessment of cardiac function by first pass technique, use 78496)

78473   multiple studies, wall motion study plus ejection fraction, at rest and stress (exercise and/or pharmacologic), with or without additional quantification

● New Code   ▲ Revised Code   + Add-On Code   ⊘ Modifier -51 Exempt

+ 78478 Myocardial perfusion study with wall motion, qualitative or quantitative study (List separately in addition to code for primary procedure)

(Use 78478 in conjunction with codes 78460, 78461, 78464, 78465)

+ 78480 Myocardial perfusion study with ejection fraction (List separately in addition to code for primary procedure)

(Use 78480 in conjunction with codes 78460, 78461, 78464, 78465)

78481 Cardiac blood pool imaging, (planar), first pass technique; single study, at rest or with stress (exercise and/or pharmacologic), wall motion study plus ejection fraction, with or without quantification

78483 multiple studies, at rest and with stress (exercise and/or pharmacologic), wall motion study plus ejection fraction, with or without quantification

(For cerebral blood flow study, use 78615)

78491 Myocardial imaging, positron emission tomography (PET), perfusion; single study at rest or stress

78492 multiple studies at rest and/or stress

78494 Cardiac blood pool imaging, gated equilibrium, SPECT, at rest, wall motion study plus ejection fraction, with or without quantitative processing

+ 78496 Cardiac blood pool imaging, gated equilibrium, single study, at rest, with right ventricular ejection fraction by first pass technique (List separately in addition to code for primary procedure)

(Use 78496 in conjunction with code 78472)

78499 Unlisted cardiovascular procedure, diagnostic nuclear medicine

(For chemical analysis, see Chemistry section)

RESPIRATORY SYSTEM

78580 Pulmonary perfusion imaging, particulate

695

 Separate Procedure

 Unlisted Procedure

 CCI Comp. Code

 Non-specific Procedure

78584 Pulmonary perfusion imaging, particulate, with ventilation; single breath

78585 rebreathing and washout, with or without single breath

78586 Pulmonary ventilation imaging, aerosol; single projection

78587 multiple projections (eg, anterior, posterior, lateral views)

78588 Pulmonary perfusion imaging, particulate, with ventilation imaging, aerosol, one or multiple projections

78591 Pulmonary ventilation imaging, gaseous, single breath, single projection

78593 Pulmonary ventilation imaging, gaseous, with rebreathing and washout with or without single breath; single projection

78594 multiple projections (eg, anterior, posterior, lateral views)

78596 Pulmonary quantitative differential function (ventilation/perfusion) study

78599 Unlisted respiratory procedure, diagnostic nuclear medicine

NERVOUS SYSTEM

78600 Brain imaging, limited procedure; static

78601 with vascular flow

78605 Brain imaging, complete study; static

78606 with vascular flow

78607 tomographic (SPECT)

78608 Brain imaging, positron emission tomography (PET); metabolic evaluation

78609 perfusion evaluation

78610 Brain imaging, vascular flow only

78615 Cerebral vascular flow

78630 Cerebrospinal fluid flow, imaging (not including introduction of material); cisternography

(For injection procedure, see 61000-61070, 62270-62319)

78635 ventriculography

(For injection procedure, see 61000-61070, 62270-62294)

78645 shunt evaluation

(For injection procedure, see 61000-61070, 62270-62294)

78647 tomographic (SPECT)

78650 Cerebrospinal fluid leakage detection and localization

(For injection procedure, see 61000-61070, 62270-62294)

78660 Radiopharmaceutical dacryocystography

78699 Unlisted nervous system procedure, diagnostic nuclear medicine

GENITOURINARY SYSTEM

78700 Kidney imaging; static only

78701 with vascular flow

78704 with function study (ie, imaging renogram)

78707 Kidney imaging with vascular flow and function; single study without pharmacological intervention

78708 single study, with pharmacological intervention (eg, angiotensin converting enzyme inhibitor and/or diuretic)

78709 multiple studies, with and without pharmacological intervention (eg, angiotensin converting enzyme inhibitor and/or diuretic)

(For introduction of radioactive substance in association with renal endoscopy, see 50559, 50578)

78710 Kidney imaging, tomographic (SPECT)

78715 Kidney vascular flow only

697

 Separate Procedure    Unlisted Procedure   CCI Comp. Code   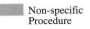 Non-specific Procedure

| 78725 | Kidney function study, non-imaging radioisotopic study |

78730 Urinary bladder residual study

(For introduction of radioactive substance in association with cystotomy or cystostomy, use 51020; in association with cystourethroscopy, use 52250)

78740 Ureteral reflux study (radiopharmaceutical voiding cystogram)

(For catheterization, see 51701-51703)

78760 Testicular imaging;

78761   with vascular flow

(For introduction of radioactive substance in association with ureteral endoscopy, see 50959, 50978)

78799 Unlisted genitourinary procedure, diagnostic nuclear medicine

(For chemical analysis, see Chemistry section)

OTHER PROCEDURES

(For specific organ, see appropriate heading)

(For radiophosphorus tumor identification, ocular, see 78800)

▲ 78800 Radiopharmaceutical localization of tumor or distribution of radiopharmaceutical agent(s); limited area

(For specific organ, see appropriate heading)

78801   multiple areas

▲ 78802   whole body, single day imaging

78803   tomographic (SPECT)

● 78804   whole body, requiring two or more days imaging

78805 Radiopharmaceutical localization of inflammatory process; limited area

78806   whole body

78807   tomographic (SPECT)

(For imaging bone infectious or inflammatory disease with a bone imaging radiopharmaceutical, see 78300, 78305, 78306)

78810 Tumor imaging, positron emission tomography (PET), metabolic evaluation

78890 Generation of automated data: interactive process involving nuclear physician and/or allied health professional personnel; simple manipulations and interpretation, not to exceed 30 minutes

78891 complex manipulations and interpretation, exceeding 30 minutes

(Use 78890 or 78891 in addition to primary procedure)

78990 Provision of diagnostic radiopharmaceutical(s)

78999 Unlisted miscellaneous procedure, diagnostic nuclear medicine

THERAPEUTIC

79000 Radiopharmaceutical therapy, hyper-thyroidism; initial, including evaluation of patient

79001 subsequent, each therapy

(For follow-up visit, see 99211-99215)

79020 Radiopharmaceutical therapy, thyroid suppression (euthyroid cardiac disease), including evaluation of patient

79030 Radiopharmaceutical ablation of gland for thyroid carcinoma

79035 Radiopharmaceutical therapy for metastases of thyroid carcinoma

▲ **79100** Radiopharmaceutical therapy, polycythemia vera, chronic leukemia, each treatment by intravenous injection

(For monoclonal antibody therapy, use 79403)

79200 Intracavitary radioactive colloid therapy

79300 Interstitial radioactive colloid therapy

699

 Separate Procedure

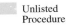 Unlisted Procedure

 CCI Comp. Code

 Non-specific Procedure

▲ **79400** Radiopharmaceutical therapy, nonthyroid, nonhematologic by intravenous injection

(Do not report 79400 in conjunction with 79403)

(For monoclonal antibody therapy, use 79403)

● **79403** Radiopharmaceutical therapy, radiolabeled monoclonal antibody by intravenous infusion

(For pre-treatment imaging, see 78802, 78804)

(Do not report 79403 in conjunction with 79400)

79420 Intravascular radiopharmaceutical therapy, particulate

79440 Intra-articular radiopharmaceutical therapy

79900 Provision of therapeutic radiopharmaceutical(s)

79999 Unlisted radiopharmaceutical therapeutic procedure

● New Code ▲ Revised Code + Add-On Code ⊘ Modifier -51 Exempt

PATHOLOGY/ LABORATORY

LABORATORY SECTION OVERVIEW

The fifth section of the CPT coding system is the laboratory section, which includes codes for pathology and laboratory services. Within each subsection, the CPT codes are arranged by the type of testing or service.

LABORATORY SUBSECTIONS

The PATHOLOGY AND LABORATORY section of CPT is divided into the following subsections:

Organ or Disease Oriented Panels	80048-80076
Drug Testing	80100-80103
Therapeutic Drug Assays	80150-80299
Evocative/Suppression Testing	80400-80440
Consultations (Clinical Pathology)	80500-80502
Urinalysis	81000-81099
Chemistry	82000-84999
Hematology and Coagulation	85002-85999
Immunology	86000-86849
Transfusion Medicine	86850-86999
Microbiology	87000-87999
Anatomic Pathology	88000-88099
Cytopathology	88104-88199
Cytogenetic Studies	88200-88299
Surgical Pathology	88300-88399
Transcutaneous Procedures	88400
Other Procedures	89050-89240
Reproductive Medicine Procedures	89250-89356

LAB 80000

LABORATORY SERVICE MODIFIERS

Pathology and laboratory services and procedures may be modified under certain circumstances. When applicable, the modifying circumstances should be identified by adding the appropriate modifier to the basic service code. The addition of modifier -22 requires a special report. Modifiers commonly used to report PATHOLOGY and LABORATORY procedures include:

-22 unusual services

-26 professional component

701

	Separate Procedure		Unlisted Procedure		CCI Comp. Code		Non-specific Procedure

-32   mandated services

-52   reduced services

-90   reference (outside) laboratory

PATHOLOGY

Pathology is that discipline of the practice of medicine that deals with the causes and nature of disease. It contributes to diagnosis, prognosis, and treatment through knowledge gained by the laboratory application of the biologic, chemical, and physical sciences to man, or materials obtained from man. Pathologists diagnose, exclude, and monitor disease by means of information gathered from the microscopic examination of tissue specimens, cells, and body fluids, and from clinical laboratory tests on body fluids and secretions. Pathologists are involved with the management of laboratories and in data processing and with new developments in high technology.

CLINICAL PATHOLOGY

Clinical Pathology focuses on microbiology (including bacteriology, mycology, parasitology, and virology), immunopathology, blood banking/transfusion medicine, chemical pathology, cytogenetics, hematology, coagulation, toxicology, medical microscopy (including urinalysis), molecular biologic techniques, and other advanced diagnostic techniques as they become available.

● New Code   ▲ Revised Code   + Add-On Code   ⃠ Modifier -51 Exempt

PATHOLOGY AND LABORATORY CODES

ORGAN OR DISEASE ORIENTED PANELS

CPT codes for organ or disease oriented panels were included in CPT due to the increased use of general screening programs by physicians, clinics, hospitals, and other health care facilities. Other codes in this section define profiles that combine laboratory tests together under a problem oriented classification.

There is a list of specific laboratory tests under each of the panel CPT codes which define the components of each panel. However, each laboratory typically establishes its own profile and provides a listing of the components of that panel performed by the laboratory with test results.

80048   Basic metabolic panel

This panel must include the following:
Calcium (82310)
Carbon dioxide (82374)
Chloride (82435)
Creatinine (82565)
Glucose (82947)
Potassium (84132)
Sodium (84295)
Urea Nitrogen (BUN) (84520)

(Do not use 80048 in addition to 80053)

▲ **80050**   General health panel

This panel must include the following:
Comprehensive metabolic panel (80053)
Blood count, complete (CBC), automated and automated
differential WBC count (85025 or 85027 and 85004)
OR
Blood count, complete (CBC), automated (85027) and
appropriate manual differential WBC count (85007 or 85009)
Thyroid stimulating hormone (TSH) (84443)

80051   Electrolyte panel

This panel must include the following:
Carbon dioxide (82374)
Chloride (82435)
Potassium (84132)
Sodium (84295)

703

 Separate
Procedure

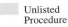 Unlisted
Procedure

 CCI Comp.
Code

 Non-specific
Procedure

80053 Comprehensive metabolic panel

This panel must include the following:
Albumin (82040)
Bilirubin, total (82247)
Calcium (82310)
Carbon dioxide (bicarbonate) (82374)
Chloride (82435)
Creatinine (82565)
Glucose (82947)
Phosphatase, alkaline (84075)
Potassium (84132)
Protein, total (84155)
Sodium (84295)
Transferase, alanine amino (ALT) (SGPT) (84460)
Transferase, aspartate amino (AST) (SGOT) (84450)
Urea Nitrogen (BUN) (84520)

(Do not use 80053 in addition to 80048, 80076)

▲ **80055** Obstetric panel

This panel must include the following:
Blood count, complete (CBC), automated and automated
    differential WBC count (85025 or 85027 and 85004)
OR
Blood count, complete (CBC), automated (85027) and
    appropriate manual differential WBC count (85007 or 85009)
Hepatitis B surface antigen (HBsAg) (87340)
Antibody, rubella (86762)
Syphilis test, qualitative (eg, VDRL, RPR, ART) (86592)
Antibody screen, RBC, each serum technique (86850)
Blood typing, ABO (86900) AND
Blood typing, Rh (D) (86901)

80061 Lipid panel

This panel must include the following:
Cholesterol, serum, total (82465)
Lipoprotein, direct measurement, high density cholesterol (HDL
    cholesterol) (83718)
Triglycerides (84478)

● New Code   ▲ Revised Code   + Add-On Code   ⊘ Modifier -51 Exempt

80069 Renal function panel

This panel must include the following:
Albumin (82040)
Calcium (82310)
Carbon dioxide (bicarbonate) (82374)
Chloride (82435)
Creatinine (82565)
Glucose (82947)
Phosphorus inorganic (phosphate) (84100)
Potassium (84132)
Sodium (84295)
Urea nitrogen (BUN) (84520)

(80073 has been deleted. To report, see codes for specific tests)

80074 Acute hepatitis panel

This panel must include the following:
Hepatitis A antibody (HAAb), IgM antibody (86709)
Hepatitis B core antibody (HbcAb), IgM antibody (86705)
Hepatitis B surface antigen (HbsAg) (87340)
Hepatitis C antibody (86803)

80076 Hepatic function panel

This panel must include the following:
Albumin (82040)
Bilirubin, total (82247)
Bilirubin, direct (82248)
Phosphatase, alkaline (84075)
Protein, total (84155)
Transferase, alanine amino (ALT) (SGPT) (84460)
Transferase, aspartate amino (AST) (SGOT) (84450)

(Do not use 80076 in addition to 80053)

(80090 deleted 2003 edition. To report, see codes for specific tests)

DRUG TESTING

80100 Drug screen, qualitative; multiple drug classes, chromatographic method, each procedure

80101 single drug class method (eg, immunoassay, enzyme assay), each drug class

80102 Drug, confirmation, each procedure

705

 Separate Procedure
 Unlisted Procedure
 CCI Comp. Code
 Non-specific Procedure

80103   Tissue preparation for drug analysis

THERAPEUTIC DRUG ASSAYS

80150   Amikacin

80152   Amitriptyline

80154   Benzodiazepines

80156   Carbamazepine; total

80157   free

80158   Cyclosporine

80160   Desipramine

80162   Digoxin

80164   Dipropylacetic acid (valproic acid)

80166   Doxepin

80168   Ethosuximide

80170   Gentamicin

80172   Gold

80173   Haloperidol

80174   Imipramine

80176   Lidocaine

80178   Lithium

80182   Nortriptyline

80184   Phenobarbital

80185   Phenytoin; total

80186   free

● New Code ▲ Revised Code ✚ Add-On Code ⊘ Modifier -51 Exempt

80188 Primidone

80190 Procainamide;

80192   with metabolites (eg, n-acetyl procainamide)

80194 Quinidine

80196 Salicylate

80197 Tacrolimus

80198 Theophylline

80200 Tobramycin

80201 Topiramate

80202 Vancomycin

80299 Quantitation of drug, not elsewhere specified

EVOCATIVE/SUPPRESSION TESTING

80400 ACTH stimulation panel; for adrenal insufficiency

This panel must include the following:
Cortisol (82533 x 2)

80402   for 21 hydroxylase deficiency

This panel must include the following:
Cortisol (82533 x 2)
17 hydroxyprogesterone (83498 x 2)

80406   for 3 beta-hydroxydehydrogenase deficiency

This panel must include the following:
Cortisol (82533 x 2)
17 hydroxypregnenolone (84143 x 2)

80408 Aldosterone suppression evaluation panel (eg, saline infusion)

This panel must include the following:
Aldosterone (82088 x 2)
Renin (84244 x 2)

707

 Separate Procedure   Unlisted Procedure   CCI Comp. Code   Non-specific Procedure

80410 Calcitonin stimulation panel (eg, calcium, pentagastrin)

This panel must include the following:
Calcitonin (82308 x 3)

80412 Corticotropic releasing hormone (CRH) stimulation panel

This panel must include the following:
Cortisol (82533 x 6)
Adrenocorticotropic hormone (ACTH) (82024 x 6)

80414 Chorionic gonadotropin stimulation panel; testosterone response.

This panel must include the following:
Testosterone (84403 x 2 on three pooled blood samples)

80415   estradiol response.

This panel must include the following:
Estradiol (82670 x 2 on three pooled blood samples)

80416 Renal vein renin stimulation panel (eg, captopril)

This panel must include the following:
Renin (84244 x 6)

80417 Peripheral vein renin stimulation panel (eg, captopril)

This panel must include the following:
Renin (84244 x 2)

80418 Combined rapid anterior pituitary evaluation panel

This panel must include the following:
Adrenocorticotropic hormone (ACTH) (82024 x 4)
Luteinizing hormone (LH) (83002 x 4)
Follicle stimulating hormone (FSH) (83001 x 4)
Prolactin (84146 x 4)
Human growth hormone (HGH)(83003 x 4)
Cortisol (82533 x 4)
Thyroid stimulating hormone (TSH) (84443 x 4)

80420 Dexamethasone suppression panel, 48 hour

This panel must include the following:
Free cortisol, urine (82530 x 2)
Cortisol (82533 x 2)
Volume measurement for timed collection (81050 x 2)

(For single dose dexamethasone, use 82533)

● New Code   ▲ Revised Code   + Add-On Code   ⊘ Modifier -51 Exempt

80422 Glucagon tolerance panel; for insulinoma

This panel must include the following:
Glucose (82947 x 3)
Insulin (83525 x 3)

80424 for pheochromocytoma.

This panel must include the following:
Catecholamines, fractionated (82384 x 2)

80426 Gonadotropin releasing hormone stimulation panel

This panel must include the following:
Follicle stimulating hormone (FSH) (83001 x 4)
Luteinizing hormone (LH)(83002 x 4)

80428 Growth hormone stimulation panel (eg, arginine infusion, l-dopa administration)

This panel must include the following:
Human growth hormone (HGH)(83003 x 4)

80430 Growth hormone suppression panel (glucose administration)

This panel must include the following:
Glucose (82947 x 3)
Human growth hormone (HGH)(83003 x 4)

80432 Insulin-induced C-peptide suppression panel

This panel must include the following:
Insulin (83525)
C-peptide (84681 x 5)
Glucose (82947 x 5)

80434 Insulin tolerance panel; for ACTH insufficiency

This panel must include the following:
Cortisol (82533 x 5)
Glucose (82947 x 5)

80435 for growth hormone deficiency

This panel must include the following:
Glucose (82947 x 5)
Human growth hormone (HGH) (83003 x 5)

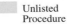 Separate Procedure   Unlisted Procedure   CCI Comp. Code   Non-specific Procedure

80436 Metyrapone panel

This panel must include the following:
Cortisol (82533 x 2)
11 deoxycortisol (82634 x 2)

80438 Thyrotropin releasing hormone (TRH) stimulation panel; one hour

This panel must include the following:
Thyroid stimulating hormone (TSH) (84443 x 3)

80439 two hour

This panel must include the following:
Thyroid stimulating hormone (TSH) (84443 x 4)

80440 for hyperprolactinemia

This panel must include the following:
Prolactin (84146 x 3)

CONSULTATIONS (CLINICAL PATHOLOGY)

80500 Clinical pathology consultation; limited, without review of patients history and medical records

80502 comprehensive, for a complex diagnostic problem, with review of patients history and medical records

(These codes may also be used for pharmacokinetic consultations)

(For consultations involving the examination and evaluation of the patient, see 99241-99275)

URINALYSIS

(For urinalysis, infectious agent detection, semi-quantitative analysis of volatile compounds, use Category III code 0041T)

81000 Urinalysis, by dip stick or tablet reagent for bilirubin, glucose, hemoglobin, ketones, leukocytes, nitrite, pH, protein, specific gravity,urobilinogen, any number of these constituents; non-automated, with microscopy

81001 automated, with microscopy

81002 non-automated, without microscopy

● New Code	▲ Revised Code	+ Add-On Code	⊘ Modifier -51 Exempt

81003   automated, without microscopy

81005   Urinalysis; qualitative or semiquantitative, except immunoassays

(For non-immunoassay reagent strip urinalysis, see 81000, 81002)

(For immunoassay, qualitative or semiquantitative, use 83518)

(For microalbumin, see 82043, 82044)

81007   bacteriuria screen, except by culture or dipstick

(For culture, see 87086-87088)

(For dipstick, use 81000 or 81002)

81015   microscopic only

81020   two or three glass test

81025   Urine pregnancy test, by visual color comparison methods

81050   Volume measurement for timed collection, each

81099   Unlisted urinalysis procedure

CHEMISTRY

82000   Acetaldehyde, blood

82003   Acetaminophen

82009   Acetone or other ketone bodies, serum; qualitative

82010   quantitative

82013   Acetylcholinesterase

(Acid, gastric, see gastric acid, 82926, 82928)

(Acid phosphatase, see 84060-84066)

82016   Acylcarnitines; qualitative, each specimen

82017   quantitative, each specimen

(For carnitine, use 82379)

711

Separate Procedure	Unlisted Procedure	CCI Comp. Code	Non-specific Procedure

82024 Adrenocorticotropic hormone (ACTH)

82030 Adenosine, 5-monophosphate, cyclic (cyclic AMP)

82040 Albumin; serum

82042   urine, quantitative, each specimen

82043   urine, microalbumin, quantitative

82044   urine, microalbumin, semiquantitative (eg, reagent strip assay)

(For prealbumin, use 84134)

82055 Alcohol (ethanol); any specimen except breath

(For other volatiles, alcohol, use 84600)

82075   breath

82085 Aldolase

82088 Aldosterone

(Alkaline phosphatase, see 84075, 84080)

82101 Alkaloids, urine, quantitative

(Alphaketoglutarate, see 82009, 82010)

(Alpha tocopherol (Vitamin E), use 84446)

82103 Alpha-1-antitrypsin; total

82104   phenotype

82105 Alpha-fetoprotein; serum

82106   amniotic fluid

82108 Aluminum

82120 Amines, vaginal fluid, qualitative

(For combined pH and amines test for vaginitis, use 82120 and 83986)

● New Code   ▲ Revised Code   + Add-On Code   ⊘ Modifier -51 Exempt

82127 Amino acids; single, qualitative, each specimen

82128 multiple, qualitative, each specimen

82131 single, quantitative, each specimen

82135 Aminolevulinic acid, delta (ALA)

82136 Amino acids, 2 to 5 amino acids, quantitative, each specimen

82139 Amino acids, 6 or more amino acids, quantitative, each specimen

82140 Ammonia

82143 Amniotic fluid scan (spectrophotometric)

(For L/S ratio, use 83661)

(Amobarbital, see 80100-80103 for qualitative analysis, 82205 for quantitative analysis)

82145 Amphetamine or methamphetamine

(For qualitative analysis, see 80100-80103)

82150 Amylase

82154 Androstanediol glucuronide

82157 Androstenedione

82160 Androsterone

82163 Angiotensin II

82164 Angiotensin I - converting enzyme (ACE)

(Antidiuretic hormone (ADH), use 84588)

(Antimony, use 83015)

(Antitrypsin, alph-1-, see 82103, 82104)

82172 Apolipoprotein, each

82175 Arsenic

713

 Separate Procedure Unlisted Procedure CCI Comp. Code 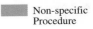 Non-specific Procedure

(For heavy metal screening, use 83015)

82180   Ascorbic acid (Vitamin C), blood

(Aspirin, see acetylsalicylic acid, 80196)

(Atherogenic index, blood, ultracentrifugation, quantitative, use 83717)

82190   Atomic absorption spectroscopy, each analyte

82205   Barbiturates, not elsewhere specified

(For qualitative analysis, see 80100-80103)

(For B-Natriuretic peptide, use 83880)

82232   Beta-2 microglobulin

(Bicarbonate, use 82374)

82239   Bile acids; total

82240   cholylglycine

(For bile pigments, urine, see 81000-81005)

82247   Bilirubin; total

82248   direct

82252   feces, qualitative

82261   Biotinidase, each specimen

82270   Blood, occult, by peroxidase activity (eg, guaiac), qualitative; feces, 1-3 simultaneous determinations

82273   other sources

(Blood urea nitrogen (BUN), see 84520, 84525)

82274   Blood, occult, by fecal hemoglobin determination by immunoassay, qualitative, feces, 1-3 simultaneous determinations

82286   Bradykinin

82300   Cadmium

● New Code   ▲ Revised Code   + Add-On Code   ⊘ Modifier -51 Exempt

82306   Calcifediol (25-OH Vitamin D-3)

82307   Calciferol (Vitamin D)

(For 1,25-Dihydroxyvitamin D, use 82652)

82308   Calcitonin

82310   Calcium; total

82330   ionized

82331   after calcium infusion test

82340   urine quantitative, timed specimen

82355   Calculus; qualitative analysis

82360   quantitative analysis, chemical

82365   infrared spectroscopy

82370   x-ray diffraction

(Carbamates, see individual listings)

82373   Carbohydrate deficient transferrin

82374   Carbon dioxide (bicarbonate)

(See also 82803)

82375   Carbon monoxide, (carboxyhemoglobin); quantitative

82376   qualitative

(To report end-tidal carbon monoxide, use Category III code 0043T)

82378   Carcinoembryonic antigen (CEA)

82379   Carnitine (total and free), quantitative, each specimen

(For acylcarnitine, see 82016, 82017)

82380   Carotene

715

 Separate Procedure   Unlisted Procedure   CCI Comp. Code   Non-specific Procedure

82382   Catecholamines; total urine

82383   blood

82384   fractionated

(For urine metabolites, see 83835, 84585)

82387   Cathepsin-D

82390   Ceruloplasmin

82397   Chemiluminescent assay

82415   Chloramphenicol

82435   Chloride; blood

82436   urine

82438   other source

(For sweat collection by iontophoresis, use 89360)

82441   Chlorinated hydrocarbons, screen

(Chlorpromazine, use 84022)

(Cholecalciferol (Vitamin D), use 82307)

82465   Cholesterol, serum or whole blood, total

(For high density lipoprotein (HDL), use 83718)

82480   Cholinesterase; serum

82482   RBC

82485   Chondroitin B sulfate, quantitative

(Chorionic gonadotropin, see gonadotropin, 84702, 84703)

82486   Chromatography, qualitative; column (eg, gas liquid or HPLC), analyte not elsewhere specified

82487   paper, 1-dimensional, analyte not elsewhere specified

82488   paper, 2-dimensional, analyte not elsewhere specified

● New Code	▲ Revised Code	+ Add-On Code	⊘ Modifier -51 Exempt

82489   thin layer, analyte not elsewhere specified

82491 Chromatography, quantitative, column (eg, gas liquid or HPLC); single analyte not elsewhere specified, single stationary and mobile phase

82492   multiple analytes, single stationary and mobile phase

82495 Chromium

82507 Citrate

82520 Cocaine or metabolite

(Cocaine, qualitative analysis, see 80100-80103)

(Codeine, qualitative analysis, see 80100-80103)

(Codeine, quantitative analysis, see 82101)

(Complement, see 86160-86162)

82523 Collagen cross links, any method

82525 Copper

(Coproporphyrin, see 84119, 84120)

(Corticosteroids, use 83491)

82528 Corticosterone

82530 Cortisol; free

82533   total

(C-peptide, use 84681)

82540 Creatine

82541 Column chromatography/mass spectrometry (eg, GC/MS, or HPLC/MS), analyte not elsewhere specified; qualitative, single stationary and mobile phase

82542   quantitative, single stationary and mobile phase

82543   stable isotope dilution, single analyte, quantitative, single stationary and mobile phase

717

Separate Procedure	Unlisted Procedure	CCI Comp. Code	Non-specific Procedure

82544   stable isotope dilution, multiple analytes, quantitative, single stationary and mobile phase

82550   Creatine kinase (CK), (CPK); total

82552   isoenzymes

82553   MB fraction only

82554   isoforms

82565   Creatinine; blood

82570   other source

82575   clearance

82585   Cryofibrinogen

82595   Cryoglobulin, qualitative or semi-quantitative (eg,cryocrit)

(For quantitative, cryoglobulin, see 82784, 82785)

(Crystals, pyrophosphate vs. urate, use 89060)

82600   Cyanide

82607   Cyanocobalamin (Vitamin B-12);

82608   unsaturated binding capacity

(Cyclic AMP, use 82030)

(Cyclic GMP, use 83008)

(Cyclosporine, use 80158)

82615   Cystine and homocystine, urine, qualitative

82626   Dehydroepiandrosterone (DHEA)

82627   Dehydroepiandrosterone-sulfate (DHEA-S)

(Delta-aminolevulinic acid (ALA), use 82135)

82633   Desoxycorticosterone, 11-

82634   Deoxycortisol, 11-

● New Code   ▲ Revised Code   + Add-On Code   ⊘ Modifier -51 Exempt

(Dexamethasone suppression test, use 80420)

(Diastase, urine, use 82150)

82638   Dibucaine number

(Dichloroethane, use 84600)

(Dichloromethane, use 84600)

(Diethylether, use 84600)

82646   Dihydrocodeinone

(For qualitative analysis, see 80100-80103)

82649   Dihydromorphinone

(For qualitative analysis, see 80100-80103)

82651   Dihydrotestosterone (DHT)

82652   Dihydroxyvitamin D, 1,25-

82654   Dimethadione

(For qualitative analysis, see 80100-80103)

(Diphenylhydantoin, use 80185)

(Dipropylacetic acid, use 80164)

(Dopamine, see 82382-82384)

(Duodenal contents, see individual enzymes; for intubation and collection, use 89100)

82657   Enzyme activity in blood cells, cultured cells, or tissue, not elsewhere specified; nonradioactive substrate, each specimen

82658   radioactive substrate, each specimen

82664   Electrophoretic technique, not elsewhere specified

(Endocrine receptor assays, see 84233-84235)`

82666   Epiandrosterone

(Epinephrine, see 82382-82384)

82668   Erythropoietin

 Separate
Procedure

 Unlisted
Procedure

CCI Comp.
Code

 Non-specific
Procedure

719

82670 Estradiol

82671 Estrogens; fractionated

82672   total

(Estrogen receptor assay, use 84233)

82677 Estriol

82679 Estrone

(Ethanol, see 82055 and 82075)

82690 Ethchlorvynol

(Ethyl alcohol, see 82055 and 82075)

82693 Ethylene glycol

82696 Etiocholanolone

(For fractionation of ketosteroids, use 83593)

82705 Fat or lipids, feces; qualitative

82710   quantitative

82715 Fat differential, feces, quantitative

82725 Fatty acids, nonesterified

82726 Very long chain fatty acids

82728 Ferritin

(Fetal hemoglobin, see hemoglobin 83030, 83033, and 85460)

(Fetoprotein, alpha-1, see 82105, 82106)

82731 Fetal fibronectin, cervicovaginal secretions, semi-quantitative

82735 Fluoride

82742 Flurazepam

(For qualitative analysis, see 80100-80103)

(Foam stability test, use 83662)

82746   Folic acid; serum

82747   RBC

(Follicle stimulating hormone (FSH), use 83001)

82757   Fructose, semen

(Fructosamine, use 82985)

(Fructose, TLC screen, use 84375)

82759   Galactokinase, RBC

82760   Galactose

82775   Galactose-1-phosphate uridyl transferase; quantitative

82776   screen

82784   Gammaglobulin; IgA, IgD, IgG, IgM, each

82785   IgE

(For allergen specific IgE, see 86003, 86005)

82787   immunoglobulin subclasses, (IgG1, 2, 3, or 4), each

(Gamma-glutamyltransferase (GGT), use 82977)

82800   Gases, blood, pH only

82803   Gases, blood, any combination of pH, pCO_2, pO_2, CO_2, HCO_3 (including calculated O_2 saturation);

(Use 82803 for two or more of the above listed analytes)

82805   with O_2 saturation, by direct measurement, except pulse oximetry

82810   Gases, blood, O_2 saturation only, by direct measurement, except pulse oximetry

(For pulse oximetry, use 94760)

 Separate Procedure   Unlisted Procedure   CCI Comp. Code   Non-specific Procedure

82820   Hemoglobin-oxygen affinity (pO_2 for 50% hemoglobin saturation with oxygen)

82926   Gastric acid, free and total, each specimen

82928   Gastric acid, free or total; each specimen

82938   Gastrin after secretin stimulation

82941   Gastrin

         (Gentamicin, use 80170)

         (GGT, use 82977)

         (GLC, gas liquid chromatography, use 82486)

82943   Glucagon

82945   Glucose, body fluid, other than blood

82946   Glucagon tolerance test

82947   Glucose; quantitative, blood, (except reagent strip)

82948   blood, reagent strip

82950   post glucose dose (includes glucose)

82951   tolerance test (GTT), three specimens (includes glucose)

82952   tolerance test, each additional beyond three specimens

82953   tolbutamide tolerance test

         (For insulin tolerance test, see 80434, 80435)

         (For leucine tolerance test, use 80428)

         (For semiquantitative urine glucose, see 81000, 81002, 81005, 81099)

82955   Glucose-6-phosphate dehydrogenase (G6PD); quantitative

82960   screen

         (For glucose tolerance test with medication, use 90784 in addition)

● New Code   ▲ Revised Code   + Add-On Code   ⊘ Modifier -51 Exempt

82962   Glucose, blood by glucose monitoring device(s) cleared by the FDA specifically for home use

82963   Glucosidase, beta

82965   Glutamate dehydrogenase

82975   Glutamine (glutamic acid amide)

82977   Glutamyltransferase, gamma (GGT)

82978   Glutathione

82979   Glutathione reductase, RBC

82980   Glutethimide

(Glycohemoglobin, use 83036)

82985   Glycated protein

(Gonadotropin, chorionic, see 84702, 84703)

83001   Gonadotropin; follicle stimulating hormone (FSH)

83002   luteinizing hormone (LH)

(For luteinizing releasing factor (LRH), use 83727)

83003   Growth hormone, human (HGH) (somatotropin)

(For antibody to human growth hormone, use 86277)

83008   Guanosine monophosphate (GMP), cyclic

83010   Haptoglobin; quantitative

83012   phenotypes

83013   Helicobacter pylori; analysis for urease activity, non-radioactive isotope

83014   drug administration and sample collection

(For H. pylori, stool, use 87338. For H. pylori, liquid scintillation counter, see 78267, 78268. For H. pylori, enzyme immunoassay, use 87339)

723

| Separate Procedure | Unlisted Procedure | CCI Comp. Code | Non-specific Procedure |

83015 Heavy metal (eg, arsenic, barium, beryllium, bismuth, antimony, mercury); screen

83018 quantitative, each

83020 Hemoglobin fractionation and quantitation; electrophoresis (eg, A2, S, C, and/or F)

83021 chromotography (eg, A2, S, C,and/or F)

83026 Hemoglobin; by copper sulfate method, non-automated

83030 F (fetal), chemical

83033 F (fetal), qualitative

83036 glycated

(For fecal hemoglobin detection by immunoassay, use 82274)

83045 methemoglobin, qualitative

83050 methemoglobin, quantitative

83051 plasma

83055 sulfhemoglobin, qualitative

83060 sulfhemoglobin, quantitative

83065 thermolabile

83068 unstable, screen

83069 urine

83070 Hemosiderin; qualitative

83071 quantitative

(Heroin, see 80100-80103)

(HIAA, use 83497)

(High performance liquid chromatography (HPLC), use 82486)

83080 b-Hexosaminidase, each assay

724

● New Code   ▲ Revised Code   **+** Add-On Code   ⊘ Modifier -51 Exempt

83088 Histamine

(Hollander test, use 91052)

83090 Homocystine

83150 Homovanillic acid (HVA)

(Hormones, see individual alphabetic listings in Chemistry section)

(Hydrogen breath test, use 91065)

83491 Hydroxycorticosteroids, 17- (17-OHCS)

(For cortisol, see 82530, 82533. For deoxycortisol, use 82634)

83497 Hydroxyindolacetic acid, 5-(HIAA)

(For urine qualitative test, use 81005)

(5-Hydroxytryptamine, use 84260)

83498 Hydroxyprogesterone, 17-d

83499 Hydroxyprogesterone, 20-

83500 Hydroxyproline; free

83505 total

83516 Immunoassay for analyte other than infectious agent antibody or infectious agent antigen, qualitative or semiquantitative; multiple step method

83518 single step method (eg, reagent strip)

83519 Immunoassay, analyte, quantitative; by radiopharmaceutical technique (eg, RIA)

83520 not otherwise specified

(For immunoassays for antibodies to infectious agent antigens, see analyte and method specific codes in the Immunology section)

(For immunoassay of tumor antigen not elsewhere specified, use 86316)

725

 Separate Procedure   Unlisted Procedure CCI Comp. Code Non-specific Procedure

CPT codes and descriptions only ©2003 American Medical Association. All rights reserved.

(Immunoglobulins, see 82784, 82785)

83525   Insulin; total

(For proinsulin, use 84206)

83527   free

83528   Intrinsic factor

(For intrinsic factor antibodies, use 86340)

83540   Iron

83550   Iron binding capacity

83570   Isocitric dehydrogenase (IDH)

(Isonicotinic acid hydrazide, INH, see code for specific method)

(Isopropyl alcohol, use 84600)

83582   Ketogenic steroids, fractionation

(Ketone bodies, for serum, see 82009, 82010; for urine, see 81000-81003)

83586   Ketosteroids, 17- (17-KS); total

83593   fractionation

83605   Lactate (lactic acid)

83615   Lactate dehydrogenase (LD), (LDH);

83625   isoenzymes, separation and quantitation

83632   Lactogen, human placental (HPL) human chorionic somatomammotropin

83633   Lactose, urine; qualitative

83634   quantitative

(For tolerance, see 82951, 82952)

(For breath hydrogen test for lactase deficiency, use 91065)

● New Code   ▲ Revised Code   ✚ Add-On Code   ⊘ Modifier -51 Exempt

83655   Lead

83661   Fetal lung maturity assessment; lecithin-sphingomyelin ratio (L/S ratio)

83662   foam stability test

83663   fluorescence polarization

83664   lamellar body density

(For phosphatidylglycerol, use 84081)

83670   Leucine aminopeptidase (LAP)

83690   Lipase

83715   Lipoprotein, blood; electrophoretic separation and quantitation

▲ **83716**   high resolution fractionation and quantitation of lipoproteins including lipoprotein subclasses when performed (eg, electrophoresis, nuclear magnetic resonance, ultracentrifugation)

83718   Lipoprotein, direct measurement; high density cholesterol (HDL cholesterol)

83719   direct measurement, VLDL cholesterol

83721   direct measurement, LDL cholesterol

(For fractionation by nuclear magnetic resonance or high resolution electrophoresis, use 83716)

(To report direct measurement, intermediate density lipoproteins (remnant lipoproteins), use Category III code 0026T)

(Luteinizing hormone (LH), use 83002)

83727   Luteinizing releasing factor (LRH)

(For qualitative analysis, see 80100-80103)

(Macroglobulins, alpha-2, use 86329)

83735   Magnesium

83775   Malate dehydrogenase

727

 Separate Procedure

 Unlisted Procedure

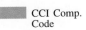 CCI Comp. Code

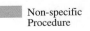 Non-specific Procedure

(Maltose tolerance, see 82951, 82952)

(Mammotropin, use 84146)

83785 Manganese

(Marijuana, see 80100-80103)

83788 Mass spectrometry and tandem mass spectrometry (MS, MS/MS), analyte not elsewhere specified; qualitative, each specimen

83789 quantitative, each specimen

83805 Meprobamate

(For qualitative analysis, see 80100-80103)

83825 Mercury, quantitative

(Mercury screen, use 83015)

83835 Metanephrines

(For catecholamines, see 82382-82384)

83840 Methadone

(For methadone qualitative analysis, see 80100-80103)

(Methamphetamine, see 80100-80103, 82145)

(Methanol, use 84600)

83857 Methemalbumin

(Methemoglobin, see hemoglobin 83045, 83050)

83858 Methsuximide

(Methyl alcohol, use 84600)

(Microalbumin, see 82043 for quantitative, see 82044 for semiquantitative)

(Microglobulin, beta-2, use 82232)

83864 Mucopolysaccharides, acid; quantitative

83866 screen

● New Code   ▲ Revised Code   + Add-On Code   ⊘ Modifier -51 Exempt

83872 Mucin, synovial fluid (Ropes test)

83873 Myelin basic protein, cerebrospinal fluid

(For oligoclonal bands, use 83916)

83874 Myoglobin

(Nalorphine, use 83925)

83880 Natriuretic peptide

83883 Nephelometry, each analyte not elsewhere specified

83885 Nickel

83887 Nicotine

(For microbial identification, see 87797, 87798)

83890 Molecular diagnostics; molecular isolation or extraction

83891 isolation or extraction of highly purified nucleic acid

83892 enzymatic digestion

83893 dot/slot blot production

83894 separation by gel electrophoresis (eg, agarose, polyacrylamide)

83896 nucleic acid probe, each

83897 nucleic acid transfer (eg, Southern, Northern)

83898 amplification of patient nucleic acid (eg, PCR, LCR), single primer pair, each primer pair

83901 amplification of patient nucleic acid, multiplex, each multiplex reaction

83902 reverse transcription

83903 mutation scanning, by physical properties (eg, single strand conformational polymorphisms (SSCP), heteroduplex, denaturing gradient gel electrophoresis (DGGE), RNA'ase A), single segment, each

| | Separate Procedure | | Unlisted Procedure | | CCI Comp. Code | | Non-specific Procedure |

729

83904	mutation identification by sequencing, single segment, each segment
83905	mutation identification by allele specific transcription, single segment, each segment
83906	mutation identification by allele specific translation, single segment, each segment
83912	interpretation and report
83915	Nucleotidase 5-
83916	Oligoclonal immune (oligoclonal bands)
83918	Organic acids; total, quantitative, each specimen
83919	qualitative, each specimen
83921	Organic acid, single; quantitative
83925	Opiates, (eg, morphine, meperidine)
83930	Osmolality; blood
83935	urine
83937	Osteocalcin (bone g1a protein)
83945	Oxalate
83950	Oncoprotein, HER-2/neu

(For tissue, see 88342, 88365)

83970 Parathormone (parathyroid hormone)

(Pesticide, quantitative, see code for specific method. For screen for chlorinated hydrocarbons, use 82441)

83986 pH, body fluid, except blood

(For blood pH, see 82800, 82803)

83992 Phencyclidine (PCP)

(For qualitative analysis, see 80100-80103)

● New Code ▲ Revised Code + Add-On Code ○ Modifier -51 Exempt

(Phenobarbital, use 80184)

84022 Phenothiazine

(For qualitative analysis, see 80100, 80101)

84030 Phenylalanine (PKU), blood

(Phenylalanine-tyrosine ratio, see 84030, 84510)

84035 Phenylketones, qualitative

84060 Phosphatase, acid; total

84061 forensic examination

84066 prostatic

84075 Phosphatase, alkaline;

84078 heat stable (total not included)

84080 isoenzymes

84081 Phosphatidylglycerol

(Phosphates inorganic, use 84100)

(Phosphates, organic, see code for specific method. For cholinesterase, see 82480, 82482)

84085 Phosphogluconate, 6-, dehydrogenase, RBC

84087 Phosphohexose isomerase

84100 Phosphorus inorganic (phosphate);

84105 urine

(Pituitary gonadotropins, see 83001-83002)

(PKU, see 84030, 84035)

84106 Porphobilinogen, urine; qualitative

84110 quantitative

84119 Porphyrins, urine; qualitative

 Separate Procedure   Unlisted Procedure   CCI Comp. Code   Non-specific Procedure

731

84120   quantitation and fractionation

84126 Porphyrins, feces; quantitative

84127   qualitative

(Porphyrin precursors, see 82135, 84106, 84110)

(For protoporphyrin, RBC, see 84202, 84203)

84132 Potassium; serum

84133   urine

84134 Prealbumin

(For microalbumin, see 82043, 82044)

84135 Pregnanediol

84138 Pregnanetriol

84140 Pregnenolone

84143 17-hydroxypregnenolone

84144 Progesterone

(Progesterone receptor assay, use 84234)

(For proinsulin, use 84206)

84146 Prolactin

84150 Prostaglandin, each

84152 Prostate specific antigen (PSA); complexed (direct measurement)

84153   total

84154   free

▲ **84155** Protein, total, except by refractometry; serum

● **84156**   urine

● **84157**   other source (eg, synovial fluid, cerebrospinal fluid)

▲ **84160**   Protein, total, by refractometry, any source

(For urine total protein by dipstick method, use 81000-81003)

▲ **84165**   Protein, electrophoretic fractionation and quantitation

84181   Western Blot, with interpretation and report, blood or other body fluid

84182   Western Blot, with interpretation and report, blood or other body fluid, immunological probe for band identification, each

(For Western Blot tissue analysis, use 88371)

84202   Protoporphyrin, RBC; quantitative

84203   screen

84206   Proinsulin

(Pseudocholinesterase, use 82480)

84207   Pyridoxal phosphate (Vitamin B-6)

84210   Pyruvate

84220   Pyruvate kinase

84228   Quinine

84233   Receptor assay; estrogen

84234   progesterone

84235   endocrine, other than estrogen or progesterone (specify hormone)

84238   non-endocrine (eg, acetylcholine) (specify receptor)

84244   Renin

84252   Riboflavin (Vitamin B-2)

(Salicylates, use 80196)

| | Separate Procedure | | Unlisted Procedure | | CCI Comp. Code | | Non-specific Procedure |

(Secretin test, see 99070, 89100 and appropriate analyses)

84255   Selenium

84260   Serotonin

(For urine metabolites (HIAA), use 83497)

84270   Sex hormone binding globulin (SHBG)

84275   Sialic acid

(Sickle hemoglobin, use 85660)

84285   Silica

84295   Sodium; serum

84300   urine

84302   other source

(Somatomammotropin, use 83632)

(Somatotropin, use 83003)

84305   Somatomedin

84307   Somatostatin

84311   Spectrophotometry, analyte not elsewhere specified

84315   Specific gravity (except urine)

(For specific gravity, urine, see 81000-81003)

(Stone analysis, see 82355-82370)

84375   Sugars, chromatographic, TLC or paper chromatography

84376   Sugars (mono, di, and oligosaccharides); single qualitative, each specimen

84377   multiple qualitative, each specimen

84378   single quantitative, each specimen

84379   multiple quantitative, each specimen

734

| ● | New Code | ▲ | Revised Code | + | Add-On Code | ⊘ | Modifier -51 Exempt |

84392   Sulfate, urine

(Sulfhemoglobin, see hemoglobin, 83055, 83060)

(T-3, see 84479-84481)

(T-4, see 84436-84439)

84402   Testosterone; free

84403   total

84425   Thiamine (Vitamin B-1)

84430   Thiocyanate

84432   Thyroglobulin

(Thyroglobulin, antibody, use 86800)

(Thyrotropin releasing hormone (TRH) test, see 80438, 80439)

84436   Thyroxine; total

84437   requiring elution (eg, neonatal)

84439   free

84442   Thyroxine binding globulin (TBG)

84443   Thyroid stimulating hormone (TSH)

84445   Thyroid stimulating immune globulins (TSI)

(Tobramycin, use 80200)

84446   Tocopherol alpha (Vitamin E)

(Tolbutamide tolerance, use 82953)

84449   Transcortin (cortisol binding globulin)

84450   Transferase; aspartate amino (AST) (SGOT)

84460   alanine amino (ALT) (SGPT)

84466   Transferrin

735

■ Separate Procedure   ■ Unlisted Procedure   ■ CCI Comp. Code   ■ Non-specific Procedure

(Iron binding capacity, use 83550)

84478 Triglycerides

84479 Thyroid hormone (T3 or T4) uptake or thyroid hormone binding ratio (THBR)

84480 Triiodothyronine T3; total (TT-3)

84481 free

84482 reverse

84484 Troponin, quantitative

(For Troponin, qualitative assay, use 84512)

84485 Trypsin; duodenal fluid

84488 feces, qualitative

84490 feces, quantitative, 24-hour collection

84510 Tyrosine

(Urate crystal identification, use 89060)

84512 Troponin, qualitative

(For Troponin, quantitative assay, use 84484)

84520 Urea nitrogen; quantitative

84525 semiquantitative (eg, reagent strip test)

84540 Urea nitrogen, urine

84545 Urea nitrogen, clearance

84550 Uric acid; blood

84560 other source

84577 Urobilinogen, feces, quantitative

84578 Urobilinogen, urine; qualitative

● New Code   ▲ Revised Code   ✚ Add-On Code   ⊘ Modifier -51 Exempt

84580   quantitative, timed specimen

84583   semiquantitative

(Uroporphyrins, use 84120)

(Valproic acid (dipropylacetic acid), ues 80164)

84585   Vanillylmandelic acid (VMA), urine

84586   Vasoactive intestinal peptide (VIP)

84588   Vasopressin (antidiuretic hormone, ADH)

84590   Vitamin A

(Vitamin B-1, use 84425)

(Vitamin B-2, use 84252)

(Vitamin B-6, use 84207)

(Vitamin B-12, use 82607)

(Vitamin B-12, absorption (Schilling), see 78270, 78271)

(Vitamin C, use 82180)

(Vitamin D, see 82306, 82307, 82652)

(Vitamin E, use 84446)

84591   Vitamin, not otherwise specified

84597   Vitamin K

(VMA, use 84585)

84600   Volatiles (eg, acetic anhydride, carbon tetrachloride, dichloroethane, dichloromethane, diethylether, isopropyl alcohol, methanol)

(For acetaldehyde, use 82000)

(Volume, blood, RISA or Cr-51, see 78110, 78111)

84620   Xylose absorption test, blood and/or urine

(For administration, use 99070)

84630   Zinc

737

 Separate Procedure    Unlisted Procedure   CCI Comp. Code   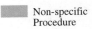 Non-specific Procedure

| 84681 | C-peptide |

84681 C-peptide

84702 Gonadotropin, chorionic (hCG); quantitative

84703   qualitative

(For urine pregnancy test by visual color comparison, use 81025)

84830 Ovulation tests, by visual color comparison methods for human luteinizing hormone

84999 Unlisted chemistry procedure

HEMATOLOGY AND COAGULATION

(For blood banking procedures, see Transfusion Medicine)

(Agglutinins, see Immunology)

(Antiplasmin, use 85410)

(Antithrombin III, see 85300, 85301)

85002 Bleeding time

85004 Blood count; automated differential WBC count

85007   blood smear, microscopic examination with manual differential WBC count

85008   blood smear, microscopic examination without manual differential WBC count

(For other fluids (eg, CSF), see 89050, 89051)

85009   manual differential WBC count, buffy coat

(Eosinophils, nasal smear, use 89190)

85013   spun microhematocrit

85014   hematocrit (Hct)

85018   hemoglobin (Hgb)

(For other hemoglobin determination, see 83020-83069)

● New Code   ▲ Revised Code   + Add-On Code   ⊘ Modifier -51 Exempt

PATHOLOGY/ LABORATORY

(For immunoassay, hemoglobin, fecal, use 86683)

(85021   deleted 2003 edition)

(85022   deleted 2003 edition)

(85023   deleted 2003 edition. To report, use 85007 and 85027)

(85024   deleted 2003 edition. To report, use 85025)

85025   complete (CBC), automated (Hgb, Hct, RBC, WBC and platelet count) and automated differential WBC count

85027   complete (CBC), automated (Hgb, Hct, RBC, WBC and platelet count)

(85031   deleted 2003 edition. To report, use 85014, 85018 and 85032)

85032   manual cell count (erythrocyte, leukocyte, or platelet) each

85041   red blood cell (RBC), automated

(Do not report code 85041 in conjunction with 85025 or 85027)

85044   reticulocyte, manual

85045   reticulocyte, automated

85046   reticulocytes, hemoglobin concentration

85048   leukocyte (WBC), automated

85049   platelet, automated

● **85055**   Reticulated platelet assay

85060   Blood smear, peripheral, interpretation by physician with written report

(85095   deleted 2002 edition. To report, use 38220)

85097   Bone marrow, smear interpretation

(For special stains, see 85540, 88312, 88313)

(85102   deleted 2002 edition. To report, use 38221)

739

Separate Procedure | Unlisted Procedure | CCI Comp. Code | Non-specific Procedure

(For bone biopsy, see 20220, 20225, 20240, 20245, 20250, 20251)

85130 Chromogenic substrate assay

(Circulating anti-coagulant screen (mixing studies), see 85611, 85732)

85170 Clot retraction

85175 Clot lysis time, whole blood dilution

(Clotting factor I (fibrinogen), see 85384, 85385)

85210 Clotting; factor II, prothrombin, specific

(See also 85610-85613)

85220 factor V (AcG or proaccelerin), labile factor

85230 factor VII (proconvertin, stable factor)

85240 factor VIII (AHG), one stage

85244 factor VIII related antigen

85245 factor VIII, VW factor, ristocetin cofactor

85246 factor VIII, VW factor antigen

85247 factor VIII, von Willebrands factor, multimetric analysis

85250 factor IX (PTC or Christmas)

85260 factor X (Stuart-Prower)

85270 factor XI (PTA)

85280 factor XII (Hageman)

85290 factor XIII (fibrin stabilizing)

85291 factor XIII (fibrin stabilizing), screen solubility

85292 prekallikrein assay (Fletcher factor assay)

740

| ● | New Code | ▲ | Revised Code | + | Add-On Code | ⊘ | Modifier -51 Exempt |

85293   high molecular weight kininogen assay (Fitzgerald factor assay)

85300   Clotting inhibitors or anticoagulants; antithrombin III, activity

85301   antithrombin III, antigen assay

85302   protein C, antigen

85303   protein C, activity

85305   protein S, total

85306   protein S, free

85307   Activated Protein C (APC) resistance assay

85335   Factor inhibitor test

85337   Thrombomodulin

(For mixing studies for inhibitors, use 85732)

85345   Coagulation time; Lee and White

85347   activated

85348   other methods

(Differential count, see 85007 et seq)

(Duke bleeding time, use 85002)

(Eosinophils, nasal smear, use 89190)

85360   Euglobulin lysis

(Fetal hemoglobin, see 83030, 83033, 85460)

85362   Fibrin(ogen) degradation (split) products (FDP)(FSP); agglutination slide, semiquantitative

(Immunoelectrophoresis, use 86320)

85366   paracoagulation

85370   quantitative

741

 Separate Procedure   Unlisted Procedure   CCI Comp. Code   Non-specific Procedure

85378 Fibrin degradation products, D-dimer; qualitative or semiquantitative

85379 quantitative

(For ultrasensitive and standard sensitivity quantitative D-dimer, use 85379)

85380 ultrasensitive (eg., for evaluation for venous thromboembolism), qualitative or semiquantitative

85384 Fibrinogen; activity

85385 antigen

85390 Fibrinolysins or coagulopathy screen, interpretation and report

● **85396** Coagulation/fibrinolysis assay, whole blood (eg, viscoelastic clot assessment), including use of any pharmacologic additive(s), as indicated, including interpretation and written report, per day

85400 Fibrinolytic factors and inhibitors; plasmin

85410 alpha-2 antiplasmin

85415 plasminogen activator

85420 plasminogen, except antigenic assay

85421 plasminogen, antigenic assay

(Fragility, red blood cell, see 85547, 85555-85557)

85441 Heinz bodies; direct

85445 induced, acetyl phenylhydrazine

(Hematocrit (PCV), see 85014)

(Hemoglobin, see 83020-83068, 85018-85027)

85460 Hemoglobin or RBCs, fetal, for fetomaternal hemorrhage; differential lysis (Kleihauer-Betke)

(See also 83030, 83033)

(Hemolysins, see 86940, 86941)

● New Code ▲ Revised Code + Add-On Code ⊘ Modifier -51 Exempt

85461   rosette

85475 Hemolysin, acid

(See also 86940, 86941)

85520 Heparin assay

85525 Heparin neutralization

85530 Heparin-protamine tolerance test

   85536 Iron stain, peripheral blood

(For iron stains on bone marrow or other tissues with physician evaluation, use 88313)

85540 Leukocyte alkaline phosphatase with count

85547 Mechanical fragility, RBC

85549 Muramidase

(Nitroblue tetrazolium dye test, use 86384)

85555 Osmotic fragility, RBC; unincubated

85557   incubated

(Packed cell volume, use 85013)

(Partial thromboplastin time, see 85730, 85732)

(Parasites, blood (eg, malaria smears), use 87207)

(Plasmin, use 85400)

(Plasminogen, use 85420)

(Plasminogen activator, use 85415)

85576 Platelet; aggregation (in vitro), each agent

(85585   deleted 2003 edition. To report, use 85008)

(85590   deleted 2003 edition. To report, use 85032)

(85595   deleted 2003 edition. To report, use 85049)

743

 Separate Procedure    Unlisted Procedure    CCI Comp. Code   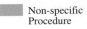 Non-specific Procedure

85597   Platelet neutralization

85610   Prothrombin time;

85611   substitution, plasma fractions, each

85612   Russell viper venom time (includes venom); undiluted

85613   diluted

(Red blood cell count, see 85025, 85027, 85041)

85635   Reptilase test

(Reticulocyte count, see 85044, 85045)

85651   Sedimentation rate, erythrocyte; non-automated

85652   automated

85660   Sickling of RBC, reduction

(Hemoglobin electrophoresis, use 83020)

(Smears (eg, for parasites, malaria), use 87207)

85670   Thrombin time; plasma

85675   titer

85705   Thromboplastin inhibition; tissue

(For individual clotting factors, see 85245-85247)

85730   Thromboplastin time, partial (PTT); plasma or whole blood

85732   substitution, plasma fractions, each

85810   Viscosity

(von Willebrand factor assay, see 85245-85247)

(WBC count, see 85025-85031, 85048, 89050)

85999   Unlisted hematology and coagulation procedure

---

744   ● New   ▲ Revised   + Add-On   ⊘ Modifier -51
            Code   Code   Code   Exempt

IMMUNOLOGY

(Acetylcholine receptor antibody, see 86255, 86256)

(Actinomyces, antibodies to, use 86602)

(Adrenal cortex antibodies, see 86255, 86256)

(For tuberculosis test, cell mediated immunity measurement of gamma interferon antigen response, use Category III code 0010T)

86000 Agglutinins, febrile (eg, Brucella, Francisella, Murine typhus, Q fever, Rocky Mountain spotted fever, scrub typhus), each antigen

(For antibodies to infectious agents, see 86602-86804)

86001 Allergen specific IgG quantitative or semiquantitative, each allergen

(Agglutinins and autohemolysins, see 86940, 86941)

86003 Allergen specific IgE; quantitative or semiquantitative, each allergen

(For total quantitative IgE, use 82785)

86005 qualitative, multiallergen screen (dipstick, paddle or disk)

(For total qualitative IgE, use 83518)

(Alpha-1 antitrypsin, see 82103, 82104)

(Alpha-1 feto-protein, see 82105, 82106)

(Anti-AChR (acetylcholine receptor) antibody titer, see 86255, 86256)

(Anticardiolipin antibody, use 86147)

(Anti-DNA, use 86225)

(Anti-deoxyribonuclease titer, use 86215)

86021 Antibody identification; leukocyte antibodies

86022 platelet antibodies

86023 platelet associated immunoglobulin assay

745

 Separate Procedure

 Unlisted Procedure

 CCI Comp. Code

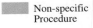 Non-specific Procedure

86038   Antinuclear antibodies (ANA);

86039   titer

(Antistreptococcal antibody, ie, anti-DNAse, use 86215)

(Antistreptokinase titer, use 86590)

86060   Antistreptolysin 0; titer

(For antibodies to infectious agents, see 86602-86804)

86063   screen

(For antibodies to infectious agents, see 86602-86804)

(Blastomyces, antibodies to, use 86612)

86077   Blood bank physician services; difficult cross match and/or evaluation of irregular antibody(s), interpretation and written report

86078   investigation of transfusion reaction including suspicion of transmissible disease, interpretation and written report

86079   authorization for deviation from standard blood banking procedures (eg, use of outdated blood, transfusion of Rh incompatible units), with written report

(Brucella, antibodies to, use 86622)

(Candida, antibodies to, use 86628. For skin testing, use 86485)

86140   C-reactive protein;

(Candidiasis, use 86628)

86141   high sensitivity (hsCRP)

86146   Beta 2 Glycoprotein 1 antibody, each

86147   Cardiolipin (phospholipid) antibody, each lg class

86148   Anti-phosphatidylserine (phospholipid) antibody

(To report antiprothrombin (phospholipid cofactor) antibody, use Category III code 0030T)

86155   Chemotaxis assay, specify method

● New Code   ▲ Revised Code   + Add-On Code   ⊘ Modifier -51 Exempt

(Clostridium difficile toxin, use 87230)

(Coccidioides, antibodies, to, see 86635. For skin testing, use 86490)

86156 Cold agglutinin; screen

86157 titer

86160 Complement; antigen, each component

86161 functional activity, each component

86162 total hemolytic (CH50)

86171 Complement fixation tests, each antigen

(Coombs test, see 86880-86886)

86185 Counterimmunoelectrophoresis, each antigen

(Cryptococcus, antibodies to, use 86641)

86215 Deoxyribonuclease, antibody

86225 Deoxyribonucleic acid (DNA) antibody; native or double stranded

(Echinococcus, antibodies to, see code for specific method)

(For HIV antibody tests, see 86701-86703)

86226 single stranded

(Anti D.S., DNA, IFA, eg, using C.Lucilae, see 86255 and 86256)

86235 Extractable nuclear antigen, antibody to, any method (eg, nRNP, SS-A, SS-B, Sm, RNP, Sc170, J01), each antibody

86243 Fc receptor

(Filaria, antibodies to, see code for specific method)

86255 Fluorescent noninfectious agent antibody; screen, each antibody

86256 titer, each antibody

747

 Separate Procedure   Unlisted Procedure   CCI Comp. Code   Non-specific Procedure

(Fluorescent technique for antigen identification in tissue, use 88346; for indirect fluorescence, use 88347)

(FTA, see 86781)

(Gel (agar) diffusion tests, use 86331)

86277   Growth hormone, human (HGH), antibody

86280   Hemagglutination inhibition test (HAI)

(For rubella, use 86762)

(For antibodies to infectious agents, see 86602-86804)

86294   Immunoassay for tumor antigen, qualitative or semiquantitative (eg, bladder tumor antigen)

86300   Immunoassay for tumor antigen, quantitative; CA 15-3 (27.29)

86301   CA 19-9

86304   CA 125

(For measurement of serum HER-2/neu oncoprotein, see 83950)

(For hepatitis delta agent, antibody, use 86692)

86308   Heterophile antibodies; screening

(For antibodies to infectious agents, see 86602-86804)

86309   titer

(For antibodies to infectious agents, see 86602-86804)

86310   titers after absorption with beef cells and guinea pig kidney

(Histoplasma, antibodies to, use 86698. For skin testing, use 86510)

(For antibodies to infectious agents, see 86602-86804)

(Human growth hormone antibody, use 86277)

86316   Immunoassay for tumor antigen ; other antigen, quantitative (eg, CA 50, 72-4, 549), each

86317   Immunoassay for infectious agent antibody, quantitative, not otherwise specified

748   ● New Code   ▲ Revised Code   ＋ Add-On Code   ⊘ Modifier -51 Exempt

(For immunoassay techniques for antigens, see 83516, 83518, 83519, 83520, 87301-87450, 87810-87899)

(For particle agglutination procedures, use 86403)

86318   Immunoassay for infectious agent antibody, qualitative or semiquantitative, single step method (eg, reagent strip)

86320   Immunoelectrophoresis; serum

86325   other fluids (eg, urine, cerebrospinal fluid) with concentration

86327   crossed (2-dimensional assay)

86329   Immunodiffusion; not elsewhere specified

86331   gel diffusion, qualitative (Ouchterlony), each antigen or antibody

86332   Immune complex assay

86334   Immunofixation electrophoresis

86336   Inhibin A

86337   Insulin antibodies

86340   Intrinsic factor antibodies

(Leptospira, antibodies to, use 86720)

(Leukoagglutinins, use 86021)

86341   Islet cell antibody

86343   Leukocyte histamine release test (LHR)

86344   Leukocyte phagocytosis

86353   Lymphocyte transformation, mitogen (phytomitogen) or antigen induced blastogenesis

(Lymphocytes immunophenotyping, use 88180 for cytometry; see 88342, 88346 for microscopic techniques)

(Malaria antibodies, use 86750)

749

 Separate Procedure   Unlisted Procedure   CCI Comp. Code   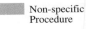 Non-specific Procedure

86359   T cells; total count

86360   absolute CD4 and CD8 count, including ratio

86361   absolute CD4 count

86376   Microsomal antibodies (eg, thyroid or liver-kidney), each

86378   Migration inhibitory factor test (MIF)

           (Mitochondrial antibody, liver, see 86255, 86256)

           (Mononucleosis, see 86308-86310)

86382   Neutralization test, viral

86384   Nitroblue tetrazolium dye test (NTD)

           (Ouchterlony diffusion, use 86331)

           (Platelet antibodies, see 86022, 86023)

86403   Particle agglutination; screen, each antibody

86406   titer, each antibody

           (Pregnancy test, see 84702, 84703)

           (Rapid plasma reagin test (RPR), see 86592, 86593)

86430   Rheumatoid factor; qualitative

86431   quantitative

           (Serologic test for syphilis, see 86592, 86593)

86485   Skin test; candida

           (For antibody, candida, use 86628)

86490   coccidioidomycosis

86510   histoplasmosis

           (For histoplasma, antibody, use 86698)

86580   tuberculosis, intradermal

86585   tuberculosis, tine test

● New Code   ▲ Revised Code   + Add-On Code   ⊘ Modifier -51 Exempt

(For tuberculosis test, cell mediated immunity measurement of gamma interferon antigen response, use Category III code 0010T)

(For skin tests for allergy, see 95010-95199)

(Smooth muscle antibody, see 86255, 86256)

(Sporothrix, antibodies to, see code for specific method)

86586   unlisted antigen, each

86590 Streptokinase, antibody

(For antibodies to infectious agents, see 86602-86804)

(Streptolysin O antibody, see antistreptolysin O, 86060, 86063)

86592 Syphilis test; qualitative (eg, VDRL, RPR, ART)

(For antibodies to infectious agents, see 86602-86804)

86593   quantitative

(For antibodies to infectious agents, see 86602-86804)

(Tetanus antibody, use 86774)

(Thyroglobulin antibody, use 86800)

(Thyroglobulin, use 84432)

(Thyroid microsomal antibody, use 86376)

(For toxoplasma antibody, see 86777-86778)

(For the detection of antibodies other than those to infectious agents, see specific antibody (eg, 86021, 86022, 86023, 86376, 86800, 86850-86870) or specific method (eg, 83516, 86255, 86256))

(For infectious agent/antigen detection, see 87260-87899)

86602 Antibody; actinomyces

86603   adenovirus

86606   Aspergillus

86609   bacterium, not elsewhere specified

86611   Bartonella

86612   Blastomyces

86615   Bordetella

86617   Borrelia burgdorferi (Lyme disease) confirmatory test (eg, Western blot or immunoblot)

86618   Borrelia burgdorferi (Lyme disease)

86619   Borrelia (relapsing fever)

86622   Brucella

86625   Campylobacter

86628   Candida

(For skin test, candida, use 86485)

86631   Chlamydia

86632   Chlamydia, IgM

(For chlamydia antigen, see 87270, 87320. For fluorescent antibody technique, see 86255, 86256)

86635   Coccidioides

86638   Coxiella Brunetii (Q fever)

86641   Cryptococcus

86644   cytomegalovirus (CMV)

86645   cytomegalovirus (CMV), IgM

86648   Diphtheria

86651   encephalitis, California (La Crosse)

86652   encephalitis, Eastern equine

86653   encephalitis, St. Louis

● New Code   ▲ Revised Code   ✛ Add-On Code   ⊘ Modifier -51 Exempt

86654   encephalitis, Western equine

86658   enterovirus (eg, coxsackie, echo, polio)

(Trichinella, antibodies to, use 86784)

(Trypanosoma, antibodies to, see code for specific method)

(Tuberculosis, use 86580 for skin testing)

(Viral antibodies, see code for specific method)

86663   Epstein-Barr (EB) virus, early antigen (EA)

86664   Epstein-Barr (EB) virus, nuclear antigen (EBNA)

86665   Epstein-Barr (EB) virus, viral capsid (VCA)

86666   Ehrlichia

86668   Francisella Tularensis

86671   fungus, not elsewhere specified

86674   Giardia Lamblia

86677   Helicobacter Pylori

86682   helminth, not elsewhere specified

(86683   has been deleted. To report, use 82274)

86684   Hemophilus influenza

86687   HTLV-I

86688   HTLV-II

86689   HTLV or HIV antibody, confirmatory test (eg, Western Blot)

86692   hepatitis, delta agent

(For hepatitis delta agent, antigen, use 87380)

86694   herpes simplex, non-specific type test

 Separate Procedure   Unlisted Procedure   CCI Comp. Code   Non-specific Procedure

86695   herpes simplex, type 1

86696   herpes simplex, type 2

86698   histoplasma

86701   HIV-1

86702   HIV-2

86703   HIV-1 and HIV-2, single assay

(For HIV-1 antigen, use 87390)

(For HIV-2 antigen, use 87391)

(For confirmatory test for HIV antibody (eg, Western Blot), use 86689)

86704 Hepatitis B core antibody (HBcAb); total

86705   IgM antibody

86706 Hepatitis B surface antibody (HBsAb)

86707 Hepatitis Be antibody (HBeAb)

86708 Hepatitis A antibody (HAAb); total

86709   IgM antibody

86710 Antibody; influenza virus

86713   Legionella

86717   Leishmania

86720   Leptospira

86723   Listeria monocytogenes

86727   lymphocytic choriomeningitis

86729   Lymphogranuloma Venereum

86732   mucormycosis

● New Code   ▲ Revised Code   **+** Add-On Code   ⊘ Modifier -51 Exempt

86735	mumps
86738	Mycoplasma
86741	Neisseria meningitidis
86744	Nocardia
86747	parvovirus
86750	Plasmodium (malaria)
86753	protozoa, not elsewhere specified
86756	respiratory syncytial virus
86757	Rickettsia
86759	rotavirus
86762	rubella
86765	rubeola
86768	Salmonella
86771	Shigella
86774	tetanus
86777	Toxoplasma
86778	Toxoplasma, IgM
86781	Treponema Pallidum, confirmatory test (eg, FTA-abs)
86784	trichinella
86787	varicella-zoster
86790	virus, not elsewhere specified
86793	Yersinia
86800	Thyroglobulin antibody

755

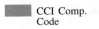 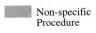

Separate Procedure   Unlisted Procedure   CCI Comp. Code   Non-specific Procedure

(For thyroglobulin, use 84432)

86803   Hepatitis C antibody;

86804   confirmatory test (eg, immunoblot)

TISSUE TYPING

(For pretransplant cross-match, see appropriate code or codes)

86805   Lymphocytotoxicity assay, visual crossmatch; with titration

86806   without titration

86807   Serum screening for cytotoxic percent reactive antibody (PRA); standard method

86808   quick method

86812   HLA typing; A, B, or C (eg, A10, B7, B27), single antigen

86813   A, B, or C, multiple antigens

86816   DR/DQ, single antigen

86817   DR/DQ, multiple antigens

86821   lymphocyte culture, mixed (MLC)

86822   lymphocyte culture, primed (PLC)

86849   Unlisted immunology procedure

TRANSFUSION MEDICINE

(For apheresis, see 36511-36512)

(For therapeutic phlebotomy, use 99195)

86850   Antibody screen, RBC, each serum technique

86860   Antibody elution (RBC), each elution

86870   Antibody identification, RBC antibodies, each panel for each serum technique

---

● New Code   ▲ Revised Code   + Add-On Code   ⊘ Modifier -51 Exempt

86880   Antihuman globulin test (Coombs test); direct, each antiserum

86885   indirect, qualitative, each antiserum

86886   indirect, titer, each antiserum

86890   Autologous blood or component, collection processing and storage; predeposited

86891   intra-or postoperative salvage

(For physician services to autologous donors, see 99201-99204)

86900   Blood typing; ABO

86901   Rh (D)

86903   antigen screening for compatible blood unit using reagent serum, per unit screened

86904   antigen screening for compatible unit using patient serum, per unit screened

86905   RBC antigens, other than ABO or Rh (D), each

86906   Rh phenotyping, complete

86910   Blood typing, for paternity testing, per individual; ABO, Rh and MN

86911   each additional antigen system

(**86915**   deleted 2003 edition. To report, use 38210-38213)

86920   Compatibility test each unit; immediate spin technique

86921   incubation technique

86922   antiglobulin technique

86927   Fresh frozen plasma, thawing, each unit

86930   Frozen blood, each unit; freezing (includes preparation)

86931   thawing

757

 Separate Procedure

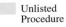 Unlisted Procedure

 CCI Comp. Code

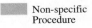 Non-specific Procedure

86932   freezing (includes preparation) and thawing

86940   Hemolysins and agglutinins; auto, screen, each

86941   incubated

86945   Irradiation of blood product, each unit

86950   Leukocyte transfusion

       (For leukapheresis, see 36511-36512)

86965   Pooling of platelets or other blood products

86970   Pretreatment of RBCs for use in RBC antibody detection, identification, and/or compatibility testing; incubation with chemical agents or drugs, each

86971   incubation with enzymes, each

86972   by density gradient separation

86975   Pretreatment of serum for use in RBC antibody identification; incubation with drugs, each

86976   by dilution

86977   incubation with inhibitors, each

86978   by differential red cell absorption using patient RBCs or RBCs of known phenotype, each absorption

86985   Splitting of blood or blood products, each unit

86999   Unlisted transfusion medicine procedure

MICROBIOLOGY

87001   Animal inoculation, small animal; with observation

87003   with observation and dissection

87015   Concentration (any type), for infectious agents

       (Do not report 87015 in conjunction with 87177)

---

758   ● New Code   ▲ Revised Code   ✛ Add-On Code   ⊘ Modifier -51 Exempt

▲ **87040**   Culture, bacterial; blood, aerobic, with isolation and presumptive identification of isolates (includes anaerobic culture, if appropriate)

▲ **87045**   stool, aerobic, with isolation and preliminary examination (eg, KIA, LIA), Salmonella and Shigella species

▲ **87046**   stool, aerobic, additional pathogens, isolation and presumptive identification of isolates

▲ **87070**   any other source except urine, blood or stool, aerobic, with isolation and presumptive identification of isolates

(For urine, use 87088)

87071   quantitative, aerobic with isolation and presumptive identification of isolates, any source except urine, blood or stool

(For urine, use 87088)

87073   quantitative, anaerobic with isolation and presumptive identification of isolates, any source except urine, blood or stool

(For definitive identification of isolates, use 87076 or 87077. for typing of isolates see 87140-87158)

▲ **87075**   any source, except blood, anaerobic with isolation and presumptive identification of isolates

87076   anaerobic isolate, additional methods required for definitive identification, each isolate

(For gas liquid chromatography (GLC) or high pressure liquid chromatography (HPLC), use 87143)

87077   aerobic isolate, additional methods required for definitive identification, each isolate

(For gas liquid chromatography (GLC) or high pressure liquid chromatography (HPLC), use 87143)

87081   Culture, presumptive, pathogenic organisms, screening only;

87084   with colony estimation from density chart

87086   Culture, bacterial; quantitative colony count, urine

759

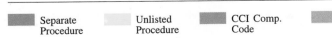

| | Separate Procedure | | Unlisted Procedure | | CCI Comp. Code | | Non-specific Procedure |

87088   with isolation and presumptive identification of isolates, urine

87101   Culture, fungi (mold or yeast) isolation, with presumptive identification of isolates; skin, hair, or nail

87102   other source (except blood)

87103   blood

87106   Culture, fungi, definitive identification, each organism; yeast

(Use 87106 in addition to codes 87101, 87102 or 87103 when appropriate)

87107   mold

87109   Culture, mycoplasma, any source

87110   Culture, chlamydia, any source

(For immunofluorescence staining of shell vials, use 87140)

87116   Culture, tubercle or other acid-fast bacilli (eg, TB, AFB, mycobacteria) any source, with isolation and presumptive identification of isolates

87118   Culture, mycobacteria, definitive identification, each isolate

(For nucleic acid probe identification, use 87149)

(For GLC or HPLC identification, use 87143)

87140   Culture, typing; immunofluorescent method, each antiserum

87143   gas liquid chromatography (GLC) or high pressure liquid chromotography (HPLC) method

87147   immunologic method, other than immunofluorescence (eg, agglutination grouping), per antiserum

87149   identification by nucleic acid probe

87152   identification by pulse field gel typing

87158   other methods

● New Code   ▲ Revised Code   + Add-On Code   ○ Modifier -51 Exempt

87164 Dark field examination, any source (eg, penile, vaginal, oral, skin); includes specimen collection

87166 without collection

87168 Macroscopic examination; arthropod

87169 parasite

87172 Pinworm exam (eg, cellophane tape prep)

87176 Homogenization, tissue, for culture

87177 Ova and parasites, direct smears, concentration and identification

(Do not report 87177 in conjunction with 87015)

(For direct smears from a primary source, use 87207)

(For coccidia or microsporidia exam, use 87207)

(For trichrome, iron hemotoxylin and other special stains, use 88313)

(For nucleic acid probes in cytologic material, use 88365)

(For molecular diagnostics, see 83890-83898, 87470-87799)

87181 Susceptibility studies, antimicrobial agent; agar diffusion method, per agent (eg, antibiotic gradient strip)

87184 disk method, per plate (12 or fewer disks)

87185 enzyme detection (eg, beta lactamase), per enzyme

87186 microdilution or agar dilution (minimum inhibitory concentration (MIC) or breakpoint), each multi-antimicrobial, per plate

+ 87187 microdilution or agar dilution, minimum lethal concentration (MLC), each plate ((List separately in addition to code for primary procedure)

(Use 87187 in conjunction with 87186 or 87188)

87188 macrobroth dilution method, each agent

87190 mycobacteria, proportion method, each agent

(For other mycobacterial susceptibility studies, see 87181, 87184, 87186, or 87188)

87197   Serum bactericidal titer (Schlicter test)

87205   Smear, primary source with interpretation; Gram or Giemsa stain for bacteria, fungi, or cell types

87206   fluorescent and/or acid fast stain for bacteria, fungi, or cell types

87207   special stain for inclusion bodies or parasites (eg, malaria, coccidia, microsporidia, trypanosomes, herpes viruses)

(For direct smears with concentration and identification, use 87177)

(For thick smear preparation, use 87015)

(For complex special stains, see 88312, 88313)

(For fat, meat, fibers, nasal eosinophils, and starch, see miscellaneous section)

87210   wet mount for infectious agents (eg, saline, India ink, KOH preps)

(For KOH examination of skin, hair or nails, see 87220)

87220   Tissue examination by KOH slide of samples from skin, hair, or nails for fungi or ectoparasite ova or mites (eg, scabies)

87230   Toxin or antitoxin assay, tissue culture (eg, Clostridium difficile toxin)

87250   Virus isolation; inoculation of embryonated eggs, or small animal, includes observation and dissection

87252   tissue culture inoculation, observation, and presumptive identification by cytopathic effect

87253   tissue culture, additional studies or definitive identification (eg, hemabsorption, neutralization, immunofluorescence stain) each isolate

(Electron microscopy, use 88348)

(Inclusion bodies in tissue sections, see 88304-88309; in smears, see 87207-87210; in fluids, use 88106)

● New Code   ▲ Revised Code   + Add-On Code   ⊘ Modifier -51 Exempt

87254	centrifuge enhanced (shell vial) technique, includes identification with immunofluorescence stain, each virus

(Report 87254 in addition to 87252 as appropriate)

87255	including identification by non-immunologic method, other than by cytopathic effect (eg., virus specific enzymatic activity)
87260	Infectious agent antigen detection by immunofluorescent technique; adenovirus
87265	Bordetella pertussis/parapertussis
87267	Enterovirus, direct fluorescent antibody (DFA)
● **87269**	giardia
87270	Chlamydia trachomatis
87271	Cytomegalovirus, direct fluorescent antibody (DFA)
▲ **87272**	cryptosporidium
87273	Herpes simplex virus type 2
87274	Herpes simplex virus 1
87275	Influenza B virus
87276	influenza A virus
87277	Legionella micdadei
87278	Legionella pneumophila
87279	Parainfluenza virus, each type
87280	respiratory syncytial virus
87281	Pneumocystis carinii
87283	Rubeola
87285	Treponema pallidum

763

Separate Procedure	Unlisted Procedure	CCI Comp. Code	Non-specific Procedure

87290   Varicella zoster virus

87299   not otherwise specified, each organism

87300   Infectious agent antigen detection by immunofluorescent technique, polyvalent for multiple organisms, each polyvalent antiserum

(For physican evaluation of infectious disease agents by immunofluorescence, use 88346)

87301   Infectious agent antigen detection by enzyme immunoassay technique, qualitative or semiquantitative, multiple step method; adenovirus enteric types 40/41

87320   Chlamydia trachomatis

87324   Clostridium difficile toxin(s)

87327   Cryptococcus neoformans

(For Cryptococcus latex agglutination, use 86403)

▲ **87328**   cryptosporidium

● **87329**   giardia

87332   cytomegalovirus

87335   Escherichia coli 0157

(For giardia antigen, use 87329)

87336   Entamoeba histolytica dispar group

87337   Entamoeba histolytica group

87338   Helicobacter pylori, stool

87339   Helicobacter pylori

(For H. pylori, stool, use 87338. For H. pylori, breath and blood by mass spectrometry, see 83013, 83014. For H. pylori, liquid scintillation counter, see 78267, 78268)

87340   hepatitis B surface antigen (HBsAg)

● New Code   ▲ Revised Code   **+** Add-On Code   ⊘ Modifier -51 Exempt

87341	hepatitis B surface antigen (HBsAg) neutralization
87350	hepatitis Be antigen (HBeAg)
87380	hepatitis, delta agent
87385	Histoplasma capsulatum
87390	HIV-1
87391	HIV-2
87400	Influenza, A or B, each
87420	respiratory syncytial virus
87425	rotavirus
87427	Shiga-like toxin
87430	Streptococcus, group A
87449	Infectious agent antigen detection by enzyme immunoassay technique qualitative or semiquantitative; multiple step method, not otherwise specified, each organism
87450	single step method, not otherwise specified, each organism
87451	multiple step method, polyvalent for multiple organisms, each polyvalent antiserum
87470	Infectious agent detection by nucleic acid (DNA or RNA); Bartonella henselae and Bartonella quintana, direct probe technique
87471	Bartonella henselae and Bartonella quintana, amplified probe technique
87472	Bartonella henselae and Bartonella quintana, quantification
87475	Borrelia burgdorferi, direct probe technique
87476	Borrelia burgdorferi, amplified probe technique
87477	Borrelia burgdorferi, quantification

765

Separate Procedure	Unlisted Procedure	CCI Comp. Code	Non-specific Procedure

87480	Candida species, direct probe technique
87481	Candida species, amplified probe technique
87482	Candida species, quantification
87485	Chlamydia pneumoniae, direct probe technique
87486	Chlamydia pneumoniae, amplified probe technique
87487	Chlamydia pneumoniae, quantification
87490	Chlamydia trachomatis, direct probe technique
87491	Chlamydia trachomatis, amplified probe technique
87492	Chlamydia trachomatis, quantification
87495	cytomegalovirus, direct probe technique
87496	cytomegalovirus, amplified probe technique
87497	cytomegalovirus, quantification
87510	Gardnerella vaginalis, direct probe technique
87511	Gardnerella vaginalis, amplified probe technique
87512	Gardnerella vaginalis, quantification
87515	hepatitis B virus, direct probe technique
87516	hepatitis B virus, amplified probe technique
87517	hepatitis B virus, quantification
87520	hepatitis C, direct probe technique
87521	hepatitis C, amplified probe technique
87522	hepatitis C, quantification
87525	hepatitis G, direct probe technique
87526	hepatitis G, amplified probe technique

● New Code   ▲ Revised Code   + Add-On Code   ⊘ Modifier -51 Exempt

87527	hepatitis G, quantification
87528	Herpes simplex virus, direct probe technique
87529	Herpes simplex virus, amplified probe technique
87530	Herpes simplex virus, quantification
87531	Herpes virus-6, direct probe technique
87532	Herpes virus-6, amplified probe technique
87533	Herpes virus-6, quantification
87534	HIV-1, direct probe technique
87535	HIV-1, amplified probe technique
87536	HIV-1, quantification
87537	HIV-2, direct probe technique
87538	HIV-2, amplified probe technique
87539	HIV-2, quantification
87540	Legionella pneumophila, direct probe technique
87541	Legionella pneumophila, amplified probe technique
87542	Legionella pneumophila, quantification
87550	Mycobacteria species, direct probe technique
87551	Mycobacteria species, amplified probe technique
87552	Mycobacteria species, quantification
87555	Mycobacteria tuberculosis, direct probe technique
87556	Mycobacteria tuberculosis, amplified probe technique
87557	Mycobacteria tuberculosis, quantification
87560	Mycobacteria avium-intracellulare, direct probe technique

87561	Mycobacteria avium-intracellulare, amplified probe technique
87562	Mycobacteria avium-intracellulare, quantification
87580	Mycoplasma pneumoniae, direct probe technique
87581	Mycoplasma pneumoniae, amplified probe technique
87582	Mycoplasma pneumoniae, quantification
87590	Neisseria gonorrhoeae, direct probe technique
87591	Neisseria gonorrhoeae, amplified probe technique
87592	Neisseria gonorrhoeae, quantification
87620	papillomavirus, human, direct probe technique
87621	papillomavirus, human, amplified probe technique
87622	papillomavirus, human, quantification
87650	Streptococcus, group A, direct probe technique
87651	Streptococcus, group A, amplified probe technique
87652	Streptococcus, group A, quantification
● 87660	Trichomonas vaginalis, direct probe technique
87797	Infectious agent detection by nucleic acid (DNA or RNA), not otherwise specified; direct probe technique, each organism
87798	amplified probe technique, each organism
87799	quantification, each organism
87800	Infectious agent detection by nucleic acid (DNA or RNA), multiple organisms; direct probe(s) technique
87801	amplified probe(s) technique
87802	Infectious agent antigen detection by immunoassay with direct optical observation; Streptococcus, group B

● New Code   ▲ Revised Code   + Add-On Code   ⊘ Modifier -51 Exempt

87803   Clostridium difficile toxin A

87804   Influenza

87810   Infectious agent detection by immunoassay with direct optical observation; Chlamydia trachomatis

87850   Neisseria gonorrhoeae

87880   Streptococcus, group A

87899   not otherwise specified

87901   Infectious agent genotype analysis by nucleic acid (DNA or RNA) HIV 1, reverse transcriptase and protease

           (For infectious agent drug susceptibility phenotype prediction for HIV-1, use Category III code 0023T)

87902   Hepatitis C virus

87903   Infectious agent phenotype analysis by nucleic acid (DNA or RNA) with drug resistance tissue culture analysis, HIV 1; first through 10 drugs tested

+ 87904   each additional 1 through 5 drugs tested (List separately in addition to code for primary procedure)

           (Use 87904 in conjunction with code 87903)

87999   Unlisted microbiology procedure

ANATOMIC PATHOLOGY

POSTMORTEM EXAMINATION

88000   Necropsy (autopsy), gross examination only; without CNS

88005   with brain

88007   with brain and spinal cord

88012   infant with brain

88014   stillborn or newborn with brain

769

▣ Separate Procedure	▣ Unlisted Procedure	▣ CCI Comp. Code	▣ Non-specific Procedure

88016   macerated stillborn

88020   Necropsy (autopsy), gross and microscopic; without CNS

88025   with brain

88027   with brain and spinal cord

88028   infant with brain

88029   stillborn or newborn with brain

88036   Necropsy (autopsy), limited, gross and/or microscopic; regional

88037   single organ

88040   Necropsy (autopsy); forensic examination

88045   coroner's call

88099   Unlisted necropsy (autopsy) procedure

CYTOPATHOLOGY

(For cervicography, see Category III code 0003T)

(For collection of cytology specimens via mammary duct catheter lavage, report 0045T-0046T)

88104   Cytopathology, fluids, washings or brushings, except cervical or vaginal; smears with interpretation

88106   filter method only with interpretation

88107   smears and filter preparation with interpretation

88108   Cytopathology, concentration technique, smears and interpretation (eg, Saccomanno technique)

(For cervical or vaginal smears, see 88150-88155)

(For gastric intubation with lavage, see 89130-89141, 91055)

(For x-ray localization, use 74340)

● New Code   ▲ Revised Code   + Add-On Code   ⊘ Modifier -51 Exempt

● **88112** Cytopathology, selective cellular enhancement technique with interpretation (eg, liquid based slide preparation method), except cervical or vaginal

(Do not report 88112 with 88108)

88125 Cytopathology, forensic (eg, sperm)

88130 Sex chromatin identification; Barr bodies

88140   peripheral blood smear, polymorphonuclear drumsticks

(For Guard stain, use 88313)

+ 88141 Cytopathology, cervical or vaginal (any reporting system); requiring interpretation by physician (List separately in addition to code for technical service)

(Use 88141 in conjunction with codes 88142-88154, 88164-88167)

88142 Cytopathology, cervical or vaginal (any reporting system), collected in preservative fluid, automated thin layer preparation; manual screening under physician supervision

88143   with manual screening and rescreening under physician supervision

(88144 deleted 2003 edition)

(88145 deleted 2003 edition)

(For automated screening of automated thin layer preparation, see 88174, 88175)

88147 Cytopathology smears, cervical or vaginal; screening by automated system under physician supervision

88148   screening by automated system with manual rescreening under physician supervision

88150 Cytopathology, slides, cervical or vaginal; manual screening under physician supervision

88152   with manual screening and computer-assisted rescreening under physician supervision

---

771

 Separate Procedure   Unlisted Procedure    CCI Comp. Code   Non-specific Procedure

88153 with manual screening and rescreening under physician supervision

88154 with manual screening and computer-assisted rescreening using cell selection and review under physician supervision

+ **88155** Cytopathology, slides, cervical or vaginal, definitive hormonal evaluation (eg, maturation index, karyopyknotic index, estrogenic index) (List separately in addition to code(s) for other technical and interpretation services)

(Use 88155 in conjunction with 88142-88154, 88164-88167)

88160 Cytopathology, smears, any other source; screening and interpretation

88161 preparation, screening and interpretation

88162 extended study involving over 5 slides and/or multiple stains

(For obtaining specimen, see percutaneous needle biopsy under individual organ in Surgery)

(For aerosol collection of sputum, use 89350)

(For special stains, see 88312-88314)

88164 Cytopathology, slides, cervical or vaginal (the Bethesda System); manual screening under physician supervision

88165 with manual screening and rescreening under physician supervision

88166 with manual screening and computer-assisted rescreening under physician supervision

88167 with manual screening and computer-assisted rescreening using cell selection and review under physician supervision

(88170 deleted 2002 edition. To report, see 10021, 10022)

(88171 deleted 2002 edition. To report, see 10021, 10022)

88172 Cytopathology, evaluation of fine needle aspirate; immediate cytohistologic study to determine adequacy of specimen(s)

88173 interpretation and report

● New Code   ▲ Revised Code   + Add-On Code   ⊘ Modifier -51 Exempt

88174 Cytopathology, cervical or vaginal (any reporting system), collected in preservative fluid, automated thin layer preparation; screening by automated system, under physician supervision

88175 with screening by automated system and manual rescreening, under physician supervision

(For manual screening, see 88142, 88143)

88180 Flow cytometry; each cell surface, cytoplasmic or nuclear marker

88182 cell cycle or DNA analysis

(For tumor morphometry and DNA and ploidy analysis by imaging techniques, use 88358)

88199 Unlisted cytopathology procedure

(For electron microscopy, see 88348, 88349)

CYTOGENETIC STUDIES

(For acetylcholinesterase, use 82013)

(For alpha-fetoprotein, serum or amniotic fluid, see 82105, 82106)

(For laser microdissection of cells from tissue sample, see 88380)

88230 Tissue culture for non-neoplastic disorders; lymphocyte

88233 skin or other solid tissue biopsy

88235 amniotic fluid or chorionic villus cells

88237 Tissue culture for neoplastic disorders; bone marrow, blood cells

88239 solid tumor

88240 Cryopreservation, freezing and storage of cells, each cell line

(For therapeutic cryopreservation and storage, use 38207)

88241 Thawing and expansion of frozen cells, each aliquot

(For therapeutic thawing of previous harvest, use 38208)

773

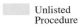 Separate Procedure   Unlisted Procedure   CCI Comp. Code   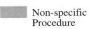 Non-specific Procedure

| 88245 | Chromosome analysis for breakage syndromes; baseline Sister Chromatid Exchange (SCE), 20-25 cells |

88245 Chromosome analysis for breakage syndromes; baseline Sister Chromatid Exchange (SCE), 20-25 cells

88248 baseline breakage, score 50-100 cells, count 20 cells, 2 karyotypes (eg, for ataxia telangiectasia, Fanconi anemia, fragile X)

88249 score 100 cells, clastogen stress (eg, diepoxybutane, mitomycin C, ionizing radiation, UV radiation)

88261 Chromosome analysis; count 5 cells, 1 karyotype, with banding

88262 count 15-20 cells, 2 karyotypes, with banding

88263 count 45 cells for mosaicism, 2 karyotypes, with banding

88264 analyze 20-25 cells

88267 Chromosome analysis, amniotic fluid or chorionic villus, count 15 cells, 1 karyotype, with banding

88269 Chromosome analysis, in situ for amniotic fluid cells, count cells from 6-12 colonies, 1 karyotype, with banding

88271 Molecular cytogenetics; DNA probe, each (eg, FISH)

88272 chromosomal in situ hybridization, analyze 3-5 cells (eg, for derivatives and markers)

88273 chromosomal in situ hybridization, analyze 10-30 cells (eg, for microdeletions)

88274 interphase in situ hybridization, analyze 25-99 cells

88275 interphase in situ hybridization, analyze 100-300 cells

88280 Chromosome analysis; additional karyotypes, each study

88283 additional specialized banding technique (eg, NOR, C-banding)

88285 additional cells counted, each study

88289 additional high resolution study

● New Code   ▲ Revised Code   + Add-On Code   ⊘ Modifier -51 Exempt

88291 Cytogenetics and molecular cytogenetics, interpretation and report

88299 Unlisted cytogenetic study

SURGICAL PATHOLOGY

88300 Level I - Surgical pathology, gross examination only

88302 Level II - Surgical pathology, gross and microscopic examination

Appendix, Incidental
Fallopian Tube, Sterilization
Fingers/Toes, Amputation, Traumatic
Foreskin, Newborn
Hernia Sac, Any Location
Hydrocele Sac
Nerve
Skin, Plastic Repair
Sympathetic Ganglion
Testis, Castration
Vaginal Mucosa, Incidental
Vas Deferens, Sterilization

88304 Level III - Surgical pathology, gross and microscopic examination

Abortion, Induced
Abscess
Aneurysm - Arterial/Ventricular
Anus, Tag
Appendix, Other than Incidental
Artery, Atheromatous Plaque
Bartholin's Gland Cyst
Bone Fragment(s), Other than Pathologic Fracture
Bursa/Synovial Cyst
Carpal Tunnel Tissue
Cartilage, Shavings
Cholesteatoma
Colon, Colostomy Stoma
Conjunctiva - Biopsy/Pterygium
Cornea
Diverticulum - Esophagus/Small Intestine
Dupuytren's Contracture Tissue
Femoral Head, Other than Fracture
Fissue/Fistula
Foreskin, Other than Newborn
Gallbladder

775

 Separate Procedure   Unlisted Procedure CCI Comp. Code   Non-specific Procedure

Ganglion Cyst
Hematoma
Hemorrhoids
Hydatid of Morgagni
Intervertebral Disc
Joint, Loose Body
Meniscus
Mucocele, Salivary
Neuroma - Morton's/Traumatic
Pilonidal Cyst/Sinus
Polyps, Inflammatory - Nasal/Sinusoidal
Skin - Cyst/Tag/Debridement
Soft Tissue, Debridement
Soft Tissue, Lipoma
Spermatocele
Tendon/Tendon Sheath
Testicular Appendage
Thrombus or Embolus
Tonsil and/or Adenoids
Varicocele
Vas Deferens, Other than Sterilizaton
Vein, Varicosity

88305 Level IV - Surgical pathology, gross and microscopic examination

Abortion - Spontaneous/Missed
Artery, Biopsy
Bone Marrow, Biopsy
Bone Exostosis
Brain/Meninges, Other than for Tumor Resection
Breast Biopsy, Not Requiring Microscopic Evaluation of Surgical Margins
Breast, Reduction Mammoplasty
Bronchus, Biopsy
Cell Block, Any Source
Cervix, Biopsy
Colon, Biopsy
Duodenum, Biopsy
Endocervix, Curettings/Biopsy
Endometrium, Currettings/Biopsy
Esophagus, Biopsy
Extremity, Amputation, Traumatic
Fallopian Tube, Biopsy
Fallopian Tube, Ectopic Pregnancy
Femoral Head, Fracture
Fingers/Toes, Amputation, Non-Traumatic
Gingiva/Oral Mucosa, Biopsy
Heart Valve
Joint, Resection

● New Code   ▲ Revised Code   + Add-On Code   ⊘ Modifier -51 Exempt

Kidney, Biopsy
Larynx, Biopsy
Leiomyoma(s), Uterine Myomectomy - without Uterus
Lip, Biopsy/Wedge Resection
Lung, Transbronchial Biopsy
Lymph Node, Biopsy
Muscle, Biopsy
Nasal Mucosa, Biopsy
Nasopharynx/Oropharynx, Biopsy
Nerve, Biopsy
Odontogenic/Dental Cyst
Omentum, Biopsy
Ovary with or without Tube, Non-neoplastic
Ovary, Biopsy/Wedge Resection
Parathyroid Gland
Peritoneum, Biopsy
Pituitary Tumor
Placenta, Other than Third Trimester
Pleura/Pericardium - Biopsy/Tissue
Polyp, Cervical/Endometrial
Polyp, Colorectal
Polyp, Stomach/Small Intestine
Prostate, Needle Biopsy
Prostate, TUR
Salivary Gland, Biopsy
Sinus, Paranasal Biopsy
Skin, Other than Cyst/Tag/Debridement/Plastic Repair
Small Intestine, Biopsy
Soft Tissue, Other than Tumor/Mass/Lipoma/Debridement
Spleen
Stomach, Biopsy
Synovium
Testis, Other than Tumor/Biopsy/Castration
Thyroglossal Duct/Brachial Cleft Cyst
Tongue, Biopsy
Tonsil, Biopsy
Trachea, Biopsy
Ureter, Biopsy
Urethra, Biopsy
Urinary Bladder, Biopsy
Uterus, with or without Tubes and Ovaries, for Prolapse
Vagina, Biopsy
Vulva/Labia, Biopsy

88307   Level V - Surgical pathology, gross and microscopic
examination

Adrenal, Resection
Bone - Biopsy/Curettings
Bone Fragment(s), Pathologic Fracture

777

	Separate Procedure		Unlisted Procedure		CCI Comp. Code		Non-specific Procedure

Brain, Biopsy
Brain/Meninges, Tumor Resection
Breast, Excision of Lesion, Requiring Microscopic Evaluation of
Surgical Margins
Breast, Mastectomy - Partial/Simple
Cervix, Conization
Colon, Segmental Resection, Other than for Tumor
Extremity, Amputation, Non-traumatic
Eye, Enucleation
Kidney, Partial/Total Nephrectomy
Larynx, Partial/Total Resection
Liver, Biopsy - Needle/Wedge
Lung, Wedge Biopsy
Lymph Nodes, Regional Resection
Mediastinum, Mass
Myocardium, Biopsy
Odontogenic Tumor
Ovary with or without Tube, Neoplastic
Pancreas, Biopsy
Placenta, Third Trimester
Prostate, Except Radical Resection
Salivary Gland
Sentinel Lymph Node
Small Intestine, Resection, Other Than for Tumor
Soft Tissue Mass (except Lipoma) - Biopsy/Simple Excision
Stomach - Subtotal/Total Resection, Other than for Tumor
Testis, Biopsy
Thymus, Biopsy
Thyroid, Total/Lobe
Ureter, Resection
Urinary Bladder, TUR
Uterus, with or without Tubes and Ovaries, Other than
Neoplastic/Prolapse

88309   Level VI - Surgical pathology, gross and microscopic
examination

Bone Resection
Breast, Mastectomy - with Regional Lymph Nodes
Colon, Segmental Resection for Tumor
Colon, Total Resection
Esophagus, Partial/Total Resection
Extremity, Disarticulation
Fetus, with Dissection
Larynx, Partial/Total Resection - with Regional Lymph Nodes
Lung - Total/Lobe/Segment Resection
Pancreas, Total/Subtotal Resection
Prostate, Radical Resection
Small Intestine, Resection for Tumor
Soft Tissue Tumor, Extensive Resection

778

● New
Code

▲ Revised
Code

✛ Add-On
Code

⊘ Modifier -51
Exempt

Stomach - Subtotal/Total Resection for Tumor
Testis, Tumor
Tongue/Tonsil - Resection for Tumor
Urinary Bladder, Partial/Total Resection
Uterus, with or without Tubes and Ovaries, Neoplastic
Vulva, Total/Subtotal Resection

(For fine needle aspiration, see 10021, 10022)

(For evaluation of fine needle aspirate, see 88172-88173)

+ 88311   Decalcification procedure (List separately in addition to code for surgical pathology examination)

▲+88312   Special stains (List separately in addition to code for primary service); Group I for microorganisms (eg, Gridley, acid fast, methenamine silver), each

+ 88313   Group II, all other, (eg, iron, trichrome), except immunocytochemistry and immunoperoxidase stains, each

(For immunocytochemistry and immunoperoxidase tissue studies, use 88342)

+ 88314   histochemical staining with frozen section(s)

88318   Determinative histochemistry to identify chemical components (eg, copper, zinc)

88319   Determinative histochemistry or cytochemistry to identify enzyme constituents, each

88321   Consultation and report on referred slides prepared elsewhere

88323   Consultation and report on referred material requiring preparation of slides

88325   Consultation, comprehensive, with review of records and specimens, with report on referred material

88329   Pathology consultation during surgery;

88331   first tissue block, with frozen section(s), single specimen

88332   each additional tissue block with frozen section(s)

▲ 88342   Immunohistochemistry (including tissue immunoperoxidase), each antibody

779

	Separate Procedure		Unlisted Procedure		CCI Comp. Code		Non-specific Procedure

(For quantitative or semiquantitative immunohistochemistry, use 88361)

88346   Immunofluorescent study, each antibody; direct method

88347   indirect method

88348   Electron microscopy; diagnostic

88349   scanning

88355   Morphometric analysis; skeletal muscle

88356   nerve

▲ **88358**   tumor (eg, DNA ploidy)

(Do not report 88358 with 88313 unless each procedure is for a different special stain)

● **88361**   tumor immunohistochemistry (eg, Her-2/neu, estrogen receptor/progesterone receptor), quantitative or semiquantitative

(Do not report 88361 with 88342 unless each procedure is for a different antibody)

(When semi-thin plastic-embedded sections are performed in conjunction with morphometric analysis, only the morphometric analysis should be coded; if performed as an independent procedure, see codes 88300-88309 for surgical pathology)

88362   Nerve teasing preparations

88365   Tissue in situ hybridization, interpretation and report

88371   Protein analysis of tissue by Western Blot, with interpretation and report;

88372   immunological probe for band identification, each

88380   Microdissection (eg, mechanical, laser capture)

88399   Unlisted surgical pathology procedure

● New Code   ▲ Revised Code   + Add-On Code   ⊘ Modifier -51 Exempt

TRANSCUTANEOUS PROCEDURES

88400 Bilirubin, total transcutaneous

OTHER PROCEDURES

(Basal metabolic rate has been deleted. If necessary to report, use 89399)

89050 Cell count, miscellaneous body fluids (eg, cerebrospinal fluid, joint fluid), except blood;

89051 with differential count

▲ **89055** Leukocyte assessment, fecal, qualitative or semiquantitative

89060 Crystal identification by light microscopy with or without polarizing lens analysis, any body fluid (except urine)

89100 Duodenal intubation and aspiration; single specimen (eg, simple bile study or afferent loop culture) plus appropriate test procedure

89105 collection of multiple fractional specimens with pancreatic or gallbladder stimulation, single or double lumen tube

(For radiological localization, use 74340)

(For chemical analyses, see Chemistry, this section)

(Electrocardiogram, see 93000-93268)

(Esophagus acid perfusion test (Bernstein), see 91030)

89125 Fat stain, feces, urine, or respiratory secretions

89130 Gastric intubation and aspiration, diagnostic, each specimen, for chemical analyses or cytopathology;

89132 after stimulation

89135 Gastric intubation, aspiration, and fractional collections (eg, gastric secretory study); one hour

89136 two hours

781

 Separate Procedure

 Unlisted Procedure

 CCI Comp. Code

 Non-specific Procedure

89140   two hours including gastric stimulation (eg, histalog, pentagastrin)

89141   three hours, including gastric stimulation

(For gastric lavage, therapeutic, use 91105)

(For radiologic localization of gastric tube, use 74340)

(For chemical analyses, see 82926, 82928)

(Joint fluid chemistry, see Chemistry, this section)

89160   Meat fibers, feces

89190   Nasal smear for eosinophils

(Occult blood, feces, use 82270)

(Paternity tests, use 86910)

● 89220   Sputum, obtaining specimen, aerosol induced technique (separate procedure)

● 89225   Starch granules, feces

● 89230   Sweat collection by iontophoresis

● 89235   Water load test

● 89240   Unlisted miscellaneous pathology test

REPRODUCTIVE MEDICINE PROCEDURES

▲ 89250   Culture of oocyte(s)/embryo(s), less than 4 days;

▲ 89251   with co-culture of oocyte(s)/embryo(s)

(For extended culture of oocyte(s)/embryo(s), see 89272)

(89252   deleted 2004 edition. To report, use 89280-89281)

89253   Assisted embryo hatching, microtechniques (any method)

89254   Oocyte identification from follicular fluid

89255   Preparation of embryo for transfer (any method)

| ● | New Code | ▲ | Revised Code | + | Add-On Code | ⊘ | Modifier -51 Exempt |

(89256   deleted 2004 edition. To report, use 89352)

89257   Sperm identification from aspiration (other than seminal fluid)

(For semen analysis, see 89300-89320)

(For sperm identification from testis tissue, use 89264)

▲ **89258**   Cryopreservation; embryo(s)

89259   sperm

(For cryopreservation of reproductive tissue, testicular, use 89335)

(For cryopreservation of reproductive tissue, ovarian, use Category III code 0058T)

(For cryopreservation of oocyte(s), use Category III code 0059T)

89260   Sperm isolation; simple prep (eg, sperm wash and swim-up) for insemination or diagnosis with semen analysis

89261   complex prep (eg, Percoll gradient, albumin gradient) for insemination or diagnosis with semen analysis

(For semen analysis without sperm wash or swim-up, use 89320)

89264   Sperm identification from testis tissue, fresh or cryopreserved

(For biopsy of testis, see 54500, 54505)

(For sperm identification from aspiration, use 89257)

(For semen analysis, see 89300-89320)

● **89268**   Insemination of oocytes

● **89272**   Extended culture of oocyte(s)/embryo(s), 4-7 days

● **89280**   Assisted oocyte fertiliation, microtechnique; less than or equal to 10 oocytes

● **89281**   greater than 10 oocytes

● **89290**   Biopsy, oocyte polar body or embryo blastomere, microtechnique (for pre-implantation genetic diagnosis); less than or equal to 5 embryos

783

	Separate Procedure		Unlisted Procedure		CCI Comp. Code		Non-specific Procedure

● **89291** greater than 5 embryos

89300 Semen analysis; presence and/or motility of sperm including Huhner test (post coital)

89310 motility and count (not including Huhner test)

89320 complete (volume, count, motility, and differential)

(Skin tests, see 86485-86585 and 95010-95199)

89321 Semen analysis, presence and/or motility of sperm

89325 Sperm antibodies

(For medicolegal identification of sperm, use 88125)

89329 Sperm evaluation; hamster penetration test

89330 cervical mucus penetration test, with or without spinnbarkeit test

● **89335** Cryopreservation, reproductive tissue, testicular

(For cryopreservation of embryo(s), use 89258. For cryopreservation of sperm, use 89259)

(For cryopreservation of reproductive tissue, ovarian, use Category III code 0058T)

(For cryopreservation of oocyte, use Category III code 0059T)

● **89342** Storage, (per year); embryo(s)

● **89343** sperm/semen

● **89344** reproductive tissue, testicular/ovarian

● **89346** oocyte

(**89350** deleted 2004 edition. To report, use 89220)

● **89352** Thawing of cryopreserved; embryo(s)

● **89353** sperm/semen, each aliquot

● **89354** reproductive tissue, testicular/ovarian

● New Code ▲ Revised Code ＋ Add-On Code ⊘ Modifier -51 Exempt

(89355   deleted 2004 edition. To report, use 89225)

● **89356**   oocytes, each aliquot

(89360   deleted 2004 edition. To report, use 89230)

(89365   deleted 2004 edition. To report, use 89235)

(89399   deleted 2004 edition. To report, use 89240)

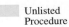 Separate Procedure   Unlisted Procedure    CCI Comp. Code   Non-specific Procedure

This page intentionally left blank.

● New
Code

▲ Revised
Code

✚ Add-On
Code

⊘ Modifier -51
Exempt

MEDICINE

MEDICINE SECTION OVERVIEW

The sixth section of the CPT coding system is the medicine section, which includes codes for immunizations, therapeutic or diagnostic injections, psychiatric services, dialysis, ophthalmology services, specialty specific diagnostic services, chemotherapy administration, physical medicine and rehabilitation services, osteopathic and chiropractic services. Within each subsection, the CPT codes are arranged by the type of service provided.

MEDICINE SUBSECTIONS

The MEDICINE section of CPT is divided into the following subsections:

Immune Globulins	90281-90399
Immunization Administration for Vaccines/Toxoids	90471-90474
Vaccines, Toxoids	90476-90749
Therapeutic or Diagnostic Infusions (excludes chemotherapy)	90780-90781
Therapeutic, Prophylactic or Diagnostic Injections	90782-90799
Psychiatry	90801-90899
Biofeedback	90900-90911
Dialysis	90918-90999
Gastroenterology	91000-91299
Ophthalmology	92002-92499
Special Otorhinolaryngologic Services	92502-92700
Cardiovascular	92950-93799
Non-Invasive Vascular Diagnostic Studies	93875-93990
Pulmonary	94010-94799
Allergy and Clinical Immunology	95004-95199
Endocrinology	95250
Neurology and Neuromuscular Procedures	95805-96004
Central Nervous System Assessments/Tests	96100-96117
Health and Behavior Assessment/Intervention	96150-96155
Chemotherapy Administration	96400-96549
Photodynamic Therapy	96567-96571
Special Dermatological Procedures	96900-96999
Physical Medicine and Rehabilitation	97001-97799
Medical Nutrition Therapy	97802-97804
Osteopathic Manipulative Treatment	98925-98929
Chiropractic Manipulative Treatment	98940-98943
Special Services, Procedures and Reports	99000-99091

MED
90000

787

 Separate Procedure   Unlisted Procedure   CCI Comp. Code   Non-specific Procedure

Qualifying Circumstances for Anesthesia	99100-99140
Sedation With or Without Analgesia	99141-99142
Other Services and Procedures	99170-99199
Home Health Procedures	99500-99602

Most of the subsections have special needs or instructions unique to that section which should be reviewed carefully before reporting.

MEDICINE SERVICES MODIFIERS

MEDICINE services and procedures may be modified under certain circumstances. When applicable, the modifying circumstance is identified by the addition of the appropriate modifier code. The following modifiers are frequently used with MEDICINE services.

-22 Unusual services

-26 Professional component

-51 Multiple procedures

   This modifier may be used to report multiple medical procedures performed at the same session, as well as a combination of medical and surgical procedures.

-52 Reduced services

-76 Repeat procedure by same physician

-77 Repeat procedure by another physician

-90 Reference (outside) laboratory

-99 Multiple modifiers

● New Code   ▲ Revised Code   ✚ Add-On Code   ⊘ Modifier -51 Exempt

MEDICINE CODES

IMMUNE GLOBULINS

Immune globulins are administered to provide protection from hepatitis B, diphtheria, rabies, respiratory viruses, tetanus and other diseases. Immune globulin CPT codes 90281-90399 identify the immune globulin product only and must be reported in addition to immunization administration CPT codes.

⊘ **90281**   Immune globulin (Ig), human, for intramuscular use

⊘ **90283**   Immune globulin (IgIV), human, for intravenous use

⊘ **90287**   Botulinum antitoxin, equine, any route

⊘ **90288**   Botulism immune globulin, human, for intravenous use

⊘ **90291**   Cytomegalovirus immune globulin (CMV-IgIV), human, for intravenous use

⊘ **90296**   Diphtheria antitoxin, equine, any route

⊘ **90371**   Hepatitis B immune globulin (HBIg), human, for intramuscular use

⊘ **90375**   Rabies immune globulin (RIg), human, for intramuscular and/or subcutaneous use

⊘ **90376**   Rabies immune globulin, heat-treated (RIg-HT), human, for intramuscular and/or subcutaneous use

⊘ **90378**   Respiratory syncytial virus immune globulin (RSV-IgIM), for intramuscular use, 50 mg, each

⊘ **90379**   Respiratory syncytial virus immune globulin (RSV-IgIV), human, for intravenous use

⊘ **90384**   Rho(D) immune globulin (RhIg), human, full-dose, for intramuscular use

⊘ **90385**   Rho(D) immune globulin (RhIg), human, mini-dose, for intramuscular use

⊘ **90386**   Rho(D) immune globulin (RhIgIV), human, for intravenous use

789

| | Separate Procedure | | Unlisted Procedure | | CCI Comp. Code | | Non-specific Procedure |

⊘ **90389** Tetanus immune globulin (TIg), human, for intramuscular use

⊘ **90393** Vaccinia immune globulin, human, for intramuscular use

⊘ **90396** Varicella-zoster immune globulin, human, for intramuscular use

⊘ **90399** Unlisted immune globulin

IMMUNIZATION ADMINISTRATION FOR VACCINES/TOXOIDS

Immunization is the administration of a vaccine or toxoid to stimulate the immune system to provide protection against disease. Immunizations are usually given in conjunction with an evaluation and management service. When an immunization is the only service performed, a minimal evaluation and management service code may be listed in addition to the injection code.

Coding Rules

1. *When an immunization is the only service provided, evaluation and management service code 99221, Minimal service, may be reported in addition to the immunization.*

2. *Immunization administration CPT codes must be reported in addition to the vaccine and toxoid CPT codes.*

3. *Supplies or equipment used to inject the vaccine or toxoid are not reported separately.*

IMMUNIZATION ADMINISTRATION

(For allergy testing, see 95004 et seq)

(For skin testing of bacterial, viral, fungal extracts, see 86485-86586)

(For therapeutic or diagnostic injections, see 90782-90799)

90471 Immunization administration (includes percutaneous, intradermal, subcutaneous, intramuscular and jet injections); one vaccine (single or combination vaccine/toxoid)

+ **90472** each additional vaccine (single or combination vaccine/toxoid) (List separately in addition to code for primary procedure)

(Use 90472 in conjunction with code 90471)

790

| ● | New Code | ▲ | Revised Code | + | Add-On Code | ⊘ | Modifier -51 Exempt |

(For administration of immune globulins, use 90780-90784, and see 90281-90399)

(For intravesical administration of BCG vaccine, use 51720, and see 90586)

90473 Immunization administration by intranasal or oral route; one vaccine (single or combination vaccine/toxoid)

+ 90474 each additional vaccine (single or combination vaccine/toxoid) (List separately in addition to code for primary procedure)

(Use 90474 in conjunction with code 90473)

VACCINES, TOXOIDS

Vaccines and toxoids are administered to provide protection from hepatitis, influenza, typhoid, measles, mumps, polio, and other diseases. Vaccine and toxoid CPT codes 90476-90749 identify the vaccine or toxoid only and must be reported in addition to immunization administration CPT codes.

(For immune globulins, see codes 90281-90399, and 90780-90784 for administration of immune globulins)

⊘ **90476** Adenovirus vaccine, type 4, live, for oral use

⊘ **90477** Adenovirus vaccine, type 7, live, for oral use

⊘ **90581** Anthrax vaccine, for subcutaneous use

⊘ **90585** Bacillus Calmette-Guerin vaccine (BCG) for tuberculosis, live, for percutaneous use

⊘ **90586** Bacillus Calmette-Guerin vaccine (BCG) for bladder cancer, live, for intravesical use

⊘ **90632** Hepatitis A vaccine, adult dosage, for intramuscular use

⊘ **90633** Hepatitis A vaccine, pediatric/adolescent dosage-2 dose schedule, for intramuscular use

⊘ **90634** Hepatitis A vaccine, pediatric/adolescent dosage-3 dose schedule, for intramuscular use

⊘ **90636** Hepatitis A and hepatitis B vaccine (HepA-HepB), adult dosage, for intramuscular use

791

 Separate Procedure Unlisted Procedure CCI Comp. Code Non-specific Procedure

⊘ **90645** Hemophilus influenza B vaccine (Hib), HbOC conjugate (4 dose schedule), for intramuscular use

⊘ **90646** Hemophilus influenza B vaccine (Hib), PRP-D conjugate, for booster use only, intramuscular use

⊘ **90647** Hemophilus influenza B vaccine (Hib), PRP-OMP conjugate (3 dose schedule), for intramuscular use

⊘ **90648** Hemophilus influenza B vaccine (Hib),PRP-T conjugate (4 dose schedule), for intramuscular use

⊘●**90655** Influenza virus vaccine, split virus, preservative free, for children 6-35 months of age, for intramuscular use

⊘▲**90657** Influenza virus vaccine, split virus, for children 6-35 months of age, for intramuscular use

⊘▲**90658** Influenza virus vaccine, split virus, for use in individuals 3 years of age and above, for intramuscular use

(90659 deleted 2004 edition. To report influenza virus vaccine, split virus, see 90657 or 90658)

⊘ **90660** Influenza virus vaccine, live, for intranasal use

⊘ **90665** Lyme disease vaccine, adult dosage, for intramuscular use

⊘ **90669** Pneumococcal conjugate vaccine, polyvalent, for children under five years, for intramuscular use

⊘ **90675** Rabies vaccine, for intramuscular use

⊘ **90676** Rabies vaccine, for intradermal use

⊘ **90680** Rotavirus vaccine, tetravalent, live, for oral use

⊘ **90690** Typhoid vaccine, live, oral

⊘ **90691** Typhoid vaccine, Vi capsular polysaccharide (ViCPs), for intramuscular use

⊘ **90692** Typhoid vaccine, heat- and phenol-inactivated (H-P), for subcutaneous or intradermal use

⊘▲**90693** Typhoid vaccine, acetone-killed, dried (AKD), for subcutaneous use (U.S. military)

| ● | New Code | ▲ | Revised Code | + | Add-On Code | ⊘ | Modifier -51 Exempt |

⊘●**90698** Diphtheria, tetanus toxoids, acellular pertussis vaccine, haemophilus influenza Type B, and poliovirus vaccine, inactivated (DTaP-Hib-IPV), for intramuscular use

⊘ **90700** Diphtheria, tetanus toxoids, and acellular pertussis vaccine (DTaP), for intramuscular use

⊘ **90701** Diphtheria, tetanus toxoids, and whole cell pertussis vaccine (DTP), for intramuscular use

⊘ **90702** Diphtheria and tetanus toxoids (DT) adsorbed for use in individuals younger than seven years, for intramuscular use

⊘▲**90703** Tetanus toxoid adsorbed, for intramuscular use

⊘▲**90704** Mumps virus vaccine, live, for subcutaneous use

⊘▲**90705** Measles virus vaccine, live, for subcutaneous use

⊘▲**90706** Rubella virus vaccine, live, for subcutaneous use

⊘▲**90707** Measles, mumps and rubella virus vaccine (MMR), live, for subcutaneous use

⊘▲**90708** Measles and rubella virus vaccine, live, for subcutaneous use

(90709   deleted 2003 edition)

⊘ **90710** Measles, mumps, rubella, and varicella vaccine (MMRV), live, for subcutaneous use

⊘ **90712** Poliovirus vaccine, (any type(s)) (OPV), live, for oral use

⊘ **90713** Poliovirus vaccine, inactivated, (IPV), for subcutaneous use

⊘●**90715** Tetanus, diphtheria toxoids and acellular pertussis vaccine (TdaP), for use in individuals seven years or older, for intramuscular use

⊘ **90716** Varicella virus vaccine, live, for subcutaneous use

⊘ **90717** Yellow fever vaccine, live, for subcutaneous use

⊘▲**90718** Tetanus and diphtheria toxoids (Td) adsorbed for use in individuals seven years or older, for intramuscular use

⊘ **90719** Diphtheria toxoid, for intramuscular use

793

| Separate Procedure | Unlisted Procedure | CCI Comp. Code | Non-specific Procedure |

⊘ **90720** Diphtheria, tetanus toxoids, and whole cell pertussis vaccine and Hemophilus influenza B vaccine (DTP-Hib), for intramuscular use

⊘ **90721** Diphtheria, tetanus toxoids, and acellular pertussis vaccine and Hemophilus influenza B vaccine (DtaP-Hib), for intramuscular use

⊘ **90723** Diphtheria, tetanus toxoids, acellular pertussis vaccine, Hepatitis B, and poliovirus vaccine, inactivated (DtaP-HepB-IPV), for intramuscular use

⊘ **90725** Cholera vaccine for injectable use

(For oral cholera, use 90592)

⊘▲**90727** Plague vaccine, for intramuscular use

⊘ **90732** Pneumococcal polysaccharide vaccine, 23-valent, adult or immunosuppressed patient dosage, for use in individuals 2 years or older, for subcutaneous or intramuscular use

⊘▲**90733** Meningococcal polysaccharide vaccine (any group(s)), for subcutaneous use

⊘●**90734** Meningococcal conjugate vaccine, serogroups A, C, Y and W-135 (tetravalent), for intramuscular use

⊘ **90735** Japanese encephalitis virus vaccine, for subcutaneous use

⊘ **90740** Hepatitis B vaccine, dialysis or immunosuppressed patient dosage (3 dose schedule), for intramuscular use

⊘ **90743** Hepatitis B vaccine, adolescent (2 dose schedule), for intramuscular use

⊘ **90744** Hepatitis B vaccine, pediatric/adolescent dosage (3 dose schedule), for intramuscular use

⊘ **90746** Hepatitis B vaccine, adult dosage, for intramuscular use

⊘ **90747** Hepatitis B vaccine, dialysis or immunosuppressed patient dosage (4 dose schedule), for intramuscular use

⊘ **90748** Hepatitis B and Hemophilus influenza B vaccine (HepB-Hib), for intramuscular use

⊘ **90749** Unlisted vaccine/toxoid

794 ● New Code   ▲ Revised Code   + Add-On Code   ⊘ Modifier -51 Exempt

THERAPEUTIC OR DIAGNOSTIC INFUSIONS (EXCLUDES CHEMOTHERAPY)

Infusion is the therapeutic introduction of a fluid, other than blood, into a vein. An infusion flows in by gravity whereas an injection is forced in by a syringe. Infusion therapy CPT codes are used to report prolonged intravenous injections requiring the presence of a physician during the infusion. These CPT codes are time specific codes covering the first hour, and each additional hour of therapy up to eight (8) hours.

Coding Rules

1. *Presence of the physician during the infusion is required.*

2. *Infusion CPT codes may not be used for chemotherapy infusions.*

3. *Infusion CPT codes may not be used for intradermal, subcutaneous, intramuscular, or routine intravenous drug injections.*

4. *Infusion CPT codes may not be reported in addition to prolonged services CPT codes.*

   90780 Intravenous infusion for therapy/diagnosis, administered by physician or under direct supervision of physician; up to one hour

   + 90781 each additional hour, up to eight (8) hours (List separately in addition to code for primary procedure)

   (Use 90781 in conjunction with code 90780)

THERAPEUTIC, PROPHYLACTIC OR DIAGNOSTIC INJECTIONS

An injection is the process of forcing a liquid, usually via a needle and syringe, into the skin, muscles, arteries or veins. Therapeutic or diagnostic injection CPT codes are used for reporting therapeutic injections of medication, via subcutaneous, intramuscular, intra-arterial or intravenous routes and for reporting intramuscular injection of antibiotics.

Coding Rules

1. *When reporting therapeutic or diagnostic injection CPT codes, the injected material should be specified.*

2. *Therapeutic or diagnostic injection CPT codes may not be used for allergen immunotherapy.*

795

| Separate Procedure | Unlisted Procedure | CCI Comp. Code | Non-specific Procedure |

3. *Use CPT therapeutic or diagnostic injection CPT codes when reporting injections to commercial health insurance companies, unless otherwise instructed by specific companies.*

4. *Use HCPCS Level II codes instead of CPT codes to report therapeutic or diagnostic injections on health insurance claims to Medicare.*

90782   Therapeutic, prophylactic or diagnostic injection (specify material injected); subcutaneous or intramuscular

(For administration of vaccines/toxoids, see 90471-90472)

90783   intra-arterial

90784   intravenous

(90782-90784 do not include injections for allergen immunotherapy. For allergen immunotherapy injections, see 95115-95117)

90788   Intramuscular injection of antibiotic (specify)

(90790-90796 have been deleted. To report, see 95990, 96408-96414, 96420-96425, 96440, 96450, 96530, 96545, 96549)

90799   Unlisted therapeutic, prophylactic or diagnostic injection

(For allergy immunizations, see 95004 et seq)

PSYCHIATRY

(For repetitive transcranial magnetic stimulation for treatment of clinical depression, use Category III code 0018T)

Psychiatry is the study, treatment and prevention of mental disorders. Psychiatric services include diagnostic and therapeutic services in the hospital, office, or other outpatient setting. Psychiatric service CPT codes are used to report general psychiatry, clinical psychiatry, and psychiatric therapeutic services and procedures. Key coding issues include the type of psychotherapy, the place of service, the face-to-face time spent with the patient during psychotherapy, and whether evaluation and management services are furnished on the same date of service as psychotherapy.

●	New Code	▲	Revised Code	+	Add-On Code	⊘ Modifier -51 Exempt

Coding Rules

1. *Attending physicians reporting hospital care services in treating a psychiatric inpatient may use the full range of hospital evaluation and management service codes.*

2. *If the physician is active in the leadership or direction of a treatment team, a code may be selected based upon the services provided that day using Case Management CPT codes from evaluation and management services codes 99361-99362.*

3. *All procedures performed in addition to hospital care, such as electroconvulsive therapy or medical psychotherapy should be listed in addition to hospital care.*

4. *Psychiatric care may be reported without time dimensions, using CPT codes 90841 or 90845, or with time dimensions, using CPT codes 90843 or 90844, based upon practices customary in the local area.*

5. *The modifiers -52, reduced service, or -22, unusual service, may be used to report services that were less or more lengthy that the time-specified CPT codes define.*

PSYCHIATRIC CONSULTATIONS

Consultation for psychiatric evaluation of a patient includes examination of a patient and exchange of information with primary physician and others, such as nurses or family members, and preparation of report.

Consultation services provided by psychiatrists are reported with evaluation and management consultation CPT codes. Psychiatric consultation services are limited to initial or follow-up evaluation and do not involve psychiatric treatment.

PSYCHIATRIC DIAGNOSTIC OR EVALUATIVE INTERVIEW PROCEDURES

90801 Psychiatric diagnostic interview examination

90802 Interactive psychiatric diagnostic interview examination using play equipment, physical devices, language interpreter, or other mechanisms of communication

 Separate Procedure   Unlisted Procedure   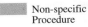 CCI Comp. Code   Non-specific Procedure

PSYCHIATRIC THERAPEUTIC PROCEDURES

OFFICE OR OTHER OUTPATIENT FACILITY

Insight Oriented, Behavior Modifying and/or Supportive Psychotherapy

90804 Individual psychotherapy, insight oriented, behavior modifying and/or supportive, in an office or outpatient facility, approximately 20 to 30 minutes face-to-face with the patient;

90805 with medical evaluation and management services

90806 Individual psychotherapy, insight oriented, behavior modifying and/or supportive, in an office or outpatient facility, approximately 45 to 50 minutes face-to-face with the patient;

90807 with medical evaluation and management services

90808 Individual psychotherapy, insight oriented, behavior modifying and/or supportive, in an office or outpatient facility, approximately 75 to 80 minutes face-to-face with the patient;

90809 with medical evaluation and management services

Interactive Psychotherapy

90810 Individual psychotherapy, interactive, using play equipment, physical devices, language interpreter, or other mechanisms of non-verbal communication, in an office or outpatient facility, approximately 20 to 30 minutes face-to-face with the patient;

90811 with medical evaluation and management services

90812 Individual psychotherapy, interactive, using play equipment, physical devices, language interpreter, or other mechanisms of non-verbal communication, in an office or outpatient facility, approximately 45 to 50 minutes face-to-face with the patient;

90813 with medical evaluation and management services

90814 Individual psychotherapy, interactive, using play equipment, physical devices, language interpreter, or other mechanisms of non-verbal communication, in an office or outpatient facility, approximately 75 to 80 minutes face-to-face with the patient;

90815 with medical evaluation and management services

● New Code   ▲ Revised Code   ✚ Add-On Code   ⊘ Modifier -51 Exempt

INPATIENT HOSPITAL, PARTIAL HOSPITAL OR RESIDENTIAL CARE FACILITY

Insight Oriented, Behavior Modifying and/or Supportive Psychotherapy

90816 Individual psychotherapy, insight oriented, behavior modifying and/or supportive, in an inpatient hospital, partial hospital or residential care setting, approximately 20 to 30 minutes face-to-face with the patient;

90817 with medical evaluation and management services

90818 Individual psychotherapy, insight oriented, behavior modifying and/or supportive, in an inpatient hospital, partial hospital or residential care setting, approximately 45 to 50 minutes face-to-face with the patient;

90819 with medical evaluation and management services

90821 Individual psychotherapy, insight oriented, behavior modifying and/or supportive, in an inpatient hospital, partial hospital or residential care setting, approximately 75 to 80 minutes face-to-face with the patient;

90822 with medical evaluation and management services

Interactive Psychotherapy

90823 Individual psychotherapy, interactive, using play equipment, physical devices, language interpreter, or other mechanisms of non-verbal communication, in an inpatient hospital, partial hospital or residential care setting, approximately 20 to 30 minutes face-to-face with the patient;

90824 with medical evaluation and management services

90826 Individual psychotherapy, interactive, using play equipment, physical devices, language interpreter, or other mechanisms of non-verbal communication, in an inpatient hospital, partial hospital or residential care setting, approximately 45 to 50 minutes face-to-face with the patient;

90827 with medical evaluation and management services

	Separate Procedure		Unlisted Procedure		CCI Comp. Code		Non-specific Procedure

90828 Individual psychotherapy, interactive, using play equipment, physical devices, language interpreter, or other mechanisms of non-verbal communication, in an inpatient hospital, partial hospital or residential care setting, approximately 75 to 80 minutes face-to-face with the patient;

90829   with medical evaluation and management services

OTHER PSYCHOTHERAPY

90845 Psychoanalysis

90846 Family psychotherapy (without the patient present)

90847 Family psychotherapy (conjoint psychotherapy) (with patient present)

90849 Multiple-family group psychotherapy

90853 Group psychotherapy (other than of a multiple-family group)

90857 Interactive group psychotherapy

OTHER PSYCHIATRIC SERVICES OR PROCEDURES

90862 Pharmacologic management, including prescription, use, and review of medication with no more than minimal medical psychotherapy

90865 Narcosynthesis for psychiatric diagnostic and therapeutic purposes (eg, sodium amobarbital (Amytal) interview)

90870 Electroconvulsive therapy (includes necessary monitoring); single seizure

90871   multiple seizures, per day

90875 Individual psychophysiological therapy incorporating biofeedback training by any modality (face-to-face with the patient), with psychotherapy (eg, insight oriented, behavior modifying or supportive psychotherapy); approximately 20-30 minutes

90876   approximately 45-50 minutes

90880 Hypnotherapy

800

● New Code   ▲ Revised Code   + Add-On Code   ⊘ Modifier -51 Exempt

90882   Environmental intervention for medical management purposes on a psychiatric patients behalf with agencies, employers, or institutions

90885   Psychiatric evaluation of hospital records, other psychiatric reports, psychometric and/or projective tests, and other accumulated data for medical diagnostic purposes

90887   Interpretation or explanation of results of psychiatric, other medical examinations and procedures, or other accumulated data to family or other responsible persons, or advising them how to assist patient

90889   Preparation of report of patient's psychiatric status, history, treatment, or progress (other than for legal or consultative purposes) for other physicians, agencies, or insurance carriers

90899   Unlisted psychiatric service or procedure

BIOFEEDBACK

Biofeedback is the process of detecting information about a patient's biological functions, eg. heart rate, breathing rate, skin temperature, and amount of muscle tension, picked up by surface electrodes (sensors) and electronically amplified to provide feedback, usually in the form of an audio-tone and/or visual read-out to the patient. Biofeedback training uses the information that has been monitored from the sensors attached to a muscle on the skin's surface, or to the skin only for thermal or other readings. With the help of a trained clinician, the patient can learn how to make voluntary changes in those biological functions and bring them under control.

(For psychophysiological therapy incorporating biofeedback training, see 90875, 90876)

90901   Biofeedback training by any modality

90911   Biofeedback training, perineal muscles, anorectal or urethral sphincter, including EMG and/or manometry

(For incontinence treatment by pulsed magnetic neuromodulation, use Category III code 0029T)

 Separate Procedure   Unlisted Procedure    CCI Comp. Code   Non-specific Procedure

DIALYSIS

Dialysis is the process of passing body fluids through a membrane to remove harmful substances. Dialysis is used in the treatment of kidney failure. Key coding issues include the type of dialysis and the location of the service.

Coding Rules

1. *All evaluation and management services related to the patient's end stage renal disease that are rendered on a day when dialysis is performed and all other patient care services that are rendered during the dialysis procedure are included in the dialysis procedure CPT codes.*

2. *All evaluation and management services unrelated to the dialysis procedure that cannot be rendered during the dialysis session may be reported in addition to the dialysis procedure.*

3. *Supplies provided to dialysis patients not considered to be included with the dialysis service or procedure are reported using CPT code 99070 or HCPCS codes E1500-E1699 for DME, and A4650-A5149 for supplies for ESRD.*

END STAGE RENAL DISEASE SERVICES

90918   End stage renal disease (ESRD) related services per full month; for patients under two years of age to include monitoring for the adequacy of nutrition, assessment of growth and development, and counseling of parents

90919   for patients between two and eleven years of age to include monitoring for the adequacy of nutrition, assessment of growth and development, and counseling of parents

90920   for patients between twelve and nineteen years of age to include monitoring for the adequacy of nutrition, assessment of growth and development, and counseling of parents

90921   for patients twenty years of age and over

90922   End stage renal disease (ESRD) related services (less than full month), per day; for patients under two years of age

90923   for patients between two and eleven years of age

90924   for patients between twelve and nineteen years of age

90925   for patients twenty years of age and over

---

802   ● New Code   ▲ Revised Code   ✛ Add-On Code   ⊘ Modifier -51 Exempt

HEMODIALYSIS

(For home visit hemodialysis services performed by a non-physician health care professional, use 99512)

(For cannula declotting, see 36831, 36833, 36860, 36861)

(For declotting of implanted vascular access device or catheter by thrombolytic agent, use 36550)

(For collection of blood specimen from a partially or completely implantable venous access device, use 36540)

(For prolonged physician attendance, see 99354-99360)

90935 Hemodialysis procedure with single physician evaluation

90937 Hemodialysis procedure requiring repeated evaluation(s) with or without substantial revision of dialysis prescription

90939 Hemodialysis access flow study to determine blood flow in grafts and arteriovenous fistulae by an indicator dilution method, hook-up; transcutaneous measurement and disconnection.

90940 measurement and disconnection

(For duplex scan of hemodialysis access, use 93990)

MISCELLANEOUS DIALYSIS PROCEDURES

(For insertion of intraperitoneal cannula or catheter, see 49420, 49421)

(For prolonged physician attendance, see 99354-99360)

90945 Dialysis procedure other than hemodialysis (eg, peritoneal, hemofiltration or other continuous replacement therapies), with single physician evaluation

(For home infusion of peritoneal dialysis, use 99559)

90947 Dialysis procedure other than hemodialysis (eg, peritoneal dialysis, hemofiltration, or other continuous renal replacement therapies) requiring repeated physician evaluations, with or without substantial revision of dialysis prescription

90989 Dialysis training, patient, including helper where applicable, any mode, completed course

803

 Separate Procedure

Unlisted Procedure

 CCI Comp. Code

 Non-specific Procedure

90993   Dialysis training, patient, including helper where applicable, any mode, course not completed, per training session

90997   Hemoperfusion (eg, with activated charcoal or resin)

90999   Unlisted dialysis procedure, inpatient or outpatient

GASTROENTEROLOGY

Gastroenterology is the study and treatment of diseases of the stomach and digestive system. CPT codes listed in this subsection are used to report diagnostic services of the esophagus and/or stomach contents, and therapeutic services such as gastric intubation and lavage. Gastroenterology services are usually performed in conjunction with an evaluation and management service, such as a consultation or visit, and should be reported separately in addition to the evaluation and management service.

(For duodenal intubation and aspiration, see 89100-89105)

(For gastrointestinal radiologic procedures, see 74210-74363)

(For esophagoscopy procedures, see 43200-43228; upper GI endoscopy 43234-43259; endoscopy, small intestine and stomal 44360-44393; proctosigmoidoscopy 45300-45321; sigmoidoscopy 45330-45339; colonscopy 45355-45385; anoscopy 46600-46615)

91000   Esophageal intubation and collection of washings for cytology, including preparation of specimens (separate procedure)

91010   Esophageal motility (manometric study of the esophagus and/or gastroesophageal junction) study;

91011   with mecholyl or similar stimulant

91012   with acid perfusion studies

91020   Gastric motility (manometric) studies

91030   Esophagus, acid perfusion (Bernstein) test for esophagitis

91032   Esophagus, acid reflux test, with intraluminal pH electrode for detection of gastroesophageal reflux;

91033   prolonged recording

---

804   ● New Code   ▲ Revised Code   + Add-On Code   ⊘ Modifier -51 Exempt

91052 Gastric analysis test with injection of stimulant of gastric secretion (eg, histamine, insulin, pentagastrin, calcium and secretin)

(For gastric biopsy by capsule, peroral, via tube, one or more specimens, use 43600)

(For gastric laboratory procedures, see also 89130-89141)

91055 Gastric intubation, washings, and preparing slides for cytology (separate procedure)

(For gastric lavage, therapeutic, use 91105)

91060 Gastric saline load test

(For biopsy by capsule, small intestine, per oral, via tube (one or more specimens), use 44100)

91065 Breath hydrogen test (eg, for detection of lactase deficiency)

91100 Intestinal bleeding tube, passage, positioning and monitoring

91105 Gastric intubation, and aspiration or lavage for treatment (eg, for ingested poisons)

(For cholangiography, see 47500, 74320)

(For abdominal paracentesis, see 49080, 49081; with instillation of medication, see 96440, 96445)

(For peritoneoscopy, use 49320; with biopsy, use 49321)

(For peritoneoscopy and guided transhepatic cholangiography, use 47560; with biopsy, use 47561)

(For splenoportography, see 38200, 75810)

● **91110** Gastrointestinal tract imaging, intraluminal (eg, capsule endoscopy), esophagus through ileum, with physician interpretation and report

(Visualization of the colon is not reported separately)

(Append modifier '-52' if the ileum is not visualized)

91122 Anorectal manometry

91123 Pulsed irrigation of fecal impaction

 Separate Procedure   Unlisted Procedure   CCI Comp. Code    Non-specific Procedure

GASTRIC PHYSIOLOGY

91132   Electrogastrography, diagnostic, transcutaneous;

91133   with provocative testing

OTHER PROCEDURES

91299 Unlisted diagnostic gastroenterology procedure

OPHTHALMOLOGY

(For surgical procedures, see Surgery, Eye and Ocular Adnexa, 65091 et seq)

Ophthalmology is the study and treatment of diseases of the eye. Ophthalmological diagnostic and treatment services are reported using CPT Medicine codes 92002-92499.

Coding Rules

1.   *Minimal, brief and limited office services, and hospital, home, extended care, emergency department and consultations are reported using appropriate evaluation and management service codes.*

2.   *Surgical procedures on the eye(s) are reported using CPT codes from the Eye and Ocular Adnexa subsection of the SURGERY section of CPT.*

3.   *To report intermediate ophthalmological services, the following must be performed and documented: a) evaluation of new or existing condition, b) complications of new diagnostic or management problems (not necessarily related to the primary diagnosis), c) history, d) general medical observation e) external ocular and adnexal examination, f) other diagnostic procedures as indicated, and g) may include the use of mydriasis. Intermediate ophthalmological services do not usually include determination of refractive state but may in an established patient under continuing active treatment.*

4.   *To report comprehensive ophthalmological services the following must be performed and documented: a) reported as a single service but may be performed at more than one session, b) history, c) general medical observation, d) external and ophthalmoscopic examination, e) gross visual fields, f) basic sensorimotor examination, g. may include, as indicated; biomicroscopy, examination with cycloplegia or mydriasis and tonometry, h) always includes initiation of diagnostic and treatment programs.*

---

806   ● New Code   ▲ Revised Code   ✚ Add-On Code   ⊘ Modifier -51 Exempt

5.   *For both intermediate and comprehensive ophthalmological services, service components, such as slip lamp examination, keratomy, ophthalmoscopy, retinoscopy, tonometry and motor evaluation are not reported separately.*

GENERAL OPHTHALMOLOGICAL SERVICES

NEW PATIENT

92002   Ophthalmological services: medical examination and evaluation with initiation of diagnostic and treatment program; intermediate, new patient

92004   comprehensive, new patient, one or more visits

ESTABLISHED PATIENT

92012   Ophthalmological services: medical examination and evaluation, with initiation or continuation of diagnostic and treatment program; intermediate, established patient

92014   comprehensive, established patient, one or more visits

(For surgical procedures, see Surgery, Eye and Ocular Adnexa, 65091 et seq)

SPECIAL OPHTHALMOLOGICAL SERVICES

Special ophthalmological services are defined as a level of service in which a special evaluation of part of the visual system is made which goes beyond the services usually included under general ophthalmological services, or in which special treatment is given. Fluorescein angioscopy, quantitative visual field examination, or extended color vision examination should be specifically reported as special ophthalmological services.

92015   Determination of refractive state

92018   Ophthalmological examination and evaluation, under general anesthesia, with or without manipulation of globe for passive range of motion or other manipulation to facilitate diagnostic examination; complete

92019   limited

92020   Gonioscopy (separate procedure)

(For gonioscopy under general anesthesia, use 92018)

 Separate Procedure
 Unlisted Procedure
 CCI Comp. Code
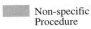 Non-specific Procedure

92060 Sensorimotor examination with multiple measurements of ocular deviation (eg, restrictive or paretic muscle with diplopia) with interpretation and report (separate procedure)

92065 Orthoptic and/or pleoptic training, with continuing medical direction and evaluation

92070 Fitting of contact lens for treatment of disease, including supply of lens

92081 Visual field examination, unilateral or bilateral, with interpretation and report; limited examination (eg, tangent screen, Autoplot, arc perimeter, or single stimulus level automated test, such as Octopus 3 or 7 equivalent)

92082 intermediate examination (eg, at least 2 isopters on Goldmann perimeter, or semiquantitative, automated suprathreshold screening program, Humphrey suprathreshold automatic diagnostic test, Octopus program 33)

92083 extended examination (eg, Goldmann visual fields with at least 3 isopters plotted and static determination within the central 30 degrees, or quantitative, automated threshold perimetry, Octopus programs G-1, 32 or 42, Humphrey visual field analyzer full threshold programs 30-2, 24-2, or 30/60-2)

(Gross visual field testing (eg, confrontation testing) is a part of general ophthalmological services and is not reported separately)

92100 Serial tonometry (separate procedure) with multiple measurements of intraocular pressure over an extended time period with interpretation and report, same day (eg, diurnal curve or medical treatment of acute elevation of intraocular pressure)

92120 Tonography with interpretation and report, recording indentation tonometer method or perilimbal suction method

92130 Tonography with water provocation

92135 Scanning computerized ophthalmic diagnostic imaging (eg, scanning laser) with interpretation and report, unilateral

92136 Ophthalmic biometry by partial coherence interferometry with intraocular lens power calculation

---

808

● New Code	▲ Revised Code	+ Add-On Code	⊘ Modifier -51 Exempt

92140   Provocative tests for glaucoma, with interpretation and report, without tonography

OPHTHALMOSCOPY

92225   Ophthalmoscopy, extended, with retinal drawing (eg, for retinal detachment, melanoma), with interpretation and report; initial

92226   subsequent

92230   Fluorescein angioscopy with interpretation and report

92235   Fluorescein angiography (includes multiframe imaging) with interpretation and report

92240   Indocyanine-green angiography (includes multiframe imaging) with interpretation and report

92250   Fundus photography with interpretation and report

92260   Ophthalmodynamometry

(For opthalmoscopy under general anesthesia, use 92018)

OTHER SPECIALIZED SERVICES

92265   Needle oculoelectromyography, one or more extraocular muscles, one or both eyes, with interpretation and report

92270   Electro-oculography with interpretation and report

92275   Electroretinography with interpretation and report

(For electronystagmography for vestibular function studies, see 92541 et seq)

(For ophthalmic echography (diagnostic ultrasound), see 76511-76529)

92283   Color vision examination, extended, eg, anomaloscope or equivalent

(Color vision testing with pseudoisochromatic plates (such as HRR or Ishihara) is not reported separately. It is included in the appropriate general or ophthalmological service, or 99172)

92284   Dark adaptation examination with interpretation and report

809

CPT PLUS! 2004

92285 External ocular photography with interpretation and report for documentation of medical progress (eg, close-up photography, slit lamp photography, goniophotography, stereo-photography)

92286 Special anterior segment photography with interpretation and report; with specular endothelial microscopy and cell count

92287 with fluorescein angiography

CONTACT LENS SERVICES

(For therapeutic or surgical use of contact lens, see 68340, 92070)

92310 Prescription of optical and physical characteristics of and fitting of contact lens, with medical supervision of adaptation; corneal lens, both eyes, except for aphakia

(For prescription and fitting of one eye, add modifier -52)

92311 corneal lens for aphakia, one eye

92312 corneal lens for aphakia, both eyes

92313 corneoscleral lens

92314 Prescription of optical and physical characteristics of contact lens, with medical supervision of adaptation and direction of fitting by independent technician; corneal lens, both eyes except for aphakia

(For prescription and fitting of one eye, add modifier -52)

92315 corneal lens for aphakia, one eye

92316 corneal lens for aphakia, both eyes

92317 corneoscleral lens

92325 Modification of contact lens (separate procedure), with medical supervision of adaptation

92326 Replacement of contact lens

● New Code ▲ Revised Code + Add-On Code ⊘ Modifier -51 Exempt

OCULAR PROSTHETICS, ARTIFICIAL EYE

92330 Prescription, fitting, and supply of ocular prosthesis (artificial eye), with medical supervision of adaptation

(If supply is not included, use modifier -26; to report supply separately, use 92393)

92335 Prescription of ocular prosthesis (artificial eye) and direction of fitting and supply by independent technician, with medical supervision of adaptation

SPECTACLE SERVICES (INCLUDING PROSTHESIS FOR APHAKIA)

92340 Fitting of spectacles, except for aphakia; monofocal

92341 bifocal

92342 multifocal, other than bifocal

92352 Fitting of spectacle prosthesis for aphakia; monofocal

92353 multifocal

92354 Fitting of spectacle mounted low vision aid; single element system

92355 telescopic or other compound lens system

92358 Prosthesis service for aphakia, temporary (disposable or loan, including materials)

92370 Repair and refitting spectacles; except for aphakia

92371 spectacle prosthesis for aphakia

SUPPLY OF MATERIALS

92390 Supply of spectacles, except prosthesis for aphakia and low vision aids

92391 Supply of contact lenses, except prosthesis for aphakia

(For supply of contact lenses reported as part of the service of fitting, see 92310-92313)

811

 Separate Procedure   Unlisted Procedure    CCI Comp. Code   Non-specific Procedure

(For replacement of contact lens, use 92326)

92392   Supply of low vision aids (A low vision aid is any lens or device used to aid or improve visual function in a person whose vision cannot be normalized by conventional spectacle correction. Includes reading additions up to 4D.)

92393   Supply of ocular prosthesis (artificial eye)

(For supply reported as part of the service of fitting, use 92330)

92395   Supply of permanent prosthesis for aphakia; spectacles

(For temporary spectacle correction, use 92358)

92396   contact lenses

(For supply reported as part of the service of fitting, see 92311, 92312)

(Use 99070 for the supply of other materials, drugs, trays, etc.)

OTHER PROCEDURES

92499   Unlisted ophthalmological service or procedure

SPECIAL OTORHINOLARYNGOLOGIC SERVICES

Otorhinolaryngology is the study and treatment of diseases of the head and neck, including the ears, nose and throat. Diagnostic or treatment procedures usually included in a comprehensive otorhinolaryngologic evaluation or office visit, are reported as an integrated medical service, using CPT evaluation and management service codes.

Coding Rules

1.   *Component procedures, such as otoscopy, rhinoscopy, tuning fork test, which may be provided as part of a comprehensive service are not reported separately.*

2.   *Special otorhinolaryngologic diagnostic or treatment services not usually included in a comprehensive otorhinolaryngologic evaluation or office visit are reported separately.*

3.   *All otorhinolaryngologic services include medical diagnostic evaluation. Technical procedures, which may or may not be performed by the physician*

● New Code   ▲ Revised Code   + Add-On Code   ⊘ Modifier -51 Exempt

personally, are often part of the service, but should not be mistaken to constitute the service itself.

(For laryngoscopy with stroboscopy, use 31579)

92502   Otolaryngologic examination under general anesthesia

92504   Binocular microscopy (separate diagnostic procedure)

92506   Evaluation of speech, language, voice, communication, auditory processing, and/or aural rehabilitation status

92507   Treatment of speech, language, voice, communication, and/or auditory processing disorder (includes aural rehabilitation); individual

92508   group, two or more individuals

92510   Aural rehabilitation following cochlear implant (includes evaluation of aural rehabilitation status and hearing, therapeutic services) with or without speech processor programming

92511   Nasopharyngoscopy with endoscope (separate procedure)

92512   Nasal function studies (eg, rhinomanometry)

92516   Facial nerve function studies (eg, electroneuronography)

92520   Laryngeal function studies

(**92525**   deleted 2003 edition. To report, see 92610-92611 for specific evaluation)

92526   Treatment of swallowing dysfunction and/or oral function for feeding

VESTIBULAR FUNCTION TESTS, WITH OBSERVATION AND EVALUATION BY PHYSICIAN, WITHOUT ELECTRICAL RECORDING

92531   Spontaneous nystagmus, including gaze

92532   Positional nystagmus test

92533   Caloric vestibular test, each irrigation (binaural, bithermal stimulation constitutes four tests)

813

 Separate Procedure   Unlisted Procedure   CCI Comp. Code   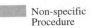 Non-specific Procedure

92534   Optokinetic nystagmus test

VESTIBULAR FUNCTION TESTS, WITH RECORDING (eg, ENG, PENG), AND MEDICAL DIAGNOSTIC EVALUATION

92541   Spontaneous nystagmus test, including gaze and fixation nystagmus, with recording

92542   Positional nystagmus test, minimum of 4 positions, with recording

92543   Caloric vestibular test, each irrigation (binaural, bithermal stimulation constitutes four tests), with recording

92544   Optokinetic nystagmus test, bidirectional, foveal or peripheral stimulation, with recording

92545   Oscillating tracking test, with recording

92546   Sinusoidal vertical axis rotational testing

+ 92547   Use of vertical electrodes (List separately in addition to code for primary procedure)

(Use 92547 in conjunction with codes 92541-92546)

(For unlisted vestibular tests, use 92700)

92548   Computerized dynamic posturography

AUDIOLOGIC FUNCTION TESTS WITH MEDICAL DIAGNOSTIC EVALUATION

(For evaluation of speech, language and/or hearing problems through observation and assessment of performance, use 92506)

92551   Screening test, pure tone, air only

92552   Pure tone audiometry (threshold); air only

92553   air and bone

92555   Speech audiometry threshold;

92556   with speech recognition

● New Code   ▲ Revised Code   + Add-On Code   ⊘ Modifier -51 Exempt

92557 Comprehensive audiometry threshold evaluation and speech recognition (92553 and 92556 combined)

(For hearing aid evaluation and selection, see 92590-92595)

92559 Audiometric testing of groups

92560 Bekesy audiometry; screening

92561 diagnostic

92562 Loudness balance test, alternate binaural or monaural

92563 Tone decay test

92564 Short increment sensitivity index (SISI)

92565 Stenger test, pure tone

92567 Tympanometry (impedance testing)

92568 Acoustic reflex testing

92569 Acoustic reflex decay test

92571 Filtered speech test

92572 Staggered spondaic word test

92573 Lombard test

92575 Sensorineural acuity level test

92576 Synthetic sentence identification test

92577 Stenger test, speech

92579 Visual reinforcement audiometry (VRA)

92582 Conditioning play audiometry

92583 Select picture audiometry

92584 Electrocochleography

 Separate Procedure   Unlisted Procedure   CCI Comp. Code   Non-specific Procedure

92585   Auditory evoked potentials for evoked response audiometry and/or testing of the central nervous system; comprehensive

92586   limited

92587   Evoked otoacoustic emissions; limited (single stimulus level, either transient or distortion products)

92588   comprehensive or diagnostic evaluation (comparison of transient and/or distortion product otoacoustic emissions at multiple levels and frequencies)

92589   Central auditory function test(s) (specify)

92590   Hearing aid examination and selection; monaural

92591   binaural

92592   Hearing aid check; monaural

92593   binaural

92594   Electroacoustic evaluation for hearing aid; monaural

92595   binaural

92596   Ear protector attenuation measurements

92597   Evaluation for use and/or fitting of voice prosthetic device to supplement oral speech

       (To report augmentative and alternative communication device services, see 92605, 92607, 92608)

(92598   deleted 2003 edition)

(92599   deleted 2003 edition. To report use 92700)

EVALUATIVE AND THERAPEUTIC SERVICES

       (For placement of cochlear implant, use 69930)

92601   Diagnostic analysis of cochlear implant, patient under 7 years of age; with programming

92602   subsequent reprogramming

● New Code	▲ Revised Code	+ Add-On Code	⊘ Modifier -51 Exempt

(Do not report 92602 in addition to 92601)

(For aural rehabilitation services following cochlear implant, including evaluation of rehabilitation status, use 92507)

92603 Diagnostic analysis of cochlear implant, age 7 years or older; with programming

92604 subsequent reprogramming

(Do not report 92604 in addition to 92603)

92605 Evaluation for prescription of non-speech-generating augmentative and alternative communication device

92606 Therapeutic service(s) for the use of non-speech-generating device, including programming and modification

92607 Evaluation for prescription for speech-generating augmentative and alternative communication device, face-to-face with the patient; first hour

(For evaluation for prescription of a non-speech-generating device, use 92605)

+ 92608 each additional 30 minutes (List separately in addition to code for primary procedure)

(Use 92608 in conjunction with 92607)

92609 Therapeutic services for the use of speech-generating device, including programming and modification

(For therapeutic service(s) for the use of a non-speech-generating device, use 92606)

92610 Evaluation of oral and pharyngeal swallowing function

(For motion fluoroscopic evaluation of swallowing function, use 92611)

(For flexible endoscopic examination, use 92612-92617)

92611 Motion fluoroscopic evaluation of swallowing function by cine or video recording

(For radiological supervision and interpretation, use 74230)

(For evaluation of oral and pharyngeal swallowing function, use 92610)

817

 Separate Procedure   Unlisted Procedure   CCI Comp. Code   Non-specific Procedure

(For flexible fiberoptic diagnostic laryngoscopy, use 31575. Do not report 31575 in conjunction with 92612-92617)

92612 Flexible fiberoptic endoscopic evaluation of swallowing by cine or video recording;

(If flexible fiberoptic or endoscopic evaluation of swallowing is performed without cine or video recording, use 92700)

92613 physician interpretation and report only

(To report an evaluation of oral and pharyngeal swallowing function, use 92610)

(To report motion fluoroscopic evaluation of swallowing function, use 92611)

92614 Flexible fiberoptic endoscopic evaluation, laryngeal sensory testing by cine or video recording;

(If flexible fiberoptic or endoscopic evaluation of swallowing is performed without cine or video recording, use 92700)

92615 physician interpretation and report only

92616 Flexible fiberoptic endoscopic evaluation of swallowing and laryngeal sensory testing by cine or video recording;

(If flexible fiberoptic or endoscopic evaluation of swallowing is performed without cine or video recording, use 92700)

92617 physician interpretation and report only

OTHER PROCEDURES

92700 Unlisted otorhinolaryngological service or procedure

CARDIOVASCULAR

Cardiovascular services refers to the study and treatment of diseases of the heart and vascular (arteries and veins) system. Cardiovascular services CPT codes are used to report therapeutic services such as cardiopulmonary resuscitation (CPR), cardioversion and percutaneous transluminal coronary angioplasty (PTCA) and diagnostic procedures such as electrocardiography, echocardiography and cardiac catheterization.

818

● New Code   ▲ Revised Code   + Add-On Code   ⊘ Modifier -51 Exempt

Coding Rules

1. *Cardiovascular services are usually performed in addition to evaluation and management services, such as a consultation or visit, and should be reported in addition to the evaluation and management service.*

2. *Many cardiovascular services fall under the Medicare Purchased Diagnostic Services guidelines, therefore reporting should be as instructed by your local Medicare carrier.*

THERAPEUTIC SERVICES

(For non-surgical septal reduction therapy (eg, alcohol ablation), use Category III code 0024T)

92950   Cardiopulmonary resuscitation (eg, in cardiac arrest)

(See also critical care services, 99291, 99292)

92953   Temporary transcutaneous pacing

(For physician direction of ambulance or rescue personnel outside the hospital, use 99288)

92960   Cardioversion, elective, electrical conversion of arrhythmia; external

92961   internal (separate procedure)

(Do not report 92961 in addition to codes 93662, 93618-93624, 93631, 93640-93642, 93650-93652, 93741-93744)

92970   Cardioassist-method of circulatory assist; internal

92971   external

(For balloon atrial-septostomy, use 92992)

(For placement of catheters for use in circulatory assist devices such as intra-aortic balloon pump, use 33970)

+ 92973   Percutaneous transluminal coronary thrombectomy (List separately in addition to code for primary procedure)

(Use 92973 in conjunction with codes 92980, 92982)

+ 92974   Transcatheter placement of radiation delivery device for subsequent coronary intravascular brachytherapy (List separately in addition to code for primary procedure)

819

 Separate Procedure   Unlisted Procedure   CCI Comp. Code   Non-specific Procedure

(Use 92974 in conjunction with codes 92980, 92982, 92995, 93508)

(For intravascular radioelement application, see 77781-77784)

92975 Thrombolysis, coronary; by intracoronary infusion, including selective coronary angiography

92977 by intravenous infusion

(For thrombolysis of vessels other than coronary, see 37201, 75896)

(For cerebral thrombolysis, use 37195)

+ **92978** Intravascular ultrasound (coronary vessel or graft) during diagnostic evaluation and/or therapeutic intervention including imaging supervision, interpretation and report; initial vessel (List separately in addition to code for primary procedure)

+ **92979** each additional vessel (List separately in addition to code for primary procedure)

(Use 92979 in conjunction with code 92978)

(Intravascular ultrasound services include all transducer manipulations and repositioning within the specific vessel being examined, both before and after therapeutic intervention (eg, stent placement)

92980 Transcatheter placement of an intracoronary stent(s), percutaneous, with or without other therapeutic intervention, any method; single vessel

+ **92981** each additional vessel (List separately in addition to code for primary procedure)

(Use 92981 in conjunction with code 92980)

(To report additional vessels treated by angioplasty or atherectomy only during the same session, see 92984, 92996)

(To report transcatheter placement of radiation delivery device for coronary intravascular brachytherapy, use 92974)

(For intravascular radioelement application, see 77781-77784)

92982 Percutaneous transluminal coronary balloon angioplasty; single vessel

| ● | New Code | ▲ | Revised Code | + | Add-On Code | ⊘ | Modifier -51 Exempt |

+ 92984   each additional vessel (List separately in addition to code for primary procedure)

(Use 92984 in conjunction with codes 92980, 92982, 92995)

(For stent placement following completion of angioplasty or atherectomy, see 92980, 92981)

(To report transcatheter placement of radiation delivery device for coronary intravascular brachytherapy, use 92974)

(For intravascular radioelement application, see 77781-77784)

92986   Percutaneous balloon valvuloplasty; aortic valve

92987   mitral valve

92990   pulmonary valve

92992   Atrial septectomy or septostomy; transvenous method, balloon (eg, Rashkind type) (includes cardiac catheterization)

92993   blade method (Park septostomy) (includes cardiac catheterization)

92995   Percutaneous transluminal coronary atherectomy, by mechanical or other method, with or without balloon angioplasty; single vessel

+ 92996   each additional vessel (List separately in addition to code for primary procedure)

(Use 92996 in conjunction with code(s) 92980, 92982, 92995)

(For stent placement following completion of angioplasty or atherectomy, see 92980, 92981)

(To report additional vessels treated by angioplasty only during the same session, use 92984)

92997   Percutaneous transluminal pulmonary artery balloon angioplasty; single vessel

+ 92998   each additional vessel (List separately in addition to code for primary procedure)

(Use 92998 in conjunction with code 92997)

821

 Separate Procedure   Unlisted Procedure   CCI Comp. Code   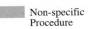 Non-specific Procedure

CARDIOGRAPHY

(For echocardiography, see 93303-93350)

93000 Electrocardiogram, routine ECG with at least 12 leads; with interpretation and report

93005 tracing only, without interpretation and report

93010 interpretation and report only

(For ECG monitoring, see 99354-99360)

93012 Telephonic transmission of post-symptom electrocardiogram rhythm strip(s), 24-hour attended monitoring, per 30 day period of time; tracing only

93014 physician review with interpretation and report only

93015 Cardiovascular stress test using maximal or submaximal treadmill or bicycle exercise, continuous electrocardiographic monitoring, and/or pharmacological stress; with physician supervision, with interpretation and report

93016 physician supervision only, without interpretation and report

93017 tracing only, without interpretation and report

93018 interpretation and report only

93024 Ergonovine provocation test

93025 Microvolt T-wave alternans for assessment of ventricular arrhythmias

93040 Rhythm ECG, one to three leads; with interpretation and report

93041 tracing only without interpretation and report

93042 interpretation and report only

93224 Electrocardiographic monitoring for 24 hours by continuous original ECG waveform recording and storage, with visual superimposition scanning; includes recording, scanning analysis with report, physician review and interpretation

93225 recording (includes hook-up, recording, and disconnection)

822

● New Code   ▲ Revised Code   ✚ Add-On Code   ⊘ Modifier -51 Exempt

93226   scanning analysis with report

93227   physician review and interpretation

93230   Electrocardiographic monitoring for 24 hours by continuous original ECG waveform recording and storage without superimposition scanning utilizing a device capable of producing a full miniaturized printout; includes recording, microprocessor-based analysis with report, physician review and interpretation

93231   recording (includes hook-up, recording, and disconnection)

93232   microprocessor-based analysis with report

93233   physician review and interpretation

93235   Electrocardiographic monitoring for 24 hours by continuous computerized monitoring and non-continuous recording, and real-time data analysis utilizing a device capable of producing intermittent full-sized waveform tracings, possibly patient activated; includes monitoring and real-time data analysis with report, physician review and interpretation

93236   monitoring and real-time data analysis with report

93237   physician review and interpretation

93268   Patient demand single or multiple event recording with presymptom memory loop, 24-hour attended monitoring, per 30 day period of time; includes transmission, physician review and interpretation

93270   recording (includes hook-up, recording, and disconnection)

93271   monitoring, receipt of transmissions, and analysis

93272   physician review and interpretation only

(For postsymptom recording, see 93012, 93014)

(For implanted patient activated cardiac event recording, see 33282, 93727)

93278   Signal-averaged electrocardiography (SAECG), with or without ECG

823

 Separate Procedure   Unlisted Procedure    CCI Comp. Code   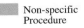 Non-specific Procedure

(For interpretation and report only, use 93278 with modifier -26)

(For unlisted cardiographic procedure, use 93799)

ECHOCARDIOGRAPHY

(For fetal echocardiography, see 76825-76828)

93303   Transthoracic echocardiography for congenital cardiac anomalies; complete

93304   follow-up or limited study

93307   Echocardiography, transthoracic, real-time with image documentation (2D) with or without M-mode recording; complete

93308   follow-up or limited study

93312   Echocardiography, transesophageal, real time with image documentation (2D) (with or without M-mode recording); including probe placement, image acquisition, interpretation and report

93313   placement of transesophageal probe only

93314   image acquisition, interpretation and report only

93315   Transesophageal echocardiography for congenital cardiac anomalies; including probe placement, image acquisition, interpretation and report

93316   placement of transesophageal probe only

93317   image acquisition, interpretation and report only

93318   Echocardiography, transesophageal (TEE) for monitoring purposes, including probe placement, real time 2-dimensional image acquisition and interpretation leading to ongoing (continuous) assessment of (dynamically changing) cardiac pumping function and to therapeutic measures on an immediate time basis

+ 93320   Doppler echocardiography, pulsed wave and/or continuous wave with spectral display (List separately in addition to codes for echocardiographic imaging); complete

---

824   ● New Code   ▲ Revised Code   **+** Add-On Code   ⊘ Modifier -51 Exempt

(Use 93320 in conjunction with codes 93303, 93304, 93307, 93308, 93312, 93314, 93315, 93317, 93350)

+ **93321** follow-up or limited study (List separately in addition to codes for echocardiographic imaging)

(Use 93321 in conjunction with codes 93303, 93304, 93307, 93308, 93312, 93314, 93315, 93317, 93350)

+ **93325** Doppler echocardiography color flow velocity mapping (List separately in addition to codes for echocardiography)

(Use 93325 in conjunction with codes 76825, 76826, 76827, 76828, 93303, 93304, 93307, 93308, 93312, 93314, 93315, 93317, 93320, 93321, 93350)

93350 Echocardiography, transthoracic, real-time with image documentation (2D), with or without M-mode recording, during rest and cardiovascular stress test using treadmill, bicycle exercise and/or pharmacologically induced stress, with interpretation and report

(The appropriate stress testing code from the 93015-93018 series should be reported in addition to 93350 to capture the exercise stress portion of the study)

CARDIAC CATHETERIZATION

⊘ **93501** Right heart catheterization

(For bundle of His recording, use 93600)

⊘ **93503** Insertion and placement of flow directed catheter (eg, Swan-Ganz) for monitoring purposes

(For subsequent monitoring, see 99356-99357)

⊘ **93505** Endomyocardial biopsy

⊘ **93508** Catheter placement in coronary artery(s), arterial coronary conduit(s), and/or venous coronary bypass graft(s) for coronary angiography without concomitant left heart catheterization

(93508 is to be used only when left heart catheterization 93510, 93511, 93524, 93526 is not performed)

(93508 is to be used only once per procedure)

(To report transcatheter placement of radiation delivery device for coronary intravascular brachytherapy, use 92974)

825

 Separate Procedure   Unlisted Procedure   CCI Comp. Code   Non-specific Procedure

(For intravascular radioelement application, see 77781-77784)

⊘ **93510** Left heart catheterization, retrograde, from the brachial artery, axillary artery or femoral artery; percutaneous

⊘ **93511** by cutdown

⊘ **93514** Left heart catheterization by left ventricular puncture

⊘ **93524** Combined transseptal and retrograde left heart catheterization

⊘ **93526** Combined right heart catheterization and retrograde left heart catheterization

⊘ **93527** Combined right heart catheterization and transseptal left heart catheterization through intact septum (with or without retrograde left heart catheterization)

⊘ **93528** Combined right heart catheterization with left ventricular puncture (with or without retrograde left heart catheterization)

⊘ **93529** Combined right heart catheterization and left heart catheterization through existing septal opening (with or without retrograde left heart catheterization)

⊘ **93530** Right heart catheterization, for congenital cardiac anomalies

⊘ **93531** Combined right heart catheterization and retrograde left heart catheterization, for congenital cardiac anomalies

⊘ **93532** Combined right heart catheterization and transseptal left heart catheterization through intact septum with or without retrograde left heart catheterization, for congenital cardiac anomalies

⊘ **93533** Combined right heart catheterization and transseptal left heart catheterization through existing septal opening, with or without retrograde left heart catheterization, for congenital cardiac anomalies

(93535 deleted. To report, see 33971)

(93536 deleted 2002 edition. To report, use 33967)

(When injection procedures are performed in conjunction with cardiac catheterization, these services do not include introduction of catheters but do include repositioning of catheters when necessary and use of automatic power injectors. Injection procedures 93539-93545 represent separate identifiable services and may be coded in conjunction with one another

● New Code   ▲ Revised Code   + Add-On Code   ⊘ Modifier -51 Exempt

when appropriate. The technical details of angiography, supervision of filming and processing, interpretation and report are not included. To report imaging supervision, interpretation and report, use 93555 and/or 93556. Modifier -51 should not be appended to 93539-93556)

⊘ **93539** Injection procedure during cardiac catheterization; for selective opacification of arterial conduits (eg, internal mammary), whether native or used for bypass

⊘ **93540** for selective opacification of aortocoronary venous bypass grafts, one or more coronary arteries

⊘ **93541** for pulmonary angiography

⊘ **93542** for selective right ventricular or right atrial angiography

⊘ **93543** for selective left ventricular or left atrial angiography

⊘ **93544** for aortography

⊘ **93545** for selective coronary angiography (injection of radiopaque material may be by hand)

(To report imaging supervision and interpretation, use 93555)

⊘ **93555** Imaging supervision, interpretation and report for injection procedure(s) during cardiac catheterization; ventricular and/or atrial angiography

⊘ **93556** pulmonary angiography, aortography, and/or selective coronary angiography including venous bypass grafts and arterial conduits (whether native or used in bypass)

(Codes 93561 and 93562 are not to be used with cardiac catheterization codes)

93561 Indicator dilution studies such as dye or thermal dilution, including arterial and/or venous catheterization; with cardiac output measurement (separate procedure)

93562 subsequent measurement of cardiac output

(For radioisotope method of cardiac output, see 78472, 78473 or 78481)

827

 Separate Procedure

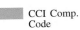 Unlisted Procedure   CCI Comp. Code

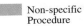 Non-specific Procedure

+ 93571 Intravascular doppler velocity and/or pressure derived coronary flow reserve measurement (coronary vessel or graft) during coronary angiography including pharmacologically induced stress; initial vessel (List separately in addition to code for primary procedure)

+ 93572 each additional vessel (List separately in addition to code for primary procedure)

(Intravascular distal coronary blood flow velocity measurements include all Doppler transducer manipulations and repositioning within the specific vessel being examined, during coronary angiography or therapeutic intervention (eg, angioplasty))

(For unlisted cardiac catheterization procedure, use 93799)

REPAIR OF SEPTAL DEFECT

93580 Percutaneous transcatheter closure of congenital interatrial communication (i.e., fontan fenestration, atrial septal defect) with implant

(Percutaneous transcatheter closure of atrial septal defect includes a right hear catheterization procedure. Code 93580 includes injection of contrast for atrial and ventricular angiograms. Codes 93501, 93529-93533, 93539, 93543, 93555 should not be reported separately in addition to code 93580)

93581 Percutaneous transcatheter closure of a congenital ventricular septal defect with implant

(Percutaneous transcatheter closure of ventricular septal defect (i.e., fontan fenestration) includes a right heart catheterization procedure. Code 93581 includes injection of contrast for atrial and ventricular angiograms. Codes 93501, 93529-93533, 93539, 93543, 93555 should not be reported separately in addition to 93581)

(For echocardiographic services performed in addition to 93580, 93581, see 93303-93317 as appropriate)

INTRACARDIAC ELECTROPHYSIOLOGICAL PROCEDURES/STUDIES

⊘ **93600** Bundle of His recording

⊘ **93602** Intra-atrial recording

⊘ **93603** Right ventricular recording

● New Code   ▲ Revised Code   + Add-On Code   ⊘ Modifier -51 Exempt

(93604, 93606 have been deleted. To report, see 93603, 93609 and 93622 as appropriate)

(93607   deleted 2002 edition. To report, use 93622)

+ **93609**   Intraventricular and/or intra-atrial mapping of tachycardia site(s) with catheter manipulation to record from multiple sites to identify origin of tachycardia (List separately in addition to code for primary procedure)

(Use 93609 in conjunction with codes 93620, 93651, 93652)

(Do not report 93609 in addition to 93613)

⊘ **93610**   Intra-atrial pacing

⊘ **93612**   Intraventricular pacing

(Do not report 93612 in conjunction with codes 93620-93622)

+ **93613**   Intracardiac electrophysiologic 3-dimensional mapping (List separately in addition to code for primary procedure)

(Use 93613 in conjunction with codes 93620, 93651, 93652)

(Do not report 93613 in addition to 93609)

⊘ **93615**   Esophageal recording of atrial electrogram with or without ventricular electrogram(s);

⊘ **93616**   with pacing

⊘ **93618**   Induction of arrhythmia by electrical pacing

(For intracardiac phonocardiogram, use 93799)

⊘ **93619**   Comprehensive electrophysiologic evaluation with right atrial pacing and recording, right ventricular pacing and recording, His bundle recording, including insertion and repositioning of multiple electrode catheters without induction or attempted induction of arrhythmia

(Do not report 93619 in conjunction with codes 93600, 93602, 93610, 93612, 93618 or 93620-93622)

⊘ **93620**   Comprehensive electrophysiologic evaluation including insertion and repositioning of multiple electrode catheters with induction or attempted induction of arrhythmia; with right atrial pacing and recording, right ventricular pacing and recording, His bundle recording

829

 Separate Procedure   Unlisted Procedure   CCI Comp. Code   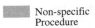 Non-specific Procedure

(Do not report 93620 in conjunction with codes 93600, 93602, 93610, 93612, 93618 or 93619)

+ 93621   with left atrial pacing and recording from coronary sinus or left atrium (List separately in addition to code for primary procedure)

(Use 93621 in conjunction with code 93620)

+ 93622   with left ventricular pacing and recording (List separately in addition to code for primary procedure)

(Use 93622 in conjunction with code 93620)

+ 93623 Programmed stimulation and pacing after intravenous drug infusion (List separately in addition to code for primary procedure)

(Use 93623 in conjunction with codes 93619, 93620)

⊘ 93624 Electrophysiologic follow-up study with pacing and recording to test effectiveness of therapy, including induction or attempted induction of arrhythmia

⊘ 93631 Intra-operative epicardial and endocardial pacing and mapping to localize the site of tachycardia or zone of slow conduction for surgical correction

⊘ 93640 Electrophysiologic evaluation of single or dual chamber pacing cardioverter-defibrillator leads including defibrillation threshold evaluation (induction of arrhythmia, evaluation of sensing and pacing for arrhythmia termination) at time of initial implantation or replacement;

⊘ 93641   with testing of single or dual chamber pacing cardioverter-defibrillator pulse generator

(For subsequent or periodic electronic analysis and/or reprogramming of single or dual chamber pacing cardioverter-defibrillators, see 93642, 93741-93744)

⊘ 93642 Electrophysiologic evaluation of single or dual chamber pacing cardioverter-defibrillator (includes defibrillation threshold evaluation, induction of arrhythmia, evaluation of sensing and pacing for arrhythmia termination, and programming or reprogramming of sensing or therapeutic parameters)

⊘ 93650 Intracardiac catheter ablation of atrioventricular node function, atrioventricular conduction for creation of complete heart block, with or without temporary pacemaker placement

830   ● New
Code   ▲ Revised
Code   + Add-On
Code   ⊘ Modifier -51
Exempt

⊘ **93651**   Intracardiac catheter ablation of arrhythmogenic focus; for treatment of supraventricular tachycardia by ablation of fast or slow atrioventricular pathways, accessory atrioventricular connections or other atrial foci, singly or in combination

⊘ **93652**   for treatment of ventricular tachycardia

⊘ **93660**   Evaluation of cardiovascular function with tilt table evaluation, with continuous ECG monitoring and intermittent blood pressure monitoring, with or without pharmacological intervention

(For testing of autonomic nervous system function, see 95921-95923)

+ **93662**   Intracardiac echocardiography during therapeutic/diagnostic intervention, including imaging supervision and interpretation (List separately in addition to code for primary procedure)

(Use 93662 in conjunction with codes 93621, 93622, 93651 or 93652, as appropriate)

(Do not report 92961 in addition to 93662)

PERIPHERAL ARTERIAL DISEASE REHABILITATION

93668   Peripheral arterial disease (PAD) rehabilitation, per session

OTHER VASCULAR STUDIES

(For arterial cannulization and recording of direct arterial pressure, use 36620)

(For radiographic injection procedures, see 36000-36299)

(For vascular cannulization for hemodialysis, see 36800-36821)

(For chemotherapy for malignant disease, see 96408-96549)

(For penile plethysmography, use 54240)

93701   Bioimpedance, thoracic, electrical

93720   Plethysmography, total body; with interpretation and report

93721   tracing only, without interpretation and report

93722   interpretation and report only

(For regional plethysmography, see 93875-93931)

831

	Separate Procedure		Unlisted Procedure		CCI Comp. Code		Non-specific Procedure

93724 Electronic analysis of antitachycardia pacemaker system (includes electrocardiographic recording, programming of device, induction and termination of tachycardia via implanted pacemaker, and interpretation of recordings)

93727 Electronic analysis of implantable loop recorder (ILR) system (includes retrieval of recorded and stored ECG data, physician review and interpretation of retrieved ECG data and reprogramming)

93731 Electronic analysis of dual-chamber pacemaker system (includes evaluation of programmable parameters at rest and during activity where applicable, using electrocardiographic recording and interpretation of recordings at rest and during exercise, analysis of event markers and device response); without reprogramming

93732 with reprogramming

93733 Electronic analysis of dual chamber internal pacemaker system (may include rate, pulse amplitude and duration, configuration of wave form, and/or testing of sensory function of pacemaker), telephonic analysis

93734 Electronic analysis of single chamber pacemaker system (includes evaluation of programmable parameters at rest and during activity where applicable, using electrocardiographic recording and interpretation of recordings at rest and during exercise, analysis of event markers and device response); without reprogramming

93735 with reprogramming

93736 Electronic analysis of single chamber internal pacemaker system (may include rate, pulse amplitude and duration, configuration of wave form, and/or testing of sensory function of pacemaker), telephonic analysis

(93737 deleted 2002 edition. To report, use 93741 or 93743)

(93738 deleted 2002 edition. To report, use 93742 or 93744)

93740 Temperature gradient studies

● New Code ▲ Revised Code + Add-On Code ⊘ Modifier -51 Exempt

93741 Electronic analysis of pacing cardioverter-defibrillator (includes interrogation, evaluation of pulse generator status, evaluation of programmable parameters at rest and during activity where applicable, using electrocardiographic recording and interpretation of recordings at rest and during exercise, analysis of event markers and device response); single chamber, without reprogramming

93742 single chamber, with reprogramming

93743 dual chamber, without reprogramming

93744 dual chamber, with reprogramming

93760 Thermogram; cephalic

93762 peripheral

93770 Determination of venous pressure

(For central venous cannulization see 36555-36556, 36500)

93784 Ambulatory blood pressure monitoring, utilizing a system such as magnetic tape and/or computer disk, for 24 hours or longer; including recording, scanning analysis, interpretation and report

93786 recording only

93788 scanning analysis with report

93790 physician review with interpretation and report

OTHER PROCEDURES

93797 Physician services for outpatient cardiac rehabilitation; without continuous ECG monitoring (per session)

93798 with continuous ECG monitoring (per session)

93799 Unlisted cardiovascular service or procedure

Separate Procedure	Unlisted Procedure	CCI Comp. Code	Non-specific Procedure

NON-INVASIVE VASCULAR DIAGNOSTIC STUDIES

Vascular studies refers to diagnostic procedures performed to determine blood flow and/or the condition of arteries and/or veins. Vascular studies include patient care required to perform the studies, supervision of the studies and interpretation of the study results with copies for patient records of hard copy output with analysis of all data, including bi-directional vascular flow or imaging when provided.

The use of a simple hand-held or other Doppler device that does not produce hard copy output, or that produces a record that does not permit analysis of bi-directional vascular flow, is considered to be part of the physical examination of the vascular system and is not reported separately. To report unilateral non-invasive diagnostic studies, add modifier -52 to the basic code.

A Duplex Scan is defined as "An ultrasonic scanning procedure with display of both two-dimensional structure and motion with time and Doppler ultrasonic signal documentation with spectral analysis and/or color flow velocity mapping or imaging.

Coding Rules

1. *Non-invasive vascular studies are usually performed in addition to evaluation and management service, such as a consultation or visit, and should be reported separately in addition to the evaluation and management service.*

2. *All of the non-invasive vascular services fall under the Medicare Purchased Diagnostic Services guidelines; therefore, reporting should be as instructed by your local Medicare carrier.*

CEREBROVASCULAR ARTERIAL STUDIES

93875 Non-invasive physiologic studies of extracranial arteries, complete bilateral study (eg, periorbital flow direction with arterial compression, ocular pneumoplethysmography, Doppler ultrasound spectral analysis)

93880 Duplex scan of extracranial arteries; complete bilateral study

93882 unilateral or limited study

93886 Transcranial Doppler study of the intracranial arteries; complete study

93888 limited study

EXTREMITY ARTERIAL STUDIES (INCLUDING DIGITS)

93922 Non-invasive physiologic studies of upper or lower extremity arteries, single level, bilateral (eg, ankle/brachial indices, Doppler waveform analysis, volume plethysmography, transcutaneous oxygen tension measurement)

93923 Non-invasive physiologic studies of upper or lower extremity arteries, multiple levels or with provocative functional maneuvers, complete bilateral study (eg, segmental blood pressure measurements, segmental Doppler waveform analysis, segmental volume plethysmography, segmental transcutaneous oxygen tension measurements, measurements with postural provocative tests, measurements with reactive hyperemia)

93924 Non-invasive physiologic studies of lower extremity arteries, at rest and following treadmill stress testing, complete bilateral study

93925 Duplex scan of lower extremity arteries or arterial bypass grafts; complete bilateral study

93926 unilateral or limited study

93930 Duplex scan of upper extremity arteries or arterial bypass grafts; complete bilateral study

93931 unilateral or limited study

EXTREMITY VENOUS STUDIES (INCLUDING DIGITS)

93965 Non-invasive physiologic studies of extremity veins, complete bilateral study (eg, Doppler waveform analysis with responses to compression and other maneuvers, phleborheography, impedance plethysmography)

93970 Duplex scan of extremity veins including responses to compression and other maneuvers; complete bilateral study

93971 unilateral or limited study

VISCERAL AND PENILE VASCULAR STUDIES

93975 Duplex scan of arterial inflow and venous outflow of abdominal, pelvic, scrotal contents and/or retroperitoneal organs; complete study

835

Separate Procedure | Unlisted Procedure | CCI Comp. Code | Non-specific Procedure

| 93976 | limited study |

| 93978 | Duplex scan of aorta, inferior vena cava, iliac vasculature, or bypass grafts; complete study |

| **93979** | unilateral or limited study |

| 93980 | Duplex scan of arterial inflow and venous outflow of penile vessels; complete study |

| **93981** | follow-up or limited study |

EXTREMITY ARTERIAL-VENOUS STUDIES

| 93990 | Duplex scan of hemodialysis access (including arterial inflow, body of access and venous outflow) |

(For measurement of hemodialysis access flow using indicator dilution methods, use 90940)

PULMONARY

Pulmonary disease is concerned with diseases of the lungs and airways. The Pulmonologist diagnoses and treats pneumonia, cancer, pleurisy, asthma, occupational diseases, bronchitis, sleep disorders, emphysema, and other complex disorders of the lungs. Pulmonologists test lung functions in many ways, endoscope the bronchial airways and prescribe and monitor mechanical assistance to ventilation. Many pulmonary disease physicians are also expert in critical care.

Pulmonary services refer to diagnostic procedures performed to determine air flow, blood gases, and the condition of the lungs and respiratory system. Pulmonary services include the laboratory procedure(s), interpretation, and physician's services (except surgical and anesthesia services) unless otherwise stated. It is common for pulmonologists to provide interpretation services only, under contract to medical facilities.

CODING RULES

1. *Pulmonary services are usually performed in addition to evaluation and management service, such as a consultation or visit, and should be coded separately in addition to the evaluation and management service.*

2. *When reporting physician interpretation only for pulmonary services include the modifier -26 "Professional Component".*

| ● New Code | ▲ Revised Code | + Add-On Code | ⊘ Modifier -51 Exempt |

3. *Most of the pulmonary services fall under the Medicare Purchased Diagnostic Services guidelines; therefore reporting should be as instructed by your local Medicare carrier.*

94010 Spirometry, including graphic record, total and timed vital capacity, expiratory flow rate measurement(s), with or without maximal voluntary ventilation

94014 Patient-initiated spirometric recording per 30-day period of time; includes reinforced education, transmission of spirometric tracing, data capture, analysis of transmitted data, periodic recalibration and physician review and interpretation

94015 recording (includes hook-up, reinforced education, data transmission, data capture, trend analysis, and periodic recalibration)

94016 physician review and interpretation only

94060 Bronchospasm evaluation: spirometry as in 94010, before and after bronchodilator (aerosol or parenteral)

(For prolonged exercise test for bronchospasm with pre- and post-spirometry, use 94620)

94070 Prolonged postexposure evaluation of bronchospasm with multiple spirometric determinations after antigen, cold air, methacholine or other chemical agent, with subsequent spirometrics

94150 Vital capacity, total (separate procedure)

94200 Maximum breathing capacity, maximal voluntary ventilation

94240 Functional residual capacity or residual volume: helium method, nitrogen open circuit method, or other method

94250 Expired gas collection, quantitative, single procedure (separate procedure)

94260 Thoracic gas volume

(For plethysmography, see 93720-93722)

94350 Determination of maldistribution of inspired gas: multiple breath nitrogen washout curve including alveolar nitrogen or helium equilibration time

837

 Separate Procedure Unlisted Procedure CCI Comp. Code Non-specific Procedure

94360 Determination of resistance to airflow, oscillatory or plethysmographic methods

94370 Determination of airway closing volume, single breath tests

94375 Respiratory flow volume loop

94400 Breathing response to CO2 (CO2 response curve)

94450 Breathing response to hypoxia (hypoxia response curve)

94620 Pulmonary stress testing; simple (eg, prolonged exercise test for bronchospasm with pre- and post-spirometry)

94621 complex (including measurements of CO2 production, O2 uptake, and electrocardiographic recordings)

94640 Pressurized or nonpressurized inhalation treatment for acute airway obstruction or for sputum induction for diagnostic purposes (eg., with an aerosol generator, nebulizer, metered dose inhaler or intermittent positive pressure breathing (IPPB) device)

(For more than one inhalation treatment performed on the same date, append modifier -76)

94642 Aerosol inhalation of pentamidine for pneumocystis carinii pneumonia treatment or prophylaxis

(94650   deleted 2003 edition)

(94651   deleted 2003 edition)

(94652   deleted 2003 edition)

94656 Ventilation assist and management, initiation of pressure or volume preset ventilators for assisted or controlled breathing; first day

94657 subsequent days

94660 Continuous positive airway pressure ventilation (CPAP), initiation and management

94662 Continuous negative pressure ventilation (CNP), initiation and management

94664   Demonstration and/or evaluation of patient utilization of an aerosol generator, nebulizer, metered dose inhaler or IPPB device

(94664 can be reported one time only per day of service)

(**94665**   deleted 2003 edition)

94667   Manipulation chest wall, such as cupping, percussing, and vibration to facilitate lung function; initial demonstration and/or evaluation

94668   subsequent

94680   Oxygen uptake, expired gas analysis; rest and exercise, direct, simple

94681   including CO2 output, percentage oxygen extracted

94690   rest, indirect (separate procedure)

(For single arterial puncture, use 36600)

94720   Carbon monoxide diffusing capacity (eg, single breath, steady state)

94725   Membrane diffusion capacity

94750   Pulmonary compliance study (eg, plethysmography, volume and pressure measurements)

94760   Noninvasive ear or pulse oximetry for oxygen saturation; single determination

(For blood gases, see 82803-82810)

94761   multiple determinations (eg, during exercise)

94762   by continuous overnight monitoring (separate procedure)

94770   Carbon dioxide, expired gas determination by infrared analyzer

(For bronchoscopy, see 31622-31656)

(For placement of flow directed catheter, use 93503)

(For venipuncture, use 36410)

(For central venous catheter placement, see 36488-36491)

839

	Separate Procedure		Unlisted Procedure		CCI Comp. Code		Non-specific Procedure

(For arterial puncture, use 36600)

(For arterial catheterization, use 36620)

(For thoracentesis, use 32000)

(For phlebotomy, therapeutic, use 99195)

(For lung biopsy, needle, use 32405)

(For intubation, orotracheal or nasotracheal, use 31500)

94772   Circadian respiratory pattern recording (pediatric pneumogram), 12 to 24 hour continuous recording, infant

(Separate procedure codes for electromyograms, EEG, ECG, and recordings of respiration are excluded when 94772 is reported)

94799   Unlisted pulmonary service or procedure

ALLERGY AND CLINICAL IMMUNOLOGY

Allergy and Immunology refers to diagnostic services performed to determine a patient's sensitivity to specific substances, the treatment of patients with allergens by the administration or allergenic extracts, and/or medical conference services.

Coding Rules

1. *Allergy and immunology services are usually performed in addition to evaluation and management service, such as a consultation or visit, and should be reported separately in addition to the evaluation and management service.*

2. *Summary or therapeutic conferences following completion of the diagnostic workup, including discussion, avoidance, elimination, symptomatic treatment and immunotherapy should be reported with evaluation and management service codes 99241-99245.*

3. *Prolonged conferences should be reported with evaluation and management Case Management CPT codes.*

ALLERGY TESTING

95004   Percutaneous tests (scratch, puncture, prick) with allergenic extracts, immediate type reaction, specify number of tests

● New Code   ▲ Revised Code   + Add-On Code   ⊘ Modifier -51 Exempt

95010 Percutaneous tests (scratch, puncture, prick) sequential and incremental, with drugs, biologicals or venoms, immediate type reaction, specify number of tests

95015 Intracutaneous (intradermal) tests, sequential and incremental, with drugs, biologicals, or venoms, immediate type reaction, specify number of tests

95024 Intracutaneous (intradermal) tests with allergenic extracts, immediate type reaction, specify number of tests

95027 Intracutaneous (intradermal) tests, sequential and incremental, with allergenic extracts for airborne allergens, immediate type reaction, specify number of tests

95028 Intracutaneous (intradermal) tests with allergenic extracts, delayed type reaction, including reading, specify number of tests

95044 Patch or application test(s) (specify number of tests)

95052 Photo patch test(s) (specify number of tests)

95056 Photo tests

95060 Ophthalmic mucous membrane tests

95065 Direct nasal mucous membrane test

95070 Inhalation bronchial challenge testing (not including necessary pulmonary function tests); with histamine, methacholine, or similar compounds

95071 with antigens or gases, specify

(For pulmonary function tests, see 94060, 94070)

95075 Ingestion challenge test (sequential and incremental ingestion of test items, eg, food, drug or other substance such as metabisulfite)

95078 Provocative testing (eg, Rinkel test)

(For allergy laboratory tests, see 86000-86999)

(For intravenous therapy, for severe or intractable allergic disease, see 90780, 90781, 90784)

841

 Separate Procedure

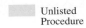 Unlisted Procedure

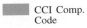 CCI Comp. Code

 Non-specific Procedure

ALLERGEN IMMUNOTHERAPY

Allergen immunotherapy CPT codes include the professional services necessary for allergen immunotherapy. Evaluation and management service codes may be reported in addition to allergen immunotherapy if other identifiable services are provided at the same time.

95115 Professional services for allergen immunotherapy not including provision of allergenic extracts; single injection

95117 two or more injections

95120 Professional services for allergen immunotherapy in prescribing physicians office or institution, including provision of allergenic extract; single injection

95125 two or more injections

95130 single stinging insect venom

95131 two stinging insect venoms

95132 three stinging insect venoms

95133 four stinging insect venoms

95134 five stinging insect venoms

95144 Professional services for the supervision of preparation and provision of antigens for allergen immunotherapy; single dose vials(s) (specify number of vials)

(A single dose vial contains a single dose of antigen administered in one injection)

95145 Professional services for the supervision of preparation and provision of antigens for allergen immunotherapy (specify number of doses); single stinging insect venom

95146 two single stinging insect venoms

95147 three single stinging insect venoms

95148 four single stinging insect venoms

95149 five single stinging insect venoms

●	New Code	▲	Revised Code	+	Add-On Code	⊘	Modifier -51 Exempt

95165 Professional services for the supervision of preparation and provision of antigens for allergen immunotherapy; single or multiple antigens (specify number of doses)

95170 whole body extract of biting insect or other arthropod (specify number of doses)

(For allergy immunotherapy reporting, a dose is the amount of antigen(s) administered in a single injection from a multiple dose vial)

95180 Rapid desensitization procedure, each hour (eg, insulin, penicillin, equine serum)

95199 Unlisted allergy/clinical immunologic service or procedure

(For skin testing of bacterial, viral, fungal extracts, see 95028, 86485-86586)

(For special reports on allergy patients, use 99080)

(For testing procedures such as radioallergosorbent testing (RAST), rat mast cell technique (RMCT), mast cell degranulation test (MCDT), lymphocytic transformation test (LTT), leukocyte histamine release (LHR), migration inhibitory factor test (MIF), transfer factor test (TFT), nitroblue tetrazolium dye test (NTD), see Immunology section in Pathology or use 95199)

ENDOCRINOLOGY

95250 Glucose monitoring for up to 72 hours by continuous recording and storage of glucose values from interstitial tissue fluid via a subcutaneous sensor (includes hook-up, calibration, patient initiation and training, recording, disconnection, downloading with printout of data)

(Do not report 95250 in conjunction with 99091)

(To report physician review, interpretation and written report associated with code 95250, see Evaluation and Management services codes)

Separate Procedure | Unlisted Procedure | CCI Comp. Code | Non-specific Procedure

NEUROLOGY AND NEUROMUSCULAR PROCEDURES

Neurology refers to the study and treatment of the nervous system. Neurology services are usually performed in conjunction with a medical consultation. The consultation should be reported separately using the appropriate evaluation and management consultation code.

Coding Rules

1. *All EEG services listed include the tracing, interpretation and report.*

2. *For interpretation of EEG only, add modifier -26 to the basic procedure code.*

3. *Most of the neurology and neuromuscular procedures fall under the Medicare Purchased Diagnostic Services guidelines; therefore, reporting should be as instructed by your local Medicare carrier.*

> (For repetitive transcranial magnetic stimulation for treatment of clinical depression, use Category III code 0018T)
>
> (Do not report codes 95860-95875 in addition to 96000-96004)

SLEEP TESTING

> (Report with a -52 modifier if less than 6 hours of recording or in other cases of reduced services as appropriate)
>
> (For unattended sleep study, use 95806)

95805   Multiple sleep latency or maintenance of wakefulness testing, recording, analysis and interpretation of physiological measurements of sleep during multiple trials to assess sleepiness

95806   Sleep study, simultaneous recording of ventilation, respiratory effort, ECG or heart rate, and oxygen saturation, unattended by a technologist

95807   Sleep study, simultaneous recording of ventilation, respiratory effort, ECG or heart rate, and oxygen saturation, attended by a technologist

95808   Polysomnography; sleep staging with 1-3 additional parameters of sleep, attended by a technologist

95810   sleep staging with 4 or more additional parameters of sleep, attended by a technologist

● New Code   ▲ Revised Code   + Add-On Code   ⊘ Modifier -51 Exempt

95811   sleep staging with 4 or more additional parameters of sleep, with initiation of continuous positive airway pressure therapy or bilevel ventilation, attended by a technologist

ROUTINE ELECTROENCEPHALOGRAPHY (EEG)

95812   Electroencephalogram (EEG) extended monitoring; 41-60 minutes

95813   greater than one hour

95816   Electroencephalogram (EEG) including recording awake and drowsy

95819   including recording awake and asleep

95822   recording in coma or sleep only

95824   cerebral death evaluation only

95827   all night recording

(For 24-hour EEG monitoring, see 95950-95953 or 95956)

(For EEG during nonintracranial surgery, use 95955)

(For Wada test, use 95958)

(For digital analysis of EEG, use 95957)

95829   Electrocorticogram at surgery (separate procedure)

95830   Insertion by physician of sphenoidal electrodes for electroencephalographic (EEG) recording

MUSCLE AND RANGE OF MOTION TESTING

95831   Muscle testing, manual (separate procedure) with report; extremity (excluding hand) or trunk

95832   hand, with or without comparison with normal side

95833   total evaluation of body, excluding hands

95834   total evaluation of body, including hands

845

Separate Procedure	Unlisted Procedure	CCI Comp. Code	Non-specific Procedure

95851 Range of motion measurements and report (separate procedure); each extremity (excluding hand) or each trunk section (spine)

95852 hand, with or without comparison with normal side

95857 Tensilon test for myasthenia gravis;

95858 with electromyographic recording

ELECTROMYOGRAPHY AND NERVE CONDUCTION TESTS

95860 Needle electromyography; one extremity with or without related paraspinal areas

95861 two extremities with or without related paraspinal areas

(For dynamic electromyography performed during motion analysis studies, see 96002-96003)

95863 three extremities with or without related paraspinal areas

95864 four extremities with or without related paraspinal areas

95867 cranial nerve supplied muscle(s), unilateral

95868 cranial nerve supplied muscles, bilateral

95869 thoracic paraspinal muscles (excluding T1 or T12)

95870 limited study of muscles in one extremity or non-limb (axial) muscles (unilateral or bilateral), other than thoracic paraspinal, cranial nerve supplied muscles, or sphincters

(To report a complete study of the extremities, see 95860-95864)

(For anal or urethral sphincter, detrusor, urethra, perineum musculature, see 51785-51792)

(For eye muscles, use 92265)

95872 Needle electromyography using single fiber electrode, with quantitative measurement of jitter, blocking and/or fiber density, any/all sites of each muscle studied

● New Code   ▲ Revised Code   + Add-On Code   ⊘ Modifier -51 Exempt

95875 Ischemic limb exercise test with serial specimen(s) acquisition for muscle(s) metabolite(s)

⊘ **95900** Nerve conduction, amplitude and latency/velocity study, each nerve; motor, without F-wave study

⊘ **95903** motor, with F-wave study

⊘ **95904** sensory

(Report 95900, 95903, and/or 95904 only once when multiple sites on the same nerve are stimulated or recorded)

INTRAOPERATIVE NEUROSPHYSIOLOGY

+ 95920 Intraoperative neurophysiology testing, per hour (List separately in addition to code for primary procedure)

(Use code 95920 in conjunction with the study performed, 92585, 95822, 95860, 95861, 95867, 95868, 95900, 95904, 95925, 95926, 95927, 95930, 95933, 95934, 95936, 95937)

(Code 95920 describes ongoing electrophysiologic testing and monitoring performed during surgical procedures. Code 95920 is reported per hour of service, and includes only the ongoing electrophysiologic monitoring time distinct from performance of specific type(s) of baseline electrophysiologic study(ies) (95860, 95861, 95867, 95868, 95900, 95904, 95933, 95934, 95936, 95937) or interpretation of specific type(s) of baseline electrophysiologic study(ies) (92585, 95822, 95925, 95926, 95927, 95930). The time spent performing or interpreting the baseline electrophysiologic study(ies) should not be counted as intraoperative monitoring, but represents separately reportable procedures. Code 95920 should be used once per hour even if multiple electrophysiologic studies are performed. The baseline electrophysiologic study(ies) should be used once per operative session.)

(For electrocorticography, use 95829)

(For intraoperative EEG during nonintracranial surgery, use 95955)

(For intraoperative functional cortical or subcortical mapping, see 95961-95962)

(For intraoperative neurostimulator programming and analysis, see 95970-95975)

Separate Procedure   Unlisted Procedure   CCI Comp. Code   Non-specific Procedure

AUTONOMIC FUNCTION TESTS

95921 Testing of autonomic nervous system function; cardiovagal innervation (parasympathetic function), including two or more of the following: heart rate response to deep breathing with recorded R-R interval, Valsalva ratio, and 30:15 ratio

95922 vasomotor adrenergic innervation (sympathetic adrenergic function), including beat-to-beat blood pressure and R-R interval changes during Valsalva maneuver and at least five minutes of passive tilt

95923 sudomotor, including one or more of the following: quantitative sudomotor axon reflex test (QSART), silastic sweat imprint, thermoregulatory sweat test, and changes in sympathetic skin potential

EVOKED POTENTIALS AND REFLEX TESTS

95925 Short-latency somatosensory evoked potential study, stimulation of any/all peripheral nerves or skin sites, recording from the central nervous system; in upper limbs

95926 in lower limbs

95927 in the trunk or head

(To report a unilateral study, use modifier -52)

(For auditory evoked potentials, use 92585)

95930 Visual evoked potential (VEP) testing central nervous system, checkerboard or flash

95933 Orbicularis oculi (blink) reflex, by electrodiagnostic testing

95934 H-reflex, amplitude and latency study; record gastrocnemius/soleus muscle

95936 record muscle other than gastrocnemius/soleus muscle

(To report a bilateral study, use modifier -50)

95937 Neuromuscular junction testing (repetitive stimulation, paired stimuli), each nerve, any one method

---

848 ● New Code ▲ Revised Code **+** Add-On Code ⊘ Modifier -51 Exempt

SPECIAL EEG TESTS

95950 Monitoring for identification and lateralization of cerebral seizure focus, electroencephalographic (eg, 8 channel EEG) recording and interpretation, each 24 hours

95951 Monitoring for localization of cerebral seizure focus by cable or radio, 16 or more channel telemetry, combined electroencephalographic (EEG) and video recording and interpretation (eg, for presurgical localization), each 24 hours

95953 Monitoring for localization of cerebral seizure focus by computerized portable 16 or more channel EEG, electroencephalographic (EEG) recording and interpretation, each 24 hours

95954 Pharmacological or physical activation requiring physician attendance during EEG recording of activation phase (eg, thiopental activation test)

95955 Electroencephalogram (EEG) during nonintracranial surgery (eg, carotid surgery)

95956 Monitoring for localization of cerebral seizure focus by cable or radio,16 or more channel telemetry, electroencephalographic (EEG) recording and interpretation, each 24 hours

95957 Digital analysis of electroencephalogram (EEG) (eg, for epileptic spike analysis)

95958 Wada activation test for hemispheric function, including electroencephalographic (EEG) monitoring

95961 Functional cortical and subcortical mapping by stimulation and/or recording of electrodes on brain surface, or of depth electrodes, to provoke seizures or identify vital brain structures; initial hour of physician attendance

+ 95962 each additional hour of physician attendance (List separately in addition to code for primary procedure)

(Use 95962 in conjunction with code 95961)

95965 Magnetoencephalography (MEG), recording and analysis; for spontaneous brain magnetic activity (eg, epileptic cerebral cortex localization)

849

| | Separate Procedure | | Unlisted Procedure | | CCI Comp. Code | | Non-specific Procedure |

95966   for evoked magnetic fields, single modality (eg, sensory, motor, language, or visual cortex localization)

+ 95967   for evoked magnetic fields, each additional modality (eg, sensory, motor, language, or visual cortex localization) (List separately in addition to code for primary procedure)

(Use 95967 in conjunction with code 95966)

(For electroencephalography performed in addition to magnetoencephalography, see 95812-95827)

(For somatosensory evoked potentials, auditory evoked potentials, and visual evoked potentials performed in addition to magnetic evoked field responses, see 92585, 95925, 95926, and/or 95930)

(For computerized tomography performed in addition to magnetoencephalography, see 70450-70470, 70496)

(For magnetic resonance imaging performed in addition to magnetoencephalography, see 70551-70553)

NEUROSTIMULATORS, ANALYSIS-PROGRAMMING

(For insertion of neurostimulator pulse generator, see 61885, 63685, 63688, 64590)

(For revision or removal of neurostimulator pulse generator or receiver, see 61888, 63688, 64595)

(For implantation of neurostimulator electrodes, see 61850-61875, 63650-63655, 64553-64580. For revision or removal of neurostimulator electrodes, see 61880, 63660, 64585)

95970   Electronic analysis of implanted neurostimulator pulse generator system (eg, rate, pulse amplitude and duration, configuration of wave form, battery status, electrode selectability, output modulation, cycling, impedance and patient compliance measurements); simple or complex brain, spinal cord, or peripheral (ie, cranial nerve, peripheral nerve, autonomic nerve, neuromuscular) neurostimulator pulse generator/transmitter, without reprogramming

95971   simple brain, spinal cord, or peripheral (ie, peripheral nerve, autonomic nerve, neuromuscular) neurostimulator pulse generator/transmitter, with intraoperative or subsequent programming

● New Code   ▲ Revised Code   + Add-On Code   ⊘ Modifier -51 Exempt

95972   complex brain, spinal cord, or peripheral (except cranial nerve) neurostimulator pulse generator/transmitter, with intraoperative or subsequent programming, first hour

+ 95973   complex brain, spinal cord, or peripheral (except cranial nerve) neurostimulator pulse generator/transmitter, with intraoperative or subsequent programming, each additional 30 minutes after first hour (List separately in addition to code for primary procedure)

(Use 95973 in conjunction with code 95972)

95974   complex cranial nerve neurostimulator pulse generator/transmitter, with intraoperative or subsequent programming, with or without nerve interface testing, first hour

+ 95975   complex cranial nerve neurostimulator pulse generator/transmitter, with intraoperative or subsequent programming, each additional 30 minutes after first hour (List separately in addition to code for primary procedure)

(Use 95975 in conjuntion with code 95974)

OTHER PROCEDURES

95990   Refilling and maintenance of implantable pump or reservoir for drug delivery, spinal (intrathecal, epidural) or brain (intraventricular);

(For analysis and/or reprogramming of implantable infusion pump, see 62367-62368)

(For refill and maintenance of implanted infusion pump or reservoir for systemic drug therapy (eg., chemotherapy or insulin) use 96530)

● **95991**   administered by physician

95999   Unlisted neurological or neuromuscular diagnostic procedure

MOTION ANALYSIS

(For performance of needle electromyography procedures, see 95860-95875)

(For gait training, use 97116)

851

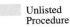 Separate Procedure   Unlisted Procedure   CCI Comp. Code   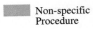 Non-specific Procedure

96000 Comprehensive computer-based motion analysis by video-taping and 3-D kinematics;

96001   with dynamic plantar pressure measurements during walking

96002 Dynamic surface electromyography, during walking or other functional activities, 1-12 muscles

96003 Dynamic fine wire electromyography, during walking or other functional activities, 1 muscle

(Do not report codes 95860-95875 in addition to 96002, 96003)

96004 Physician review and interpretation of comprehensive computer based motion analysis, dynamic plantar pressure measurements, dynamic surface electromyography during walking or other functional activities, and dynamic fine wire electromyography, with written report

CENTRAL NERVOUS SYSTEM ASSESSMENTS/TESTS

(For development of cognitive skills, see 97532, 97533)

96100 Psychological testing (includes psychodiagnostic assessment of personality, psychopathology, emotionality, intellectual abilities, eg, WAIS-R, Rorschach, MMPI) with interpretation and report, per hour

96105 Assessment of aphasia (includes assessment of expressive and receptive speech and language function, language comprehension, speech production ability, reading, spelling, writing, eg, by Boston Diagnostic Aphasia Examination) with interpretation and report, per hour

96110 Developmental testing; limited (eg, Developmental Screening Test II, Early Language Milestone Screen), with interpretation and report

96111   extended (includes assessment of motor, language, social, adaptive and/or cognitive functioning by standardized developmental instruments, eg, Bayley Scales of Infant Development) with interpretation and report, per hour

● New Code   ▲ Revised Code   + Add-On Code   ⊘ Modifier -51 Exempt

96115   Neurobehavioral status exam (clinical assessment of thinking, reasoning and judgment, eg, acquired knowledge, attention, memory, visual spatial abilities, language functions, planning) with interpretation and report, per hour

(For mini-mental status examination performed by a physician, see Evaluation and Management services codes)

96117   Neuropsychological testing battery (eg, Halstead-Reitan, Luria, WAIS-R) with interpretation and report, per hour

HEALTH AND BEHAVIOR ASSESSMENT/INTERVENTION

(For health and behavior assessment and/or intervention performed by a physician, see Evaluation and Management or Preventive Medicine servuces codes)

96150   Health and behavior assessment (eg, health-focused clinical interview, behavioral observations, psychophysicological monitoring, health-oriented questionnaires), each 15 minutes face-to-face with the patient; intial assessment

96151   re-assessment

96152   Health and behavior intervention, each 15 minutes, face-to-face; individual

96153   group (2 or more patients)

96154   family (with the patient present)

96155   family (without the patient present),

CHEMOTHERAPY ADMINISTRATION

Chemotherapy is the process of treating cancer with chemicals formulated to harm or destroy the cancer cells. Chemotherapy agents are administered via intravenous or infusion methods. Chemotherapy administration may be coded when administered by a physician or a qualified assistant under the supervision of a physician, excluding chemotherapy administered by hospital or home health agency personnel.

853

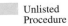 Separate Procedure

 Unlisted Procedure

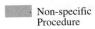 CCI Comp. Code

Non-specific Procedure

Coding Rules

1. *Chemotherapy administration is independent of the patient's office visit.*

2. *The injection procedures may occur independently, or on the same day as an office visit.*

3. *Visit services should be reported using the appropriate evaluation and management service code in addition to the chemotherapy administration code.*

4. *Regional (isolation) chemotherapy perfusion should be reported using existing CPT codes for arterial infusion.*

5. *Placement of the intra-arterial catheter should be reported using the appropriate code from the Cardiovascular Surgery section.*

CHEMOTHERAPY DRUGS

Chemotherapy administration CPT codes do not include provision of the chemotherapy agent. CPT code 96545 is used to report provision of the chemotherapy agent for non-Medicare patients. For Medicare patients, choose HCPCS codes from the series J9000-J9999 to report chemotherapy drugs.

Preparation of chemotherapy agent(s) is included in the service for administration of the agent. Report separate CPT codes for each parenteral method of administration employed when chemotherapy is administered by different techniques.

CHEMOTHERAPY ADMINISTRATION

96400 Chemotherapy administration, subcutaneous or intramuscular, with or without local anesthesia

96405 Chemotherapy administration, intralesional; up to and including 7 lesions

96406 more than 7 lesions

96408 Chemotherapy administration, intravenous; push technique

96410 infusion technique, up to one hour

+ **96412** infusion technique, one to 8 hours, each additional hour (List separately in addition to code for primary procedure)

(Use 96412 in conjunction with code 96410)

● New Code ▲ Revised Code + Add-On Code ⊘ Modifier -51 Exempt

96414 infusion technique, initiation of prolonged infusion (more than 8 hours), requiring the use of a portable or implantable pump

(For refilling and maintenance of a portable pump or an implantable infusion pump or reservoir for drug delivery, see 96520, 96530)

96420 Chemotherapy administration, intra-arterial; push technique

96422 infusion technique, up to one hour

+ 96423 infusion technique, one to 8 hours, each additional hour (List separately in addition to code for primary procedure)

(Use 96423 in conjunction with code 96422)

(For regional chemotherapy perfusion via membrane oxygenator perfusion pump to an extremity, use 36823)

96425 infusion technique, initiation of prolonged infusion (more than 8 hours), requiring the use of a portable or implantable pump

(For refilling and maintenance of a portable pump or an implantable infusion pump or reservoir for drug delivery, see 96520, 96530)

96440 Chemotherapy administration into pleural cavity, requiring and including thoracentesis

96445 Chemotherapy administration into peritoneal cavity, requiring and including peritoneocentesis

96450 Chemotherapy administration, into CNS (eg, intrathecal), requiring and including spinal puncture

(For intravesical (bladder) chemotherapy administration, use 51720)

(For insertion of subarachnoid catheter and reservoir for infusion of drug, see 62350, 62351, 62360, 62361, 62362; for insertion of intraventricular catherter and reservoir, see 61210, 61215)

96520 Refilling and maintenance of portable pump

96530 Refilling and maintenance of implantable pump or reservoir for drug delivery, systemic (eg., intravenous, intra-arterial)

855

 Separate Procedure   Unlisted Procedure   CCI Comp. Code   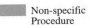 Non-specific Procedure

(For refilling and maintenance of an implantable infusion pump for spinal or brain drug infusion, use 95990)

(For collection of blood specimen from a partially or completely implantable venous access device, use 36540)

96542 Chemotherapy injection, subarachnoid or intraventricular via subcutaneous reservoir, single or multiple agents

96545 Provision of chemotherapy agent

(For radioactive isotope therapy, see 79000-79999)

96549 Unlisted chemotherapy procedure

PHOTODYNAMIC THERAPY

Photodynamic therapy (PDT) is a two-part treatment for esophageal cancer, gastric cancer, and lung cancer using a photosensitizing drug activated by red, non-thermal laser light.

(To report ocular photodynamic therapy, use 67221)

96567 Photodynamic therapy by external application of light to destroy premalignant and/or malignant lesions of the skin and adjacent mucosa (eg, lip) by activation of photosensitive drug(s), each phototherapy exposure session

+ **96570** Photodynamic therapy by endoscopic application of light to ablate abnormal tissue via activation of photosensitive drug(s); first 30 minutes (List separately in addition to code for endoscopy or bronchoscopy procedures of lung and esophagus)

+ **96571** each additional 15 minutes (List separately in addition to code for endoscopy or bronchoscopy procedures of lung and esophagus)

(96570, 96571 are to be used in addition to bronchoscopy, endoscopy codes)

(Use 96570, 96571 in conjunction with codes 31641, 43228 as appropriate)

SPECIAL DERMATOLOGICAL PROCEDURES

(For whole body photography, see Category III code 0044T)

(For intralesional injections, see 11900, 11901)

● New Code ▲ Revised Code + Add-On Code ⊘ Modifier -51 Exempt

(For Tzanck smear, use 87207)

96900 Actinotherapy (ultraviolet light)

96902 Microscopic examination of hairs plucked or clipped by the examiner (excluding hair collected by the patient) to determine telogen and anagen counts, or structural hair shaft abnormality

96910 Photochemotherapy; tar and ultraviolet B (Goeckerman treatment) or petrolatum and ultraviolet B

96912 psoralens and ultraviolet A (PUVA)

96913 Photochemotherapy (Goeckerman and/or PUVA) for severe photoresponsive dermatoses requiring at least four to eight hours of care under direct supervision of the physician (includes application of medication and dressings)

96920 Laser treatment for inflammatory skin disease (psoriasis); total area less than 250 sq cm

96921 250 sq cm to 500 sq cm

96922 over 500 sq cm

96999 Unlisted special dermatological service or procedure

PHYSICAL MEDICINE AND REHABILITATION

Physical medicine is the diagnosis, treatment, and prevention of disease with the aid of physical agents such as light, heat, cold, water, electricity or with mechanical devices. Physical medicine services may be provided by physicians or physical therapists. Physical medicine and rehabilitation CPT codes are divided into three sections: Modalities, Procedures and Tests and Measurements. Other services performed by medical professionals specializing in physical medicine and/or physical therapy include: muscle testing, range of joint motion, electromyography, biofeedback training by EMG, and transcutaneous nerve stimulation (TNS).

Coding Rules

1. *The physician or therapist is required to be in constant attendance when reporting CPT codes for modalities and procedures.*

2. *The physical medicine procedure CPT codes specify treatment to one area, initial 30 minutes, and provide CPT codes to report each additional 15 minutes of treatment.*

857

	Separate Procedure		Unlisted Procedure		CCI Comp. Code		Non-specific Procedure

SPECIAL PHYSICAL MEDICINE CODING ISSUES

Many worker's compensation and casualty insurance companies use pre-CPT coding systems, such as CRVS, and do not use any form of diagnostic coding, relying instead on special reports to justify the procedures performed and services provided. As the majority of physical medicine services are performed for accidents and injuries, many work related, the medical professional performing these services must be informed of the specific reporting requirements in the area that they practice.

PHYSICAL MEDICINE AND REHABILITATION SERVICES

(For muscle testing, range of joint motion, electromyography, see 95831 et seq)

(For biofeedback training by EMG, use 90901)

(For transcutaneous nerve stimulation (TNS), use 64550)

97001 Physical therapy evaluation

97002 Physical therapy re-evaluation

97003 Occupational therapy evaluation

97004 Occupational therapy re-evaluation

97005 Athletic training evaluation

97006 Athletic training re-evaluation

MODALITIES

Supervised

97010 Application of a modality to one or more areas; hot or cold packs

97012 traction, mechanical

97014 electrical stimulation (unattended)

(For acupuncture with electrical stimulation, use 97781)

97016 vasopneumatic devices

● New Code   ▲ Revised Code   ✛ Add-On Code   ⃠ Modifier -51 Exempt

97018 paraffin bath

97020 microwave

97022 whirlpool

97024 diathermy

97026 infrared

97028 ultraviolet

Constant Attendance

97032 Application of a modality to one or more areas; electrical stimulation (manual), each 15 minutes

97033 iontophoresis, each 15 minutes

97034 contrast baths, each 15 minutes

97035 ultrasound, each 15 minutes

97036 Hubbard tank, each 15 minutes

97039 Unlisted modality (specify type and time if constant attendance)

THERAPEUTIC PROCEDURES

97110 Therapeutic procedure, one or more areas, each 15 minutes; therapeutic exercises to develop strength and endurance, range of motion and flexibility

97112 neuromuscular reeducation of movement, balance, coordination, kinesthetic sense, posture, and/or proprioception for sitting and/or standing activities

97113 aquatic therapy with therapeutic exercises

97116 gait training (includes stair climbing)

(Use 96000-96003 to report comprehensive gait and motion analysis procedures)

97124 massage, including effleurage, petrissage and/or tapotement (stroking, compression, percussion)

859

 Separate Procedure    Unlisted Procedure   CCI Comp. Code   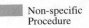 Non-specific Procedure

(For myofascial release, use 97140)

97139 Unlisted therapeutic procedure (specify)

97140 Manual therapy techniques (eg, mobilization/ manipulation, manual lymphatic drainage, manual traction), one or more regions, each 15 minutes

97150 Therapeutic procedure(s), group (2 or more individuals)

(Report 97150 for each member of group)

(Group therapy procedures involve constant attendance of the physician or therapist, but by definition do not require one-on-one patient contact by the physician or therapist)

(For manipulation under general anesthesia, see appropriate anatomic section in Musculoskeletal System)

(For osteopathic manipulative treatment (OMT), see 98925-98929)

97504 Orthotic(s) fitting and training, upper extremity(ies), lower extremity(ies), and/or trunk, each 15 minutes

(Code 97504 should not be reported with 97116)

(For casting and strapping of fracture, injury or dislocation, see 29000, 29590)

97520 Prosthetic training, upper and/or lower extremities, each 15 minutes

97530 Therapeutic activities, direct (one-on-one) patient contact by the provider (use of dynamic activities to improve functional performance), each 15 minutes

97532 Development of cognitive skills to improve attention, memory, problem solving, (includes compensatory training), direct (one-on-one) patient contact by the provider, each 15 minutes

97533 Sensory integrative techniques to enhance sensory processing and promote adaptive responses to environmental demands, direct (one-on-one) patient contact by the provider, each 15 minutes

● New Code   ▲ Revised Code   + Add-On Code   ⊘ Modifier -51 Exempt

97535 Self-care/home management training (eg, activities of daily living (ADL) and compensatory training, meal preparation, safety procedures, and instructions in use of assistive technology devices/adaptive equipment) direct one-on-one contact by provider, each 15 minutes

▲ **97537** Community/work reintegration training (eg, shopping, transportation, money management, avocational activities and/or work environment/modification analysis, work task analysis, use of assistive technology device/adaptive equipment), direct one-on-one contact by provider, each 15 minutes

(For wheelchair management/propulsion training, use 97542)

97542 Wheelchair management/propulsion training, each 15 minutes

97545 Work hardening/conditioning; initial 2 hours

+ **97546** each additional hour (List separately in addition to code for primary procedure)

(Use 97546 in conjunction with code 97545)

ACTIVE WOUND CARE MANAGEMENT

(Do not report 97601, 97602 in addition to 11040-11044)

97601 Removal of devitalized tissue from wound(s); selective debridement, without anesthesia (eg, high pressure waterjet, sharp selective debridement with scissors, scalpel and tweezers), including topical application(s), wound assessment, and instruction(s) for ongoing care, per session

97602 non-selective debridement, without anesthesia (eg, wet-to-moist dressing, enzymatic, abrasion), including topical application(w), wound assessment, and instruction(s) for ongoing care, per session

TESTS AND MEASUREMENTS

(For muscle testing, manual or electrical, joint range of motion, electromyography or nerve velocity determination, see 95831-95904)

97703 Checkout for orthotic/prosthetic use, established patient, each 15 minutes

97750 Physical performance test or measurement (eg, musculo-skeletal, functional capacity), with written report, each 15 minutes

● **97755** Assistive technology assessment (eg, to restore, augment or compensate for existing function, optimize functional tasks and/or maximize environmental accessibility), direct one-on-one contact by provider, with written report, each 15 minutes

(To report augmentative and alternative communication devices, use 92605 or 92607)

OTHER PROCEDURES

(For extracorporeal shock wave musculoskeletal therapy, use Category III code 0019T)

97780 Acupuncture, one or more needles; without electrical stimulation

97781 with electrical stimulation

97799 Unlisted physical medicine/rehabilitation service or procedure

MEDICAL NUTRITION THERAPY

Medical nutrition therapy (MNT) is the assessment of nutritional status followed by nutritional therapy. The nutrition assessment includes review and analysis of 1) medical, nutrition and medication histories, 2) physical examination, 3) anthropometric measurements, and 4) laboratory test values. Nutrition therapy may include 1) diet modification, 2) counseling and education, 3) disease self-management skills training, and 4) administration of specialized therapies such as medical foods, intravenous or tube feedings.

MEDICAL NUTRITION THERAPY CODES

97802 Medical nutrition therapy; initial assessment and intervention, individual, face-to-face with the patient, each 15 minutes

97803 re-assessment and intervention, individual, face-to-face with the patient, each 15 minutes

97804 group (2 or more individual(s)), each 30 minutes

(For medical nutrition therapy assessment and/or intervention performed by a physician, see Evaluation and Management or Preventive Medicine service codes)

| ● | New Code | ▲ | Revised Code | + | Add-On Code | ⊘ | Modifier -51 Exempt |

OSTEOPATHIC MANIPULATIVE TREATMENT

Osteopathic medicine is a system of therapy based on the theory that the body is capable of making its own remedies against disease and other toxic conditions when it is in normal structural relationship and has favorable environmental conditions and adequate nutrition. Osteopathic manipulative treatment (OMT) is a form of manual treatment applied by a physician to eliminate or alleviate somatic dysfunction and related disorders. This treatment may be accomplished by a variety of techniques.

Coding Rules

1. *Evaluation and management services may be reported separately, if, and only if the patient's condition requires a significant separately identifiable evaluation and management service, above and beyond the usual pre-service and post service work associated with the osteopathic manipulation.*

2. *CPT codes in this section are used to report OMT services provided in any location.*

OSTEOPATHIC MANIPULATIVE TREATMENT CODES

98925 Osteopathic manipulative treatment (OMT); one to two body regions involved

98926 three to four body regions involved

98927 five to six body regions involved

98928 seven to eight body regions involved

98929 nine to ten body regions involved

CHIROPRACTIC MANIPULATIVE TREATMENT

Chiropractic medicine is a system of diagnosis and treatment based on the theory that irritation of the nervous system by mechanical, chemical or psychic factors is the cause of disease. Chiropractic services may include office visits, diagnostic tests, physical therapy, and/or chiropractic manipulation. Chiropractic manipulation treatment (CMT) is a form of manual treatment applied by a chiropractic physician to eliminate or alleviate somatic dysfunction and related disorders.

863

 Separate Procedure   Unlisted Procedure   CCI Comp. Code   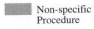 Non-specific Procedure

Coding Rules

1. *Chiropractic manipulation treatment includes a pre-manipulation patient assessment.*

2. *Evaluation and management services provided in conjunction with CMT may be reported separately with the addition of CPT modifier -25, along with any diagnostic tests or other therapy provided.*

REPORTING CHIROPRACTIC MANIPULATION TO MEDICARE

Medicare restricts the number of times the CMT code may be reported, provides a maximum reimbursement amount per year, and requires extensive supporting documentation as described below.

Documentation of Treatment Phase

Proper documentation of the treatment phase is extremely important when submitting claims for chiropractic services to Medicare. The treatment phase consists of the date the course of treatment was initiated and the number of treatments rendered to date. Proper documentation enables Medicare to process your claims quickly and accurately. For payment of chiropractic claims, the following information must be on the CMS1500 claim form:

1. *The service must be manual manipulation of the spine. This service is reported by CPT codes 98940-98943.*

2. *The primary diagnosis must be subluxation of the spine, either so stated or identified by a term descriptive of the subluxation. The following diagnoses are acceptable because they would always involve a subluxation:*

Intervertebral disc disorders	*722.0-722.9*
Curvatures of the spine	*737.0-737.9*
Spondylolisthesis	*738.4,756.12*
Nonallopathic lesions	*739.1-739.4*
Spondylolysis	*756.11*

3. *The level of subluxation must be stated.*

4. *The symptoms related to the level of subluxation must be given.*

5. *The date of the confirming x-ray must be on the claim. Note that the x-ray must have been taken within 12 months prior to or 3 months after the course of treatment was initiated.*

6. *The date this course of treatment was initiated and the number of treatments rendered since the start of this course must be on the claim.*

---

864 ● New Code ▲ Revised Code ＋ Add-On Code ⃠ Modifier -51 Exempt

Special Situations

If a patient returns with a new condition or injury, this represents a new treatment phase. The treatment phase information should reflect when you first saw the patient for this condition. Do not use the date you first saw the patient for an earlier course of treatment. Note on your CMS1500 claim form that this is a new condition. Remember that a new documenting x-ray may be required.

In the case of chronic conditions, an x-ray older than 12 months may be acceptable. For coverage of chronic conditions such as scoliosis, spondylolysis, and spondylolisthesis, there must be a reasonable expectation that there is a restorative potential. Remember that maintenance care is not covered by Medicare.

CHIROPRACTIC MANIPULATIVE TREATMENT CODES

98940 Chiropractic manipulative treatment (CMT); spinal, one to two regions

98941 spinal, three to four regions

98942 spinal, five regions

98943 extraspinal, one or more regions

SPECIAL SERVICES, PROCEDURES AND REPORTS

The MEDICINE section of CPT includes a subsection Special Services and Reports, with CPT codes 99000-99090 which provides the reporting physician with a means of identifying the completion of special reports and services that are an adjunct to the basic services rendered. The specific special services code reported indicates the special circumstances under which a basic procedure is performed.

The proper use of Special Services CPT codes can result in a significant increase in reimbursement. Most codes in this section are "add on" codes which means that they are used in addition to whatever other CPT codes describe the procedures or services performed.

MISCELLANEOUS SERVICES

99000 Handling and/or conveyance of specimen for transfer from the physician's office to a laboratory

99001 Handling and/or conveyance of specimen for transfer from the patient in other than a physician's office to a laboratory (distance may be indicated)

865

Separate Procedure | Unlisted Procedure | CCI Comp. Code | Non-specific Procedure

99002 Handling, conveyance, and/or any other service in connection with the implementation of an order involving devices (eg, designing, fitting, packaging, handling, delivery or mailing) when devices such as orthotics, protectives, prosthetics are fabricated by an outside laboratory or shop but which items have been designed, and are to be fitted and adjusted by the attending physician

(For routine collection of venous blood, use 36415)

▲ **99024** Postoperative follow-up visit, normally included in the surgical package, to indicate that an evaluation and management service was performed during a postoperative period for a reason(s) related to the origianl procedure

(As a component of a surgical "package," see Surgery guidelines)

(**99025** deleted 2004 edition.)

99026 Hospital mandated on call service; in-hospital, each hour

99027 out-of-hospital, each hour

(For physician standby services requiring prolonged physician attendance, use 99360, as appropriate. Time spent performing separately reportable procedure(s) or service(s) should not be included in the time reported as mandated on call service)

▲ **99050** Services requested after posted office hours in addition to basic service

99052 Services requested between 10:00 PM and 8:00 AM in addition to basic service

99054 Services requested on Sundays and holidays in addition to basic service

99056 Services provided at request of patient in a location other than physician's office which are normally provided in the office

99058 Office services provided on an emergency basis

99070 Supplies and materials (except spectacles), provided by the physician over and above those usually included with the office visit or other services rendered (list drugs, trays, supplies, or materials provided)

(For spectacles, see 92390-92395)

● New Code   ▲ Revised Code   + Add-On Code   ⊘ Modifier -51 Exempt

99071   Educational supplies, such as books, tapes, and pamphlets, provided by the physician for the patient's education at cost to physician

99075   Medical testimony

99078   Physician educational services rendered to patients in a group setting (eg, prenatal, obesity, or diabetic instructions)

99080   Special reports such as insurance forms, more than the information conveyed in the usual medical communications or standard reporting form

(Do not report 99080 in conjunction with 99455, 99456 for the completion of Workmen's Compensation forms)

99082   Unusual travel (eg, transportation and escort of patient)

99090   Analysis of clinical data stored in computers (eg, ECGs, blood pressures, hematologic data)

(For physician/health care professional collection and interpretation of physiologic data stored/transmitted by patient/caregiver, see 99091)

(Do not report 99090 if other more specific CPT codes exist, eg, 93014, 93227, 93233, 93272 for cardiographic services; 95250 for continuous glucose monitoring, 97750 for musculoskeletal function testing)

99091   Collection and interpretation of physiologic data (eg, ECG, blood pressure, glucose monitoring) digitally stored and/or transmitted by the patient and/or caregiver to the physician or other qualified health care professional, requiring a minimum of 30 minutes of time

QUALIFYING CIRCUMSTANCES FOR ANESTHESIA

(For explanation of these services, see Anesthesia guidelines)

+ 99100   Anesthesia for patient of extreme age, under 1 year and over 70 (List separately in addition to code for primary anesthesia procedure)

(For procedures performed on infants less than 1 year of age at time of surgery, see 00833, 00834)

867

 Separate Procedure   Unlisted Procedure   CCI Comp. Code   Non-specific Procedure

+ 99116   Anesthesia complicated by utilization of total body hypothermia (List separately in addition to code for primary anesthesia procedure)

+ 99135   Anesthesia complicated by utilization of controlled hypotension (List separately in addition to code for primary anesthesia procedure)

+ 99140   Anesthesia complicated by emergency conditions (specify) (List separately in addition to code for primary anesthesia procedure)

(An emergency is defined as existing when delay in treatment of the patient would lead to a significant increase in the threat to life or body part)

SEDATION WITH OR WITHOUT ANALGESIA (CONSCIOUS SEDATION)

(If the sedation with or without analgesia (conscious sedation) is administered in support of a procedure provided by another physician, see Anesthesia section)

⊘ **99141**   Sedation with or without analgesia (conscious sedation); intravenous, intramuscular or inhalation

(94760-94762 may not be reported in addition to 99141)

⊘ **99142**   oral, rectal and/or intranasal

(94760-94762 may not be reported in addition to 99142)

OTHER SERVICES AND PROCEDURES

99170   Anogenital examination with colposcopic magnification in childhood for suspected trauma

(For conscious sedation, use 99141, 99142)

99172   Visual function screening, automated or semi-automated bilateral quantitative determination of visual acuity, ocular alignment, color vision by pseudoisochromatic plates, and field of vision (may include all or some screening of the determination(s) for contrast sensitivity, vision under glare)

(This service must employ graduated visual acuity stimuli that allow a quantitative determination of visual acuity (eg, Snellen chart). This service may not be used in addition to a gernal ophthalmological service or an E/M service)

● New Code   ▲ Revised Code   + Add-On Code   ⊘ Modifier -51 Exempt

(Do not report 99172 in conjunction with code 99173)

99173   Screening test of visual acuity, quantitative, bilateral

(The screening test used must employ graduated visual acuity stimuli that allow a quantitative estimate of visual acuity (eg, Snellen chart). Other identifiable services unrelated to this screening test provided at the same time may be reported separately (eg, preventive medicine services). When acuity is measured as part of a general ophthalmological service or of an E/M service of the eye, it is a diagnostic examination and not a screening test.)

(Do not report 99173 in conjunction with code 99172)

99175   Ipecac or similar administration for individual emesis and continued observation until stomach adequately emptied of poison

(For diagnostic intubation, see 82926-82928, 89130-89141)

(For gastric lavage for diagnostic purposes, see 91055)

99183   Physician attendance and supervision of hyperbaric oxygen therapy, per session

(Evaluation and Management services and/or procedures (eg, wound debridement) provided in a hyperbaric oxygen treatment facility in conjunction with a hyperbaric oxygen therapy session should be reported separately)

99185   Hypothermia; regional

99186   total body

99190   Assembly and operation of pump with oxygenator or heat exchanger (with or without ECG and/or pressure monitoring); each hour

99191   3/4 hour

99192   1/2 hour

99195   Phlebotomy, therapeutic (separate procedure)

99199   Unlisted special service, procedure or report

| | Separate Procedure | | Unlisted Procedure | | CCI Comp. Code | | Non-specific Procedure |

HOME HEALTH PROCEDURES/SERVICES

Home health procedures/services codes are used by non-physician health care professionals to report services provided in the patient's residence.

99500   Home visit for prenatal monitoring and assessment to include fetal heart rate, non-stress test, uterine monitoring, and gestational diabetes monitoring

99501   Home visit for postnatal assessment and follow-up care

99502   Home visit for newborn care and assessment

99503   Home visit for respiratory therapy care (eg, bronchodilator, oxygen therapy, respiratory assessment, apnea evaluation)

99504   Home visit for mechanical ventilation care

99505   Home visit for stoma care and maintenance including colostomy and cystostomy

99506   Home visit for intramuscular injections

99507   Home visit for care and maintenance of catheter(s) (eg, urinary, drainage, and enteral)

(**99508**   deleted 2003 edition. To report, see 95806-95811)

99509   Home visit for assistance with activities of daily living and personal care

(To report self-care/home management training, see 97535)

(To report home medical nutrition assessment and intervention services, see 97802-97804)

(To report home speech therapy services, see 92507-92508)

99510   Home visit for individual, family, or marriage counseling

99511   Home visit for fecal impaction management and enema administration

▲ **99512**   Home visit for hemodialysis

(For home infusion of peritoneal dialysis, use 99601, 99602)

(**99539**   deleted 2003 edition. To report, use 99600)

870

● New Code   ▲ Revised Code   + Add-On Code   ⊘ Modifier -51 Exempt

(99551   deleted 2004 edition. To report, see 99601-99602)

(99552   deleted 2004 edition. To report, see 99601-99602)

(99553   deleted 2004 edition. To report, see 99601-99602)

(99554   deleted 2004 edition. To report, see 99601-99602)

(99555   deleted 2004 edition. To report, see 99601-99602)

(99556   deleted 2004 edition. To report, see 99601-99602)

(99557   deleted 2004 edition. To report, see 99601-99602)

(99558   deleted 2004 edition. To report, see 99601-99602)

(99559   deleted 2004 edition. To report, see 99601-99602)

(99560   deleted 2004 edition. To report, see 99601-99602)

(99561   deleted 2004 edition. To report, see 99601-99602)

(99562   deleted 2004 edition. To report, see 99601-99602)

(99563   deleted 2004 edition. To report, see 99601-99602)

(99564   deleted 2004 edition. To report, see 99601-99602)

(99565   deleted 2004 edition. To report, see 99601-99602)

(99566   deleted 2004 edition. To report, see 99601-99602)

(99567   deleted 2004 edition. To report, see 99601-99602)

(99568   deleted 2004 edition. To report, see 99601-99602)

(99569   deleted 2004 edition. To report, see 99601-99602)

99600   Unlisted home visit service or procedure

871

 Separate Procedure   Unlisted Procedure   CCI Comp. Code   Non-specific Procedure

HOME INFUSION PROCEDURES/SERVICES

Home infusion procedures codes are used to report per diem home visits for the purpose of administering infusions. With the exception of the infusion drug; all materials, equipments and supplies are included in the basic code. Drugs used for the infusion are coded separately.

- **99601** Home infusion/specialty drug administration, per visit (up to 2 hours)

- **+99602** each additional hour (List separately in addition to code for primary procedure)

    (Use 99602 in conjunction with 99601)

● New Code   ▲ Revised Code   ✚ Add-On Code   ⊘ Modifier -51 Exempt

CATEGORY II CODES

This section of the CPT coding system is the Category II Performance Measurement section. The primary purpose of this section is to provide classification codes which will allow the collection of data for performance measurement.

The assignment of a Category II code to a given service or procedure does not mean that the particular service or procedure is endorsed, approved, safe or has applicability to clinical practice. The Category II code simply provides a mechanism to identify and review performance measurements.

Category II codes consist of four numbers followed by the letter "F."

- **0001F**   Blood pressure, measured

- **0002F**   Tobacco use, smoking, assessed

- **0003F**   Tobacco use, non-smoking, assessed

- **0004F**   Tobacco use cessation intervention, counseling

- **0005F**   Tobacco use cessation intervention, pharmacologic therapy

- **0006F**   Statin therapy, prescribed

- **0007F**   Beta-blocker therapy, prescribed

- **0008F**   ACE inhibitor therapy, prescribed

- **0009F**   Anginal symptoms and level of activity, assessed

- **0010F**   Anginal symptoms and level of activity, assessed using a standardized instrument (eg, Canadian Cardiovascular Society Classification-CCSC-System, Seattle Angina Questionnaire-SAQ)

- **0011F**   Oral antiplatelet therapy; prescribed (eg, aspirin, clopidogrel/Plavix, or combination of aspirin and dipyridamole/Aggrenox)

	Separate Procedure		Unlisted Procedure		CCI Comp. Code		Non-specific Procedure

This page intentionally left blank.

● New
Code

▲ Revised
Code

✚ Add-On
Code

⊘ Modifier -51
Exempt

CATEGORY III CODES

CATEGORY III SECTION OVERVIEW

The eighth section of the CPT coding system is the Category III Emerging Technology section. The primary purpose of this section is to provide classification codes which will allow the collection of data on emerging technology services and procedures.

The assignment of a Category III code to a given service or procedure does not mean that the particular service or procedure is endorsed, approved, safe or has applicability to clinical practice. The Category III code simply provides a mechanism to identify and review emerging services and procedures.

Category III codes consist of four numbers followed by a letter. These is no particular organization to the codes listed in this section.

CATEGORY III CODES

0001T   Endovascular repair of infrarenal abdominal aortic aneurysm or dissection; modular bifurcated prosthesis (two docking limbs)

(For radiological supervision and interpretation, use 75952 in conjunction with 0001T)

(**0002T**   deleted 2004 edition. To report, use 34805)

0003T   Cervicography

(0004T has been deleted. To report, use 88380)

0005T   Transcatheter placement of extracranial cerebrovascular artery stent(s), percutaneous; initial vessel

+ 0006T   each additional vessel (List separately in addition to code for primary procedure)

(Use 0006T in conjunction with code 0005T)

(For radiological supervision and interpretation, use 0007T)

0007T   Transcatheter placement of extracranial cerebrovascular artery stent(s), percutaneous, radiological supervision and interpretation, each vessel

(For procedure, see 0005T, 0006T)

875

 Separate Procedure

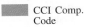 Unlisted Procedure

CCI Comp. Code

 Non-specific Procedure

0008T Upper gastrointestinal endoscopy including esophagus, stomach, and either the duodenum and/or jejunum as appropriate, with suturing of the esophagogastric junction

0009T Endometrial cryoablation with ultrasonic guidance

0010T Tuberculosis test, cell mediated immunity measurement of gamma interferon antigen response

0012T Arthroscopy, knee, surgical, implantation of osteochondral graft(s) for treatment of articular surface defect; autografts

0013T   allografts

0014T Meniscal transplantation, medial or lateral, knee (any method)

0016T Destruction of localized lesion of choroid (eg, choroidal neovascularization), transpupillary thermotherapy

0017T Destruction of macular drusen, photocoagulation

0018T Delivery of high power, focal magnetic pulses for direct stimulation to cortical neurons

0019T Extracorporeal shock wave therapy; involving musculoskeletal system

0020T   involving plantar fascia

0021T Insertion of transcervical or transvaginal fetal oximetry sensor

0023T Infectious agent drug susceptibility phenotype prediction using genotypic comparison to known genotypic/phenotypic database, HIV 1

0024T Non-surgical septal reduction therapy (eg, alcohol ablation), for hypertrophic obstructive cardiomyopathy, with coronary arteriograms, with or without temporary pacemaker

(0025T   deleted 2004 edition. To report, use 76514)

0026T Lipoprotein, direct measurement, intermediate density lipoproteins (IDL) (remnant lipoproteins)

---

876   ● New
      Code

▲ Revised
   Code

+ Add-On
   Code

⊘ Modifier -51
   Exempt

0027T   Endoscopic lysis of epidural adhesions with direct visualization using mechanical means (eg., spinal endoscopic catheter system) or solution injection (eg., normal saline) including radiologic localization and epidurography

(For diagnostic epidurography, use 64999)

0028T   Dual energy x-ray absorptiometry (DEXA) body composition study, one or more sites

0029T   Treatment(s) for incontinence, pulsed magnetic neuromodulation, per day

0030T   Antiprothrombin (phospholipid cofactor) antibody, each Ig class

0031T   Speculoscopy;

0032T   with directed sampling

0033T   Endovascular repair of descending thoracic aortic aneurysm, pseudoaneurysm or dissection; involving coverage of left subclavian artery origin, initial endoprosthesis

(For radiological supervision and interpretation, use 0038T)

0034T   not involving coverage of left subclavian artery origin, initial endoprosthesis

(For radiological supervision and interpretation, use 0038T)

0035T   Placement of proximal or distal extension prosthesis for endovascular repair of descending thoracic aortic aneurysm, pseudoaneurysm or dissection; initial extension

(For radiological supervision and interpretation, use 0040T)

(Do not report 0034T and 0035T when placement of extension converts repair to cover left subclavian origin, use only 0033T)

+ 0036T   each additional extension (List separately in addition to code for primary procedure)

(Use 0036T in conjunction with code 0035T)

(For radiological supervision and interpretation, use 0040T)

0037T   Open subclavian to carotid artery transposition performed in conjunction with endovascular thoracic aneurysm repair, by neck incision, unilateral

---

877

 Separate Procedure   Unlisted Procedure   CCI Comp. Code   Non-specific Procedure

(For bilateral procedure, use modifier -50)

(Do not report 0037T in addition to 35694)

0038T Endovascular repair of descending thoracic aortic aneurysm, pseudoaneurysm or dissection involving coverage of left subclavian artery origin, initial endoprosthesis, radiological supervision and interpretation

(For implantation of endovascular graft, use 0033T)

0039T Endovascular repair of descending thoracic aortic aneurysm, pseudoaneurysm or dissection not involving coverage of left subclavian artery origin, initial endoprosthesis, radiological supervision and interpretation

(For implantation of endovascular graft, use 0034T)

0040T Placement of proximal or distal extension prosthesis for endovascular repair of descending thoracic aortic aneurysm, pseudoaneurysm or dissection, each extension, radiological supervision and interpretation

(For implantation of endovascular graft extensions, see 0035T, 0036T)

0041T Urinalysis infectious agent detection, semi-quantitative analysis of volatile compounds

0042T Cerebral perfusion analysis using computed tomography with contrast administration, including post-processing of parametric maps with determination of cerebral blood flow, cerebral blood volume, and mean transit time

0043T Carbon monoxide, expired gas analsysis (eg., ETCOc/hemolysis breath test)

0044T Whole body integumentary photography, at request of a physician, for monitoring of high-risk patients; with dysplastic nevus syndrome or familial melanoma

● **0045T** with history of dysplastic nevi or personal history of melanoma

● **0046T** Catheter lavage of a mammary duct(s) for collection of cytology specimen(s), in high risk individuals (GAIL risk scoring or prior personal history of breast cancer), each breast; single duct

● **0047T** each additional duct

● **0048T** Implantation of a ventricular assist device, extracorporeal, percutaneous transseptal access, single or dual cannulation

●+**0049T** Prolonged extracorporeal percutaneous transseptal ventricular assist device, greater than 24 hours, each subsequent 24 hour period (List separately in addition to code for primary procedure)

(Use 0049T in conjunction with 0048T)

● **0050T** Removal of a ventricular assist device, extracorporeal, percutaneous transseptal access, single or dual cannulation

● **0051T** Implantation of a total replacement heart system (artificial heart) with recipient cardiectomy

(For implantation of heart assist or ventricular assist device, see 33975, 33976)

● **0052T** Replacement or repair of thoracic unit of a total replacement heart system (artificial heart)

(For replacement or repair of other implantable components in a total replacement heart system (artificial heart), use 0053T)

● **0053T** Replacement or repair of implantable component or components of total replacement heart system (artificial heart), excluding thoracic unit

(For replacement or repair of a thoracic unit of a total replacement heart system (artificial heart), use 0052T)

●+**0054T** Computer assisted musculoskeletal surgical navigational orthopedic procedure, with image-guidance based on fluoroscopic images (List separately in addition to code for primary procedure)

●+**0055T** Computer assisted musculoskeletal surgical navigational orthopedic procedure, with image-guidance based on CT and MRI images (List separately in addition to code for primary procedure)

●+**0056T** Computer assisted musculoskeletal surgical navigational orthopedic procedure, image-less (List separately in addition to code for priary procedure)

879

 Separate Procedure   Unlisted Procedure   CCI Comp. Code   Non-specific Procedure

● **0057T** Upper gastrointestinal endoscopy, including esophagus, stomach, and either the duodenum and/or jejunum as appropriate, with deliver yof thermal energy to the muscle of the lower esophageal sphincter and/or gastric cardia, for treatment of gastroesophageal reflux disease

● **0058T** Cryopreservation; reproductive tissue, ovarian

● **0059T**   oocyte(s)

(For cryopreservation of embryo(s), sperm and testicular reproductive tissue, see 89258, 89259, 89335)

● **0060T** Electrical impedance scan of the breast, bilateral (risk assessment device for breast cancer)

● **0061T** Destruction/reduction of malignant breast tumor including breast carcinoma cells in the margins, microwave phased array thermotherapy, disposable catheter with combined temperature monitoring probe and microwave sensor, externally applied microwave energy, including interstitial placement of sensor

(For imaging guidance performed inconjunction with 0061T, see 76942, 76986)

ALPHABETICAL INDEX

The alphabetical index includes listings by procedure, CPT® headings and sub-headings and anatomic site. Procedures and services commonly known by their acronyms, eponyms, homonyms or other designations are also included. The alphabetical index of CPT® PLUS is unique in that both indexes to specific page numbers and indexes to CPT code numbers are included.

HOW TO USE THE ALPHABETICAL INDEX

When using the alphabetical index to locate CPT codes, use the following search sequence:

- Look for the CPT HEADING for the general category of surgical procedure(s) or medical service(s) or TOPIC for instructional and/or explanatory information.

- Look for the CPT Sub-heading for the organ system(s) involved or service(s) performed or the TOPIC sub-heading for the instructional or explanatory issue. Scan the index listings to determine if the specific procedure or service or topic is listed.

- For CPT codes, use the thumb-tab indexes to locate the appropriate CPT code section. If the specific procedure or service was listed in the index, locate the procedure or service in the CPT code section and verify the full description of the CPT code before using. If the specific procedure or service was not listed in the index, first locate the organ system and/or medical service sub-heading and then review the CPT code section until you locate the specific procedure and/or service.

- For instructional and/or explanatory topics, turn to the page number specified in the alphabetical index.

- Alternately, look for SYNONYMS, HOMONYMS, EPONYMS or ACRONYMS.

ORGANIZATION OF THE ALPHABETICAL INDEX

When using the alphabetical index, it is important to understand how entries to the index have been made. Index entries fall into one or more of the general categories described below.

1. MAIN TERMS:

SURGERY SERVICES CODES *10000-69999*
  Auditory system 69000-69979
  Cardiovascular system 33000-397799
  Digestive system 40490-49999
  Endocrine system 60000-60699
  Eye and ocular adnexa 65091-68899
Surgical pathology, gross examination only 88300
Surgical preparation or creation recipient site 15000-15001
Surgical treatment
  anal fistula 46270-46285
  ectopic pregnancy 59120-59140
  ....

2. PROCEDURE OR SERVICE:

Destruction
  benign or premalignant lesions 17000-17250
  celiac pleaxus by neurolytic agent 64680
  cervical spinal muscles by neurolytic agent 64613
  ciliary body 66700-66740
  cutaneous vascular proliferative lesions 17106-17108
  cyst or lesion, iris or ciliary body 66770
  hemorrhoids 46934-46936
  intercostal nerve by neurolytic agent 64620
  ....

Note that in the two above examples, the CPT code categories and procedures/services are listed as the heading and a "range" of CPT codes follows. The range of CPT codes directs the coder to the appropriate CPT section where additional information on the procedure(s) or service(s) may be located. All CPT code sections and individual sub-headings are listed in **BOLD UPPER CASE**.

3. TOPIC:

RADIOLOGY SERVICES 641-702
  Bilateral procedure codes 662
  Complete procedures 641
  Medicare considerations 643
  Modifiers 642
  Services overview 641
  Subsections 641
  Supervision and interpretation only 641
  ....

In the above example, the CPT headings and subheadings are listed and a page or range of page numbers follows. The page number(s) directs the coder to the specific page(s) where additional information on the topic(s) may be located. Note that all listings providing page numbers are underlined, so that they will not be confused with index listings that provide CPT code(s). All topics referring to CPT code sections or chapter headings are listed in **BOLD UPPER CASE.**

4) SYNONYMS, EPONYMS AND ACRONYMS:

Bankart procedure (capsulorrhaphy, anterior with labral repair) 23455

BCG 90585

Belsey IV procedure (esophagogastric fundoplasty) 43324

Bennett type procedure (quadricepsplasty) 27430

PSA 84153

T3 84480

Torkildsen type operation (ventriculocisternostomy) 62180

5) SECTIONS

Sections of the book are referenced by page number(s) instead of CPT code number(s). Such listings are underlined.

This page intentionally left blank.

A

Abdominal
   hysterectomy total   58150-58200
   paracentesis   49080-49081
Abdomino-vaginal vesical neck suspension   51845
Ablation
   operative
      supraventricular arrhythmogenic focus   33250-33251
      ventricular arrhythmogenic focus   33261
   of liver tumors   47380-47382
   tissue
      CT guidance for   76362
      MR guidance for   76394
      ultrasound guidance for   76940
Abrasion   15786-15787
Acetabuloplasty   27120-27122
Acetaldehyde, blood   82000
Acetaminophen   82003
Acetone   82009-82010
Acetylcholinesterase   82013
Acne surgery   10040
Acoustic reflex
   decay test   92569
   testing   92568
Acromionectomy   23130
Acromioplasty   23130, 23415-23420
ACTH   82024
   stimulation panel   80400-80406
Actinotherapy   96900
Acupuncture   97780-97781
Acute
   gastrointestinal blood loss imaging   78278
   venous thrombosis imaging   78456
Acylcarnitines   82016-82017
Adenoidectomy   42820-42821, 42830-42836
Adenosine, 5-monophosphate, cyclic (cyclic amp)   82030
Adenovirus vaccine   90476-90477
Adjustment external fixation system   20693
Adjuvant techniques   35685-35686
Administration and interpretation health risk assessment instrument   99420
Adrenal imaging cortex medulla   78075
Adrenalectomy   60540-60545, 60650
Adrenocorticotropic hormone (ACTH)   82024
Aerosol inhalation pentamidine   94642
Agglutinins, febrile   86000
Albumin
   serum   82040
   urine   82042
Alcohol (ethyl)   82055-82075
Aldolase   82085
Aldosterone   82088
Alkaloids, urine   82101

885

Allergen immunotherapy
   professional services 95115-95134
   supervision and provision antigens 95144-95170
Allergen-specific
    IgE 86003-86005
    IgG 86001
ALLERGY AND CLINICAL IMMUNOLOGY SERVICES *95004-95199*
Allograft spine surgery 20930-20931
Alpha-1-antitrypsin 82103-82104
Alpha-fetoprotein 82105-82106
Aluminum 82108
Alveolectomy 41830
Alveoloplasty 41874
Ambulatory blood pressure monitoring 93784-93790
Amines vaginal fluid 82120
Amino acids 82127-82139
Ammonia 82140
Amniocentesis 59000-59001
Amniotic fluid scan 82143
Amphetamine or methamphetamine 82145
Amputation
   ankle 27888
   arm through humerus 24900-24935
   finger/thumb 26910-26952
   foot 28800-28805
   forearm 25900-25909, 25915
   interpelviabdominal 27290
   leg, lower 27598, 27880-27886
   metacarpal 26910
   metatarsal 28810
   penis 54120-54135
   thigh 27290-27295, 27594-27596
   toe 28810-28825
Amylase 82150
Analysis information/data stored in computers 99090
Anastomosis
   arterial, extracranial-intracranial 61711
   choledochal cyst 47716
   extrahepatic biliary ducts and gastrointestinal tract 47760, 47780
   facial-
     hypoglossal 64868
     phrenic 64870
     spinal accessory 64866
   intrahepatic ducts and gastrointestinal tract 47765
   pancreatic cyst to gastrointestinal tract 48180, 48520-48540
   pulmonary artery to aorta (Damus-Kaye-Stansel procedure) 33606
   Roux-en-Y 47780-47785
ANATOMIC PATHOLOGY SERVICES *88000-88099*
Anatomical illustrations 37-85
Androstanediol glucuronide 82154
Androstenedione 82157
Androsterone 82160

887

Anesthesia services for—continued
  clavicle and scapula 00450-00454
  cleft lip 00102
  complicated
    by emergency conditions 99140
    controlled hypotension 99135
    total body hypothermia 99116
  ear 00120-00126
  electroconvulsive therapy 00104
  esophagus 00500
  extraperitoneal procedures lower abdomen 00860-00870
  eye 00140-00148
  eyelid 00103
  facial bones 00190-00192
  femur 01220-01234
  forearm
    wrist, and hand 01810
    wrist/hand cast 01860
  head, neck, and posterior trunk 00300
  heart
    pericardium, and great vessels of chest 00560-00563
    transplant or heart/lung transplant 00580
  hernia repairs
    lower abdomen 00830-00832
    upper abdomen 00750-00756
  hip joint 01200-01214
  humerus and elbow 01730-01760
  injection procedure
    diskography, cervical 01905
    diskography, lumbar 01905
    myelography, cervical 01905
    myelography, lumbar 01905
    myelography, posterior fossa 01905
    pneumoencephalography 01905
  integumentary system 00400-00410
  interpelviabdominal amputation 01140
  intracranial procedures 00210-00222
  intraoral procedures 00170-00176
  intraperitoneal procedures
    lower abdomen 00840-00851
    upper abdomen 00790-00796
  knee
    joint 01380-01404
    popliteal area 01320
  lithotripsy, extracorporeal shock wave 00872-00873
  lower
    anterior abdominal wall 00800-00802
    femur 01340-01360
    intestinal endoscopic procedures 00810
    leg, ankle, and foot 01465, 01470-01474
    leg cast 01490
    posterior abdominal wall 00820
  lumbar region 00630-00635

Anesthesia services for—continued
   major
      abdominal blood vessels 00770
      lower abdominal vessels 00880-00882, 01930
      vessels neck 00350-00352
   male external genitalia 00920-00938
   neck 00320-00322
   non-invasive imaging/radiation therapy 01922
   nose and accessory sinuses 00160-00164
   obesity, morbid 00797
   obturator neurectomy 01180-01190
   pacemaker insertion 00530
   partial rib resection 00470-00474
   patient extreme age 99100
   perineal integumentary system 00900-00908
   physiological support harvesting organ(s) 01990
   radical tumor pelvis 01150
   radius, ulna, wrist, or hand bones 01820-01832
   regional IV administration local anesthetic agent 01995
   repair arterio-venous (A-V) fistula 01784
   salivary glands 00100
   shoulder
      and axilla 01610
      cast application 01680-01682
   spine and spinal cord procedures 00670
   symphysis pubis/sacroiliac joint 01160-01170
   thoracic spine and cord 00620-00622
   thoracotomy procedures 00540-00548
   tibia, fibula, patella 01390-01392
   transurethral procedures 00910-00918
   upper
      anterior abdominal wall 00700-00702
      arm and elbow 01710-01716
      gastrointestinal endoscopic procedures 00740
      leg 01250
      posterior abdominal wall 00730
   vaginal procedures 00940-00952
   vascular shunt, or shunt revision 01844
   veins
      forearm, wrist, and hand 01850-01852
      knee and popliteal area 01430-01432
      lower leg 01520-01522
      shoulder and axilla 01670
      upper arm and elbow 01780-01782
      upper leg 01260
Angiogram through existing catheter 75898
Angiography
   adrenal 75731-75733
   arteriovenous shunt 75790
   brachial 75658
   carotid 75660-75680
   cervicocerebral 75650

Angiography—continued
  extremity
    bilateral 75716
    lower 73725
    unilateral 75710
    upper 73225
  internal mammary 75756
  pelvic 72198, 75736
  pulmonary 75741-75746
  renal 75722-75724
  selective 75774
  spinal 75705
  vertebral 75685
  visceral 75726
Angioplasty, pulmonary artery 92997-92998
Angioscopy therapeutic intervention 35400
Angiotensin converting enzyme (ACE) 82164
Animal inoculation 87001-87003, 87250
Ankle disarticulation 27889
Anogenital examination 99170
Anoplasty 46700-46705
Anorectal
  manometry 91122
  myomectomy 45108
Anoscopy 46600-46615
Antepartum care 59425-59426, 59510
Anterior
  colporrhaphy 57240, 57289
  vesicourethropexy 51841
    Marshall-Marchetti-Krantz, Burch 51840
Anthrax vaccine 90581
Anti-phosphatidylserine antibody 86148
Antibody
  actinomyces 86602
  adenovirus 86603
  aspergillus 86606
  bacterium 86609
  blastomyces 86612
  bordetella 86615
  borrelia 86618-86619
  brucella 86622
  campylobacter 86625
  candida 86628
  chlamydia 86631-86632
  coccidioides 86635
  coxiella brunetii (Q fever) 86638
  cryptococcus 86641
  cytomegalovirus (CMV) 86644-86645
  diphtheria 86648
  encephalitis
    California (La crosse) 86651
    Eastern equine 86652
    St. Louis 86653
    Western equine 86654

Antibody—continued
  enterovirus 86658
  Epstein-Barr (EB) virus 86663-86665
  francisella tularensis 86668
  fungus, not elsewhere specified 86671
  giardia lamblia 86674
  helicobacter pylori 86677
  helminth 86682
  hemophilus influenza 86684
  hepatitis
      A 86708-86709
      B 86704-86707
      C 86803-86804
      delta agent 86692
  herpes simplex 86694-86695
  histoplasma 86698
  HIV-1 86701
      and HIV-2 86702-86703
  HTLV/HIV antibody, confirmatory test 86689
  HTLV-I 86687
  HTLV-II 86688
  influenza virus 86710
  legionella 86713
  leishmania 86717
  leptospira 86720
  listeria monocytogenes 86723
  Lyme disease 86617
  lymphocytic choriomeningitis 86727
  lymphogranuloma venereum 86729
  mucormycosis 86732
  mumps 86735
  mycoplasma 86738
  neisseria meningitidis 86741
  nocardia 86744
  parvovirus 86747
  plasmodium (malaria) 86750
  protozoa, not elsewhere specified 86753
  red blood cell 86850-86870
  respiratory syncytial virus 86756
  rotavirus 86759
  rubella 86762
  rubeola 86765
  salmonella 86768
  shigella 86771
  tetanus 86774
  toxoplasma 86777-86778
  treponema pallidum 86781
  trichinella 86784
  varicella-zoster 86787
  virus not elsewhere specified 86790
  yersinia 86793
Antihuman globulin test (Coombs test) 86880-86886
Antinuclear antibodies (ANA) 86038-86039
Antistreptolysin O 86060-86063
Aortic suspension 33800

891

Aortography
    abdominal   75625-75630
    thoracic   75600-75605
Aortoplasty, supravalvular stenosis   33417
Apheresis, therapeutic   36511-36516
    plasma   36514
    platelets   36513
    red blood cells   36512
    white blood cells   36511
Apolipoprotein   82172
Appendectomy   44950-44960, 44970
Application
    allograft, skin   15350-15351
    cranial tongs, caliper, stereotactic frame   20660
    halo   20661-20664
    halo type appliance   21100
    interdental fixation device   21110
    intervertebral biomechanical device(s)   22851
    multiplane   20692
    neurostimulator   64550
    uniplane   20690
    xenograft skin   15400-15401
Aqueous shunt to extraocular reservoir   66180
Arrest, epiphyseal
    combined distal femur, proximal tibia and fibula   27479
    distal
        femur   27475
        fibula   27732
        tibia   27730
        tibia and fibula   27734
    proximal and distal tibia and fibula   27740-27742
    tibia and fibula   27477
Arrest hemiepiphyseal
    distal femur, proximal tibia/fibula   27485
Arsenic   82175
Arterial
    catheterization   36620-36625
    occlusion, temporary balloon   61623
    puncture   36600
Arteriovenous anastomosis   36819-36820
Arthrocentesis aspiration
    intermediate joint   20605
    major joint   20610
    small joint   20600
Arthrodesis
    additional interspace   22585
    ankle   27870
    atlas-axis   22595
    carpometacarpal joint
        digits   26843-26844
        thumb   26841-26842
    cervical   22554
    craniocervical   22590
    elbow joint   24800-24802

Arthrodesis—continued
    glenohumeral joint 23800-23802
    great toe 28750
    hip joint 27284-27286
    interphalangeal joint 26860-26863
    knee 27580
    lumbar 22558
    metacarpophalangeal joint 26850-26852
    midtarsal
        navicular-cuneiform (eg, Miller type procedure) 28737
        tarsometatarsal 28730-28740
    odontoid process 22548
    pantalar 28705
    radioulnar joint 25830
    sacroiliac joint 27280
    single interspace
        additional interspace 22632
        lumbar 22630
    single level
        cervical 22600
        lumbar 22612
        thoracic 22610
    spinal deformity
        anterior 22808-22812
        posterior 22800-22804
    subtalar 28725
    symphysis pubis 27282
    thoracic 22556
    tibiofibular joint 27871
    triple 28715
    wrist 25800-25810
Arthroplasty
    ankle 27700-27703
    elbow 24360-24363
    femoral prosthetic replacement 27130
    glenohumeral joint 23470-23472
    intercarpal/carpometacarpal joints 25447
    interphalangeal joint 26535-26536
    knee
        condyle and plateau 27446-27447
        femoral condyles/tibial plateau(s) 27442-27443
        hinge prosthesis (eg, Walldius type) 27445
        tibial plateau 27440-27441
    metacarpophalangeal joint 26530-26531
    patella 27437-27438
    prosthetic replacement
        distal radius 25441-25446
        distal ulna 25442
        lunate 25444
        scaphoid 25443
        trapezium 25445
    radial head 24365-24366
    temporomandibular joint 21240-21243
    wrist 25332

Arthroscopic
   repair, cruciate ligament   29888-29889
   treatment, fracture
      intercondylar spine(s) knee   29850-29851
      tibia   29855-29856
Arthroscopy
   ankle   29891-29899
   elbow
      diagnostic   29830
      surgical   29834-29838
   hip   29860-29863
   knee   29870-29889
   metacarpophalangeal joint   29900-29902
   shoulder
      diagnostic   29805
      surgical   29806-29827
   temporomandibular joint   29800, 29804
   unlisted   29999
   wrist
      diagnostic   29840
      surgical   29843-29848
Arthrotomy
   acromioclavicular, sternoclavicular joint   23044
   ankle   27610-27612, 27620
   biopsy
      hip joint   27052
      sacroiliac joint   27050
   carpometacarpal joint   26070, 26100
   distal radioulnar joint   25107
   elbow   24000-24102
   glenohumeral joint   23040, 23044, 23105-23107
   hip   27030-27033, 27054
   interphalangeal joint   26080, 26110
   intertarsal/tarsometatarsal joint   28020, 28050
   knee   27310, 27330-27335, 27403
   meniscus repair, knee   27403
   metacarpophalangeal joint   26075, 26105
   radiocarpal/midcarpal joint   25040
   sternoclavicular joint   23044, 23101, 23106
   synovectomy, hip joint   27054
   temporomandibular joint   21010
   wrist joint   25040, 25100-25105
Artificial insemination   58321-58323, 58976
Arytenoidectomy or arytenoidopexy   31400, 31560
Arytenoidopexy   31400
Ascending aorta graft   33860-33863
Ascorbic acid (vitamin C)   82180
Aspiration
   bladder   51000-51010
   bone cyst   20615
   bone marrow   38220
   cyst/pelvis   50390
   decompression procedure   62287
   fine needle   10021-10022

Binocular microscopy 92504
BIOFEEDBACK *90901-90911*
Biopsy
  abdominal 49000
  anorectal wall 45100
  bone 20220-20245
  bone marrow 38221
  brain stem 61575-61576
  breast 19100-19103
  cervix 57454-57455, 57460, 57500, 57520
  conjunctiva 68100
  cornea 65410
  epididymis 54800-54820
  external auditory canal 69105
  external ear 69100
  extraocular muscle 67350
  eyelid 67810
  floor mouth 41108
  hypopharynx 42802
  intestine 44020, 44100
  intranasal 30100
  lacrimal gland 68510
  lacrimal sac 68525
  lip 40490
  liver 47000-47001, 47100
  lung/mediastinum 32405, 32095-32100
  lymph node(s) 38500-38530
  muscle 20200-20206
  nail unit 11755
  nasopharynx 42804-42806
  nerve 64795
  oropharynx 42800
  ovary 58900
  palate uvula 42100
  pancreas 48100
  penis 54100-54105
  pleura 32400-32402
  prostate 55700-55705
  salivary gland 42405
  skin/subcutaneous tissue, mucous membrane 11100-11101
  soft tissue
    back/flank 21920-21925
    forearm wrist 25065-25066
    leg/ankle area 27613-27614
    neck/thorax 21550
    pelvis and hip area 27040-27041
    shoulder 23065-23066
    thigh/knee area 27323-27324
    upper arm/elbow area 24065-24066
  spinal cord, percutaneous 62269
  stomach 43600-43605
  testis 54500-54505
  thyroid 60100
  tongue 41100-41105

Biopsy—continued
  urethra 53200
  vaginal mucosa 57100-57105, 57421
  vertebral body 20250-20251
  vestibule mouth 40808
  vulva perineum 56605-56606, 56821
Biotinidase 82261
Bladder instillation
  anticarcinogenic agent 51720
  irrigation 51700
Blalock-taussig type operation (shunt subclavian to pulmonary artery) 33737-33750
Bleeding time 85002
Blepharoplasty 15820-15823
Blepharotomy drainage abscess eyelid 67700
Blood bank, physician services 86077-86079
Blood count
  blood smear examination 85007-85008
  differential WBC count 85004-85007, 85009
  hematocrit 85014
  hemoglobin 85018
  hemogram
    automated 85025-85027
    manual 85012, 85032
  red blood cell (RBC) 85032-85041
  reticulocyte count 85044-85046
  white blood cell (WBC) 85032, 85048
Blood gases 82803
Blood smear, peripheral, interpretation by physician 85060
Blood typing
  ABO 86900
  antigen screening compatible blood unit 86903-86904
  paternity testing 86910-86911
  RBC antigens, other than ABO/RH (D) 86905
  RH (D) 86901
  RH phenotyping 86906
Blood-derived peripheral stem cell harvesting 38205-38206
Bone age studies 76020
Bone density study 78350-78351
Bone graft
  cranial 61316, 62148
  femoral head, neck, intertrochanteric/subtrochanteric area 27170
  harvesting 20900-20902
  microvascular anastomosis
    fibula 20955
    other than fibula 20962
Bone imaging 78300-78320
Bone length studies (orthoroentgenogram, scanogram) 76040
Bone marrow
  aspiration 38220
  biopsy 38221
  harvesting 38230
  imaging 78102-78104
  smear interpretation 85097
  transplantation 38240-38242

Botulinum antitoxin   90287
Botulism immune globulin   90288
Bowel imaging   78290
Brachytherapy isodose calculation   77328
Bradykinin   82286
Brain imaging
   CT scan   0042T, 70450-70470, 70496
   MRI   70551-70553
   nuclear medicine   78600-78607, 78610
   PET   78608-78609
   x-ray with contrast   70010-70015
Brain implantation, chemotherapy agent   61517
Breast reconstruction   19357-19369
Breath hydrogen test   91065
Breathing response
   CO_2 response curve   94400
Bronchography   71040-71060
Bronchoplasty   31770-31775, 32501
Bronchoscopy
   biopsy   31625-31629, 31632-31633
   bronchial alveolar lavage   31624
   brushing/protected brushings   31623
   destruction tumor/relief stenosis   31641
   diagnostic   31622
   excision tumor   31640
   injection contrast material segmental bronchography   31656
   placement catheter(s) radioelement application   31643
   removal foreign body   31635
   therapeutic aspiration tracheobronchial tree   31645-31646
   tracheal dilation and placement tracheal stent   31631
   tracheal/bronchial dilation/closed reduction fracture   31630
   transbronchial biopsy   31628, 31632
     needle aspiration biopsy   31629, 31633
Bronchospasm evaluation   94060
Bundle his recording   93600
Burr hole(s)   61156-61210
   drainage hematoma   61154-61156
   exploration
     infratentorial   61253
     supratentorial   61250
   ventricular puncture, injection contrast media   61120
Bypass graft
   autogenous composite   35682-25683,
   composite, prosthetic and vein   35681
   with other than vein   35601-35671
   with vein   35501-35571

C

C-peptide   80432, 84681
C-reactive protein   86140-86141
Cadmium   82300
Calcifediol   82306

898

Calciferol (vitamin D)   82307
Calcitonin   82308
Calcium   82310-82340
Calculus   82355-82370
Caloric vestibular test   92533
Campbell type procedure (reconstruction dislocating patella)   27422
Cannulation, thoracic duct   38794
Canthoplasty   67950
Canthotomy   67715
Capsular contracture release (eg, Sever type procedure)   23020
Capsulectomy
   breast   19371
   interphalangeal joint   26525
   metacarpophalangeal joint   26520
Capsulodesis metacarpophalangeal joint   26516-26518
Capsulorrhaphy
   anterior   23450-23462
   anterior with labral repair   23455
   glenohumeral joint   23465-23466
   reconstruction, wrist   25320
Capsulotomy
   breast   19370
   foot   28260-28262
   hip   27036
   interphalangeal joint   26525, 28272
   knee   27435
   metacarpophalangeal joint   26520, 28270
   wrist   25085
Carbon dioxide   82374
   expired gas determination   94770
Carbon monoxide   82375-82376
   diffusing capacity   94720
Carcinoembryonic antigen (CEA)   82378
Cardiac
   blood pool imaging
      gated equilibrium   78472-78473, 78494-78496
      planar   78481-78483
   magnetic resonance imaging   75552-75556
   shunt detection   78428
Cardioassist method, circulatory assist   92970-92971
Cardiolipin (phospholipid) antibody   86147
Cardiopulmonary resuscitation   92950
Cardiotomy exploratory   33310-33315
Cardiovascular stress test   93015-93018
***CARDIOVASCULAR SYSTEM MEDICAL SERVICES**   92950-93799*
***CARDIOVASCULAR SYSTEM SURGICAL PROCEDURES**   33000-39599*
Cardioversion   92960-92961
Carnitine   82379
Carotene   82380
Carpectomy   25210-25215
Cartilage graft harvesting   20910-20912
***CASE MANAGEMENT SERVICES**   99361-99373*

Cast application
  body, shoulder to hips *29035-29046*
  elbow to finger *29075*
  hand and lower forearm *29085*
  shoulder to hand *29065*
  clubfoot *29450*
  cylinder *29365*
  finger
     cast *29086*
     splint *29130-29131*
  halo type body cast *29000*
  hip *29305-29325*
  long arm
     cast *29065*
     splint *29105*
  long leg
     cast *29345-29355, 29365, 29450*
     splint *29505*
  patellar tendon bearing (PTB) cast *29435*
  plaster
     figure-of-eight *29049*
     velpeau *29058*
  rigid total contact leg cast *29445*
  Risser jacket *29010-29015*
  short arm
     cast *29075*
     splint *29125-29126*
  short leg
     cast *29405-29435, 29450*
     splint *29515*
  shoulder spica *29055*
  turnbuckle jacket *29020-29025*
Cataract removal 66830-66990
Catecholamines 80424, 82382-82384
Cathepsin-D 82387
Catheter
  introduction
     aorta *36200*
     right heart/main pulmonary artery *36013*
  nasotracheal aspiration *31720*
  placement
     arterial system *36215-36248*
     coronary artery(s) *93508*
     pulmonary artery *36014-36015*
     venous system *36011-36012*
  tracheobronchial aspiration *31725*
Catheterization
  bronchial brush biopsy *31717*
  bronchography *31710*
  combined endoscopic *74330*
  sonohystergraphy/hysterosalpingography *58340*
  transglottic *31700*
  umbilical artery *36660*
  umbilical vein *36510*
  urethra *51701-51703*

900

Cauterization
 ablation, mucosa turbinates 30801-30802
 cervix 57510-57513
 nose, hemorrhage 30901-30906
Cell count, miscellaneous body fluids 89050-89051
Central auditory function test(s) 92589
CENTRAL NERVOUS SYSTEM ASSESSMENTS/TESTS* *96100-96177
Cephalogram, orthodontic 70350
Cerclage
 cervix during pregnancy 59320-59325
 uterine cervix 57700
Cerebral blood flow 78615
Cerebrospinal fluid flow, imaging 78630-78647
Ceruloplasmin 82390
Cervical puncture 61050-61055
Cervicoplasty 15819
Cesarean delivery 59514
Change
 biliary drainage catheter, percutaneous 47525
 cystostomy tube 51705-51710
 nephrostomy/pyelostomy tube 50398
 percutaneous tube/drainage catheter 75984
 ureterostomy tube 50688
Checkout orthotic/prosthetic use 97703
Chelatable iron, estimation total body iron 78172
Chemical
 cauterization 17250
 exfoliation 17360
 peel 15788-15793
 pleurodesis 32005
Chemiluminescent assay 82397
***CHEMISTRY* 82000-84999**
Chemodenervation extraocular muscle 67345
Chemosurgery, Mohs technique 17304-17310
Chemotaxis assay 86155
***CHEMOTHERAPY ADMINISTRATION* 96400-96549**
Chemotherapy implantation, brain 61517
***CHIROPRACTIC MANIPULATIVE TREATMENT (CMT)* 98940-98943**
Chloramphenicol 82415
Chloride 82435-82438
Chlorinated hydrocarbons 82441
Cholangiography, percutaneous 74320
Cholangiopancreatography 43260-43269
Cholecystectomy 47562-47564, 47600-47620
Cholecystoenterostomy 47570, 47720-47741
Cholecystography 74290-74291
Cholecystostomy percutaneous 47490
Choledochotomy/choledochostomy 47420-47425
Cholera vaccine 90725
Cholesterol, serum 82465
Cholinesterase 82480-82482
Chondroitin B sulfate 82485
Chopart type procedure (amputation, foot) 28800-28805
Chorionic villus sampling 59015
Chromatography 82486, 82491-82492

901

Chromium 82495
Chromogenic substrate assay 85130
Chromosome analysis 88280-88289
   amniotic fluid/chorionic villus 88267
   breakage syndromes 88245-88249
   in situ amniotic fluid cells 88269
Chromotubation oviduct 58350
Cineplasty 24940
Cineradiography 76120-76125
Circadian respiratory pattern recording 94772
Circumcision 54150-54161
Cisternography, positive contrast 70015
Citrate 82507
Clagett type procedure (closure chest wall) 32810
Claviculectomy 23120-23125
Clayton type procedure (ostectomy all metatarsal heads) 28114
Clinical pathology consultation 80500-80502
Clitoroplasty intersex state 56805
Closure
   anal fistula 46288
   aortico-left ventricular tunnel 33722
   atrioventricular valve 33600
   bladder exstrophy 51940
   chest wall (Clagett type procedure) 32810
   cystostomy 51880
   enteroenteric/enterocolic fistula 44650
   enterostomy 44620-44626
   enterovesical fistula 44660-44661
   esophagostomy/fistula 43420-43425
   gastrocolic fistula 43880
   gastrostomy surgical 43870
   intestinal cutaneous fistula 44640
   laceration vestibule mouth 40830-40831
   lacrimal
     fistula 68770
     punctum 68760-68761
   nephrocutaneous/pyelocutaneous fistula 50520
   nephrovisceral fistula 50525-50526
   postauricular fistula, mastoid 69700
   rectourethral fistula 45820-45825
   rectovaginal fistula 57300-57308
   rectovesical fistula 45800-45805
   salivary fistula 42600
   semilunar valve 33602
   sternotomy separation 21750
   ureterocutaneous fistula 50920
   ureterovisceral fistula 50930
   urethrocutaneous fistula 53520
   urethrostomy 53520
   urethrovaginal fistula 57310-57311
   ventricular septal defect 33681-33688
   vesicouterine fistula 51920-51925
   vesicovaginal fistula 51900
Clot lysis time 85175

903

Community/work reintegration training 97537
Compatibility test 86920
Complement
    antigen 86160
    fixation tests 86171
    functional activity 86161
    total hemolytic 86162
Computed tomography (CT scan)
    abdomen 74150-74175, 75635
    bone mineral density study 76070-76071
    cervical spine 72125-72127
    follow-up study 76380
    guidance
        needle biopsy 76360
        placement radiation therapy fields 76370
        stereotactic localization 76355
        visceral tissue ablation 76362
    head/brain 70450-70470, 70496, 0042T
    lower extremity 73700-73706, 75635
    lumbar spine 72131-72133
    maxillofacial area 70486-70488
    pelvis 72191-72194
    soft tissue neck 70490-70492, 70498
    thoracic spine 72128-72130
    thorax 71250-71275
    upper extremity 73200-73206
Computerized dynamic posturography 92548
Concentration parasites, ova, or tubercle bacillus (TB, AFB) 87015
Conditioning play audiometry 92582
Condylectomy, temporomandibular joint 21050
Conization cervix 57461, 57520-57522
Conjunctival flap 68360-68362
Conjunctivoplasty 68320-68330
Conjunctivorhinostomy 68745-68750
Construction
    apical-aortic conduit 33404
    artificial vagina 57291-57292
    bladder 51596
    intermarginal adhesions 67880-67882
    tracheoesophageal fistula 31611
CONSULTATIONS 99241-99275
CONSULTATIONS CLINICAL PATHOLOGY 80500-80502
Consultations
    medical
        confirmatory 99271-99275
        inpatient, initial 99251-99255
        inpatient, follow-up 99261-99263
        office 99241-99245
    pathology
        comprehensive 88321-88325
        during surgery 88329-88332
    radiology
        medical physics 77336-77370
        X-ray examination 76140

Contact laser vaporization 52648
Contact lens 92070, 92310-92317, 92325-92326, 92391, 92396
Continent
   diversion 50825
   ileostomy (Kock procedure) 44316
Continuous
   negative pressure (CNP) ventilation 94662
   positive airway pressure (CPAP) ventilation 94660
Contrast injection assessment abscess/cyst 49424
Control
   nasal hemorrhage
      anterior 30901-30903
      posterior 30905-30906
   nasopharyngeal hemorrhage 42970-42972
   oropharyngeal hemorrhage 42960-42962
Coombs test 86880
Copper 82525
Coracoacromial ligament release 23415
Cordocentesis 59012
Corneal
   relaxing incision 65772
   wedge resection 65775
Coronary
   angioplasty, balloon percutaneous transluminal 92982-92984
   artery bypass graft (CABG)
      arterial graft(s) 33533-33536
      vein only 33510-33516
      venous graft(s) and arterial graft(s) 33517-33523
   endarterectomy 33572
Coronoidectomy 21070
Corpora cavernosa
   corpus spongiosum shunt 54430
   glans penis fistulization 54435
   saphenous vein shunt 54420
Corpora cavernosography 74445
Correction/repair
   claw finger 26499
   cock-up fifth toe 28286
   everted punctum, cautery 68705
   hallux valgus 28290-28299
   hallux valgus (Keller, Mcbride, Mayo procedure) 28292
   hammertoe 28285
   inverted nipples 19355
   lid retraction 67911
   malrotation 44055
   trichiasis 67820-67835
Corticosterone 82528
Corticotropic releasing hormone (CRH) 80412
Cortisol 80412, 82533
Costotransversectomy 21610
Counterimmunoelectrophoresis 86185
CPAP (continuous positive airway pressure) ventilation 94660
CPK (creatine kinase) total 82550-82552

Craniotomy—continued
  treatment
    intracranial hypertension 61322-61323
    penetrating wound brain 61571
Creatine 82540
  kinase (CK), (CPK) 82550-82554
Creatinine 82565-82575
Creation
  arteriovenous fistula 36825
  lesion spinal cord by stereotactic method 63600
  pericardial window 32659
  shunt, cerebrospinal fluid 62200
Cricopharyngeal myotomy 43030
CRITICAL CARE SERVICES *99291-99292*
Cross intrinsic transfer 26510
Cryofibrinogen 82585
Cryoglobulin 82595
Cryopreservation
  embryo 89258
  freezing and storage cells 38207, 88240
  sperm 89259
Cryosurgery, rectal tumor 46937-46938
Cryotherapy, acne 17340
Cryptectomy 46210-46211
Crystal identification by light microscopy 89060
CSF leakage detection and localization 78650
Culture
  and fertilization oocyte(s) 89250-89251
  bacterial 87040-87088
  chlamydia 87110
  fungus 87101-87106
  mycobacteria 87116-87118
  mycoplasma 87109
  pathogen 87084
  tubercle/acid-fast bacilli 87116
  typing 87140-87158
Curettage
  cauterization anal fissure 46940-46942
  postpartum 59160
Cutaneous
  appendico-vesicostomy 50845
  vesicostomy 51980
Cyanide 82600
Cyanocobalamin (vitamin B-12) 82607-82608
Cystectomy
  complete 51570-51596
  partial 51550-51565
Cystine and homocystine, urine 82615
Cystography 74430
Cystolithotomy cystotomy with removal calculus 51050
Cystometrogram 51725-51726
Cystoplasty, cystourethroplasty 51800
Cystorrhaphy suture bladder wound, injury/rupture 51860-51865

Cystotomy
    excision
        bladder diverticulum 51525
        bladder tumor 51530
        ureterocele repair 51535
        vesical neck 51520
    insertion radioactive material 51020-51030
    insertion ureteral catheter or stent 51045
    stone basket extraction 51065
    with drainage 51040
Cystourethroplasty 51800-51820
Cystourethroscopy 52000-52355, 52647-52648
CYTOGENETIC STUDIES *88271-88275, 88291, 88299*
Cytogenetics and molecular cytogenetics 88291
Cytomegalovirus
    antibody 86644-86645
    immune globulin (CMV-IgIV) 90291
CYTOPATHOLOGY *88104-88199*
    cervical or vaginal 88141-88143
    slides cervical or vaginal 88150-88155, 88164-88167
    smears
        cervical or vaginal 88147-88148
        other source 88160-88162

D

Dacryocystography nasolacrimal duct 68850, 70170
Dacryocystorhinostomy 68720
Damus-Kaye-Stansel procedure (anastomosis pulmonary artery to aorta) 33606
Dark
    adaptation examination 92284
    field examination 87164-87166
Debridement
    mastoid cavity 69220-69222
    nail(s) 11720-11721
    open fracture(s) dislocation(s), skin 11010-11012
    skin 11040-11044
        infected 11000-11001
Decalcification procedure 88311
Declotting vascular access device or catheter 36550
Decompression
    facial nerve 61950, 69720-69725, 69740-69745, 69955
    fasciotomy
        forearm 24495
        forearm wrist 25020-25025
    fingers, hand 26035
    internal auditory canal 69960
    lesion, brain stem or upper spinal cord 61575-61576
    orbit 61330
    plantar digital nerve 64726
    spinal cord equina nerve root(s) 63055-63057

Decompression—continued
  spinal cord nerve root(s) 63064-63066
  unspecified nerve(s) 64722
Decompressive fasciotomy hand 26037
Decortication
  and parietal pleurectomy 32320
  pulmonary 32220-32225, 32651-32652
Dehydroepiandrosterone (DHEA) 82626
  -sulfate (DHEA-S) 82627
Delay flap or sectioning flap
  eyelids, nose, ears, or lips 15630
  forehead, cheeks, chin, neck, axillae, genitalia, hands, or feet 15620
  scalp, arms, or legs 15610
  trunk 15600
Deligation, ureter 50940
Delivery placenta 59414
Denervation hip joint 27035
Denis-Browne splint strapping 29590
Deoxycortisol 80436, 82634
Deoxyribonuclease antibody 86215
Deoxyribonucleic acid (DNA) antibody 86225-86226
Dermabrasion 15780-15783
***DERMATOLOGY MEDICAL PROCEDURES** 96900-96999*
Descending thoracic aorta graft 33875
Desoxycorticosterone 82633
Destruction
  benign or premalignant lesions, skin 17000-17250
  celiac plexus by neurolytic agent 64680
  cervical spinal muscles by neurolytic agent 64613
  ciliary body 66700-66740
  cutaneous vascular proliferative lesions 17106-17108
  cyst or lesion, iris or ciliary body 66770
  hemorrhoids 46934-46936
  intercostal nerve by neurolytic agent 64620
  lesion
    anus 46900-46924
    choroid 67220-67225, 0016T
    conjunctiva 68135
    cornea 65450
    dentoalveolar structures 41850
    lid margin 67850
    palate or uvula 42160
    penis 54050-54065
    retina 67208-67218, 67227-67228, 0017T
    vestibule mouth 40820
    vulva 56501-56515
  malignant lesion
    face, ears, eyelids, nose, lips, mucous membrane 17280-17286
    scalp, neck, hands, feet, genitalia 17270-17276
    trunk, arms or legs 17260-17266
  nerve joint
    cervical or thoracic by neurolytic agent 64626-64627
    lumbar or sacral by neurolytic agent 64622-64623
    other peripheral nerve or branch by neurolytic agent 64640

909

Destruction —continued
    pudendal nerve by neurolytic agent 64630
  rectal tumor 45190, 46937-46938
  retinopathy 67227-67228
  superior hypogastric plexus 64681
  trigeminal nerve by neurolytic agent 64600-64610
  vaginal lesion(s) 57061-57065
  warts, molluscum contagiosum, or milia 17110-17111
Determination of
  airway closing volume 94370
  central c-v hemodynamics 78414
  maldistribution inspired gas 94350
  refractive state 92015
  resistance to airflow 94360
  venous pressure 93770
Determinative histochemistry 88318-88319
Development cognitive skills 97532
Developmental testing 96110-96111
DIAGNOSTIC RADIOLOGY SERVICES 70010-76499
DIAGNOSTIC ULTRASOUND SERVICES 76506-76999
DIALYSIS SERVICES 90918-90999
Dialysis
  hemodialysis 90935-90940
  peritoneal 90945-90947
  training 90989-90993
Diaphragm or cervical cap fitting 57170
Dibucaine number 82638
DIGESTIVE SYSTEM SURGICAL PROCEDURES 40490-49999
Digital analysis electroencephalogram (EEG) 95957
Dihydrocodeinone 82646
Dihydromorphinone 82486, 82649
Dihydrotestosterone (DHT) 82651
Dihydroxyvitamin D 82652
Dilation
  and curettage (D&C), corpus uteri 58120
  anal sphincter 45905
  biliary duct stricture, percutaneous transhepatic 74363
  catheterization, salivary duct 42660
  cervical canal 57800
  cervical stump 57820
  esophagus 43450-43458
  lacrimal punctum 68801
  rectal sphincter 45910
  salivary duct 42650
  urethra 53660-53665
  urethral stricture 52281, 53600-53621
  vagina 57400
Dimethadione 82654
Diphtheria
  and tetanus toxoids (DT) 90702
  antibody 86648
  antitoxin 90296
  tetanus toxoids and acellular pertussis vaccine (DTaP) 90700

Diphtheria—continued
  tetanus toxoids and acellular pertussis vaccine and hemophilus influenza B vaccine (DTaP-HiB) 90721
  tetanus toxoids and whole cell pertussis vaccine and hemophilus influenza B vaccine (DTP-HiB) 90720
  tetanus toxoids and whole cell pertussis vaccine (DTP) 90701
  toxoid 90719
Direct nasal mucous membrane test 95065
Direct or patch closure, sinus venosus 33645
Disarticulation
  hip 27295
  knee 27598
  shoulder 23920-23921
  wrist 25920-25924
Discission
  secondary membranous cataract 66820-66821
  vitreous strands 67030
Diskectomy 63075-63078
Diskography 72285-72295
Dislocation
  acromioclavicular, open treatment 23550-23552
  acute shoulder, open treatment 23660
  ankle
    closed treatment 27840-27842
    open treatment 27846-27848
  anterior pelvic ring, open treatment 27217
  carpometacarpal other than thumb
    closed treatment 26676-26676
    open treatment 26685-26686
    percutaneous skeletal fixation 26676
  carpometacarpal thumb, closed treatment 26641-26645
  distal radioulnar
    closed treatment 25675
    open treatment 25676
  elbow
    closed treatment 24600-24605, 24640
    open treatment 24615
  fracture, trans-scaphoperilunar type
    closed treatment 25680
    open treatment 25685
  hip
    arthroplasty, closed treatment 27265-27266
    closed treatment 27250-27252
    open treatment 27253-27254, 27258-27259
  interphalangeal joint
    closed treatment 26770-26775, 28660-28665
    open treatment 26785, 28675
    percutaneous skeletal fixation 26770-26776, 28666
  knee
    closed treatment 27550-27552
    open treatment 27556-27558
  lunate
    closed treatment 25690
    open treatment 25695

DOCUMENTATION OF EXAMINATIONS—continued
   Hematologic, lymphatic and/or immunologic examination 133
   Musculoskeletal examination 136
   Neurological examination 139
   Psychiatric examination 142
   Respiratory examination 145
   Skin examination 148
Documentation of medical decision making 151
Documentation of counseling or coordination of care 154
DOMICILIARY, REST HOME, CUSTODIAL CARE SERVICES *99321-99333*
Donor procedures
   cardiectomy 33940
   cardiectomy-pneumonectomy 33930
   hepatectomy 47133, 47140-47142
   nephrectomy 50300-50320
   pancreatectomy 48550
   pneumonectomy 32850
Doppler echocardiography 93320-93350
   fetal 76827-76828
Douglas type procedure (suture tongue to lip micrognathia) 41510
Drainage
   abscess
      dentoalveolar structures 41800
      external auditory canal 69020
      finger 26010-26011
      hematoma external ear 69000-69005
      hematoma, nasal 30000
      hematoma, nasal septum 30020
      lymph node or lymphadenitis 38300-38305
      ovary 58823
      palate, uvula 42000
      parotid 42300-42305
      perirenal or renal 50020-50021
      peritoneal or localized peritonitis 49020-49021
      periurethral 53040
      perivesical or prevesical space 51080
      retroperitoneal 49060-49061
      scrotal wall 55100
      subdiaphragmatic or subphrenic 49040-49041
      submaxillary or sublingual, intraoral 42310
      submaxillary, external 42320
      vestibule mouth 40800-40801
   extraperitoneal lymphocele to peritoneal cavity 49062
   ovarian cyst(s) 58800-58805
   palmar bursa 26025-26030
   pelvic abscess 58823
   perineal, urinary extravasation 53080-53085
   pseudocyst, pancreas 48510-48511
   skene's gland, abscess or cyst 53060
   tendon sheath, digit palm 26020
Dressing change under anesthesia 15852
   burns 16010-16030
Drug analysis, tissue preparation 80103

Drug assay
    amikacin 80150
    amitriptyline 80152
    benzodiazepine 80154
    carbamazepine 80156-80157
    cyclosporine 80158
    desipramine 80160
    digoxin 80162
    dipropylacetic acid (valproic acid) 80164
    doxepin 80166
    ethosuximide 80168
    gentamicin 80170
    gold 80172
    haloperidol 80173
    imipramine 80174
    lidocaine 80176
    lithium 80178
    nortriptyline 80182
    phenobarbital 80184
    phenytoin 80185-80186
    primidone 80188
    procainamide 80190-80192
    quantitation drug, not elsewhere specified 80299
    quinidine 80194
    salicylate 80196
    tacrolimus 80197
    theophylline 80198
    tobramycin 80200
    topiramate 80201
    vancomycin 80202
Drug confirmation 80102
Drug implant(s) 11981-11983
Drug screens 80100-80101, 82486
***DRUG TESTING** 80100-80103*
DT 90702
DTaP 90700
DTP 90701, 90720
Dual energy x-ray absorptiometry (DEXA), bone density study 76075-76076, 0028T
Duodenal
    exclusion with gastrojejunostomy 48547
    intubation and aspiration 89100-89105
Duodenography, hypotonic 74260
Duodenotomy 44010
Duplex scan
    abdominal pelvic, scrotal contents, retroperitoneal organs 93975-93979
    aorta, inferior vena cava, iliac vasculature, or bypass grafts 93978-93979
    extracranial arteries 93880-93882
    extremity veins 93970-93971
    hemodialysis access 93990
    lower extremity arteries or arterial bypass grafts 93925-93926
    penile vessels 93980-93981
    upper extremity arteries or arterial bypass grafts 93930-93931
Dural graft, spinal 63710
Dwyer type procedure (osteotomy calcaneus) 28300
Dynamic cavernosometry 54231

E

Ear
    piercing   69090
    protector attenuation measurements   92596
Echocardiography
    fetal   76825-76826
    transesophageal   93312-93314
    transthoracic   93307-93308
Echoencephalography   76506
Echography
    abdominal   76700-76705
    breast(s)   76645
    chest   76604
    extremity   76880
    infant, hips   76885-76886
    intraoperative   76986
    pelvic   76856-76857
    placement radiation therapy fields   76950
    pregnant uterus   76805-76816
    retroperitoneal   76770-76775
    scrotum   76870
    soft tissues head and neck   76536
    spinal canal and contents   76800
    transplanted kidney   76778
    transrectal   76872-76873
    transvaginal   76817, 76830
Educational supplies   99071
Egger's type procedure (transfer tendon/muscle, hamstrings to femur)   27400
Electrical stimulation to aid bone healing   20974-20975
Electro-oculography   92270
Electrocardiographic monitoring   93224-93237
Electrocochleography   92584
Electroconvulsive therapy   90870-90871
Electrocorticogram at surgery   95829
Electroejaculation   55870
Electroencephalogram (EEG)   95812-95830, 95950-95958
    during nonintracranial surgery   95955
Electrolysis epilation   17380
Electromyography
    motion analysis   96002, 96003
    needle   95860-95872
    studies (EMG) anal or urethral sphincter   51784
Electron microscopy   88348-88349
Electronic analysis
    antitachycardia pacemaker system   93724
    dual chamber
        internal pacemaker system   93733
        pacemaker system   93731-93732
    implantable loop recorder (ILR) system   93727
    implanted neurostimulator pulse generator system   95970-95975

Electronic analysis—continued
   pacing cardioverter-defibrillator 93741-93744
   programmable implanted pump 62367-62368
   single chamber
      internal pacemaker system 93736
      pacemaker system 93734-93735
Electrophoretic technique 82664
Electrophysiologic evaluation
   comprehensive 93619-93622
   pacing cardioverter-defibrillator 93642
      leads 93640-93641
   study with pacing and recording 93624
Electroretinography 92275
Elevation depressed skull fracture 62000-62010
Embolectomy
   axillary, brachial, innominate, subclavian artery 34101
   carotid, subclavian or innominate artery 34001
   femoropopliteal, aortoiliac artery 34201
   innominate, subclavian artery 34051
   popliteal-tibio-peroneal artery 34203
   pulmonary artery 33910
   radial or ulnar artery 34111
   renal, celiac, mesentery, aortoiliac artery 34151
Embryo transfer intrauterine 58974
EMERGENCY DEPARTMENT SERVICES 99281-99288
End stage renal disease (ESRD)
   full month 90918-90921
   less than full month 90922-90925
Endocervical curettage 57505
ENDOCRINE SYSTEM SURGICAL PROCEDURES 60000-60699
Endolymphatic sac operation 69805-69806
Endometrial sampling 58100
Endomyocardial biopsy 93505
Endoscopic
   catheterization 74328-74329
   evaluation small intestinal pouch 44385-44386
   flexible fiberoptic evaluation, swallowing 92612-92617
   injection implant material submucosal tissues 51715
   plantar fasciotomy 29893
   retrograde cholangiopancreatography (ERCP) 43260-43272
Endoscopy
   biliary 47550-47556
   coronary artery bypass 33508
   ophthalmic 66990
   vascular 37500-37501
   wrist, surgical 29848
Endovascular repair, iliac aneurysm 34900
Enterectomy resection small intestine 44120-44128, 44202
Enteroclysis tube, percutaneous placement 74355
Enterocystoplasty 51960
Enteroenterostomy anastomosis intestine 44130
Enterolysis 44005
Enterostomy
   or cecostomy, tube 44300
   small bowel 44020-44021

916

Enterovirus
  antibody 86658
  antigen detection 87267
Enucleation
  excision external thrombotic hemorrhoid 46320
  eye 65101-65105
Environmental intervention medical management purposes 90882
Enzyme activity 82657-82658
Epiandrosterone 82666
Epicardial and endocardial pacing and mapping, intra-operative 93631
Epididymectomy 54860-54861
Epididymovasostomy 54900-54901
Epidurography 72275
Epiglottidectomy 31420
Epikeratoplasty 65767
Epiphyseal arrest
  distal radius and ulna 25455
  distal radius or ulna 25450
  greater trochanter 27185
Episiotomy or vaginal repair 59300
Ergonovine provocation test 93024
Erythropoietin 82668
Escharotomy 16035-16036
Esophageal
  intubation and collection washings 91000
  motility 78258
  motility study 91010-91012
  recording atrial electrogram 93615-93616
Esophagectomy
  cervical partial 43116
  distal two-thirds, partial 43117-43121
  thoracoabdominal or abdominal approach, partial 43122-43123
  total 43107-43113
  total or partial 43124
Esophagogastric fundoplasty
  Collis 43326
  Nissen, Belsey IV, Hill procedures 43324
  Thal-Nissen procedure 43325
Esophagogastric tamponade 43460
Esophagogastrostomy (cardioplasty) 43320
Esophagojejunostomy abdominal approach 43340-43341
Esophagomyotomy (Heller type) 43330-43331
Esophagoplasty 43300-43314
Esophagoscopy
  ablation tumor(s), polyp(s), or other lesion(s) 43228
  balloon dilation 43220
  band ligation esophageal varices 43205
  biopsy 43202
  control bleeding 43227
  diagnostic 43200
  injection sclerosis esophageal varices 43204
  insertion
    guide wire 43226
    plastic tube or stent 43219

EVALUATION AND MANAGEMENT SERVICES CODES—continued
   Hospital services 99217-99239
   Intensive (non-critical) low birthweight services 99298-99299
   Neonatal critical care 99295-99296
   Newborn care 99431-99440
   Nursing facility services 99301-99316
   Office or other outpatient services 99201-99215
   Pediatric critical care 99293-99294
   Pediatric critical care patient transport 99289-99290
   Preventive medicine services 99381-99429
   Prolonged services 99354-99360
   Unlisted E/M services 99499
Evaluation
   cardiovascular function with tilt table evaluation 93660
   fine needle aspirate 88172-88173
   hearing aid, electroacoustic 92594-92595
   speech 92506
   swallowing and oral function 92610-92613
   voice prosthetic communication device 92597
Evisceration ocular contents 65091-65093
EVOCATIVE/SUPPRESSION TESTING *80400-80440*
Evoked
   otoacoustic emissions 92587-92588
   potentials and reflex tests 95925-95937
Exchange
   abscess or cyst drainage catheter 49423
   arterial catheter during thrombolytic therapy 37209
   intraocular lens 66986
   previously placed arterial catheter 75900
   transfusion blood 36450-36455
Excision
   abdominal wall tumor 22900
   ampulla of vater 48148
   and repair eyelid 67961-67966
   aural
     glomus tumor 69550-69554
     polyp 69540
   Bartholin's gland or cyst 56740
   benign cyst or tumor, mandible 21040
   benign lesion
     arms or legs 11400-11406
     face, ears, eyelids, nose, lips, mucous membrane 11440-11446
     scalp, neck, hands, feet, genitalia 11420-11426
   benign tumor
     carpal bones 25130-25136
     clavicle or scapula 23140-23146
     cranial bone 61563-61564
     facial bone 21029
     femur 27355-27358
     humerus 24110-24116, 24116
     mandible 21046-21047
     maxilla 21048-21049
     metacarpal 26200-26205

CPT PLUS! 2004

Excision—continued
    benign tumor—continued
        phalanx finger   26210-26215
        proximal humerus   23150-23156
        radius or olecranon process   24120-24126
        radius or ulna   25120-25126
    bile duct tumor   47711-47712
    bone
        clavicle   23180
        facial bone(s)   21026
        femur, tibia fibula partial   27360
        fibula   27641
        humerus   24140
        mandible   21025
        metacarpal partial   26230
        olecranon process   24147
        phalanx finger partial   26235-26236
        phalanx toe   28124
        proximal humerus   23184
        radial head or neck   24145
        radius   25151
        scapula   23182
        talus or calcaneus   28120
        tarsal or metatarsal bone   28122
        tibia   27640
        ulna   25150
    bone cyst
        carpal bones   25130-25136
        clavicle or scapula   23140-23146
        femur   27355-27358
        humerus   24110-24116
        metacarpal   26200-26205
        phalanx finger   26210-26215
        proximal humerus   23150-23156
        radius or olecranon process   24120-24126
        radius or ulna   25120-25126
    bone cyst or benign tumor   27065-27067
        humerus   24110
        phalanges foot   28108
        proximal humerus   23150-23156
        talus or calcaneus   28100-28103
        tarsal or metatarsal bones 28104-28107
        tibia or fibula   27635-27638
    branchial cleft cyst   42810-42815
    breast lesion   19125-19126
    bulbourethral gland (Cowper's gland)   53250
    carotid body tumor   60600-60605
    cervical
        rib   21615-21616
        stump   57540-57556
    chalazion   67800-67808
    chest wall tumor
        including ribs   19260
        involving ribs   19271-19272

920

Excision—continued
  choledochal cyst 47715
  coarctation aorta 33840-33851
  coccygeal pressure ulcer 15920-15922
  constricting ring, finger 26596
  cyst or adenoma, thyroid 60200
  cyst(s) kidney 50280
  cystic hygroma 38550-38555
  dermoid cyst, nose 30124-30125
  distal ulna 25240
  epiphyseal bar 20150
  excessive skin and subcutaneous tissue
    abdomen 15831
    arm 15836
    buttock 15835
    forearm or hand 15837
    hip 15834
    leg 15833
    other area 15839
    submental fat pad 15838
    thigh 15832
  exostosis(es), external auditory canal 69140
  extensor tendon, hand or finger 26415
  external ear 69110-69120
  fibroadenoma breast tissue 19120
  fibrous tuberosities, dentoalveolar structures 41822
  flexor tendon implantation, prosthetic rod 26390
  foot lesion tendon, tendon sheath, or capsule 28090
  frenum labial or buccal 40819
  fulguration
    carcinoma urethra 53220
    skene's glands 53270
    urethral caruncle 53265
    urethral polyp(s) 53260
    urethral prolapse 53275
  ganglion wrist 25111-25112
  hemorrhoid tags 46230
  hydrocele 55040-55041
    spermatic cord 55500
  hyperplastic alveolar mucosa 41828
  infected graft
    abdomen 35907
    extremity 35903
    neck 35901
    thorax 35905
  interdigital neuroma 28080
  intra-abdominal or retroperitoneal tumors 49200-49201
  intracardiac tumor 33120
  intranasal lesion 30117-30118
  ischial bursa 27060
  ischial pressure ulcer 15940-15946
  lacrimal gland 68500-68505
    tumor 68540-68550
  lacrimal sac 68520

Excision—continued
   lactiferous duct fistula 19112
   lesion
      conjunctiva 68110-68130
      cornea 65400
      epididymis 54830
      esophagus 43100-43101
      eyelid 67840
      floor mouth 41116
      meniscus or capsule knee 27347
      mesentery 44820
      palate, uvula 42104-42107
      pancreas 48120
      pharynx 42808
      sclera 66130
      small or large bowel 44110-44111
      spermatic cord 55520
      tendon sheath or capsule 26160
      tendon sheath or capsule leg ankle 27630
      tendon sheath, forearm wrist 25110
      testis 54512
      tongue 41110-41114
      tumor dentoalveolar structures 41825-41827
      vestibule mouth 40810-40816
   lingual
      frenum 41115
      tonsil 42870
   lip 40510-40527
   lymph node(s) 38500
   malignant lesion
      face, ears, eyelids, nose, lips 11640-11646
      scalp, neck, hands, feet, genitalia 11620-11626
      trunk, arms, or legs 11600-11606
   malignant tumor
      facial bone 21034
      mandible 21044-21045
      stomach 43611
   maxillary torus palatinus 21032
   meckel's diverticulum 44800
   mediastinal
      cyst 39200
      tumor 39220
   mucosa vestibule mouth 40818
   Mullerian duct cyst 55680
   nail and nail matrix 11750-11752
   nasal polyp(s) 30110-30115
   neurofibroma
      cutaneous nerve 64788
      extensive 64792
      major peripheral nerve 64790
   neuroma
      cutaneous nerve 64774
      digital nerve 64776-64778
      hand or foot 64782-64783

Excision—continued
   neuroma—continued
      major peripheral nerve 64784
      sciatic nerve 64786
   olecranon bursa 24105
   osseous tuberosities, dentoalveolar structures 41823
   parotid tumor or gland 42410-42426
   penile plaque 54110-54112
   pericardial cyst or tumor 33050
   perinephric cyst 50290
   pilonidal cyst 11770-11772
   pituitary tumor 61546
   posterior vertebral component intrinsic bony lesion 22100-22103
   prepatellar bursa 27340
   presacral or sacrococcygeal tumor 49215
   pterygium 65420-65426
   radial head 24130
   rectal
      procidentia 45130-45135
      tumor 45160-45170
   rib 21600
   sacral pressure ulcer 15931-15937
   skin and subcutaneous tissue hidradenitis 11450-11471
   soft tissue
      lesion, external auditory canal 69145
      tumor, shoulder 23075-23076
   spermatocele 54840
   sublingual
      gland 42450
      salivary cyst 42408
   submandibular (submaxillary) gland 42440
   surgical planing skin nose rhinophyma 30120
   synovial cyst, popliteal space (eg, Baker's cyst) 27345
   tendon
      finger 26180
      palm 26170
   thyroglossal duct cyst or sinus 60280-60281
   toe lesion tendon, tendon sheath, or capsule 28092
   tonsil tags 42860
   torus mandibularis 21031
   tracheal
      stenosis and anastomosis 31780-31781
      tumor or carcinoma 31785-31786
   trochanteric
      bursa or calcification 27062
      pressure ulcer 15950-15958
   tumor
      foot 28043-28045
      forearm wrist area 25075-25076
      hand or finger 26115-26116
      leg or ankle area 27618-27619
      pelvis and hip area 27047-27048
      soft tissue back or flank 21930
      soft tissue neck or thorax 21555-21556

Excision—continued
  tumor—continued
    thigh or knee area 27327-27328
    upper arm or elbow area 24075-24076
  turbinate 30130
  ulcer or benign tumor, stomach 43610
  urachal cyst or sinus 51500
  urethral diverticulum 53230-53235
  vaginal
    cyst or tumor 57135
    septum 57130
  varicocele or ligation spermatic veins varicocele 55530-55540
  vertebral body, intrinsic bony lesion 22110-22116
Exclusion small bowel from pelvis 44700
Exenteration orbit 65110-65114
Expired gas collection 94250, 0043T
Exploration
  carotid artery 35701
  congenital atresia bile ducts 47700
  epididymis 54820
  femoral artery 35721
  forearm or wrist, with removal foreign body 25248
  middle ear 69440
  orbit with
    biopsy 61332
    removal foreign body 61334
    removal lesion 61333
  other vessels 35761
  penetrating wound
    abdomen/flank/back 20102
    chest 20101
    extremity 20103
    neck 20100
  popliteal artery 35741
  postoperative hemorrhage, thrombosis or infection
    abdomen 35840
    chest 35820
    extremity 35860
    neck 35800
  repair and drainage rectal injury 45562-45563
  retroperitoneal area 49010
  spinal fusion 22830
  undescended testis 54550-54560
Exploratory laparotomy, exploratory celiotomy 49000
Exposure prostate 55860-55865
Expression conjunctival follicles 68040
Extensive craniectomy multiple cranial suture craniosynostosis 61558-61559
External
  cannula declotting 36860-36861
  cephalic version 59412
  ocular photography 92285
Extracapsular cataract removal 66984
Extractable nuclear antigen, antibody to 86235
Extrapleural enucleation empyema 32540
***EYE AND OCULAR ADNEXA SURGICAL PROCEDURES** 65091-68899*

F

Facial nerve
   decompression, repair total 69955
   function studies 92516
Factor inhibitor test 85335
Family psychotherapy 90846-90847, 99510
Fascia lata graft 20920-20922
Fasciectomy 26121-26125
   plantar fascia 28060-28062
Fasciotomy
   elbow lateral or medial 24350-24356
   foot toe 28008
   hip or thigh 27025
   iliotibial, open 27305
   leg 27600-27602, 27892-27894
   palmar 26040-26045
   thigh, knee decompression 27496-27499, 27892-27894
Fat
   differential, feces 82715
   or lipids, feces 82705-82710
   stain, feces, urine, or sputum 89125
Fatty acids 82725
Fc receptor 86243
FEMALE GENITAL SYSTEM SURGICAL PROCEDURES 56405-58999
Fenestration semicircular canal 69820
Ferritin 82728
Fetal
   biophysical profile 76818-76819
   contraction stress test 59020
   fibronectin 82731
   monitoring 59050-59051
   non-stress test 59025
   scalp blood sampling 59030
Fibrin degradation products, d-dimer 85378-85380
Fibrin(ogen) degradation products (fdp)(fsp) 85362-85370
Fibrinogen 85384-85385
Fibrinolysins or coagulopathy screen 85390
Fibrinolysis assay 85396
Fibrinolytic factors and inhibitors 85400-85421
Filleted finger or toe flap 14350
Filtered speech test 92571
Fimbrioplasty 58760
Fine needle aspiration 10021-10022
   orbital contents 67415
Fissurectomy 46200
Fistulization
   sclera glaucoma 66150-66172
   sublingual salivary cyst 42325-42326
Fitting
   contact lens 92070, 92310-92313
   diaphragm or cervical cap 87170

925

Fitting—continued
   insertion pessary 57160
   low vision aid 92354-92355
     spectacle prosthesis 92352-92353
     spectacles 92340-92342
Fixation
   contralateral testis 54620
   spinal internal by wiring 22841
   tongue mechanical 41500
Flap
   island pedicle 15740
   neurovascular pedicle 15750
   omental 49904-49906
Flexor origin slide forearm wrist 25315-25316
Flexor-plasty elbow 24330-24331
Flow cytometry 88180-88182
Fluorescein
   angiography 92235
   angioscopy 92230
Fluorescent noninfectious agent antibody 86255-86256
Fluoride 82735
Fluoroscopic
   guidance 76003
   localization needle biopsy 76005
Fluoroscopy, physician time 76001
Flurazepam 82742
Focal application phase control substance 69410
Folic acid 82746-82747
Follicle puncture 58970
Foreign body
   brain 61570
   dentoalveolar structures 41805
   esophagus 74235
   external auditory canal 69200
   external eye 65205
   eyelid 67938
   foot 28190
   intraocular 65235
   intravascular 75961
   lacrimal passages 68530
   localization ophthalmic ultrasonic 76529
   muscle or tendon sheath removal 20520
   pelvis or hip 27086
   penis 54115
   peritoneal cavity 49085
   pharynx 42809
   scrotum 55120
   shoulder 23330
   subcutaneous tissues incision and removal 10120
   upper arm or elbow area 24200
   vagina 57415
   vestibule mouth 40804
Foreskin manipulation 54450

Formation pedicle   *15570-15576*
Fracture
  acetabulum
    closed treatment   *27220-27222*
    open treatment   *27226-27228*
  articular
    closed treatment   *26740-26742*
    open treatment   *26746*
  bimalleolar ankle
    closed treatment   *27808-27810*
    open treatment   *27814*
  calcaneal
    closed treatment   *28400-28405*
    open treatment   *28415-28420*
    percutaneous skeletal fixation   *28406*
  carpal bone
    closed treatment   *25630-25635*
    open treatment   *25645*
  carpal scaphoid
    closed treatment   *25622-25624*
    open treatment   *25628*
  carpometacarpal thumb
    closed treatment   *26641-26645*
    open treatment   *26665*
    percutaneous skeletal fixation   *26650*
  clavicular
    closed treatment   *23500-23505*
    open treatment   *23515*
  coccygeal
    closed treatment   *27200*
    open treatment   *27202*
  complicated
    frontal sinus, open treatment   *21344*
    mandible, open treatment   *21470*
  depressed
    frontal sinus, open treatment   *21343*
    malar, open treatment   *21360*
    zygomatic arch, open treatment   *21356*
  distal fibular
    closed treatment   *27786-27788*
    open treatment   *27792*
  distal phalangeal finger or thumb
    closed treatment   *26750-26755*
    open treatment   *26765*
    percutaneous skeletal fixation   *26756*
  distal radial
    closed treatment   *25600-25605*
    open treatment   *25620*
    percutaneous skeletal fixation   *25611*
  femoral shaft
    closed treatment   *27500-27503, 27508*
    open treatment   *27506-27507*

Fracture—continued
  femur
      closed treatment *27238-27245*
      distal end, medial or lateral condyle, open treatment *27514*
      epiphyseal separation, closed treatment *27516-27517*
      epiphyseal separation, open treatment *27519*
      neck, closed treatment *27230-27232*
      open treatment *27236, 27513*
      percutaneous skeletal fixation *27235, 27509*
  great toe phalanx or phalanges
      closed treatment *28490-28495*
      open treatment *28505*
      percutaneous skeletal fixation *28496*
  greater humerus tuberosity
      closed treatment *23620-23625*
      open treatment *23630*
  greater trochanteric
      closed treatment *27246*
      open treatment *27248*
  humerus
      closed treatment *23600*
      condylar, closed treatment *24576-24577*
      condylar, open treatment *24579*
      condylar, percutaneous skeletal fixation *24582*
      epicondylar, closed treatment *24560-24565*
      epicondylar, open treatment *24575*
      epicondylar, percutaneous skeletal fixation *24566*
      percutaneous skeletal fixation *24538*
  humerus shaft
      closed treatment *24500-24505*
      open treatment *24515-24516*
  humerus supracondylar or transcondylar
      closed treatment *24530-24535*
      open treatment *24545-24546*
  hyoid
      closed treatment *21493-21494*
      open treatment *21495*
  iliac spine, open treatment 27215
  intercondylar spine(s) knee
      closed treatment *27538*
      open treatment *27540*
  interdental wiring 21497
  larynx, closed treatment 31585-31586
  malar area
      open treatment *21365-21366*
      percutaneous treatment *21355*
  mandible
      condylar, open treatment *21465*
      external fixation, open treatment *21454*
      interdental fixation, closed treatment *21453*
      interdental fixation, open treatment *21462*

Fracture—continued
  mandible—continued
    manipulation, closed treatment 21451
    maxillary alveolar ridge, closed treatment 21440
    maxillary alveolar ridge, open treatment 21445
    percutaneous treatment 21452
    without interdental fixation, open treatment 21461
    without manipulation, closed treatment 21450
  medial malleolus
    closed treatment 27760-27762
    open treatment 27766
  metacarpal
    closed treatment 26600-26607
    open treatment 26615
    percutaneous skeletal fixation 26608
  metatarsal
    closed treatment 28470-28475
    open treatment 28485
    percutaneous skeletal fixation 28476
  nasal
    bone, closed treatment 21310-21320
    open treatment 21325-21335
    septal, closed treatment 21337
    septal, open treatment 21336
    turbinate(s) 30930
  nasoethmoid
    complex, percutaneous treatment 21340
    open treatment 21338-21339
  nasomaxillary complex (Lefort II type)
    closed treatment 21345
    open treatment 21346-21348
  odontoid, open treatment 22318-22319
  orbit
    closed treatment 21400-21401
    open treatment 21406-21408
  orbital floor blowout, open treatment 21385-21395
  palatal or maxillary (Lefort I type)
    closed treatment 21421
    open treatment 21422-21423
  patellar
    closed treatment 27520
    open treatment 27524
  pelvic ring
    closed treatment 27193-27194
    percutaneous skeletal fixation 27216
  periarticular elbow, open treatment 24586-24587
  phalangeal finger or thumb, open treatment 26765
  phalangeal shaft
    closed treatment 26720-26725
    open treatment 26735
    percutaneous skeletal 26727
  phalanx or phalanges, other than great toe
    closed treatment 28510-28515
    open treatment 28525

Fracture —continued
  proximal fibula or shaft
    closed treatment 27780-27781
    open treatment 27784
  proximal humerus
    closed treatment 23600-23605
    open treatment 23615-23616
  radial and ulnar shaft
    closed treatment 25560-25565
    open treatment 25574-25575
  radial head or neck
    closed treatment 24650-24655
    open treatment 24665-24666
  radial shaft
    closed treatment 25500-25505, 25520
    open treatment 25515, 25525-25526
  rib
    closed treatment 21800
    open treatment 21805
  scapular
    closed treatment 23570-23575
    open treatment 23585
  sesamoid
    closed treatment 28530
    open treatment 28531
  skull, closed treatment 21300
  sternum
    closed treatment 21820
    open treatment 21825
  talus
    closed treatment 28430-28435
    open treatment 28445
    percutaneous skeletal fixation 28436
  tarsal bone
    open treatment 28465
    percutaneous skeletal fixation 28456
    treatment 28450-28455
  tibia
    closed treatment 27824-27825
    open treatment 27826-27828
  tibia proximal
    closed treatment 27530-27532
    open treatment 27535-27536
  tibial shaft
    closed treatment 27750-27752
    open treatment 27758-27759
    percutaneous skeletal fixation 27756
  treatment rib requiring external fixation 21810
  trimalleolar ankle
    closed treatment 27816-27818
    open treatment 27822-27823
  ulna
    closed treatment 24670-24675
    open treatment 24685

Fracture—continued
  ulnar shaft
    closed treatment 25530-25535
    open treatment 25545
  ulnar styloid
    closed treatment 25650
    open treatment 25652
  vertebra, open treatment 22325-22328
  vertebral
    body, closed treatment 22310
    closed treatment 22315
    process, closed treatment 22305
Fredet-Ramstedt type operation (pyloromyotomy) 43520
Free
  fascial flap 15758
  flap
    fascial 15758
    muscle 15756
    omental 49904-49906
    skin 15757
  jejunum transfer with microvascular anastomosis 43496
  muscle flap 15756
  omental flap with microvascular anastomosis 49906
  osteocutaneous flap with microvascular anastomosis
    great toe 20973
    iliac crest 20970
    metatarsal 20972
  skin flap 15757
Frenoplasty 41520
Fresh frozen plasma 86927
Frost suture (temporary closure eyelids by suture) 67875
Frozen blood preparation 86930-86932
Fructose 82757, 84375
Fsh 83001
Functional
  cortical and subcortical mapping 95961-95962
  residual capacity 94240
Fundus photography 92250
Fusion thumb with autogenous graft 26820

G

Galactokinase, RBC 82759
Galactose 82760
  Galactose-1-phosphate uridyl transferase 82775-82776
Gamete, zygote, or embryo intrafallopian transfer 58976
Gammaglobulin
  IgA, IgD, IgG, IgM 82784
  IgE 82785
  immunoglobulin subclasses, (IgGL, 2, 3, and 4) 82787
Ganglion cyst, aspiration 20612

Gases
  blood, any combination pH, pCO$_2$, pO$_2$, CO, HCO$_3$ 82803-82805
  blood, O$_2$ saturation 82810
  blood, pH only 82800
Gastrectomy 43620-43639
Gastric
  acid 82926-82928
  analysis test 91052
  emptying study 78264
  intubation aspiration
    diagnostic 89130-89132
    fractional collections 89135-89141
    lavage treatment 91105
  intubation washings, and preparing slides cytology 91055
  motility studies 91020
  mucosa imaging 78261
  restrictive procedure, with gastric bypass 43846-43847
    without gastric bypass 43842-43843
  saline load test 91060
Gastrin 82941
  after secretin stimulation 82938
Gastrocnemius recession (eg, Strayer procedure) 27687
Gastroduodenostomy 43810, 43850-43855
GASTROENTEROLOGY MEDICAL PROCEDURES *91000-91299*
Gastroesophageal reflux study 78262
Gastrointestinal
  endoscopic ultrasound 76975
  protein loss 78282
  reconstruction previous esophagectomy 43360-43361
  tract imaging 91110
Gastrojejunostomy 43820-43825, 43860-43865
Gastrorrhaphy 43840
Gastrostomy 43830-43832
  tube change 43760
  tube, percutaneous placement 43750
Gastrotomy 43500-43510
  tube, percutaneous placement 74350
Generation automated data 78890-78891
Genioplasty 21120-21123
Gingivectomy 41820
Gingivoplasty 41872
Glossectomy 41120-41155
Glucagon 82943
  tolerance panel 80422-80424
  tolerance test 82946
Glucose 80422-80424, 80430-80435, 82945, 82947-82953
  blood by glucose monitoring device(s) 82962
  monitoring 95250
Glucose-6-phosphate dehydrogenase (G6PD) 82955-82960
Glucosidase, beta 82963
Glutamate dehydrogenase 82965
Glutamine (glutamic acid amide) 82975
Glutamyltransferase, gamma (GGT) 82977

Glutathione   82978
  reductase, RBC   82979
Glutethimide   82980
Glycated protein   82985
Goldwaite type procedure (reconstruction dislocating patella)   27422
Gonadotropin
  chorionic (HCG)   84702-84703
  follicle stimulating hormone (FSH)   83001
  luteinizing hormone (LH)   83002
  releasing hormone stimulation panel   80426
Gonioscopy   92020
Goniotomy   65820
Graft
  bone
    cranial   61316
    mandible   21215
    nasal maxillary or malar areas   21210
  composite   15760
  derma-fat-fascia   15770
  ear cartilage   21235
  facial nerve paralysis
    free fascia graft   15840
    free muscle graft   15841-15842
    regional muscle transfer   15845
  forehead, cheeks, chin, mouth, neck, axillae, genitalia, hands, feet   15240-15241
  nose, ears, eyelids, lips   15260-15261
  rectal incontinence prolapse   46753
  rib cartilage   21230
  scalp, arms, legs   15220-15221
  trunk   15200-15201
Gross type operation (repair omphalocele)   49610-49611
Group psychotherapy   90853
Growth hormone
  human (HGH) (somatotropin)   83003
  human (HGH), antibody   86277
  stimulation panel   80428
  suppression panel   80430
Guanosine monophosphate (GMP), cyclic   83008

H

H-reflex, amplitude and latency study   95934-95936
Hallux rigidus correction first metatarsophalangeal joint   28289
Handling conveyance specimen   99000-99002
Haptoglobin   83010-83012
Harrington rod technique (posterior non-segmental instrumentation)   22840
Harvest
  femoropopliteal vein   35572
  upper extremity vein   35500
Hauser type procedure (reconstruction dislocating patella)   27420
HEALTH AND BEHAVIOR ASSESSMENT/INTERVENTION   96150-96155

Hearing aid
   check   92592-92593
   examination and selection   92590-92591
Heart catheterization, combined
   right and
      left heart   93529
         retrograde left heart   93526-93531
         transseptal left heart   93527-93533
      right with left ventricular puncture   93528
      transseptal and retrograde left heart   93524
Heart transplant   33945
Heart-lung transplant   33935
Heavy metal   83015-83018
Heinz bodies   85441-85445
Helicobacter pylori, breath test analysis   78267-78268, 83013-83014
Heller type procedure (esophagomyotomy)   43330
Hemagglutination inhibition test (HAI)   86280
HEMATOLOGY AND COAGULATION   *85002-85999*
Hematopoietic progenitor cell(s)
   donor   38204
   harvesting   38205-38206
   transplant preparation   38207-38215
Hemiarthroplasty hip   27125
HEMIC AND LYMPHATIC SYSTEMS SURGICAL PROCEDURES   *38100-38999*
Hemiepiphyseal arrest   24470
Hemiphalangectomy or interphalangeal joint excision, toe   28160
Hemodialysis procedure   90935-90937
Hemoglobin   83026-83069
   fractionation and quantitation   83020-83021
   or RBCs, fetal   85460-85461
Hemolysin
   acid   85475
   and agglutinins   86940-86941
Hemoperfusion   90997
Hemophilus influenza B vaccine (HIB)   90645-90648
Hemorrhage management liver   47350-47362
Hemorrhoidectomy   46221-46262
Hemosiderin   83070-83071
Heparin
   assay   85520
   neutralization   85525
   -protamine tolerance test   85530
Hepatectomy   47120-47133, 47140-47142
Hepatic venography   75889-75891
Hepaticotomy or hepaticostomy   47400
Hepatitis
   A and hepatitis B vaccine (hepA-hepB)   90636
   A antibody (haab)   86708-86709
   A vaccine   90632-90634
   B and hemophilus influenza B vaccine (hepb-hib)   90748
   B core antibody (hbcab)   86704-86705
   B immune globulin (hbig)   90371
   B surface antibody (hbsab)   86706
   B vaccine   90744-90747

Hepatitis—continued
  Be antibody (hbeab)   86707
  C antibody   86803-86804
Hepatobiliary ductal system imaging   78223
Hepatotomy   47010-47011
Heterophile antibodies   86308-86310
Heyman type procedure (capsulotomy, midtarsal)   28264
Hib (hemophilus influenza B vaccine)   90645
His bundle recording   93600
Histamine   83088
History and examination normal newborn infant   99431, 99435
HLA typing
  A, B, or C   86812-86813
  dr/dq   86816-86817
  lymphocyte culture   86821-86822
HOME HEALTH PROCEDURES   99500-99600
HOME INFUSION PROCEDURES   99601-99602
HOME SERVICES   99341-99350
Home visit
  established patient   99347-99350
  new patient   99341-99345
Homovanillic acid (HVA)   83150
Hospital care
  initial   99221-99223
  subsequent   99231-99233
Hospital discharge day management   99238-99239
HOSPITAL SERVICES   99217-99239
Hydroxycorticosteroids   83491
Hydroxyindolacetic acid   83497
Hydroxyprogesterone   80402-80406, 83498-83499
Hydroxyproline   83500-83505
Hymenectomy partial   56700
Hymenotomy   56720
Hyperbaric oxygen therapy   99183
Hyperthermia   77600-77620
Hypnotherapy   90880
Hypophysectomy or excision pituitary tumor   61548
Hypothermia   99185-99186
Hysterectomy   58150-58294, 58550-58554
Hysteroplasty   58540
Hysterorrhaphy   58520
  ruptured uterus   59350
Hysterosalpingography   74740
Hysteroscopy   58555-58563
Hysterosonography   76831
Hysterotomy, abdominal   59100

I

Ileoscopy through stoma   44380-44383
Ileostomy or jejunostomy, non-tube   44310
Imaging lymphatics and lymph nodes   78195

Imbrication diaphragm   39545
Immune complex assay   86332
IMMUNE GLOBULINS   *90281-90399*
IMMUNIZATION ADMINISTRATION VACCINES/TOXOIDS   *90471-90474*
Immunoassay   83516-83520
   infectious agent antibody   86317-86318, 87449-87451
   tumor antigen   86294, 86316
Immunocytochemistry   88342
Immunodiffusion   86329-86331
Immunoelectrophoresis   86320-86327, 86334
Immunofixation electrophoresis   86334
Immunofluorescent study   88346-88347
IMMUNOLOGY   *86000-86849*
Implant
  non-biodegradeable drug
    insertion   11981
    removal   11982
    removal and reinsertion   11983
  removal
    elbow joint   24160
    radial head   24164
Implantation
  cardiac event recorder   33282
  device intrathecal or epidural drug infusion   62360-62362
  electromagnetic bone conduction hearing device   69710
  intracavitary chemotherapy agent   61517
  intrathecal or epidural catheter   62350-62351
  intravitreal drug delivery system   67027
  mesh or other prosthesis   49568
  nerve end into bone or muscle   64787
  neurostimulator electrode array, percutaneous   63650
  neurostimulator electrodes
    autonomic nerve   64560
    cranial nerve   64553
    neuromuscular   64565
    peripheral nerve   64555
  ventricular assist device   33975-33976, 33979
Impression
  auricular prosthesis   21086
  definitive obturator prosthesis   21080
  facial prosthesis   21088
  interim obturator prosthesis   21079
  mandibular resection prosthesis   21081
  nasal prosthesis   21087
  oral surgical splint   21085
  orbital prosthesis   21077
  palatal
    augmentation prosthesis   21082
    lift prosthesis   21083
  speech aid prosthesis   21084
  surgical obturator prosthesis   21076
In-situ vein bypass   35582-35587

Incision
  abscess soft tissue   20000-20005
  anal septum   46070
  bone cortex
    femur or knee   27303
    foot   28005
    forearm OR wrist   25035
    hand or finger   26034
    humerus or elbow   23935
    pelvis hip joint   26992
    shoulder area   23035
    thorax   21510
  cataract   66820-66821
  conjunctiva, drainage cyst   68020
  cornea, astigmatism   65772
  drainage
    lacrimal gland   68400
    lacrimal sac   68420
  extensor tendon sheath, wrist   25000
  femoral artery   34812-34813
  frontal lobe   61490
  gallbladder   47490
  hemorrhoids, external   46083
  hymenotomy   56720
  iliac artery, exposure   34820, 34833
  implantation neurostimulator electrodes
    autonomic nerve   64577
    cranial nerve   64573
    neuromuscular   64580
    peripheral nerve   64575
  iris   66500-66505
  kidney   50010, 50045
  labial frenum   40806
  lacrimal punctum   68440
  larynx   31300-31320
  leg or ankle   27607
  lingual frenum   41010
  lung, biopsy   32095-32100
  mitral valve   33420-33422
  nerve
    root   63185-63190
    sacral   64581
    vagus   43640-43641
  pericardium   33015-33020
  prostate, transurethral   52450
  skin   10040-10180
  spinal cord   63200
  synovectomy   26140
  thrombosed hemorrhoid   46083
  trachea, emergency 31603-31605
  ureter   50600

Incision and drainage
  abscess 10060-10061
    appendiceal 44900-44901
    floor mouth 41015-41018
    intramural, intramuscular, or submucosal 46045
    ischiorectal or intramural 46060
    ischiorectal perirectal 46040
    neck or thorax 21501-21502
    perianal abscess 46050
    rectum 45005-45020
    retropharyngeal or parapharyngeal 42720-42725
    supralevator, pelvirectal, or retrorectal 45020
    thigh or knee region 27301
    tongue/floor mouth 41000-41009
    vulva or perineum 56405
  Bartholin's gland abscess 56420
  bursa, foot 28001
  epididymis, testis scrotal space 54700
  foot 28002-28003
  forearm wrist 25028-25031
  hematoma 10140
  leg or ankle 27603-27604
  pelvis or hip joint area 26990-26991
  penis 54015
  perianal abscess 46050
  peritonsillar abscess 42700
  pilonidal cyst 10080-10081
  postoperative wound infection 10180
  shoulder area 23030-23031
  thyroglossal cyst 60000
  upper arm or elbow area 23930-23931
Incision and placement
  cranial neurostimulator pulse generator 61885-61886
  peripheral neurostimulator pulse generator 64590
  spinal neurostimulator pulse generator 63685
Incision and reconstruction atria operative 33253
Incision and removal foreign body, subcutaneous tissues 10120-10121
Incontinence treatment, pulsed magnetic neuromodulation 0029T
Indicator dilution studies 93561-93562
Indocyanine-green angiography 92240
Induced abortion 59840-59857
Induction arrhythmia by electrical pacing 93618
Infectious agent
  antigen detection
    enzyme immunoassay technique 87301-87430
    immunofluorescent technique 87260-87299
  detection
    immunoassay direct optical observation 87810-87899
    nucleic acid (DNA or RNA) 87470-87660
Influenza virus vaccine 90655-90660
Infratemporal
  post-auricular approach to middle cranial fossa 61591
  pre-auricular approach to middle cranial fossa 61590
Infusion or instillation radioelement solution 77750

Ingestion challenge test 95075
Inhalation bronchial challenge testing 95070-95071
Injection
   air or contrast into peritoneal cavity 49400
   anterior chamber 66020-66030
   contrast medium dacryocystography 68850
   corpora cavernosa 54235
   epidural blood or clot patch 62273
   including catheter placement 62318-62319
   infusion neurolytic substance 62280-62282
   intralesional 11900-11901
   sinus tract 20500-20501
   tendon sheath ligament 20550-20551
   therapeutic
      agent into tenon's capsule 67515
      prophylactic or diagnostic 90782-90784
   turbinate(s) 30200
   vitreous substitute 67025
Injection anesthetic agent
   axillary nerve 64417
   brachial plexus 64415-64416
   carotid sinus 64508
   celiac plexus 64530
   cervical plexus 64413
   facial nerve 64402
   femoral nerve 64447-64448
   greater occipital nerve 64405
   ilioinguinal, iliohypogastric nerves 64425
   intercostal nerve(s)
      single 64420
      multiple, regional block 64421
   lumbar or thoracic 64520
   lumbar plexus 64449
   paracervical (uterine) nerve 64435
   paravertebral facet joint nerve 64470-64476
   peripheral nerve or branch 64450
   phrenic nerve 64410
   pudendal nerve 64430
   sciatic nerve 64445-64446
   sphenopalatine ganglion 64505
   spinal accessory nerve 64412
   stellate ganglion 64510
   superhypogastric plexus 64517
   suprascapular nerve 64418
   transforaminal epidural 64479-64484
   trigeminal nerve, any division or branch 64400
   vagus nerve 64408
Injection procedure
   ankle arthrography 27648
   cardiac catheterization 93539-93545
   chemonucleolysis 62292
   cholangiography 47505
      percutaneous transhepatic 47500
   contrast venography 36005

Injection procedure—continued
   corpora cavernosography 54230
   cystography or voiding urethrocystography 51600
   diskography 62290-62291
   elbow arthrography 24220
   evaluation previously placed peritoneal-venous shunt 49427
   hip arthrography 27093-27095
   identification sentinel node 38792
   intraoperative pancreatography 48400
   knee arthrography 27370
   lymphangiography 38790
   mammary ductogram or galactogram 19030
   myelography computerized axial tomography, spinal 62284
   occlusion arteriovenous malformation, spinal 62294
   peyronie disease 54200-54205
   placement chain contrast chain urethrocystography 51605
   pyelography 50394
   retrograde urethrocystography 51610
   sacroiliac joint 27096
   shoulder arthrography 23350
   sialography 42550
   splenoportography 38200
   temporomandibular joint arthrography 21116
   ureterography 50684
   ureteropyelography 50684
   visualization ileal conduit ureteropyelography 50690
   wrist arthrography 25246
Injection sclerosing solution 36470-36471
   hemorrhoids 46500
   spider veins
     face 36469
     limb or trunk 36468
Insertion
   arterial and venous cannula 36823
   bladder catheter, non-indwelling 51701
     indwelling 51702-51703
   breast prosthesis 19340-19342
   cannula
     hemodialysis 36800-36815
     prolonged extracorporeal circulation 36822
   cardioverter-defibrillator
     electrodes 33245
     pulse generator 33240, 33246
   central venous catheter
     non-tunneled 36555-36556
     tunneled 36557-36558
   central venous access device
     subcutaneous port 36560-36561, 36570-36571
     subcutaneous pump 36563
     with catheters 36565-36566
     without port or pump 36568-36569
   cervical dilator 59200
   drug delivery implant, non-biodegradable 11981
   electrode lead(s) 33249

940

Insertion—continued
  flow directed catheter (eg, Swan-Ganz) 93503
  graft aorta or great vessels 33330-33335
  implantable contraceptive capsules 11975
  intra-arterial infusion pump 36260
  intra-aortic balloon
    assist device 33970, 33973
    catheter, percutaneous 33967
  intraocular lens prosthesis 66985
  intraperitoneal cannula or catheter 49419-49421
  intrauterine device (IUD) 58300
  nasal septal prosthesis 30220
  ocular implant 65130-65140
  pacemaker
    pulse generator only 33212-33213
    fluoroscopy and radiography 71090
  pacing electrode, cardiac venous system 33224, 33225
  penile prosthesis 54400-54405
  peritoneal-venous shunt 49425
  permanent pacemaker 33200-33208
  pin-retained palatal prosthesis 42281
  sphenoidal electrodes 95830
  subcutaneous reservoir, pump or infusion system 61215
  temporary
    cardiac electrode or pacemaker catheter 33210
    pacing electrodes 33211
  testicular prosthesis 54660
  thomas shunt 36835
  tissue expander(s) 11960
  transvenous intrahepatic portosystemic shunt 37182
  wire or pin with application skeletal traction 20650
Instillation contrast material laryngography or bronchography 31708
Instrumentation
  anterior 22845-22847
  posterior
    non-segmental (eg, Harrington rod technique) 22840
    segmental 22842-22844
Insulin 80422, 80432-80435, 83525-83527
  antibodies 86337
  tolerance panel 80434
INTEGUMENTARY SYSTEM SURGICAL PROCEDURES 10040-19499
Intensity modulated radiotherapy 77301, 77418
Intensive (non-critical) low birth weight services 99298-99299
Interactive group psychotherapy 90857
Interruption inferior vena cava 37620
INTERSEX SURGICAL PROCEDURES 55970-55980
Interstitial
  radioactive colloid therapy 79300
  radioelement application 77776-77778
Interthoracoscapular amputation 23900
Intervention, health and behavior 96152-96155
Intestinal
  bleeding tube, passage, positioning and monitoring 91100
  plication 44680
  stricturoplasty 44615

941

Intra-articular radiopharmaceutical therapy 79440
Intra-atrial
  pacing 93610
  recording 93602
Intracapsular cataract extraction 66983
Intracardiac catheter ablation
  arrhythmogenic focus 93651-93652
  atrioventricular node function 93650
Intracavitary
  radioactive colloid therapy 79200
  radioelement application 77761-77763
Intracutaneous tests 95015-95028
Intraluminal dilation strictures obstructions 74360
Intramuscular injection antibiotic 90788
Intravascular
  coronary flow reserve measurement 93571-93572
  radiopharmaceutical therapy 79420
  ultrasound 37250-37251
Intravenous injection agent to test blood flow 15860
Intraventricular
  intra-atrial mapping tachycardia site(s) 93609
  pacing 93612
Intravitreal injection pharmacologic agent 67028
Intrinsic factor 83528
  antibodies 86340
Introduction
  catheter, superior or inferior vena cava 36010
  guide, renal pelvis ureter 50395
  hemostatic agent or pack, vaginal hemorrhage 57180
  intracatheter or catheter, renal pelvis 50392-74475
  long gastrointestinal tube (eg, Miller-Abbott) 44500-74340
  needle
    aortic translumbar 36160
    arteriovenous shunt 36145
    brachial artery 36120
    carotid or vertebral artery 36100
    extremity artery 36140
    vein 36000
  transhepatic
    catheter, percutaneous 47510
    stent, percutaneous 47511
  ureteral catheter 50393-74480
Intubation endotracheal, emergency procedure 31500
Ipecac administration 99175
Iridectomy 66600-66635
Iridoplasty by photocoagulation 66762
Iridotomy
  laser surgery 66761
  stab incision 66500-66505
Iron 83540
  binding capacity 83550
  stain (RBC or bone marrow smears) 85536
Irradiation blood product 86945

L

Labeled red cell sequestration 78140
Laboratory panel
    ACTH stimulation panel 80400
    acute hepatitis panel 80074
    basic metabolic panel 80048
    comprehensive metabolic panel 80053
    corticotropic releasing hormone (CRH) stimulation panel 80412
    electrolyte panel 80051
    general health panel 80050
    glucagon tolerance panel 80422-80424
    gonadotropin releasing hormone stimulation panel 80426
    growth hormone
        stimulation panel 80428
        suppression panel 80430
    hepatic function panel 80076
    insulin
        tolerance panel 80434-80435
        -induced C-peptide suppression panel 80432
    lipid panel 80061
    metyrapone panel 80436
    obstetric panel 80055
    renal function 80069
    thyrotropin releasing hormone (trh) stimulation panel 80438-80440
LABORATORY SERVICES CODES 80000-89999
    Anatomic pathology 88000-88099
    Chemistry 82000-84999
    Consultations clinical pathology 80500-80502
    Cytogenetic studies 88230-88299
    Cytopathology 88104-88199
    Drug testing 80100-80103
    Evocative/suppression testing 80400-80440
    Hematology and coagulation 85002-85999
    Immunology 86000-86849
    Microbiology 87001-87999
    Organ or disease oriented panels 80048-80076
    Other pathology and laboratory procedures 89050-89240
    Reproductive medicine procedures 89250-89356
    Surgical pathology 88300-88399
    Therapeutic drug assays 80150-80299
    Transcutaneous procedures 88400
    Transfusion medicine 86850-86999
    Urinalysis 81000-81099
Labyrinthectomy 69905-69910
Labyrinthotomy 69801-69802
Lactate (lactic acid) 83605
    dehydrogenase (ld), (ldh) 83615-83625
Lactogen 83632
Lactose 83633-83634

Laminectomy
  biopsy/excision, intraspinal neoplasm 63275-63290
  cordotomy 63194-63199
  drainage, intramedullary cyst/syrinx 63172-63173
  excision
    arteriovenous malformation spinal cord 63250-63252
    intraspinal lesion, intradural 63270-63273
    intraspinal lesion neoplasm 63265-63268
  exploration decompression spinal cord 63001-63011, 63015-63017
  facetectomy and foraminotomy 63045-63048
  implantation neurostimulator electrodes 63655
  myelotomy 63170
  release tethered spinal cord 63200
  removal abnormal facets pars inter-articularis 63012
  rhizotomy 63185-63190
  section
    dentate ligaments 63180-63182
    spinal accessory nerve 63191
Laminotomy decompression nerve root(s) 63020-63044
Laparoscopic treatment ectopic pregnancy 59150-59151
Laparoscopically assisted nephroureterectomy 50548
Laparoscopy
  abdomen, peritoneum, and omentum 49320-49323
  ablation renal cysts 50541-50542
  adrenalectomy 60650
  appendectomy 44970
  cholecystectomy 47562
    with cholangiography 47563
    with exploration common duct 47564
  cholecystoenterostomy 47570
  donor nephrectomy 50547
  enterolysis 44200
  esophagogastric fundoplasty (eg, Nissen, Toupet procedures) 43280
  fimbrioplasty 58672
  fulguration oviducts 58670
  gastrostomy 43653
  hysterectomy 58550-58554
  intestinal resection 44202
  jejunostomy 44201
  ligation spermatic veins varicocele 55550
  liver 47370-47379
  lymphatic system 38570-38572
  lysis adhesions 58660
  myomectomy 58545-58546
  nephrectomy 50543, 50546
  occlusion oviducts by device 58671
  orchiectomy 54690
  orchiopexy 54692
  pyeloplasty 50544
  removal
    adnexal structures 58661
    leiomyomata 58561
  salpingostomy 58673
  sling operation 51992

Laparoscopy—continued
   splenectomy 38120
   transection vagus nerves 43651-43652
   transhepatic cholangiography 47560-47561
   ureterolithotomy 50945
   urethral suspension 51990
   vaginal hysterectomy 58550
Laparotomy 58960
   hepatic parasitic cyst(s) or abscess(es) 47015
Lapidus type procedure (correction hallux valgus) 28297
Laryngeal
   function studies 92520
   reinnervation 31590
   sensory testing 92614-92617
Laryngectomy
   partial 31367-31382
   subtotal 31367-31368
   total 31360-31382
Laryngography contrast 31708, 70373
Laryngoplasty 31580-31588
   cricoid split 31587
   not otherwise specified 31588
Laryngoscopy
   direct 31515-31571
   flexible fiberoptic 31575-31578
   flexible or rigid fiberoptic 31579
   indirect 31505-31513
Laryngotomy 31300-31320, 31360-31368
Laser treatment for skin disease (psoriasis) 96920-96922
Lateral
   canthopexy 21282
   retinacular release 27425
Lavage
   by cannulation
      maxillary sinus 31000
      sphenoid sinus 31002
   colonic 44701
   peritoneal 49080
Layer closure wounds
   face, ears, eyelids, nose, lips mucous membranes 12051-12057
   neck, hands, feet external genitalia 12041-12047
   scalp, axillae, trunk extremities 12031-12037
LDH 83615-83625
Lead 83655
Lecithin-sphingomyelin ratio (l/s ratio) 83661-83662
Left
   heart catheterization 93510-93514
   ventricular pacing and recording 93622
Lengthening
   hamstring tendon 27393-27395
   palate
      and pharyngeal flap 42226
      with island flap 42227

Lengthening—continued
   shortening
      flexor or extensor tendon, forearm wrist 25280
      tendon, leg or ankle 27685-27686
   tendon
      extensor, hand or finger 26476
      flexor, hand or finger 26478
Leucine aminopeptidase (lap) 83670
Leukocyte
   alkaline phosphatase with count 85540
   count
      automated 85004, 85025, 85027, 85048
      differential 85004-85009, 85025
      fecal 89055
      manual 85007, 85009, 85032
   histamine release test (lhr) 86343
   phagocytosis 86344
   transfusion 86950
Ligation
   arteries
      ethmoidal 30915
      internal maxillary artery 30920
   banding angioaccess arteriovenous fistula 37607
   biopsy, temporal artery 37609
   common iliac vein 37660
   division
      and stripping, saphenous veins 37720-37735
      long saphenous vein 37700
      short saphenous vein 37780
   esophageal varices 43400
   external carotid artery 37600-37606
   femoral vein 37650
   internal
      hemorrhoids 46945-46946
      jugular vein 37565
      or common carotid artery 37605-37606
   major artery
      abdomen 37617
      chest 37616
      extremity 37618
      neck 37615
   perforators, subfascial, radical (Linton type) 37760
   peritoneal-venous shunt 49428
   salivary duct, intraoral 42665
   stapling at gastroesophageal junction 43405
   takedown systemic-to-pulmonary artery shunt 33924
   transection fallopian tube(s) 58600-58611, 58670
   varicose veins 37785
   vas deferens 55450
Linton type procedure (ligation perforators) 37760

Lipase   83690
Lipectomy, suction assisted
    head and neck   15876
    lower extremity   15879
    trunk   15877
    upper extremity   15878
Lipoprotein   83715-83721
Lithotripsy extracorporeal shock wave   50590
Liver
    allotransplantation   47135-47136
    function study   78220
    imaging   78201-78202
        SPECT   78205-78206
    laparoscopy   47370-47379
    -spleen imaging   78215-78216
    tumor ablation   47380-47382
Lombard test   92573
Loudness balance test   92562
Low
    birth weight services, intensive (non-critical)   99298-99299
    intensity ultrasound stimulation   20979
Lung
    lavage total   32997
    transplant   32851-32854, 33935
Luteinizing releasing factor (lrh)   83727
Lyme disease vaccine   90665
Lymphadenectomy
    abdominal   38747
    axillary   38740-38745
    cervical   38720-38724
    inguinofemoral   38760-38765
    limited staging   38562-38564
    pelvic   38770
    retroperitoneal transabdominal   38780
    suprahyoid   38700
    thoracic   38746
Lymphangiography
    extremity   75801-75803
    pelvic/abdominal   75805-75807
Lymphangiotomy lymphatic channels   38308
Lymphocyte transformation   86353
Lymphocytotoxicity assay   86805-86806
Lysis
    englobulin   85360
    epidural adhesions using solution injection   62263-62264
    intranasal synechia   30560
    labial adhesions   56441
Lysozyme   85549

M

Magnesium 83735
Magnetic resonance angiography
   abdomen 74185
   chest 71555
   lower extremity 73725
   pelvis 72198
   spinal canal 72159
   upper extremity 73225
Magnetic resonance imaging (MRI)
   abdomen 74181-74183
   ankle 73721-73723
   bone marrow blood supply 76400
   brain 70551-70553, 70557-70559
   breast 76093-76094
   chest 71550-71552
   foot and foot joints 73718-73723
   knee 73721-73723
   leg 73718-73720
   orbit, face, and neck 70540-70543
   pelvis 72195-72197
   spinal canal 72141-72158
   temporomandibular joint 70336
   upper extremity 73218-73223
Magnetic resonance spectroscopy 76390
Magnetoencephalography (MEG) 95965-95967
Magnuson type operation (capsulorrhaphy, anterior) 23450
Major reconstruction chest wall 32820
Malar augmentation/reconstruction 21270
Malate dehydrogenase 83775
MALE GENITAL SYSTEM SURGICAL PROCEDURES *54000-55899*
Mammaplasty augmentation 19324-19325
Mammary ductogram or galactogram 76086-76088
Mammography 76090-76092
Manganese 83785
Manipulation
   ankle 27810, 27818, 27860
   chest wall 94667-94668
   clavical 23505
   elbow 24300, 24640
   finger 26725-26726, 26742, 26755
   foreskin 54450
   hip joint 27275
   knee joint 27570
   metacarpal (hand) 26605-26607
   metacarpophalangeal 26340, 26700-26706, 26742
   shoulder joint 23700
   spine with anesthesia 22505
   vertebral 22315
   wrist 25259, 25624, 25635, 25660, 25675, 25680, 25690
Manometric studies (ureter) 50686
   through nephrostomy or pyelostomy tube 50396

Manual therapy techniques   97140
Maquet type procedure (anterior tibial tubercleplasty)   27418
Marshall-Marchetti-Krantz procedure (anterior vesicourethropexy)   51840-51841, 51852,
    58267, 58293
Marsupialization   10040
    Bartholin's gland cyst   56440
    cyst or abscess, liver   47300
    cyst, pancreas   48500
    sublingual salivary cyst   42409
    urethral diverticulum   53240
Mass spectrometry and tandem mass spectrometry (ms, ms/ms)   83788-83789
Massage
    cardiac   32160
    therapy   97124
Mastectomy
    gynecomastia   19140
    modified radical   19240
    partial   19160-19162
    radical   19200-19220
    simple   19180
    subcutaneous   19182
Mastoid obliteration   69670
Mastoidectomy   69501-69511, 69601-69603
Mastopexy   19316
Mastotomy   19020
MATERNITY CARE AND DELIVERY PROCEDURES   *59000-59899*
Maxillectomy   31225-31230
Maxillofacial fixation, halo type   21100
Maxillofacial prosthetics   21076-21089
Maximum breathing capacity   94200
Measles
    and rubella virus vaccine   90708
    mumps and rubella virus vaccine (MMR)   90707
    mumps, rubella, and varicella vaccine (MMRV)   90710
    virus vaccine   90705
Meat fibers, feces   89160
Meatoplasty   69310
Meatotomy   53020-53025
Mechanical fragility, RBC   85547
Medial canthopexy   21280
Mediastinoscopy   39400
Mediastinotomy   39000-39010
MEDIASTINUM AND DIAPHRAGM SURGICAL PROCEDURES   *39000-39599*
Medical conference by physician   99361-99362
Medical disability evaluation   99455-99456
MEDICAL NUTRITION THERAPY   *97802-97804*
Medical testimony   99075
MEDICINE SERVICES   *787-872*
    Modifiers   788
    Overview   787
    Subsections   787
MEDICINE SERVICES CODES   *90281-99602*
    Allergy and clinical immunology   95004-95199
    Biofeedback   90901-90911

MEDICINE SERVICES CODES—continued
   Cardiovascular *92950-93799*
   Central nervous system assessments/tests *96100-96117*
   Chemotherapy administration *96400-96549*
   Chiropractic manipulative treatment *98940-98943*
   Dermatological procedures *96900-96999*
   Dialysis *90918-90999*
   Endocrinology, glucose monitoring *95250*
   Gastroenterology *91000-91299*
   Health and behavior assessment *96150-96155*
   Home health procedures *99500-99602*
   Immune globulins *90281-90399*
   Immunization administration for vaccines/toxoids *90471-90474*
   Medical nutrition therapy *97802-97804*
   Motion analysis *96000-96004*
   Neurology and neuromuscular medical procedures *95805-95999*
   Non-invasive vascular diagnostic studies *93875-93990*
   Ophthalmology *92002-92499*
   Osteopathic manipulative treatment (OMT) *98925-98929*
   Other services and procedures *99170-99199*
   Otorhinolaryngologic services *92502-92700*
   Photodynamic therapy *96567-96571*
   Physical medicine and rehabilitation *97001-97799*
   Psychiatry *90801-90899*
   Pulmonary *94010-94799*
   Qualifying circumstances for anesthesia *99100-99140*
   Sedation with or without analgesia *99141-99142*
   Special services, procedures and reports *99000-99091*
   Therapeutic or diagnostic infusions *90780-90781*
   Therapeutic, prophylactic or diagnostic injections *90782-90799*
   Vaccines, toxoids *90476-90749*
Membrane diffusion capacity *94725*
Meningococcal polysaccharide vaccine *90733*
Meningococcal conjugate vaccine *90734*
Meniscectomy
   knee joint *27332-27333*
   temporomandibular joint *21060*
Meprobamate *83805*
Mercury *83015, 83825*
Metobolite *82520*
Metanephrines *83835*
Metatarsectomy *28140*
Methadone *83840*
Methemalbumin *83857*
Methemglobulin *83045-83050*
Methenamine silver stain *88312*
Methsuximide *83858*
MICROBIOLOGY *0023T, 87001-87999*
Microscopic examination, hairs *96902*
Microsomal antibodies *86376*
Migration inhibitory factor (MIF) test *86378*
Miller type procedure (arthrodesis, midtarsal navicular-cuneiform) *28737*
Millet-Abbott intubation *44500, 74340*
Minerva cast *29035, 29710*

Miscarriage
  incomplete abortion 59812
  missed abortion 59820-59821
  septic abortion 59830
Mitchell procedure (correction hallux valgus) 28296
MMR 90707
MMRV 90710
Mobilization splenic flexure 44139
Modification
  contact lens 92325
  ocular implant 65125
Mohs micrographic technique 17304-17310
Molecular
  cytogenetics 88271-88275, 88291
  diagnostics 83890-83912
Molluscum contagiosum destruction 17110-17111, 54050-54065
Monitoring
  blood pressure, 24 hour 93784-93790
  fetal, during labor 59050-59051, 99500
  glucose 95250
  interstitial fluid pressure 20950
  localization of cerebral seizure focus 95950-95956
Morphometric analysis 88355-88361
Motility study 91010-91012
Motion analysis 96000-96004
Mucin, synovial fluid (ropes test) 83872
Mucocele, sinusotomy 31075
Mucopolysaccharides 83864-83866
MUGA (multiple gated aquisition) 78472-78478, 78483
Multifetal pregnancy reduction(s) (MPR) 59866
Mumps virus vaccine 90704
Muramidase 85549
Muscle
  biopsy 20200-20206
  flaps 15732-15738
  grafts 15841-15845
  testing, manual 95831-95834
  transfer, shoulder or upper arm 23395-23397, 24301, 24320
MUSCULOSKELETAL SYSTEM SURGICAL PROCEDURES *20000-29999*
Mustard type operation (repair transposition great arteries) 33774
Myelin basic protein, CSF 83873
Myelography 72240-72270
  posterior fossa 70010
Myocardial
  imaging
    infarct avid, planar 78466-78469
    positron emission tomography (PET) 78459
    positron emission tomography (PET) perfusion 78491-78492
  perfusion
    imaging 78460-78465
    study 78478-78480
  resection 33542
Myoglobin 83874

Myomectomy   58140-58146, 58545-58546
Myringoplasty   69620
Myringotomy   69420-69421

N

Narcosynthesis psychiatric diagnostic and therapeutic purposes   90865
Nasal
    deformity repair   40700-40761
    endoscopy   31231-31294
    function studies   92512
    prosthesis impression 21087
    sinus endoscopy   31233-31294
    smear eosinophils   89190
Nasogastric tube placement   43752
Nasomaxillary fracture   21345-21348
Nasopharyngoscopy   92511
Natriuretic peptide   83880
Neck
    angiography   70457-70459, 70498
    biopsy   21550
    CT scan   70490-70492, 70498
    MRI   70540-70543
    tumor excision   21555-21557
    ultrasound   76536
    wound exploration   20100
    x-ray   70360
Necropsy (autopsy)   88000-88045, 88099
Needle biopsy
    abdomen   49180
    bone   20220-20225
    bone marrow   38221
    breast   19100
    gastrointestinal endoscopy   43238, 43242
    kidney   50200
    liver   47000-47001
    mediastinum   32405
    muscle   20206
    pancreas   48102
    pleura   32460
    prostate   55700
    spinal cord   62269
    thyroid gland   60100
    transbronchial   31629, 31633
Needle localization, breast   19125-19126, 19290-19291
Neisseria gonorrhea   87590-87592, 87850
Neobladder construction   51596
Neonatal critical care
    initial   99295
    subsequent   99296
Nephelometry   83883
Nephrectomy   50220-50240, 50543, 50546-50548

Nephrolithotomy   50060-50075
Nephropexy   50400-50405
Nephrorrhaphy   50500
Nephrostolithotomy, percutaneous   50080-50081
Nephrostomy   50040
   change tube   50398
   endoscopic   50562-50570
   percutaneous   52334
Nephrotomy   50045
Nerve
   conduction study   95900-95904
   graft   64885-64907
   teasing preparations   88362
NERVOUS SYSTEM SURGICAL PROCEDURES   *61000-64999*
Neuraxial analgesia/anesthesia in labor   01967-01969
Neurectomy
   hamstring muscle   27315
   intrinsic musculature foot   28030
   popliteal   27320
   tympanic   69676
Neurobehavioral status exam   96115
Neuroendoscopy   62160-62165
NEUROLOGY AND NEUROMUSCULAR MEDICAL PROCEDURES   *95805-96004*
Neurolysis   64704-64708, 64727
Neuroma, excision   64774-64786
Neuromuscular junction testing   95937
Neurophysiology testing, intraoperative   95920
Neuroplasty
   cranial nerve   64716
   digital nerve   64702-64704
   nerve, hand or foot   64704
   peripheral nerve, arm or leg   64708-64714
   ulnar nerve
      at elbow   64718
      at wrist   64719
Neuropsychological testing   96117
Neurorrhaphy   64831-64876
   with graft   64885-64907
Neurostimulators   64590, 64595, 95970-95975
Neutralization test, viral   86382
Newborn
   care   99431-99440, 99502
   resuscitation   99440
Nickel   83885
Nicotine   83887
Nipple
   exploration   19110
   reconstruction   19350
Nissen procedure (laparoscopy esophagogastric fundoplasty)   43280
Nitroblue tetrazolium dye test (NTD)   86384
Nocturnal penile tumescence rigidity test   54250
Non-cardiac vascular flow imaging   78445
Non-contact laser coagulation, prostate   52647
Non-invasive ear or pulse oximetry (oxygen saturation)   94760-94762

Non-invasive physiologic studies
  extracranial arteries 93875
  extremity veins 93965
  lower extremity arteries 93924
  upper or lower extremity arteries 93922-93923
NON-INVASIVE VASCULAR DIAGNOSTIC STUDIES *93875-93990*
Non-pressurized inhalation treatment 94640
Non-stress test, fetal 50925
Non-union repair
  femur 27470-27442
  tarsal, metatarsal 28320-28322
Norepinephrine 82383-82384
Nose
  abscess 30000-30020
  biopsy 30100
  excision 30150-30160
  hemorrhage cauterization 30901-30906
  removal, foreign body 30300
Nose reconstruction
  primary 30400-30420
  secondary 30430-30450
  septum 30520
NUCLEAR MEDICINE SERVICES *78000-79999*
Nucleotidase 83915
NURSING FACILITY SERVICES *99301-99316*
  assessment 99301-99303
  care plan oversight services 99379-99380
  discharge day management 99315-99316
  subsequent care 99311-99313
Nuss procedure 21742, 21743

O

Obliteration
  aortopulmonary septal defect 33813-33814
  arteriovenous malformation 61613
  carotid aneurysm 61613
  carotid-cavernous fistula 61613
  mastoid 69670
Observation care, hospital 99217-99220
Observation or inpatient hospital care 99234-99236
Obstetrical care 59000-59899
Obturator nerve 64763-64766
Occiptal nerve 64744
Occlusion fallopian tube(s) by device 58615
Occult blood 82270
Occupational therapy
  evaluation 97003
  re-evaluation 97004
Ocular implant 65125-65175
Ocular prosthesis 21077, 65770, 66928-66985, 92330-92335, 92358, 92393

OFFICE VISIT SERVICES *99201-99215*
  after hours 99050-99054
  provided on an emergency basis 99058
Office visit
  established patient 99211-99215
  new patient 99201-99205
Oligoclonal immunoglobulin 83916
Omental flap 49904-49906
Omentectomy 49255, 58950-58954
Oocyte
  biopsy 89290-89291
  cryopreservation 0059T
  identification with follicular fluid 89254
  insemination 89268
  retrieval, in-vitro fertilization 58970
  storage 89346
  thawing 89356
Oophorectomy 58262-58263, 58291-58292, 58552, 58554, 58661, 58940-58943
Open closure major bronchial fistula 32815
Operating microscope 69990
Operculectomy 41821
Ophthalmic
  biometry 76516-76519
  mucous membrane tests 95060
  ultrasonic foreign body localization 76529
  ultrasound 76511-76514
Ophthalmodynamometry 92260
Ophthalmology examination under general anesthesia 92018-92019
OPHTHALMOLOGY MEDICAL SERVICES *92002-92499*
Ophthalmoscopy 92225-92226
Opiates 83925
Opponensplasty 26490-26496
Optic nerve decompression 67570
Optokinetic nystagmus test 92534, 92544
OPV (oral polio virus) 90712
Orbicularis oculi (blink) reflex 95933
Orbital implant
  insertion 67550
  removal or revision 67560
  repositioning, periorbital osteotomies 21267-21268
Orbitocranial
  approach to anterior cranial fossa 61584-61585
  zygomatic approach to middle cranial fossa 61592
Orbitotomy
  with bone flap or window 67420-67450
  without bone flap 67400-67414
Orchiectomy 54520-54535, 54690
Orchiopexy 54640-54650
ORGAN OR DISEASE ORIENTED PANELS *80048-80076*
Organic acids 83918-83921
Orogastric tube placement 43752
Oropharynx biopsy 42800
Orthodontic cephalogram 70350
Orthopantogram 70355

Orthoptic training 92065
Orthotics fitting and training 97504
Oscillating tracking test 92545
Osmolality 83930-83935
Osmotic fragility, RBC 85555-85557
Ostectomy
    calcaneus 28118-28119
    metacarpal 26250-26255
    metatarsal head(s) 28288
        complete excision 28111-28113
        complete excision (eg, Clayton type procedure) 28114
        partial excision 28110
    scapula 23190
    sternum 21620
    tarsal coalition excision 28116
Osteocalcin 83937
OSTEOPATHIC MANIPULATIVE TREATMENT (OMT) 98925-98929
Osteoplasty
    carpal bone 25394
    facial bones 21208-21209
    femur 27465-27468
    humerus 24420
    metacarpal or phalanges 26568
    radius and ulna 25390-25393
    tibia and fibula, lengthening 27715
Osteotomy
    calcaneus (eg, Dwyer or Chambers type procedure) 28300
    clavicle 23480-23485
    femur 27140, 27151
        neck 27161
        shaft or supracondylar without fixation 27448-27450
        transfer greater trochanter 27140
    fibula 27707-27712
    hip 27146-27151, 27156
    humerus 24400-24410
    mandible 21198-21199
    maxilla 21206
    metacarpal 26565
    metatarsal 28306-28309
    pelvis bilateral 27158
    phalanges finger 26567
    radius 25350-25355
        and ulna 25365, 25375
    spine
        anterior 22220-22226
        posterior or posterolateral 22210-22216
    talus 28302
    tarsal bones 28304-28305
        Fowler type 28305
    tibia 27705
        and fibula 27709
    toes 28299, 28310-28312
    ulna 25360
Otolaryngology exam 92502

Otoplasty, protruding ear 69300
OTORHINOLARYNGOLOGIC MEDICAL SERVICES *92502-92597*
Outflow tract augmentation (gusset) 33478
Ova, smears 87177
Ovarian cystectomy 58925
Ovulation tests, by visual color comparison methods 84830
Oxalate 83945
Oxygen saturation 82805-82810
Oxygen uptake, expired gas analysis 94680-94690

P

Pacemaker (heart)
  conversion 33214
  insertion 33200-33208
  removal 33233-33237
  replacement, pulse generator 33212-33213
  repositioning, electrode 33215, 33226
  telephonic analysis 93733, 93736
Packing, nasal hemorrhage 30901-30906
Palate and uvula procedures 42000-42299
Palatopharyngoplasty 42145
Palatoplasty cleft palate 42200-42225
Pancreatectomy 48140-48160
Pancreaticojejunostomy 48180
Pancreatorrhaphy 48545
Pap smears 88141-88155, 88164-88167, 88174-88175
Papillectomy or excision single tag, anus 46220
Papilloma destruction 54050-54065
Paracentesis anterior chamber eye 65800-65815
Parathormone 83970
Parathyroid
  autotransplantation 60512
  imaging 78070
  procedures 60500-60505
Parathyroidectomy 60500-60505
Paravaginal defect repair 57284
Paring benign hyperkeratotic lesion(s) 11055-11057
Parotid duct diversion 42507-42510
Particle agglutination 86403-86406
Patch allergy test(s) 95044
Patellectomy or hemipatellectomy 27350
PATHOLOGY AND LABORATORY SERVICES *705-790*
  Modifiers 705-706
  Subsections 705
PATHOLOGY AND LABORATORY SERVICES CODES *80000-89999*
  Anatomic pathology 88000-88099
  Chemistry 82000-84999
  Consultations (clinical pathology) 80500-80502
  Cytogenetic studies 88230-88299
  Cytopathology 88104-88199
  Drug testing 80100-80103

958

PATHOLOGY AND LABORATORY SERVICES CODES—continued
   Evocative/suppression testing 80400-80440
   Hematology and coagulation 85002-85999
   Immunology 86000-86849
   Microbiology 87001-87999
   Molecular diagnostics 83890-83912
   Organ or disease oriented panels 80048-80076
   Other procedures 89050-89240
   Reproductive medicine 89250-89356
   Surgical pathology 88300-88399
   Therapeutic drug assays 80150-80299
   Transcutaneous procedures 88400
   Transfusion medicine 86850-86999
   Urinalysis 81000-81099
Pathology consultation during surgery 88329-88332
Patient demand single or multiple event recording 93268-93272
Patient-initiated spirometric recording 94014-94016
Pediatric critical care patient transport 99289-99290
Pediatric critical care services 99293-99294
   patient transport 99289-99290
Pelvic
   examination 57410
   exenteration 51597
   fixation 22848
   lymphadenectomy 58240
Pelvimetry 74710
Penile
   plethysmography 54240
   prosthesis 54400-54417
   revascularization 37788
   rigidity test 54250
   venous occlusive procedure 37790
   venous studies 93980-93981
Percutaneous needle biopsy
   abdominal mass 49180
   liver 47000-47001
   lung 32405
   muscle 20206
   pancreas 48102
   pleura 32400
   salivary gland 42400
   spinal cord 62269
   thyroid 60100
Percutaneous transluminal angioplasty
   aortic 35472
   brachiocephalic 35474
   coronary 92982-92984
   femoral-popliteal 35474
   iliac 35473
   pulmonary 92997-92998
   renal 35471
   venous 35476
   visceral 35471
Pereyra procedure 51845, 57289, 58267, 58293

Pericardiectomy   32660, 33030-33031
Pericardiocentesis   33010-33011
Pericardiotomy   33020
Perineogram   74775
Perineoplasty   56810
Periodontal mucosal grafting   41870
Periorbital osteotomies   21260-21263, 21267-21268
Perirectal injection sclerosing solution   45520
Peritoneal dialysis   90945-90947
Peritoneocentesis, abdominal paracentesis, or peritoneal lavage   49080-49081
Peritoneogram   74190
Pessary insertion   57160
Petrous apicectomy   69530
pH body fluid, except blood   83986
Phalangectomy toe   28150-28160
Pharmacologic management   90862
Pharyngectomy 42890
Pharyngoesophageal repair   42953
Pharyngolaryngectomy   31390-31395
Pharyngoplasty   42950
Pharyngostomy   42955
Phencyclidine (PCP)   83992
Phenobarbital 82205
    assay   80184
Phenothiazine   84022
Phenylalanine (PKU), blood   84030
Phenylketones, qualitative   84035
Phenytoin assay   80185-80186
Phlebotomy   99195
Phosphatase   84060-84080
Phosphatidylglycerol   84081
Phosphogluconate, 6-, dehydrogenase, RBC   84085
Phosphohexose isomerase   84087
Phosphorus inorganic   84100-84105
Photo
    patch test(s)   95052
    tests   95056
Photochemotherapy   96910-96913
    endoscopic light   96570-96571
PHOTODYNAMIC THERAPY 96567-96571
Photopheresis, extracorporeal   36522
Photosensitivity testing   95056
PHYSICAL MEDICINE AND REHABILITATION SERVICES   97001-97799
Physical performance test or measurement   97750
Physical therapy
    evaluation   97001-97002
    modality
        contrast baths   97034
        diathermy   97024
        electrical stimulation   97014-97032
        hot or cold packs   97010
        Hubbard tank   97036
        infrared   97026
        iontophoresis   97033

Physical therapy—continued
  modality—continued
    microwave 97020
    paraffin bath 97018
    traction, mechanical 97012
    ultrasound 97035
    ultraviolet 97028
    unlisted procedure 97039
    vasopneumatic devices 97016
    whirlpool 97022
  osteopathic manipulation 98925-98929
  procedure
    aquatic therapy 97113
    gait training 97116
    massage 97124
    neuromuscular reeducation movement 97112
    therapeutic exercises 97110
    traction 97140
  re-evaluation 97002
  wheelchair management 97542
Physician services
  attendance and supervision hyperbaric oxygen therapy 99183
  direction, advanced life support 99288
  educational services 99078
  outpatient cardiac rehabilitation 93797-93798
  standby service 99360
  supervision care plan oversight 99374-99380
Pierce ears 69090
Pilondial cyst
  excision 11770-11772
  incision 10080-10081
Pinch graft 15050
Plague vaccine 90727
Plasma
  frozen preparation 86927
  radioiron disappearance (turnover) rate 78160
  volume 78110-78111
Plasmin 85400
Plasminogen 85420-85421
Plasmodium anitbody 86750
Plastic repair
  arteriovenous aneurysm 36834
  canaliculi 68700
  cleft lip/nasal deformity 40700-40761
  introitus 56800
  salivary duct, sialodochoplasty 42500-42505
  urethrocele 57230
Platelet
  aggregation 85576
  antibody 86022-86023
  assay 85055
  blood 85025
  count, automated 85049
  neutralization 85597
  survival study 78190-78191

Plethysmography
   extremities 93922-93923
   penis 54240
   total body 93720-93722
   veins 93965
Pleural scarification 32215
Pleurectomy 32310-32320, 32656
Pleurodesis 32005, 32650
Pneumocentesis, lung 32420
Pneumococcal
   conjugate vaccine 90669
   polysaccharide vaccine 90732
Pneumonectomy 32440-32500
   donor 32850, 33930
Pneumonolysis extraperiosteal 32940
Pneumonostomy 32200-32201
Poliovirus vaccine
   live, for oral use (OPV) 90712
   inactivated, (IPV) 90713
Pollicization digit 26550
Polysomnography 95808-95811
Pooling platelets 86965
Porphobilinogen 84106-84110
Porphyrins 84119-84127
Portoenterostomy (eg, Kasai procedure) 47701
Positional nystagmus 92532
Positron emission tomography (PET)
   brain 78608-78609
   heart 78459
   myocardial perfusion 78491-78492
   tumor 78810
Posterior colporrhaphy 57250
Postoperative
   biliary duct stone removal 74327
   follow-up visit 99024
   wound infection 10180
Postpartum care 59430
Potassium 84132-84133
Potts-Smith operation (shunt descending aorta to pulmonary artery) 33762
Prealbumin 84134
Pregnancy test 81025, 84702-84703
Pregnanediol 84135
Pregnanetriol 84138
Pregnenolone 84140
Prenatal testing
   amniocentesis 59000-59001
   chorionic villus sampling (CVS) 59015
   cordocentesis 59012
   fetal blood 59030
   fetal monitoring 59050
   non-stress test 59025, 99500
   oxytocin stress test 59020
   ultrasound 76801-76819, 76825

Preparation
  cryopreserved embryos thawing 89352
  embryo transfer 89255
  moulage for custom breast implant 19396
  report of psychiatric status 90889
Prescription
  contact lens 92310-92317
  ocular prosthesis 92330-92335
Pretreatment
  RBCs 86970-86972
  serum 86975-86978
PREVENTIVE MEDICINE SERVICES *99381-99429*
Preventive medicine
  counseling
      individual 99401-99404
      individuals, group setting 99411-99412
    evaluation, new patient, initial 99381-99387
    periodic reevaluation, established patient 99391-99397
Probing
  lacrimal canaliculi 68840
  nasolacrimal duct 68810-68815
Proctectomy 45110-45123
Proctopexy 45540-45541, 45550
Proctoplasty 45500-45505
Proctosigmoidoscopy 45300-45321
Proetz type procedure (displacement therapy) 30210
Progesterone 84144
Programmed stimulation and pacing 93623
Proinsulin 84206
Prolactin 80418, 80440, 84146
Prolonged physician services
  inpatient 99356-99357
  office/outpatient 99354-99355
  standby 99360
  without direct (face-to-face) contact 99358-99359
PROLONGED SERVICES *99354-99360*
Prophylactic treatment
  clavicle 23490
  femur 27495
  humeral shaft 24498
  proximal humerus 23491
  radius 25490
      and ulna 25492
  tibia 27745
  ulna 25491-25492
Prophylaxis retinal detachment 67141-67145
Prostaglandin 84150
Prostate specific antigen (PSA) 84152-84154
Prostatectomy 52601, 52612-52614, 55801-55845
  laparoscopic 55866
Prostatotomy 55720-55725
Prosthesis
  breast 19328-19342, 19396
  cornea 65770
  facial 21088

Prosthesis—continued
    knee   27438, 27445
    nasal   21087
    orbital   21077
    penile   54400-54417
Prosthetic training   97520
Protein   84155-84182
    western blot   84181-84182, 88371-88372
Prothrombin time   85610-85611
Proton beam delivery   77520-77525
Protoporphyrin, RBC   84202-84203
Provision of
    chemotherapy agent   96545
    diagnostic radiopharmaceutical(s)   78990
    therapeutic radiopharmaceutical(s)   79900
Provocative testing
    allergy   95078
    glaucoma   92140
Psychiatric
    diagnostic interview examination   90801-90802
    interventional evaluation   90802
    psychological testing   96100
***PSYCHIATRY MEDICINE SERVICES**   90801-90899*
Psychoanalysis   90845
Psychological testing   96100
Psychotherapy
    individual   90804-90829
    multiple-family, group   90846-90849, 90853-90857, 99510
Pterygomaxillary fossa surgery   31040
Pulmonary
    artery embolectomy   33910-33916
    compliance study   94750
    endarterectomy   33916
    perfusion imaging   78580-78585, 78588
    quantitative differential function   78596
    stress testing   94620
    value procedures   33470-33475
    ventilation imaging   78586-78587, 78591-78594
***PULMONARY MEDICAL SERVICES**   94010-94799*
Pump
    implantable, refilling and maintenance of   96530
    portable, refilling and maintenance of   96520
Punch graft hair transplant   15775-15776
Puncture(s)
    artery   36600
    aspiration
        abscess   10160
        cyst, breast   19000-19001
        hydrocele, tunica vaginalis   55000
    chest drainage   32000-32002
    lung   32420
    pericardium   33010-33011
    skull 61000-61055
    shunt   61070
    spinal cord   62270

Push transfusion   36440
Putti-platt procedure (capsulorrhaphy, anterior)   23450
Pyeloplasty   50400-50405, 50544
Pyelostolithotomy, percutaneous   50080-50081
Pyelostomy   50125, 50400-50405
Pyelotomy   50120-50135
   endoscopic   50570
Pyloromyotomy (Fredet-Ramstedt type operation)   43520
Pyloroplasty   43800
Pyridoxal phosphate (vitamin B-6)   84207
Pyruvate   84210
   kinase   84220

Q

Q fever   86000, 86638
Quadricepsplasty (eg, Bennett or Thompson type)   27430
QUALIFYING CIRCUMSTANCES FOR ANESTHESIA   99100-99140
Quinine   84228

R

Rabies
   immune globulin   90375-90376
   vaccine   90675-90676
Radial
   keratotomy   65771
   styloidectomy   25230
Radiation dosimetry calculation   77300
Radiation therapy management   77431
Radiation treatment
   delivery   77401-77418
   management   77427-77499
Radical abdominal hysterectomy   58210
Radical excision
   bursa, synovia wrist, or forearm tendon sheaths   25115-25116
   lesion, external auditory canal   69150-69155
Radical resection
   abdomen   51597
   elbow   24149
   humerus   23220-23222
   metacarpal   26250-26255
   phalanx finger   26260-26262
   radius   25170
   sternum   21630-21632
   tonsil   42842-42845
   tumor
      back or flank   21935
      bone   28171-28175

965

Radical resection—continued
   tumor—continued
      clavicle 23200
      face or scalp 21015
      femur or knee 27365
      fibula 27646
      foot 28046
      forearm wrist area 25077
      hand or finger 26115-26117
      hip 27075-27079
      leg or ankle area 27615
      pelvis and hip area 27049
      radial head or neck 24152-24153
      radius or ulna 25170
      scapula 23210
      shaft or distal humerus 24150-24151
      shoulder 23077
      talus or calcaneus 27647
      thigh or knee area 27329
      tibia 27645
      tissue neck or thorax 21557
      upper arm 24150-24153
      upper arm or elbow 24077
Radical trachelectomy 57531
Radiographic absorptiometry (photodensitometry) 76078
Radioiron
   oral absorption 78162
   red cell utilization 78170
RADIOLOGY SERVICES 641-702
   Bilateral procedure codes 642
   Complete procedures 641
   Medicare considerations 643
   Modifiers 642
   Services overview 641
   Subsections 641
   Supervision and interpretation only 641
RADIOLOGY SERVICES CODES 70010-79999
   Diagnostic radiology 70010-76499
   Diagnostic ultrasound 76506-76999
   Nuclear medicine 78000-79999
   Radiation oncology 77261-77799
Radiopharmaceutical
   ablation 79030
   dacryocystography 78660
   localization
      abscess 78805-78807
      tumor 78800-78804
   therapy 79000-79100, 79400-79900
Range of motion testing 92018-92019, 95851-95858
Rapid desensitization procedure 95180
Raskind procedure 33735-33737
Rastelli type operation (total repair, truncus arteriosus) 33786
Receptor assay 84233-84238

Reconstruction
   angular deformity, toe 28313
   chest wall 32820
   cleft foot 28360
   collateral ligament
      interphalangeal joint 26545
      metacarpophalangeal joint 26541-26542
   cranial bones extracranial 21181-21184
   dislocating patella 27424
      Campbell, Goldwaite type procedure 27422
      Hauser type procedure 27420
   external auditory canal 69310-69320
   eyelid 67971-67975
   forehead 21172-21180, 21182-21184
   knee, ligamentous 27427-27429
   mandible 21244
      or maxilla 21245-21249
   mandibular
      condyle 21247
      rami 21193-21196
   midface
      Lefort I 21141-21147
      Lefort II 21150-21151
      Lefort III 21154-21160
      osteotomies and bone grafts 21188
   nail bed 11762
   orbit with osteotomies 21256
   orbital
      rims 21172-21180
      walls and rims 21182-21184
   pectus excavatum or carinatum 21740-21743
   posterior tibial tendon (eg, Kidner type procedure) 28238
   shoulder rotator cuff avulsion 23420
   supernumerary digit 26587
   tendon pulley 26500-26504
   toe
      macrodactyly 28340-28341
      polydactyly 26587, 28344
      syndactyly 28345
   ulna or radioulnar joint 25337
   vena cava 34502
   zygomatic arch and glenoid fossa 21255
Rectocele repair 45560
Red blood cell (RBC)
   count 85032-85041
   hematocrit 85014
   platelet estimation 85007
   survival study 78130-78135
   volume determination 78120-78121
Reduction
   craniomegalic skull 62115-62117
   forehead 21137-21139
   lung volume 32491
   mammaplasty 19318

Reduction—continued
   masseter muscle and bone 21295-21296
   overcorrection of ptosis 67909
   pregnancy, multi-fetal 59866
   procidentia 45900
   torsion of testis 54600
   volvulus intussusception, internal hernia 44050
Reimplantation
   arteries 35691-35697
   kidney 50380
   ovary 58825
   pulmonary artery 33788
   ureter, to bladder 50780-50785
   ureters 51565
Reinsertion
   drug delivery implant 11983
   ocular implant 65150-65155
   ruptured biceps or triceps tendon 24342
   spinal fixation device 22849
Release
   encircling material 67115
   extensive scar tissue 67343
   hamstring proximal 27097
   intrinsic muscles, hand 26593
   tarsal tunnel 28035
   thenar muscle(s) 26508
Removal
   anal seton, other marker 46030
   ankle implant 27704
   anterior spinal instrumentation 22855
   benign tumor facial bone 21029
   blood clot anterior segment eye 65930
   bone flap or prosthetic plate skull 62142
   cardiac event recorder 33284
   cardioverter-defibrillator
     electrode(s) 33243-33244
     pulse generator 33241
   cast 29700-29715
   cataract 66830-66984
   catheter
     central venous 36589
     fractured 75961
     peritoneum 49422
     spinal cord 62355
   cerclage suture under anesthesia 59871
   corneal epithelium 65435-65436
   CSF shunt system brain 62256-62258
   drug implant 11982-11983
   embedded foreign body, eyelid 67938
   epithelial downgrowth, anterior chamber eye 65900
   external fixation system 20694
   fecal impaction or foreign body, rectum 45915
   fixation device 20670-20680

Removal—continued
 foreign body
   dentoalveolar structures 41805-41806
   esophageal 43020, 43045, 43215, 74235
   external auditory canal 69200-69205
   external eye 65205
   foot 28190-28193
   intraocular 65235
   lacrimal passages 68530
   mouth 40804-40805
   muscle or tendon sheath 20520-20525
   nose 30300-30320
   orbit 61334, 67413, 67430
   pelvis or hip 27086-27087
   penis 54115
   pharynx 42809
   scrotum 55120
   shoulder 23040-23044, 23330-23332
   upper arm or elbow area 24200-24201
   upper leg or knee area 27372
 halo 20665
 hematoma, brain 61312-61315
 impacted
   cerumen 69210
   vaginal foreign body 57415
 implant
   breast 19328-19330
   contraceptive capsules 11976-11977
   non-biodegradeable drug 11982-11983
   finger or hand 26320
 implanted material
   anterior segment of eve 65920
   posterior segment of eve 67120-67121
 infusion pump
   intra-arterial 36262
   intravenous 36590
   spinal cord 62365
 intra-aortic balloon assist device 33968-33974
 intraluminal (intracatheter) obstructive material 36537
 intrathecal or epidural catheter 62355
 intrauterine device (IUD) 58301
 lens material 66840-66940
 lung
   other than total pneumonectomy 32480-32500
   total pneumonectomy 32440-32445
 mammary implant 19328-19330
 ocular implant 65175, 65920
 pacemaker
   and electrodes 33236-33237
   electrode(s) 33234-33235
   pulse generator 33233
 pancreatic calculus 48020
 penile prosthesis 54406, 54410-54417
 pericatheter obstructive material (eg, fibrin sheath) 36536

Removal—continued
  perineal prosthesis 53442
  peritoneal
      foreign body 49085
      shunt 49429
  permanent intraperitoneal cannula or catheter 49422
  posterior
      nonsegmental spinal instrumentation 22850
      segmental spinal instrumentation 22852
  prosthesis
      hip 27090-27091
      knee 27488
      penis 54406, 54410-54417
      skull 62142
      urethral sphincter 53446-53447
      wrist 25250-25251
  secondary membranous cataract 66830
  shunt system, spine 63746
  skin tags 11200-11201
  subcutaneous reservoir or pump 62365
  subdeltoid calcareous deposits 23000
  sutures under anesthesia 15850-15851
  Thiersch wire or suture, anal canal 46754
  tissue expander(s) 11971
  tongs or halo applied by another physician 20665
  transplanted
      pancreatic allograft 48556
      renal allograft 50370
  transvenous electrode(s) 33238
  tumor, temporal bone 69970
  turnbuckle jacket 29715
  ventricular assist device 33977-33978, 33980
  vitreous, anterior approach 67005-67010
  wrist prosthesis 25250-25251
Renal
  allotransplantation 50360-50365
  biopsy 50200-50205
  endoscopy 50551-50580
  exploration 50010
Renin 80408, 80416, 84244
Reoperation
  carotid thromboendarterectomy 35390
  coronary artery bypass procedure or valve procedure 33530
Repair
  achilles tendon 27650-27654
  anal fistula 46288, 46706-46716
  aneurysm 35001-35162
      aorta 0001T, 0033T-0040T, 33877, 34800-34805, 34825-34832, 75952-75953
      arteriovenous 36834
      iliac artery 75954
      intracranial artery 61697-61708
  ankle
      ligament 27695-27698
      tendon 27612, 27650-27654, 27680-27687

Repair—continued
  anomalous
    coronary artery 33502-33506
    venous return 33730
  anterior palate, including vomer flap 42235
  aortic arch 33852-33853
  arteriovenous fistula
    extremities 35184, 35190
    head and neck 35180, 35188
    thorax and abdomen 35182, 35189
  atrial septal defect 33641
    and ventricular septal defect 33813-33814, 33647
  atrioventricular canal 33660-33670
  bifid digit 26587
  blepharoptosis 67901-67908
  blood vessel
    hand, finger 35207
    intra-abdominal 35221, 35251, 35281
    intrathoracic 35211-35216, 35241-35246, 35271, 35276
    lower extremity 35226, 35256, 35286
    neck 35201, 35231, 35261
    upper extremity 35206, 35236, 35266
  brow ptosis 67900
  cardiac wound 33300-33305
  choanal atresia 30540-30545
  cleft hand 26580
  cloacal anomaly 46744-46748
  collateral ligament, metacarpophalangeal or interphalangeal joint 26540
  complex
    cardiac anomaly(ies) 33608-33610, 33615-33617
    eyelids, nose, ears, lips 13150-13153
    forehead, cheeks, chin, mouth, neck, axillae, genitalia, hands, feet 13131-13133
    scalp, arms,, legs 13120-13122
    trunk 13100-13102
  cor triatriatum or supravalvular mitral ring 33732
  coronary arteriovenous or arteriocardiac chamber fistula 33500-33501
  diaphragmatic hernia 39502-39541
  dislocating peroneal tendons 27675-27676
  double outlet right ventricle 33611-33612
  dupuytren's contracture 26040
  dural/CSF leak 63707, 63709
  ectropion 67914-67917
  elbow ligament 24343-24346
  encephalocele, skull vault 62120
  enterocele 57268-57270
  entropion 67921-67924
  epigastric hernia 49570-49572
  extensor tendon
    central slip 26426-26428
    distal insertion 26433-26434
    finger 26418-26420
    hand 26410-26412
    insertion, closed treatment 26432
    leg 27664-27665

Repair—continued
  fascial defect leg 27656
  femur nonunion or malunion distal to head and neck 27470-27472
  finger, volar plate, interphalangeal joint 26548
  fistula
    anal 46706
    oromaxillary 30580
    oronasal 30600
  flexor tendon 26350-26358
    leg 27658-27659
  graft-enteric fistula 35870
  hernia 50728
    abdominal 49565, 49590
    epigastric 49570, 49572
    femoral 49550-59557
    inguinal 49491-49521
    intestinal 44025-44050
    umbilical 44580-44587
  high imperforate anus 46730-46742
  hypospadias
    complications 54340-54348
    cripple 54352
    one stage, distal 54322-54328
    one stage, perineal 54336
    one stage, proximal penile or penoscrotal 54332
  inguinal hernia 49491-49507, 49650-49651
    sliding 49525
  initial
    femoral hernia 49550-49553
    incisional or ventral hernia 49560-49561
    inguinal hernia 49491-49507
  intrinsic muscles hand 26591
  iris ciliary body 66680
  laceration
    conjunctiva 65270-65273
    cornea 65275
    cornea sclera 65280-65286
    diaphragm 39501
    floor mouth tongue 41250
    palate 42180-42182
    tongue 41251
    tongue floor mouth 41252
  large omphalocele or gastroschisis 49605-49606
  left ventricular outflow tract obstruction 33414
  lip 40650-40654
  low imperforate anus 46715-46716
  lumbar hernia 49540
  lung hernia through chest wall 32800
  macrodactylia 26590
  meningocele 63700-63702
  metatarsal nonunion or malunion 28322
  mitral valve 33420-33427
  myelomeningocele 63704-63706
  nail bed 11760

Repair—continued
  nasal septal perforations 30630
  nasolabial fistula 42260
  neonatal diaphragmatic hernia 39503
  nerve 64876
    graft 64885-64907
    suture 64831-64876
  nonunion, metacarpal or phalanx 26546
  nonunion or malunion
    humerus 24430-24435
    radius and ulna 25415-25420
    radius or ulna 25400-25405
    scaphoid bone 25440
  omphalocele (Gross type operation) 49600-49611
  oval window fistula 69666
  pacemaker 33218-33220
  paraesophageal hiatus hernia 39502
  patent ductus arteriosus 33820-33824
  perineum 56810
  pleura 32215
  postinfarction ventricular septal defect 33545
  profundus tendon 26370-26373
  prosthetic valve dysfunction 33496
  pulmonary
    artery stenosis 33917
    atresia 33918-33920
  rectocele 45560
  recurrent
    femoral hernia 49555-49557
    incisional or ventral hernia 49565-49566
    inguinal hernia 49520-49521
  retinal detachment 67101-67112
  round window fistula 69667
  ruptured
    musculotendinous cuff 23410-23412
    spleen 38115
  scleral staphyloma 66220-66225
  scrotum 55175-55180
  septal defect 93580-93581
  single
    transvenous electrode 33218
    ventricle 33619
  sinus valsalva
    aneurysm 33720
    fistula 33702-33710
  skin wound
    complex 13100-13160
    simple 12020-12021
  small omphalocele 49600
  spectacles 92370-92371
  spica body cast or jacket 29720
  spigelian hernia 49590
  spleen 38115

Repair—continued
  superficial wounds
    face, ears, eyelids, nose, lips mucous membranes 12011-12018
    scalp, neck, axillae, external genitalia, trunk, extremities 12001-12007
  symblepharon 68330-68340
  syndactyly 26560-26562
  tarsal bones, nonunion or malunion 28320
  tendon
    foot 28200-28210
    or muscle, forearm, wrist 25260-25275
    or muscle, upper arm or elbow 24341
  testis 54600-54670
  tetralogy fallot 33692-33697
  thoracoabdominal aortic aneurysm 33877
  tibia
    congenital pseudarthrosis 27727
    nonunion or malunion 27720-27725
  torn ligament, capsule, knee 27405-27409
  trachea
    fistula 31755
    stenosis 31780-31781
    wound 31800-31805
  transposition great arteries 33770-33781
  tricuspid valve 33463-33465
  truncus arteriosus (Rastelli type operation) 33786
  tunica vaginalis hydrocele (bottle type) 55060
  two transvenous electrodes 33220
  umbilical hernia 49580-49587
  urethral sphincter 57220
  uterus, rupture 58520, 59350
  vulva, post partum 59300
  wound, extraocular muscle, tendon, tenon's capsule 65290
Replacement
  aortic valve 33405-33413
  bone flap or prosthetic plate skull 62143
  contact lens 92326
  irrigation, subarachnoid/subdural catheter 62194
  lumbosubarachnoid shunt 63744
  mitral valve 33430
  pulmonary valve 33475
  revision CSF shunt 62230
  tissue expander 11970
  tricuspid valve 33465
  ureter by bowel segment 50840
  ventricular catheter 62225, 62160
Replantation
  arm 20802
  digit 20816-20822
  foot 20838
  forearm 20805
  hand 20808
  thumb 20824-20827

Repositioning
    cardiac venous system 33226
    central venous catheter 36597
    gastric feeding tube 43761
    intraocular lens prosthesis 66825
    pacemaker electrode 33215
    pacing cardioverter-defibrillator electrode 33215
Reproductive medicine procedures 89250-89356
Reptilase test 85635
Resection
    bronchus (bronchoplasty) 32501
    condyle(s), phalanx 28153
    diaphragm 39560-39561
    elbow joint 24155
    external cardiac tumor 33130
    humeral head 23195
    incision subvalvular tissue 33415
    lateral pharyngeal wall or pyriform sinus 42892
    lesion
        base anterior cranial fossa 61600-61601
        infratemporal fossa, parapharyngeal space, petrous apex 61605-61606
        parasellar area, cavernous sinus, clivus or midline skull base 61607-61608
    lip 40530
    lung 32520-32525
    ovarian malignancy 58950-58952
    palate 42120
    pancreas and peripancreatic tissue 48005
    phalangeal base 28126
    pharyngeal wall 42894
    ribs extrapleural 32900
    scrotum 55150
    temporal bone 69535
    transplantation long tendon biceps 23440
Respiratory
    flow volume loop 94375
    syncytial virus immune globulin (RSV-IgIM) 90378
    syncytial virus immune globulin (RSV-IgIV) 90379
***RESPIRATORY SYSTEM SURGICAL PROCEDURES** 30000-32999*
Rest home visit
    established patient 99331-99333
    new patient 99321-99323
Reticulocyte 85044-85045
Retinopathy 67227-67228
Retrobulbar injection
    alcohol 67505
    medication 67500
Retroperitoneal fibrosis 50715
Revision
    aqueous shunt to extraocular reservoir 66185
    arteriovenous fistula 36832-36833
    arthroplasty wrist joint 25449
    colostomy 44340-44346
    fenestration operation 69840
    gastric restrictive procedure 43848

975

Revision—continued
  gastroduodenal anastomosis 43850-43855
  gastrojejunal anastomosis 43860-43865
  ileostomy 44312-44314
  infusion pump, intra-arterial 36261
  lower extremity arterial bypass 35879-35881
  mastoidectomy 69601-69605
  operative wound, anterior segment 66250
  orbitocraniofacial reconstruction 21275
  peritoneal-venous shunt 49426
  reconstructed breast 19380
  reinsertion transhepatic tube 47530
  removal
    cranial neurostimulator pulse generator or receiver 61888
    implanted spinal neurostimulator pulse generator 63688
    intracranial neurostimulator electrodes 61880
    peripheral neurostimulator electrodes 64585
    peripheral neurostimulator pulse generator 64595
    spinal neurostimulator electrode 63660
  skin pocket 33223
    pacemaker 33222
  stapedectomy or stapedotomy 69662
  total
    hip arthroplasty 27134-27138
    knee arthroplasty 27486-27487
  tracheostomy scar 31830
  transvenous intrahepatic shunt 37183
  urinary-cutaneous anastomosis 50727-50728
Rheumatoid factor 86430-86431
Rhinectomy 30150-30160
Rhinoplasty
  nasal deformity 30460-30462
  primary 30400-30420
  secondary 30430-30450
Rho(D) immune globulin (RhIg) 90384-90385
Rho(D) immune globulin (RhIgIV) 90386
Rhythm ECG, one to three leads 93040-93042
Rhytidectomy
  cheek, chin, and neck 15828
  forehead 15824
  glabellar frown lines 15826
  neck 15825
  superficial musculoaponeurotic system (SMAS) flap 15829
Riboflavin (vitamin B-2) 84252
Right heart
  catheterization 93501
  congenital cardiac anomalies 93530
Right ventricular
  recording 93603
  resection 33476
Rinkel test (provocative testing) 95078
Rorschach test 96100
Ross procedure 33413
Rotavirus vaccine 90680

Routine
    electroencephalography 95812-95827
    obstetric care 59400, 59618
Rubella virus vaccine 90706
Ruiz-mora type procedure (correction cock-up toe(s)) 28286
Russell viper venom time 85612-85613

S

Sacral nerve 64561, 64581
Sacrospinous ligament fixation 57282
Salabrasion 15810-15811
Salivary gland
    function study 78232
    imaging 78230-78231
Salpingectomy 58700
Salpingo-oophorectomy 58720, 58950-58954
Salpingostomy 58673, 58770
Saphenopopliteal vein anastomosis 34530
Scanning computerized ophthalmic diagnostic imaging 92135
Scapulopexy 23400
Schilling test (vitamin B absorption study) 78270
Schlicter test (serum bactericidal titer) 87197
Scleral reinforcement 67250-67255
Scraping cornea, diagnostic 65430
Screening
    mammography 76092
    test
        pure tone, air only 92551
        visual acuity 99173
Scrotal exploration 55110
Scrotoplasty 55175-55180
Secondary
    closure surgical wound or dehiscence 13160
    repair dura CSF leak 61618-61619
Section recurrent laryngeal nerve 31595
***SEDATION WITH OR WITHOUT ANALGESIA* *99141-99142**
Seddon-Brookes type procedure (tenoplasty, with muscle transfer) 24320
Sedimentation rate 85651-85652
Select picture audiometry 92583
Selenium 84255
Self care/home management training 97535, 99509
Selverstone-Crutchfield type procedure (surgery intracranial aneurysm) 61703
Semen analysis 89300-89321
Senning type operation (repair transposition great arteries) 33774-33777
Sensorimotor examination 92060
Sensorineural acuity level test 92575
Septal
    defect, repair 93580-93581
    or other intranasal dermatoplasty 30620
Septoplasty or submucous resection 30520

Sequestrectomy
   clavicle 23170
   forearm, wrist 25145
   humeral head to surgical neck 23174
   olecranon process 24138
   radial head or neck 24136, 25145
   scapula 23172
   shaft or distal humerus 24134
Serial tonometry 92100
Serotonin 84260
Serum
   bactericidal titer (Schlicter test) 87197
   screening cytotoxic percent reactive antibody (PRA) 86807-86808
Services
   provided in location other than physician's office 99056
   requested
      after office hours 99050
      between 10:00 pm and 8:00 am 99052
      on sundays and holidays 99054
Sesamoidectomy 28315
   thumb or finger 26185
Sever type procedure (capsular contracture release) 23020
Severing
   adhesions anterior segment eye 65860-65880
   tarsorrhaphy 67710
Sex chromatin identification
   Barr bodies 88130
   peripheral blood smear 88140
Sex hormone binding globulin (SHBG) 84270
SGOT 84450
SGPT 84460
Shaving lesion
   face, ears, eyelids, nose, lips, mucous membrane 11310-11313
   scalp, neck, hands, feet, genitalia 11305-11308
   trunk, arms or legs 11300-11303
Shigella antibody 86771
Short increment sensitivity index (SISI) 92564
Shortening tendon
   extensor, hand or finger 26477
   flexor, hand or finger 26479
Shunt
   ascending aorta to pulmonary artery (Waterston type operation) 33755
   central 33764
   descending aorta to pulmonary artery (Potts-Smith type operation) 33762
   subclavian to pulmonary artery (Blalock-Taussig type operation) 33750
   superior vena cava to pulmonary artery 33766-33767
Shuntogram 75809
Sialic acid 84275
Sialodochoplasty 42500-42505
Sialography 70390
Sialolithotomy 42330-42340
Sickling RBC, reduction 85660
Sigmoidoscopy 45330-45345
Signal-averaged electrocardiography (SAECG) 93278
Silica 84285

Silver type procedure hallux valgus 28290
Simple
   cystometrogram (CMG) 51725
   uroflowmetry (UFR) 51736
Single event recording patient demand 93268
Sinusoidal vertical axis rotational testing 92546
Sinuscopy 31233-31235
Sinusotomy
   frontal 31070-31087
   maxillary 31020-31032
   sphenoid 31050-31051
   unilateral 31090
SISI test 92564
Skene's gland 53060, 53270
Skin
   abrasion 15786-15787
   biopsy 11100-11101
   debridement 11000-11044
   grafts 15000-15400, 15757
   skin tags 11200-11201
Skin graft and flap
   allograft 15350-15351
   composite graft 15760-15770
   formation 15570-15576
   microvascular anastomosis 15756-15758
   muscle 15732-15738, 15842
   splint 15100-15121
   tissue transfer 14000-14350
   xenograft 15400-15401
Skin test
   candida 86485
   coccidioidomycosis 86490
   histoplasmosis 86510
   tuberculosis 86580-86585
   unlisted antigen 86586
Sleep
   latency or maintenance wakefulness testing 95805
   study 95806-95807
Sling operation 57288
Slipped femur epiphysis
   open treatment 27177-27181
   treatment 27175-27176
Slitting prepuce 54000-54001
Small intestinal endoscopy, enteroscopy 44360-44379
Smear primary source, with interpretation 87205-87210
Snip incision lacrimal punctum 68440
Sodium
   serum 84295
   other source 84302
   urine 84300
Sofield type procedure, osteotomy
   femoral shaft 27454
   humeral shaft 24410
   multiple 27712
Somatomedin 84305

Somatosensory evoked potential study 95925-95927
Somatostatin 84307
Special
    anterior segment photography 92286-92287
    dosimetry 77331
    medical radiation physics consultation 77370
    reports 99080
    stains 88312-88314
    treatment procedure 77470
SPECIAL SERVICES, PROCEDURES AND REPORTS 99000-99091
Specific gravity 84315
Spectacles 92340-92390
Spectrophotometry 84311
Speculoscopy 0013T-0032T
Speech
    evaluation 70371-92506
    generating communication device 92607-92609, 92597
    treatment 92507-92508
Sperm
    antibodies 89325
    evaluation 89329-89330
    identification 89264
      from aspiration 89257
    isolation 89260-89261
    storage 89343
    thawing 89353
    washing artificial insemination 58323
Sphincteroplasty, anal 46750-46762
Sphincterotomy anal 46080
Spinal puncture
    lumbar 62270
    therapeutic 62272
Spirometry 94010-94070
Spleen imaging only 78185
Splenectomy 38100-38102
Splenoportography 75810
Split graft trunk, arms, legs 15100-15101
Splitting blood or blood products 86985
Spontaneous nystagmus 92531
    test 92541
Sputum specimen 89220
Staggered spondaic word test 92572
Staging celiotomy Hodgkins disease or lymphoma 49220
Stand by services 99360
Stapedectomy or stapedotomy 69660-69662
Stapes mobilization 69650
Starch granules, feces 89225
Steindler stripping (division plantar fascia and muscle) 28250
Stem cell
    cryopreservation 38207, 88240
    depletion 38210-38214
    harvesting 38205-38206
    transplantation 38240-38242

Stenger test
  pure tone 92565
  speech 92577
Stereotactic
  biopsy
      aspiration, or excision lesion, spinal cord 63615
      intracranial lesion 61750-61751
  computer assisted volumetric (navigational) procedure 61795
  implantation depth electrodes into the cerebrum 61760
  localization 61770
      breast biopsy 76095
  radiation treatment, management cerebral lesion(s) 77432
  radiosurgery 61793
  stimulation spinal cord 63610
Sternal debridement 21627
Stimulus evoked response 51792
Storage
  embryo 89342
  oocyte 89346
  reproductive tissue 89344
  sperm 89343
Strabismus surgery 67311-67318, 67331-67340
Strapping
  ankle 29540
  elbow or wrist 29260
  hand or finger 29280
  hip 29520
  knee 29530
  low back 29220
  shoulder 29240
  thorax 29200
  toes 29550
  unna boot 29580
Strayer procedure (gastrocnemius recession) 27687
Streptokinase, antibody 86590
Stump elongation, upper extremity 24935
Subconjunctival injection 68200
Subcutaneous
  hormone pellet implantation 11980
  injection filling material 11950-11954
Subdural
  implantation strip electrodes 61531
  tap 61000-61001
Subluxation radial head in child, closed treatment 24640
Submucous resection turbinate 30140
Subsequent hospital care normal newborn 99433
Subtotal or total hysterectomy after cesarean delivery 59525
Subtraction in conjunction with contrast studies 76350
Sugars 84376-84379
  chromatographic 84375
Sulfate, urine 84392
Supplies and materials provided by physician 99070

Supply
   contact lenses   92391, 92396
   low vision aids   92392
   ocular prosthesis   92393
   permanent prosthesis   92395-92396
   spectacles   92390
Supracervical abdominal hysterectomy   58180
Surface application radioelement   77789
SURGERY SERVICES   *221-640*
   Add-on codes   226
   Global surgical package   221
   Modifiers   224-225
   Multiple surgical procedures   222
   Separate procedure   224
   Special report   222
   Starred procedures   226-227
   Subsections   224
   Surgical supplies   227
SURGERY SERVICES CODES   *10000-69999*
   Auditory system   69000-69979
   Cardiovascular system   33000-37799
   Digestive system   40490-49999
   Endocrine system   60000-60699
   Eye and ocular adnexa   65091-68899
   Female genital system   56405-58999
   Hemic and lymphatic systems   38100-38999
   Integumentary system   10000-19999
   Intersex surgery   55970-55980
   Male genital system   54000-55899
   Maternity care and delivery   59000-59899
   Mediastinum and diaphragm   39000-39599
   Musculoskeletal system   20000-29999
   Nervous system   61000-64999
   Respiratory system   30000-32999
   Urinary system   50010-53899
Surgical closure tracheostomy or fistula   31820-31825
Surgical correction hydraulic abnormality
   inflatable prosthesis   54408
   inflatable sphincter device   53449
SURGICAL PATHOLOGY   *88300-88399*
   gross and microscopic examination   88302-88309
   gross examination only   88300
Surgical preparation or creation recipient site   15000-15001
Surgical treatment
   anal fistula   46270-46285
   ectopic pregnancy   59120-59140
Susceptibility studies   87181-87190
Suture
   abdominal wall evisceration or dehiscence   49900
   additional
      major peripheral nerve   64859
      nerve, hand or foot   64837
   brachial plexus   64861
   digital nerve, hand or foot   64831-64832

Suture—continued
   esophageal wound or injury 43410-43415
   extrahepatic biliary duct 47900
   facial nerve 69740-69745
     extracranial 64864
     infratemporal 64865
   infrapatellar tendon 27380-27381
   iris ciliary body 66682
   large intestine 44604-44605
   ligation thoracic duct 38380-38382
   lumbar plexus 64862
   major peripheral nerve, arm or leg 64856-64857
   mesentery 44850
   nerve 64872-64876
     hand or foot 64834-64836
   pharynx wound or injury 42900
   posterior tibial nerve 64840
   quadriceps or hamstring muscle rupture 27385-27386
   recent wound, eyelid 67930-67935
   removal under anesthesia 15850
   repair aorta or great vessels 33320-33322
   sciatic nerve 64858
   small intestine 44602-44603
   testicular injury 54670
   tongue to lip micrognathia (Douglas type procedure) 41510
   tracheal wound or injury 31800-31805
Swallowing function
   evaluation of 92610-92613
   pharynx, esophagus 74230
Swan-ganz catheter insertion and placement 93503
Swanson type cavus foot procedure (osteotomy, metatarsal) 28309
Sweat collection 89230
Sympathectomy
   cervical 64802
   cervicothoracic 64804
   digital arteries 64820
   lumbar 64818
   radial artery 64821
   superficial palmar arch 64823
   thoracolumbar 64809
   ulnar artery 64822
Symphysiotomy horseshoe kidney 50540
Syndactylization, toes 28280
Synovectomy
   carpometacarpal joint 26130
   interphalangeal joint 26140
   metacarpophalangeal joint 26135
   tendon sheath
     foot 28086-28088
     radical flexor tendon 26145
     wrist 25118-25119, 25105
Synthetic sentence identification test 92576
Syphilis test 86592-86593

T

T3   84480
T-cells   86359-86361
Talectomy (astragalectomy)   28130
Tarsal strip procedure   67917-67924
Tattooing   11920-11922
TB test   86580-86585
Telephone call by physician   99371-99373
Telephonic transmission electrocardiogram rhythm strip(s)   93012-93014
Teletherapy isodose plan   77305-77315
Temperature gradient studies   93740
Temporary
    closure eyelids by suture (eg, Frost suture)   67875
    transcutaneous pacing   92953
Temporomandibular joint arthrography   70328-70332
Tendon
    graft   20924
    lengthening, upper arm or elbow   24305
    sheath incision   26055
    transplantation forearm, wrist   25310-25312
Tennis elbow   24350-24356
Tenodesis
    biceps tendon   24340
    distal joint   26474
    long tendon biceps   23430
    proximal interphalangeal joint   26471
    wrist   25300-25301
Tenolysis
    complex extensor tendon, finger   26449
    extensor tendon
        foot   28220-28226
        hand or finger   26445
    flexor or extensor tendon
        forearm, wrist   25295
        leg, ankle   27680-27681
    flexor tendon
        foot   28220-28222
        palm and finger   26442
        palm or finger   26440
    triceps, 24332
Tenoplasty with muscle transfer   24320
Tenotomy
    abductor hallucis muscle   28240
    abductors, extensor(s) hip, open   27006
    achilles tendon, percutaneous   27605-27606
    adductor
        hip   27000-27003
        or hamstring, percutaneous   27306-27307
        subcutaneous   27003
    elbow to shoulder, open   24310
    extensor hand or finger, open   26460

Tenotomy—continued
  flexor
    finger, open 26455
    palm, open 26450
  hip flexor(s), open 27005
  open
    extensor, foot or toe 28234
    flexor or extensor tendon, forearm, wrist 25290
    hamstring, knee to hip 27390-27392
    tendon flexor, foot 28230
    tendon flexor, toe 28232
  percutaneous 26060
    toe 28010-28011
  shoulder area 23405-23406
Tensilon test myasthenia gravis 95857-95858
Testicular imaging 78760-78761
Testing autonomic nervous system function 95921-95923
Testosterone 84402-84403
Tetanus 86280
  antibody 86774
  and diphtheria toxoids (TD) 90718
  immune globulin (TIG) 90389
  toxoid adsorbed 90703
Thal-nissen procedure (esophagogastric fundoplasty) 43325
Thawing
  and expansion frozen cells 88241
  cryopreserved
    embryo 89352
    oocytes 89356
    reproductive tissue 89354
    sperm 89353
  previously frozen cells 38208-38209
Therapeutic
  activities 97530
  apheresis 36511-36516
  enema 74283
THERAPEUTIC DRUG ASSAYS 80150-80299
THERAPEUTIC OR DIAGNOSTIC INFUSIONS 90780-90781
THERAPEUTIC PROPHYLACTIC OR DIAGNOSTIC INJECTIONS 90782-90799
Therapeutic radiology
  port film(s) 77417
  simulation-aided field setting 77280-77295
  treatment planning 77261-77263
Thermogram
  cephalic 93760
  peripheral 93762
Thiamine (vitamin B-1) 84425
Thiersch procedure 15050
Thiocyanate 84430
Thompson type procedure (quadricepsplasty) 27430
Thoracentesis
  puncture pleural cavity aspiration 32000
  with insertion tube 32002
Thoracic gas volume 94260

985

Thoracoplasty Schede type or extrapleural 32905-32906
Thoracoscopy
   diagnostic 32601-32606
   surgical 32650-32665
   with
      open flap drainage 32036
      rib resection 32035
Thoracostomy 32020, 32035-32036
Thoracotomy
   anesthesia for 00540-00548
   biopsy lung or pleura 32095
   cardiac massage 32160
   control traumatic hemorrhage, repair lung tear 32110
   cyst(s) removal 32140
   excision-plication bullae 32141
   exploration and biopsy 32100
   open intrapleural pneumonolysis 32124
   postoperative complications 32120
   removal
      intrapleural foreign body or fibrin deposit 32150
      intrapulmonary foreign body 32151
Thrombectomy
   arterial or venous graft 35875-35876
   arteriovenous fistula 36831
   axillary
      and subclavian vein 34490
      brachial, innominate, subclavian artery 34101
   carotid subclavian or innominate artery 34001
   femoropopliteal, aortoiliac artery 34201, 34421-34451
   innominate subclavian artery 34051, 34061-34101
   popliteal-tibio-peroneal artery 34203
   radial or ulnar artery 34111
   renal celiac, mesentery, aortoiliac artery 34151
   subclavian vein 34471
   vena cava 34401-34451
Thrombin time
   plasma 85670
   titer 85675
Thromboendarterectomy 35301-35381
Thrombolysis
   cerebral 37195
   coronary 92975-92977
Thrombomodulin 85337
Thromboplastin
   inhibition 85705
   time, partial (PTT) 85730-85732
Thymectomy 60520-60522
Thyroglobulin 84432
   antibody 86800
Thyroglossal excision 60280-60281
Thyroid
   carcinoma metastases
      imaging 78015-78018
      uptake 78020

Tracheostoma revision 31613-31614
Tracheostomy
   emergency procedure 31603-31605
   fenestration procedure 31610
   planned 31600-31601
Tracheotomy tube change 31502
Training
   biofeedback 90901-90911
   cognitive skills 98532
   community/work reintegration 97537
   home management 97535, 99509
   orthoptic/pleoptic 92065
   prosthetics 97520
   walking (physicial therapy) 97116
   wheelchair management 97542
Transcatheter
   biopsy 37200
   introduction intravascular stent(s) 75960
   occlusion or embolization 37204
     central nervous system 61624
     non-central nervous system 61626
   placement
     intracoronary stent(s) 92980-92981
     intravascular stent(s) 37205-37208, 0005T-0007T
     intravascular foreign body 37203
     intravascular foreign body, percutaneous 75961
   therapy 75894-75896
Transcervical
   catheterization fallopian tube 74742
   introduction fallopian tube catheter 58345
Transcochlear approach to posterior cranial fossa 61596
Transcondylar lateral) approach to posterior cranial fossa 61597
Transcortin (cortisol binding globulin) 84449
Transcranial doppler study the intracranial arteries 93886-93888
Transduodenal sphincterotomy or sphincteroplasty 47460
Transcortin 84449
Transection
   carotid artery in
     cavernous sinus 61609-61610
     petrous canal 61611-61612
   esophagus with repair 43401
   facial nerve 64742
   greater occipital nerve 64744
   inferior alveolar nerve 64738
   infraorbital nerve 64734
   lingual nerve 64740
   mental nerve 64736
   obturator nerve 64763-64766
   other
     cranial nerve 64771
     spinal nerve 64772
   phrenic nerve 64746
   pudendal nerve 64761
   pulmonary artery 33922

Transection—continued
  repositioning aberrant renal vessels 50100
  supraorbital nerve 64732
  vagi 64755
  vagus nerve
    abdominal 64760
    transthoracic 64752
Transesophageal echocardiography 93312-93318
Transfer
  adductor to ischium 27098
  external oblique muscle to greater trochanter 27100
  finger to another position 26555
  free toe joint 26556
  iliopsoas to
    femoral neck 27111
    greater trochanter 27110
  paraspinal muscle to hip 27105
  pedicle flap 15650
  tendon
    hand 26480-26483
    muscle, hamstrings to femur (eg, Egger's type procedure) 27400
    palmar 26485-26489
    to restore intrinsic function 26497-26498
  toe-to-hand 26551-26554
  transplant tendon 27690-27692
Transferase
  alanine amino (ALT) (SGPT) 84460
  aspartate amino (AST) (SGOT) 84450
Transferrin 84466
Transfusion
  blood or blood components 36430
  intrauterine, fetal 36460
TRANSFUSION MEDICINE 86850-86999
Transhepatic portography, percutaneous 75885-75887
Transluminal
  atherectomy 75992-75996
  balloon angioplasty 35450-35460
  peripheral atherectomy 35480-35495
Transmastoid antrotomy 69501
Transmetacarpal amputation 25927-25931
Transmyocardial laser revascularization 33140-33141
Transperineal placement needles or catheters into prostate 55859
Transpetrosal approach to posterior cranial fossa 61598
Transplant hamstring tendon to patella 27396-27397
Transplantation
  bone marrow 38240-38242
  cornea 65710-65755
  hair, graft 15775-15776
  heart 33945
    and lung 33935
  liver 47135-47136
  pancreatic allograft 48160, 48550-48556
  stem cells 38240-38242
  testis(es) to thigh 54680

989

Transport, pediatric patient 99289-99290
Transposition
    ovary(s) 58825
    procedure 67320
Transposition, reimplantation
    carotid to subclavian artery 35695
    subclavian to carotid artery 35694
    vertebral to
        carotid artery 35691
        subclavian artery 35693
Transrectal drainage pelvic abscess 45000
Transtemporal approach to posterior cranial fossa 61595
Transthoracic echocardiography 93303-93304
Transtracheal
    injection bronchography 31715
    introduction needle wire dilator/stent 31730
Transureteroureterostomy 50770
Transurethral
    balloon dilation prostatic urethra 52510
    destruction prostate tissue 53850-53853
    drainage prostatic abscess 52700
    electrosurgical resection prostate 52601
    fulguration postoperative bleeding 52606
    incision prostate 52450
    resection
        bladder neck 52500
        postoperative bladder neck contracture 52640
        prostate 52612-52614
        regrowth obstructive tissue 52630
        residual obstructive tissue 52620
Transvenous intrahepatic portosystemic shunt (TIPS) 37182-37183
Transverse arch graft 33870
Transvesical ureterolithotomy 51060
Treatment
    devices, design and construction 77332-77334
    first degree burn 16000
    incomplete abortion 59812
    missed abortion 59820-59821
    septic abortion 59830
    speech 92507-92508
    superficial wound dehiscence 12020-12021
    swallowing dysfunction 92526
Tricuspid valve repositioning 33468
Triglycerides 84478
Triiodothyronine t3 84480-84482
Trimming nondystrophic nails 11719
Troponin 84484-84512
Trypanosomiasis 86171, 86280
Trypsin 84485-84490
TSH (thyroid stimulating hormone) 84443
Tubal
    ligation 58600
    pregnancy 59121

Tube
  or needle catheter jejunostomy 44015
  pericardiostomy 33015
  thoracostomy 32020
Tuberculosis
  antigen response test 0010T
  skin test 86580-86585
  vaccine (BCG) 90585-90586
Tubotubal anastomosis 58750
Tubouterine implantation 58752
Tumor
  abdomen 49200-49201
  biliary tract 43272, 47711-47712
  bladder 52234-52240
  bone 20982
  brain 61510
  breast 19120-19126
  colon 44393, 45383
  destruction, chemosurgery 17304-17310
  esophagus 43228
  fallopian tube 58950-58954
  heart 33120-33130
  hip 27047-27049, 27065-27067
  intestines 44369
  kidney 50562, 52355
  larynx 31300
  ovary 58950-58954
  pericardia 32661, 33050
  pituitary gland 61546-61548, 62165
  spinal cord 63275-63290
  stomach 43610-43611
  testis 54530-54535
  thyroid 60200
  ulna 25120-25126, 25170
  uterus 58140-58146
  vagina 57135
Tumor imaging, positron emission tomography (PET) 78810
Tunica vaginalis 55000, 55040-55041, 55060
Tympanic
  incision 69420-69421
  membrane repair 69450, 69610
  neurectomy 69676
Tympanolysis, transcanal 69450
Tympanometry (impedance testing) 92567
Tympanoplasty
  antrotomy or mastoidotomy 69635-69637
  mastoidectomy 69641-69644
Tympanostomy 69433-69436
Typhoid vaccine 90690-90693
Tyrosine 84510
Tzank smear 87207

U

U-tube hepaticoenterostomy 47802
Ulnar nerve 64718-64719
Ultrasonic guidance
    amniocentesis 59001, 76946
    aspiration ova 76948
    chorionic villus sampling 76945
    compression repair arterial pseudo-aneurysm/arteriovenous fistulae 76936
    cyst or renal pelvis aspiration 76938
    endomyocardial biopsy 76932
    interstitial radioelement application 76965
    intrauterine fetal transfusion or cordocentesis 76941
    needle biopsy 43232, 43238, 43242, 45342, 76942
    pericardiocentesis 76930
    placement radiation therapy fields 76960
    radiation therapy 76950
    thoracentesis or abdominal paracentesis 76942
    tissue ablation 76940
Ultrasound
    bone density measurement and interpretation 76977
    intravascular 37250-37251, 92978-92979
    measurement of bladder capacity 51798
    ophthalmic 76511-76514
    pelvic, non-obstetric 76856-76857
    pregnant uterus 76801-76817
    study follow-up 76970
    transvaginal 76830
Ultraviolet light therapy
    dermatology 96900, 96910-96912
    physical medicine 97028
Umbilectomy omphalectomy, excision umbilicus 49250
Unlisted
    cytogenetic study 88299
    immune globulin 90399
    miscellaneous pathology test 89399
    service
        cardiovascular 93799
        dermatology 96999
        evaluation and management 99499
        home visit 99600
        ophthalmology 92499
        physical medicine/rehabilitation 97799
        preventive medicine 99429
        psychiatric 90899
        pulmonary 94799
        special service procedure or report 99199
    therapeutic prophylactic or diagnostic injection 90799
    vaccine/toxoid 90749

Unlisted procedure
  abdomen
    musculoskeletal system 20999, 22999
    peritoneum and omentum 49329, 49999
  accessory sinuses 31299
  allergy/clinical immunologic service 95199
  anesthesia 01999
  anterior segment eye 66999
  anus 46999
  arthroscopy 29999
  biliary tract 47999
  breast 19499
  cardiac surgery 33999
  casting or strapping 29799
  chemistry 84999
  chemotherapy 96549
  clinical brachytherapy 77799
  computed tomography 76497
  conjunctiva 68399
  craniofacial and maxillofacial 21299
  cytopathology 88199
  dentoalveolar structures 41899
  diagnostic gastroenterology 91299
  diagnostic nuclear medicine
    cardiovascular 78499
    endocrine 78099
    gastrointestinal 78299
    genitourinary 78799
    miscellaneous 78999
    musculoskeletal 78399
    nervous system 78699
    respiratory 78599
  diagnostic radiographic (x-ray) 76499
  dialysis 90999
  diaphragm 39599
  endocrine system 60699
  endoscopy, vascular 37501
  esophagus 43289, 43499
  external ear 69399
  eyelids 67999
  female genital system 58999
  femur or knee 27599
  fetal invasive 59897
  fluoroscopic 76496
  foot or toes 28899
  forearm or wrist 25999
  hands or fingers 26989
  hematology and coagulation 85999
  hemic or lymphatic system 38999
  humerus or elbow 24999
  hysteroscopy procedure, uterus 58579
  immunology 86849
  inner ear 69949
  intestine 44799, 44238

993

Unlisted procedure—continued
  lacrimal system 68899
  laparoscopy
    abdomen, peritoneum and omentum 49329
    appendix 44979
    biliary tract 47579
    endocrine system 60659
    esophagus 43289
    hernioplasty, herniorrhaphy, herniotomy 49659
    intestine (except rectum) 44238
    lymphatic system 38589
    maternity care and delivery 59898
    oviduct, ovary 58679
    rectum 44239
    renal 50549
    spermatic cord 55559
    spleen 38129
    stomach 43659
    testis 54699
    uterus 58578
  larynx 31599
  leg or ankle 27899
  lips 40799
  liver 47379, 47399
  lungs and pleura 32999
  magnetic resonance 76498
  male genital system 55899
  maternity care and delivery 59899
  maxillofacial prosthetics 21089
  Meckel's diverticulum and the mesentery 44899
  mediastinum 39499
  medical radiation physics 77399
  microbiology 87999
  middle ear 69799
  musculoskeletal system
    head 21499
    general 20999
  neck or thorax 21899
  necropsy (autopsy) 88099
  nervous system 64999
  neurological or neuromuscular diagnostic 95999
  nose 30999
  ocular muscle 67399
  orbit 67599
  otorhinolaryngology 92700
  palate, uvula 42299
  pancreas 48999
  pelvis or hip joint 27299
  pharynx, adenoids, or tonsils 42999
  physical therapy 97139, 97799
    modality 97039
  posterior segment 67299
  pressure ulcer 15999
  radiopharmaceutical therapeutic 79999

Unlisted procedure—continued
    rectum 44239, 45999
    salivary glands or ducts 42699
    shoulder 23929
    skin, mucous membrane and subcutaneous tissue 17999
    spine 22899
    stomach 43659, 43999
    surgical pathology 88399
    temporal bone, middle fossa approach 69979
    therapeutic radiology
        clinical treatment planning 77299
        treatment management 77499
    tongue, floor mouth 41599
    trachea bronchi 31899
    transfusion medicine 86999
    ultrasound 76999
    urinalysis 81099
    urinary system 53899
    vascular
        endoscopy 37501
        injection 36299
        surgery 37799
    vestibule mouth 40899
Unusual travel 99082
Upgrade pacemaker system 33214
Upper gastrointestinal endoscopy 43234-43259
Urea
    breath test 78267-78268
    nitrogen 84520-84545
Ureteral
    endoscopy 50951-50980
    reflux study 78740
Ureterectomy 50650-50660
Ureterocalycostomy 50750
Ureterocolon conduit 50815
Ureteroenterostomy 50800
Ureteroileal conduit 50820
Ureterolithotomy 50610-50630
Ureterolysis 50715-50725
Ureteroneocystostomy 50780-50785, 50830, 51565
Ureteroplasty 50700
Ureteropyelostomy 50740
Ureterorrhaphy 50900
Ureterosigmoidostomy 50810
Ureterscopy
    dilation 52344-52346
    third stage 52351
Ureterostomy 50860, 50951
Ureterotomy 50600-50605
Ureteroureterostomy 50760-50770, 50830
Urethral pressure profile studies (UPP) 51772
Urethrectomy 53210-53215
Urethrocystography 74450-74455
Urethromeatoplasty 53450-53460

Urethroplasty   46744-46748, 53400-54318
Urethrorrhaphy   53502-53515
Urethrotomy or urethrostomy   53000-53010
Uric acid   84550-84560
***URINALYSIS**   81000-81099*
  infectious agent detection   0041T
Urinary
  bladder residual study   78730
  undiversion   50830
***URINARY SYSTEM SURGICAL PROCEDURES**   50010-53899*
Urine pregnancy test   81025
Urobilinogen   84577-84583
Uroflowmetry complex   51736-51741
Urography   74400-74425
Use vertical electrodes   92547
Uterine
  evacuation and curettage, hydatidiform mole   59870
  suspension   58400-58410
Uvulectomy   42140

V

V flap procedure   54322
Vaccinia immune globulin   90393
Vaccines
  anthrax   90581
  cholera   90725
  diphtheria toxoid   90719
  diphtheria, tetanus (DT)   90702
  encephalitis   90735
  hepatitis A   90632-90634
  hepatitis A and B   90636
  hepatitis B   90740-90747
  influenza   90655-90658, 90660
  lyme disease   90665
  measles   90705
  measles, mumps and rubella (MMR)   90707
  meningococcal   90733-90734
  mumps   90704
  plague   90727
  pneumococcal   90669, 90732
  polio   90712-90713
  rabies   90675-90676
  tetanus toxoid   90703
  typhoid   90690-90693
  yellow fever   90717
***VACCINES, TOXOIDS**   90476-90749*
Vaginal
  delivery only   59409-59610
  hysterectomy   58260-58294, 58550-58554
Vaginectomy   57106-57112

Venous—continued
  sampling through catheter 75893
  thrombosis
    imaging 78457-78458
    study 78455
  valve transposition 34510
Ventilating tube removal 69424
Ventilation assist and management 94656-94657, 99504
Ventricular
  assist device 33975-33980
  puncture 61020-61026, 61105-61120
Ventriculocisternostomy 62180, 62200-62201
Ventriculomyotomy 33416
Vermilionectomy (lip shave) 40500
Vertebral corpectomy 63081-63308
Very long chain fatty acids 82726
Vesiculectomy 55650
Vesiculotomy 55600-55605
Vestibular function tests 92531-92548
Vestibular nerve section 69915-69950
Vestibuloplasty 40840-40845
Viral antibodies 86280
Virus identification 87254
Virus isolation 87250-87255
Viscosity 85810
Visual
  evoked potential (VEP) testing 95930
  field examination 92081-92083
  reinforcement audiometry (VRA) 92579
Vital capacity 94150
Vitamin
  A 84590
  B-12 82607-82608
    absorption studies combined 78272
    absorption study (eg, Schilling test) 78270-78271
  C 82180
  K 84597
Vitrectomy 67036-67040
Voiding pressure studies (VP) 51795-51797
Volatiles 84600
Volkmann contracture 25315-25316
Volume measurement timed collection 81050
Vulvectomy 56620-56640

W

Wada activation test hemispheric function 95958
Walldius type procedure (arthroplasty, knee) 27445
Warts, destruction 17110-17111
Wassmund procedure 21206
Water load test 89235
Waterston type operation (shunt ascending aorta to pulmonary artery) 33755

Wedge
  excision skin nail fold   11765
  osteotomy   21122
  resection or bisection ovary   58920
Wedging
  cast   29740
  clubfoot cast   29750
Wheelchair management/propulsion training   97542
White blood cells (WBC)   85004-85009, 85025-85027, 85048
Whitman procedure   27120
Whole blood volume determination   78122
Wilke type procedure (parotid duct diversion)   42507
Windowing cast   29730
Winter procedure   54435
Wire
  insertion   20650
  interdental   21497
Work
  hardening/conditioning   97545-97546
  -related or medical disability examination   99455-99456

XYZ

X-ray examination
  abdomen   74000-74022
  abscess, fistula or sinus tract study   76080
  acromioclavicular joints   73050
  ankle   73600-73610
  calcaneus   73650
  chest   71010-71035
  clavicle   73000
  colon   74270-74280
  complex motion body section   76101-76102
  elbow   73070-73085
  esophagus   74220
  eye   70030
  facial bones   70140-70150
  femur   73550
  finger(s)   73140
  foot   73620-73630
  forearm   73090
  gastrointestinal tract, upper   74240-74249
  hand   73120-73130
  hip   73500-73530, 73540
  humerus   73060
  internal auditory meati   70134
  knee   73560-73580
  lower extremity, infant   73592
  mandible   70100-70110
  mastoids   70120-70130
  nasal bones   70160
  neck, soft tissue   70360

X-ray examination—continued
   nose to rectum, foreign body 76010
   optic foramina 70190
   orbits 70190-70200
   osseous survey 76061-76065
   pelvis 72170-72190
     and hips, infant or child 73540
   pharynx or larynx 70370
     cervical esophagus 74210
   renal cyst study 74470
   ribs 71100-71111
   sacroiliac joint(s) 72200-72202
     arthrography 73542
   sacrum and coccyx 72220
   salivary gland calculus 70380
   scapula 73010
   sella turcica 70240
   shoulder 73020-73040, 73050
   single plane body section 76100
   sinuses 70210-70220
   skull 70250-70260
   small bowel 74250-74251
   spine 72010-72190
   sternoclavicular joint 71130
   sternum 71120-71130
   stress view(s), any joint 76006
   surgical specimen 76098
   teeth 70300-70320
   temporomandibular joint 70328-70330
   tibia and fibula 73590
   toe(s) 73660
   upper extremity, infant 73092
   wrist 73100-73115
Xenograft 15400-15401
Xeroradiography 76150
Xylose absorption test 84620
Yeast culture 87106
Yellow fever vaccine 90717
Zieglar procedure 66820
Zinc 84630
Zygote, gamete 58976